Preface

November 1995 marked the centennial of the discovery of x-rays by Roentgen. During those first 100 years, diagnostic imaging, through a variety of modalities, has greatly influenced medical diagnosis and treatment. In 1940, the management of approximately 1 in 10 patients was influenced by a radiographic study. By 1980, virtually all patients underwent some sort of diagnostic imaging study. In the new millennium, imaging is used to guide many therapeutic procedures that previously would have required surgical exposure and prolonged hospitalization.

Diagnostic radiology has undergone dramatic changes in the past four decades. Before 1970, the specialty relied primarily on radiographs that were often supplemented by various contrast examinations for clinical problem solving. A revolution in diagnostic imaging began in the early 1970s with the development of cross-sectional and longitudinal imaging using ultrasound. Almost concomitantly, computed tomography (CT) followed, and soon rapid improvements in technology afforded us the ability to directly image areas of the body that previously were accessible only to the surgeon's knife. Magnetic resonance (MR) imaging joined the diagnostic toolkit in the early 1980s and added a new dimension to the diagnosis of disorders of the central nervous and musculoskeletal systems. Molecular imaging has emerged as a method of identifying specific tissues in the body, and in the next decade, this imaging technique should move rapidly from the laboratory to practical applications.

Improvements in imaging have changed the diagnostic approach to many conditions. Invasive procedures such as bronchography, cholecystography, cholangiography, cisternography, laryngography, lymphangiography, and pneumoencephalography are, thankfully, no longer performed and have all been replaced by CT and/or MR. Many other procedures such as tomography, intravenous urography, sinus radiography, and endoscopic retrograde cholangiopancreatography are on an "endangered species" list of studies and will be replaced by CT and/or MR within the next few years.

While the newer forms of diagnostic imaging were being developed, refinements in existing technology led the way to a whole new field of endeavor for radiologists— interventional and invasive radiology. Radiologists' abilities are no longer limited to simply making diagnoses. They have now developed the tools and skills to treat many conditions such as aneurysms, gastrointestinal bleeding, tumors, recurrent pulmonary emboli, and certain joint instabilities. Furthermore, using CT guidance, radiologists can safely perform biopsies, excisions, tumor ablation procedures, and surgical screw placements.

Our specialty is in a constantly evolving state. Improvements in computer technology have produced highly detailed multiplanar and three-dimensional imaging, as well as digital imaging. Digital processing of data is now the norm, and the days of film/screen imaging are numbered as picture archiving and computer storage systems become the standard method of viewing and storing imaging studies.

In the 1990s, the general awareness of the cost of health care has caused us to seek alternative methods for making diagnoses and treating patients. In addition to the growing field of minimally invasive surgery, radiologic-guided intervention is replacing many surgical procedures. At the beginning of the new millennium, the medical profession is experiencing an increased demand for accountability. Diagnostic radiology is ready to answer that call.

This book is intended for the medical student who is beginning clinical rotations. It is a thorough revision of the second edition and reflects the many changes that have occurred in the field. Significant new material includes discussions on newer interventional techniques and cardiac imaging you are likely to encounter. As before, to avoid duplication of material, disorders of the pediatric age group are integrated into each chapter rather than considered separately. Pneumonia in a child has the same radiographic appearance as in an adult and therefore should be discussed under the topic rather than the age group. Other significant changes include the addition of nearly 200 new figure parts and the replacement of some old figures with those that reflect state-of-the-art imaging.

In writing the original edition of this book as well as its revisions, I have kept the orientation based on clinical problem solving. Many of the radiology texts for medical students list the radiographic signs of various conditions as isolated facts without attempting to correlate them with the pathophysiology that produces them. Diagnostic imaging is true detective work. The image represents the patient at a particular point in time. By knowing anatomy and observing the changes that disease has inflicted on a patient's anatomy, it is possible to identify the pathologic process(es) that produced those changes. It is my goal to show that by recognizing a radiographic *pattern*, it is possible to define the pathophysiologic process(es) producing that pattern.

The first chapter provides an overview of diagnostic imaging, listing the "menu" of imaging options available to help solve clinical problems. The physical basis for each type of imaging is briefly stated. The second chapter discusses radiographic contrast agents. The third is devoted to a growing subspecialty, interventional and invasive radiology. The remaining chapters of the book describe imaging of the lungs, heart, breast, abdomen, gastrointestinal tract, urinary tract, obstetric and gynecological systems, the musculoskeletal system, and the brain and spinal cord.

Each clinical chapter is divided into three sections covering technical considerations, anatomic considerations, and pathologic considerations. The *technical considerations* portion of each chapter includes the type of examinations performed for that area, the use of special views, and a description of how each examination may be of help in clinical problem solving. The *technical considerations* include topics such as proper identification of images with regard to the patient, laterality, an analysis of proper density, exposure parameters, and the presence of motion.

The *anatomic considerations* portion reviews pertinent anatomy of the region being studied. No attempt is made to be encyclopedic; rather, the approach is very brief but covers all the essentials. It is important for you, the reader, to recognize that the images you are viewing are two-dimensional representations of three-dimensional structures. You must remember the adage that if you know the gross appearance of a structure, you can easily predict its radiographic or other imaging appearance.

The *pathologic considerations* include those pathophysiologic alterations of normal anatomic structures that produce the abnormalities shown on the images. Logic suggests that a disease can affect an organ in a limited number of ways. Similarly, the way an organ responds to a disease process is limited. For example, in the gastrointestinal tract, a mucosal tumor appears the same whether it is located in the esophagus, stomach, small intestine, or colon. The same holds true for other lesions of this system. Furthermore, an extrapolation may be made to other tubular structures in the body—airways, urinary tract, and blood vessels. Once you recognize the *pattern* of a lesion, you will recognize it anywhere in the body, even if it is in an unusual location.

Throughout the text, you are reminded of the large variety of imaging studies that may be performed on a patient. Your choice of study should be based on your analysis of the patient's history, the physical findings, economics, and your good judgment. Any diagnostic study should be appropriate for the patient's signs and symptoms. Please remember that these studies are expensive.

You will find that the text emphasizes certain types of imaging examinations and makes little or no mention of others. My goal is to provide you with state-of-the-art imaging information. This revision reflects changes that have occurred in imaging protocols. For example, intravenous urography is less commonly used for patients with suspected urinary calculi; CT (without contrast) has become the standard study. However, because this text is also used in parts of the world where the most sophisticated imaging techniques are not available, some older studies that are still performed are mentioned and illustrated.

Each chapter ends with a list of suggested additional readings. Most of these are current textbooks in the various subspecialties of diagnostic radiology. You are referred to them for more in-depth discussions of individual topics. Most of these books should be available in the medical school library, hospital library, or radiology departmental library. Furthermore, the American College of Radiology (ACR) has published numerous documents on technical standards for diagnostic and therapeutic radiologic studies as well as on appropriateness of imaging studies. These may be accessed without cost from the ACR Web site, http://www.acr.org.

In addition, I have added an appendix that contains "diagnostic pearls"—a summary of interesting and helpful tidbits to aid the reader in diagnosis.

Finally, it is my hope that you will find the book easy to read and understand. Learning should be fun. It has been my intent to keep it that way in each edition of this book.

Richard H. Daffner, MD, FACR
Pittsburgh, Pennsylvania, 2007

Clinical Radiology
The Essentials

3RD EDITION

■ **RICHARD H. DAFFNER, MD, FACR**

Professor of Radiologic Sciences
Drexel University College of Medicine

Department of Diagnostic Radiology
Allegheny General Hospital

Adjunct Clinical Professor of Radiology
University of Pittsburgh
School of Medicine
Pittsburgh, Pennsylvania

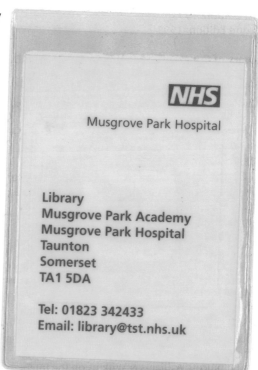

⊞ Wolters Kluwer | Lippincott Williams & Wilkins
Health
Philadelphia · Baltimore · New York · London
Bu

Acquisitions Editor: Donna Balado
Managing Editor: Cheryl W. Stringfellow
Associate Managing Editor: Liz Stalnaker
Marketing Manager: Jennifer Kuklinski
Production Editor: Gina Aiello
Designer: Theresa Mallon
Compositor: Nesbitt Graphics, Inc.
Printer: R.R. Donnelly-Willard

351 West Camden Street
Baltimore, MD 21201

530 Walnut Street
Philadelphia, PA 19106

Printed in the United States of America

First Edition, 1993
Second Edition, 1999

Library of Congress Cataloging-in-Publication Data

Daffner, Richard H., 1941-
  Clinical radiology : the essentials / Richard H. Daffner.—3rd ed.
     p. ; cm.
  Includes bibliographical references and index.
  ISBN-13: 978-0-7817-9968-3
  ISBN-10: 0-7817-9968-6
  1. Diagnostic imaging. 2. Diagnosis, Radioscopic. I. Title.
  [DNLM: 1. Diagnostic Imaging—methods—Atlases. WN 17 D124c 2007]
  RC78.7.D53D34 2007
  616.07'54—dc22

                                        2006100663

To purchase additional copies of this book, call our customer service department at **(800) 638-3030**
or fax orders to **(301) 223-2320**. International customers should call **(301) 223-2300**.

Visit Lippincott Williams & Wilkins on the Internet: http://www.LWW.com. Lippincott Williams &
Wilkins customer service representatives are available from 8:30 am to 6:00 pm, EST.

06 07 08 09 10
1 2 3 4 5 6 7 8 9 10

Acknowledgments

No book of this nature may be produced without the cooperation of a large number of contributors. The author wishes to acknowledge the following colleagues from the Department of Diagnostic Radiology at Allegheny General Hospital, who provided case material and consultation in their areas of expertise: Irwin Beckman, DO; Farhad M. Contractor, MD; Nilima Dash, MD; Melanie Fukui, MD; Kamyar Ilkhanipour, MD; Cathy Kim, MD; Paul M. Kiproff, MD; Andrew Ku, MD; Anthony R. Lupetin, MD; Elmer Nahum, MD; William Poller, MD; Jonathan M. Potts, MD; Robert L. Sciulli, MD; Akash Sharma, MD; Marc Wallace, DO; and Robert Williams, MD.

I extend my appreciation to the following experts who also provided case material for this text: H. Scott Beasley, MD, and David Epstein, MD, from the Department of Radiology, Western Pennsylvania Hospital; Carl Fuhrman, MD, of the Department of Radiology, University of Pittsburgh School of Medicine; Mihra Taljanovic, MD, of the Department of Radiology, University of Arizona; Leonard Swischuk, MD, of the University of Texas at Galveston; James M. Provenzale, MD, of the Department of Diagnostic Radiology, Duke University Medical Center; Sinda B. Dianzumba, MD, of the Division of Cardiology, Allegheny General Hospital; and John J. Crowley, MD, of the Department of Pediatric Imaging, Children's Hospital of Michigan, Detroit.

I appreciate the contributions of Patricia Prince, RT, RDMS, formerly of the Department of Obstetrics and Gynecology, Allegheny General Hospital, for the obstetrics/gynecology ultrasound cases.

I would like to thank Douglas Whitman and Donna Spillane of the Department of Communications, Allegheny General Hospital, for the photography. In addition, I would like to thank Randall S. McKenzie of McKenzie Illustrations for his superb artwork.

My thanks, too, to Maggie Cauley, Department of Diagnostic Radiology, Allegheny General Hospital, for secretarial and editorial assistance in the preparation of the manuscript.

Finally, I especially thank my wife, Alva, for her encouragement and support during the long months of preparation of this work.

In memory of
Morris M. Daffner, PhG; William F. Barry Jr, MD;
George J. Baylin, MD; and Lawrence A. Davis, MD—
teachers, scholars, friends.
Thank you for all you taught me.

Contents

Overview and Principles of Diagnostic Imaging

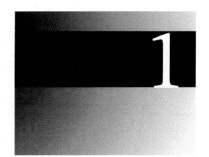

HISTORICAL PERSPECTIVES

The science of radiology had its birth in November 1895 when Wilhelm Conrad Roentgen, a Dutch physicist, discovered a form of radiation that now bears his name, the roentgen ray. He called this new form of unknown radiation—which was invisible, could penetrate objects, and caused fluorescence—*X-strahlung* (x-ray) because initially he did not understand its nature. Roentgen was experimenting with cathode ray tubes, studying their behavior in a completely darkened room. He noticed that when the tube was operating, a faint glow appeared on his laboratory table. That glow, he discovered, was caused by a fluorescent plate that he had inadvertently left on the bench. When he reached for the plate, he was shocked to see the image of the bones of his hand cast onto the plate. His meticulous work investigating his discovery provided the world with an understanding of this new form of radiation. For his monumental work, Roentgen was awarded the Nobel Prize in physics in 1901.

The first recorded diagnostic use of x-rays was in 1896. In the first decade of the discovery of the roentgen ray, the physical effects of x-rays on patients were also observed. It was not long before a new medical specialty, radiology, was born. Traditionally, radiology was divided into two distinct branches: diagnostic and therapeutic. The only common area between these disciplines was the use of ionizing radiation. As each field continued to develop and grow in complexity, it became apparent that separation of the two specialties was needed. Specialists now train in either diagnostic radiology or radiation oncology (therapy).

The last quarter of the twentieth century brought changes in diagnostic radiology that far surpassed those made in the previous 75 years. Developments made in recent decades have revolutionized medical diagnosis, making areas of the body previously inaccessible to nonsurgical examination clearly visible. Furthermore, the ability to image all areas of the body accurately made possible not only biopsy procedures but also numerous interventional techniques that use newer methods of diagnostic imaging for guidance. Previously, these procedures would have required surgical exploration. From a personal perspective, I have had the privilege of being part of the "imaging revolution" that has occurred since I began my radiology residency in 1970. Image intensification, electronic imaging, and the use of computers in radiology are taken for granted today. Unfortunately, that was not always the case. The following personal anecdote epitomizes the state of radiology 40 years ago.

I was a third-year medical student serving on my medicine rotation at the county hospital in Buffalo when we scheduled one of my patients for a fluoroscopic examination of his suspected paralyzed right hemidiaphragm. At the appointed hour of the exam, I was summoned to the radiology department in the basement of the old hospital. I was given a heavy, semirigid lead apron and a pair of red goggles, which they told me to put on. I followed the technologist into the fluoroscopy suite, where several other house staff were similarly attired in apron and goggles. As soon as the door closed, the lights were turned off, and I was suddenly blind in the pitch-blackness. I could hear the radiologist, the late Dr. George Alker, talking to the patient.

He was asking the patient to breathe and to turn in various directions. At one point he asked, "Does everybody see that?"

"Uh huh," was the reply from everyone in the room but me.

"What about you, Dr. Daffner? Did you see it?"

"Dr. Alker," I replied, "I can't see squat!"

"Good Lord, son. Take off your goggles!"

Nobody had told me that the goggles were only for helping my eyes adapt to the dark. I thought they were needed to see the fluoroscopic screen. Before image intensification became standard in radiology departments, however, that was the state of fluoroscopy.

Fortunately, the department in which I trained was state-of-the-art, and we had image intensification. However, even in the early 1970s, not all departments were so equipped. As a senior resident doing *locum tenens* work at a small hospital in eastern North Carolina, I was told to provide coverage at the private office of the radiologist, for whom I was filling in. I walked across the parking lot to his office to do an upper gastrointestinal series. I was somewhat taken aback when I learned that his office did not have image intensification and I would have to use old-fashioned "red goggle" fluoroscopy. I donned my goggles and worked with them on for about a half hour, the prescribed period for dark adaptation, before going into the fluoroscopy suite, where I removed them. I stepped on the foot pedal and looked at the screen and saw nothing but a faint green glow. I decided my eyes were not completely dark adapted, so I put the goggles back on and waited another half hour. Again, the same result in the fluoroscopy suite. I have always believed in "three times is the charm" and decided to give it one more try. This time, when I stepped on the foot pedal, I could actually see something! I had the patient drink some barium and was actually able to follow it down the esophagus, where I lost it in the denser abdomen. After the patient drank some more barium, I moved the fluoroscopic screen around and saw a curvilinear structure. "Aha! The duodenal bulb," I thought to myself. I took four spot films and then instructed the technologist to give the patient more barium and take overhead films. Fifteen minutes later the technologist came into the reading room holding a dripping wet film in a metal frame. (The hospital had no automatic processing either.) It was my spot film. I held it up to the light box and saw four perfect views of the right femoral head! How far radiology has come since then. Table 1.1, a timeline for diagnostic radiology, shows the progress made in the century since Roentgen's discovery.

The realm of diagnostic radiology encompasses various modalities of imaging that may be used individually or, more commonly, in combination to provide the clinician with enough information to aid in making a diagnosis. Diagnostic imaging includes radiography with and without contrast enhancement, computed tomography (CT), magnetic resonance (MR) imaging, diagnostic ultrasound, and nuclear imaging. The first three of these imaging forms use x-rays. Nuclear imaging also is associated with radiation and involves the detection of emissions from radioactive isotopes in various parts of the body; MR imaging and ultrasound do not use ionizing radiation. The newest frontier in diagnostic imaging, molecular imaging, makes possible the identification of certain molecules within cell structures. Although still being investigated, molecular imaging promises to be a boon for the diagnosis of cancers. A brief introduction to each type of examination will help you to understand how these modalities are used in clinical problem solving.

RADIOGRAPHY

Definition

X-rays, or *roentgen rays,* are a form of electromagnetic radiation or energy of extremely short wavelength. The spectrum of electromagnetic radiation is illustrated in Figure 1.1. X-rays in the diagnostic range (shaded area) are near the end of the spectrum of short wavelengths. The shorter the wavelength of an electromagnetic radiation form, the greater its energy and, as a rule, the greater its ability to penetrate various materials.

TABLE 1.1
DIAGNOSTIC RADIOLOGY TIMELINE

Year	Development
1895	Roentgen discovers x-rays
1896	First clinical x-ray made
1897	Bismuth used as contrast for stomach x-rays
1901	Dangers of x-rays first reported by William Rollins
1906	First retrograde pyelogram using colloidal silver nitrate (collargol)
1910	Barium used as contrast agent in gastrointestinal (GI) tract
1911	First double contrast of upper GI
1913	Modern x-ray tube invented by William Coolidge
	Stationary grid invented by Gustav Bucky
	X-ray film of nitrocellulose developed
1914	World War I begins
1915	Bucky's grid motorized by Hollis Potter
1919	First pneumoencephalogram
1921	Intensifying screens developed by Carl Patterson
	First air myelogram
1922	Iodized oil used for myelography
1923	First double-contrast barium enema
1927	First cerebral angiogram
1929	Great Depression begins
	First excretory urogram
1932	Nephrotomography developed
1937	First angiocardiogram
1938	First successful mammogram
1939	World War II begins
1941	First A-mode ultrasound of the skull
1942	Automatic processor for film developed (no pun intended)
1945	Atom bombs dropped on Hiroshima and Nagasaki
1948	First coronary artery angiogram
1949	Xerography developed
1953	Sven Seldinger introduces technique for vascular puncture
1953	Image intensifier used in radiology
1954	Diatrizoate introduced as a safer contrast medium
	Echocardiography developed
1957	Whole-body nuclear scanner developed by Hal Anger
1962	B-mode ultrasound developed
1963	President Kennedy assassinated
1964	SPECT scanning
1968	First men on the moon
1972	CT developed
1974	PET scan
1978	First brain MR image
1980	First commercial MR scanner
1985	Digital radiography, PACS
1990	Helical (spiral) CT
1998	Multislice CT
2000	Molecular imaging

CT, computed tomography; MR, magnetic resonance; PACS, picture archiving and communications system; SPECT, single photon emission computed tomography.

X-rays are described in terms of particles or packets of energy called quanta or *photons*. Photons travel at the speed of light. The amount of energy carried by each photon depends on the wavelength of the radiation. This is measured in electron volts. An electron volt is the amount of energy an electron gains as it is accelerated through a potential of 1 volt.

An atom is ionized when it loses an electron. Any photon with approximately 15 or more electron volts of energy is capable of producing ionization in atoms and molecules (*ionizing* radiation). X-rays, γ-rays, and certain types of ultraviolet radiation are all typical ionizing radiation forms.

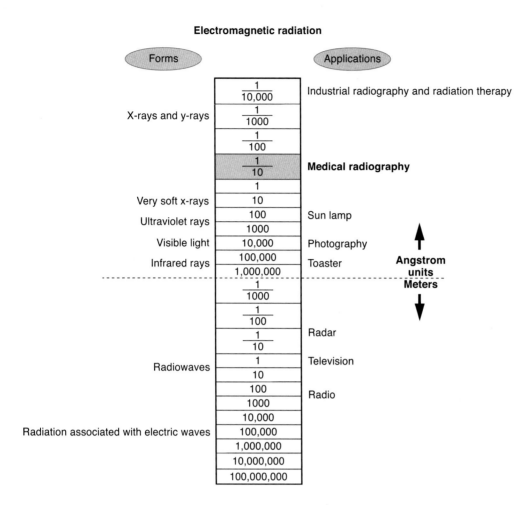

Production of X-Rays

X-rays used in diagnostic radiology require a vacuum and the presence of a high potential difference between a cathode and an anode. In the basic x-ray tube, electrons are boiled off the cathode (filament) by heating it to a very high temperature. Moving these electrons toward the anode at an energy level sufficient to produce x-rays requires a high potential—up to 125,000 volts (125 kV). When the accelerated electrons strike the tungsten anode, x-rays are produced.

Production of Images

Image production by x-rays results from *attenuation* of those x-rays by the material through which they pass. Attenuation is the process by which x-rays are removed from a beam through absorption and scatter. In general, the greater the material's density—that is, the number of grams per cubic centimeter—the greater its ability to absorb or scatter x-rays (Fig. 1.2). Absorption is also influenced by the atomic number of the structure. The denser the structure, the greater the attenuation, which results in less blackening of the film (fewer x-rays strike the film). Less-dense structures attenuate the beam to a lesser degree and result in more blackening of the film (more x-rays strike the film; Fig. 1.3).

It is important to differentiate between two types of density that you will hear mentioned when discussing radiographs with radiologists or other colleagues: physical density and radiographic density. Physical density is the type of density just described. *Radiographic density* refers to the degree of blackness of a film. *Radiographic contrast* is the difference in radiographic densities on a film. The radiographic density of a substance is related to its physical

Figure 1.2. Relationship between density and absorption of x-rays. The denser a particular material, the greater its ability to absorb x-rays. Greater absorption produces less darkening on the film; less absorption produces more darkening.

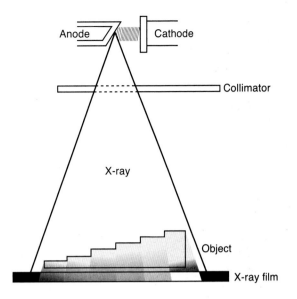

density. The effect on film or other recording media occurs paradoxically: structures of high physical density produce less radiodensity and vice versa. Structures that produce more blackening on film are referred to as being *radiolucent;* those that produce less blackening are called *radiopaque* or *radiodense*. There are four types of radiographic densities; in increasing order of physical density, these are gas (air), fat, soft tissue (water), and bone (metal). Radiographically, these appear as black, gray-black, gray, and white, respectively. Contrast material used in conjunction with radiographic studies is of high radiodensity, above that of

Figure 1.3. The level of absorption of x-rays depends on the composition of the tissue. Denser tissue absorbs more x-rays; less-dense tissue transmits more x-rays. The resulting radiographic image is essentially a "shadowgram."

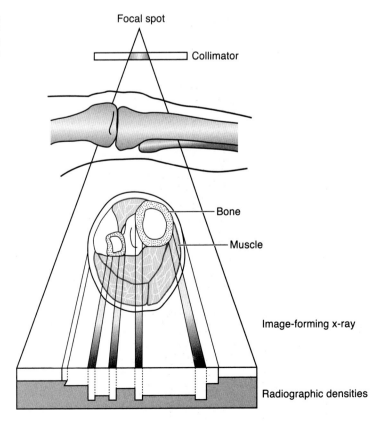

water and lower than that of bone. CT has the ability to detect minute differences in the densities of tissues and portray them in varying shades of gray. These CT densities are measured in Hounsfield units, after Godfrey Hounsfield, the father of CT. Water is arbitrarily given the value of 1.0, fat and gas densities are negative values, and bone densities are very high.

Recording Media

The most common type of recording medium used to be x-ray film. X-ray film is still used in many parts of the world. However, state-of-the art radiology departments are replacing x-ray film with electronic recording media. X-ray film consists of a plastic sheet coated with a thin emulsion that contains silver bromide and a small amount of silver iodide. This emulsion is sensitive to light and radiation. A protective coating covers the emulsion. When the film is exposed to light or to ionizing radiation and then developed, chemical changes take place within the emulsion, resulting in the deposition of metallic silver, which is black. The amount of blackening on the film depends entirely on the amount of radiation reaching the film and therefore on the amount attenuated or removed from the beam by the subject.

Other recording media include fluoroscopic screen and image intensification systems, photoelectric detector crystals, xenon detector systems, and computer-linked detectors that measure actual attenuation. The latter are linked to discs in the computer system and are described in greater detail later in the chapter.

A fluoroscopic screen is coated with a substance (phosphor) that gives off visible light (or fluoresces) when it is irradiated. The brightness of the light is proportional to the intensity of the x-ray beam striking the plate and depends on the amount of radiation removed from the beam by the object being irradiated. In its most common use today, the fluoroscopic screen is combined with an electronic device that converts the visible light into an electron stream that amplifies the image (makes it brighter) by converting the electron pattern back into visible light. This system allows the radiologist to see the image clearly without requiring dark adaptation of the eyes, as was necessary in "conventional" (non–image-enhanced) fluoroscopy, described graphically earlier in the chapter. The technology of image intensification was originally developed around 1950 for military use in nighttime security and warfare. Intensifying screens, variants of fluoroscopic screens, are used in most film cassettes to reduce the amount of radiation needed to produce an acceptable exposure.

Photons emitted by radioisotopes are detected with sodium iodide crystals. These crystals respond, when irradiated, by emitting light whose brightness is related to the energy of the photons striking them. Photodetectors convert the light into an electronic signal, which is then amplified and converted into a variety of display images. Modern systems use computer-linked detectors.

The twenty-first century is clearly the era of the computer and the age of the "information superhighway." Computers are now common fixtures in state-of-the-art radiology departments. CT and MR scanners and digital radiography units use electronic sensors that actually measure the attenuation coefficient of tissue through which the x-ray beam has passed and converts this mathematical value into a digitized shade of gray. The data are fed into a computer that plots the location of each of those measurements to produce the computer image. This is recorded on compact discs (CDs) or digital video discs (DVDs) and is displayed on a television monitor or made into a hard copy (film or paper) by a multiformat camera.

Computed radiography, a derivative of CT technology, is now replacing conventional film-screen radiography. It forms the basis for the *picture archiving and communications system* (PACS; Figs. 1.4 and 1.5) as well as for teleradiology. The typical PACS uses a photosensitive electronic plate that records the amount of radiation striking each location. This, as previously explained, depends on the density of the tissue through which the x-ray beam passes and the degree of attenuation of the beam. The radiation intensity at each site is recorded digitally to produce a digital image that can be transmitted directly to a high-resolution monitor or from which hard copies can be made. Storage is on CD or DVD.

Modern radiology departments do not have conventional view boxes. Rather, the reading stations are a series of high-quality television monitors (see Fig. 1.5). Similarly, the clinical areas of the hospital and the physicians' offices have monitors rather than view boxes. The problem of delay in transportation of x-ray films from the processing area to the file room and then to the reading areas is eliminated because the images are sent directly from the processing area to the

Figure 1.4. Outline of a picture archiving and communications system (PACS). CT, computed tomography; DR, digital radiography; DSA. digital subtraction angiography; MRI, magnetic resonance imaging; QC, quality control.

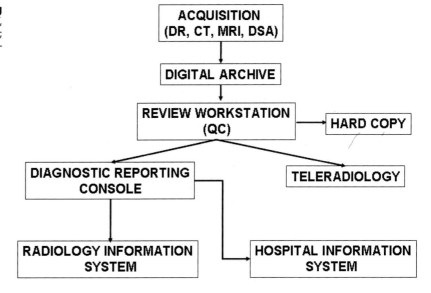

reading areas electronically. Furthermore, lost or bad films are no longer a problem. Clinicians can directly view images by having them sent directly from the central archive to their work areas. An image that is too dark or too light can be electronically manipulated at the reading station (Fig. 1.6). Finally, having the diagnostic information in digital form enables the speedy electronic transfer of data for teleradiology.

State-of-the-art medical facilities have made the transition to PACS and computerized technology. Doing so requires cooperation among members of the radiology department as well as medical records and hospital administration. In fully integrated systems, like those used at the Mayo Clinic and its satellites, the radiology information system (RIS) communicates directly with the hospital information system (HIS). The RIS is used for scheduling examinations, communicating clinical data to the radiologists, archiving studies, and reporting the interpretations of those studies. The HIS provides all the medical information that a treating or consulting physician may need when seeing a patient.

Teleradiology is a natural offshoot of electronic imaging. Early systems relied on the transmission of data over telephone lines, but the process was very slow. Improvements in communication networks, including the Internet, led to the rapid development of a new industry. Modern teleradiology systems are Web based and thus no longer rely on telephone lines. Among its many applications, teleradiology is probably most commonly used to provide after-hours ("night hawk") coverage when a department cannot have a radiologist on staff all night. Several enterprising companies have located in Sydney, Australia, or in Israel, where the time differences allow their radiologists to be working during the day while supplying information to U.S. doctors working at night. As a rule, these companies provide "preliminary" interpreta-

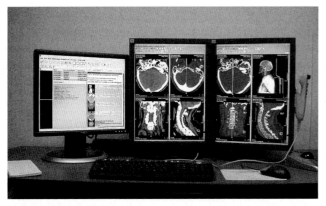

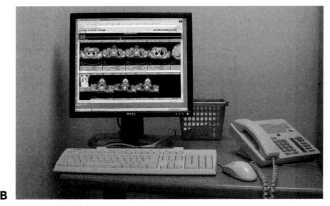

A   B

Figure 1.5. PACS reading consoles. A. Diagnostic console in the radiology department. **B.** Satellite console in an office.

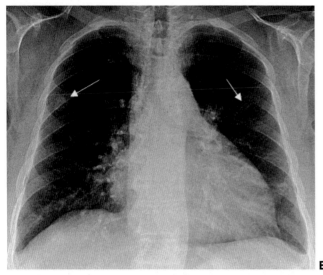

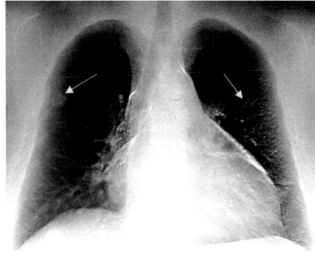

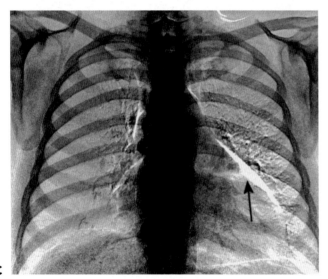

Figure 1.6. Electronic manipulations possible with PACS. A, frontal radiograph of patient with known renal carcinoma shows suspected nodules in both upper lobes (*arrows*) **B,** same image with bones electronically subtracted shows bilateral lung nodules (*arrows*). **C,** same image with lungs and heart subtracted shows the nodules also subtracted. Note the artifact over the heart due to cardiac motion (*arrow*).

tions for a set fee per study. Their staff comprise American-trained radiologists certified by the American Board of Radiology; most have also completed fellowships and are licensed in all 50 U.S. states. The second application of teleradiology is providing coverage for facilities that do not have on-site radiologists. This may involve some night and weekend work as well. In this situation, images are sent to a central "command post," usually at a university and typically staffed all night. The third use of teleradiology is for consultation. In this situation, images are sent from one facility to another for a more experienced radiologist to review. In our department, we use this mode for consultation between satellite facilities in our hospital system.

Voice recognition technology has further improved the turnaround time to produce a final report on imaging studies. Voice recognition machines produce quality reports with little need for editing by the radiologist, replacing the traditional method of dictation transcribed by a typist. When voice recognition is combined with PACS technology, final reports can be generated within minutes of the imaging study being performed.

Image Quality

Physical and geometric factors affect the radiographic image, regardless of the format. These factors include thickness of the part being irradiated, motion, scatter, magnification, and distortion.

The *thickness* of the part being imaged determines how much of the beam is removed or attenuated, as explained earlier. Thus, for adequate penetration, an obese patient requires

Figure 1.7. Grid function. A grid absorbs scattered radiation. Angling of the lead strips permits only the primary x-ray beam to pass through.

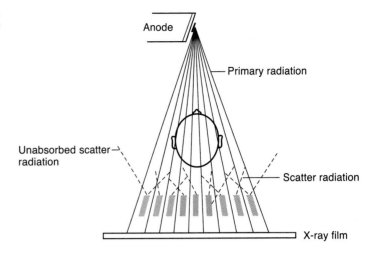

more x-rays than does a thin patient, bone requires more x-rays than does the surrounding muscle, and a limb with a cast requires more x-rays, as does a wet plaster cast (because the water attenuates the x-ray beam).

Motion of a part being radiographed results in a blurred, nondiagnostic image. Motion may be overcome by shortening the exposure time, and one way of decreasing exposure time is to enhance the effectiveness of the recording medium. This may be done by using an intensifying screen—a device coated with a fluorescent material that gives off visible light when struck by x-rays. The visible light produces the exposure. Cassettes containing screens are used for about 99% of diagnostic radiographic work. This has the advantage of reducing the exposure time during which motion can occur. Improvements in screen technology have allowed detailed examinations without increasing radiation dosage—a particular advantage for mammography. However, this technology is being replaced by digital imaging, as previously mentioned.

Scatter is produced by deflection of some of the primary radiation beam; this can produce fog on the film and is undesirable. To eliminate as much scatter as possible, a grid with alternating angled slats of very thin radiolucent material combined with thin lead strips is used (Fig. 1.7). To prevent the lead strips from casting their own shadows as they absorb radiation, the whole grid is moved very quickly during the exposure, eliminating shadow lines. This system is known as the Bucky-Potter system, after the two men who invented it.

The radiographic image is a two-dimensional representation of three-dimensional structures. Consequently, some parts will be farther from the film than others. Geometrically, x-rays behave similarly to light. Hence, *magnification* of objects will occur when they are some distance from the film. The farther an object is from the film, the greater the magnification and the less the sharpness; the closer an object is to the film, the less the magnification and the greater the sharpness (Fig. 1.8). This has considerable importance in evaluating the heart on chest radiographs. On the standard chest radiograph, the x-ray enters the back of the patient

Figure 1.8. Magnification and image sharpness. A. The object is farther from the film, resulting in a larger image. However, its margin is not distinct. **B.** The object is closer to the film, resulting in a smaller and sharper image than in A.

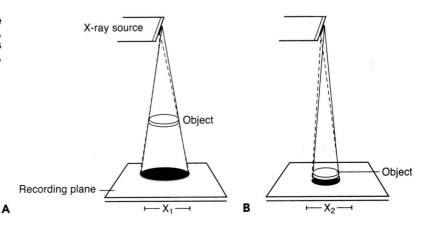

and exits the front; this is called a posterior-to-anterior (PA) radiograph. Because the heart is located anteriorly, relatively little magnification results. However, on an anterior-to-posterior (AP) radiograph of the chest, the beam enters the patient's front and exits the back. Hence, magnification of the heart is somewhat greater because of its shorter distance from the film. The best rule to follow to reduce the undesirable effect of magnification is to have the part of greatest interest closest to the film. This will produce the truest image of the region of interest.

Distortion occurs when the object being radiographed is not perfectly perpendicular to the x-ray beam. The radiographic image of an object depends on the sum of the shadows produced by that object when x-rayed. Changes in the relationship of that object to the x-ray beam may distort its radiographic image (Fig. 1.9). For diagnostic clarity, therefore, it is best to have the part of major interest as close to and as perpendicular to the film as possible.

Radiography is the bread and butter of the diagnostic radiologist. The term *plain film* refers to radiography in which no contrast material is used to enhance various body structures. In performing radiographic examinations, the natural contrast between the basic four radiodensities—air (gas), soft tissue (water), fat, and bone (metal)—is relied on to define abnormalities. Examples of plain-film studies with which you are familiar include chest, abdominal, and skeletal radiographs.

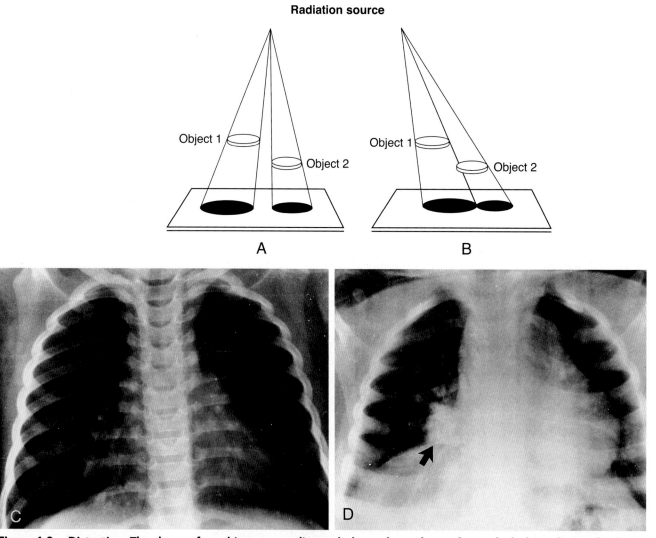

Figure 1.9.   Distortion. The shape of an object on a radiograph depends on the angle at which the radiographic beam strikes it. A. Two objects of similar size cast distinct images when the x-ray beam is nearly perpendicular. The difference in size is the result of magnification. **B.** Angling the x-ray beam while the objects remain in the same relationship to one another results in an overlapping image that is not a true representation of the actual objects. **C.** Posterior-to-anterior (P)A radiograph of the chest in a patient with right middle lobe pneumonia. **D.** Lordotic view of the same patient made with the patient bending backward toward the film. Notice the change in the appearance of the heart, ribs, and infiltrate, which now appears as a mass adjacent to the heart border on the right (*arrow*).

Radiography has its special modifications: fluoroscopy and tomography. Fluoroscopy is a useful modality for studying the diaphragm, heart motion, valve calcification within the heart, and localization of chest masses (Fig. 1.10). Despite being a fast and inexpensive way to determine the presence or absence of lung nodules, it is underutilized.

Conventional tomography is a mode of imaging in which the x-ray tube and the film move in concert to produce a blurred image. It was originally developed by scientists in five countries working independently between 1921 and 1935. The objects in the focal plane, or fulcrum, remain in sharp focus (Fig. 1.11). Tomography blurs out unwanted structures while keeping the object of interest in clearer focus. It is most useful in evaluating bony structures. Tomography improves contrast but cannot create contrast where there is none to begin with.

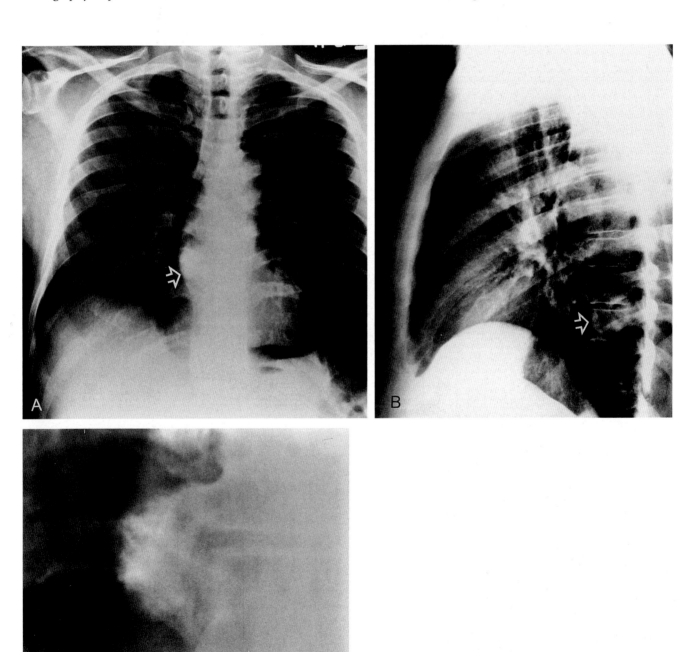

Figure 1.10.   The value of chest fluoroscopy. A. PA chest radiograph shows a "mass" through the cardiac shadow to the right of midline (*arrow*). **B.** Lateral view shows the mass to be posterior (*arrow*). **C.** Fluoroscopic spot film shows the density in question to be bone spurs bridging the thoracic vertebral bodies. There was no tumor.

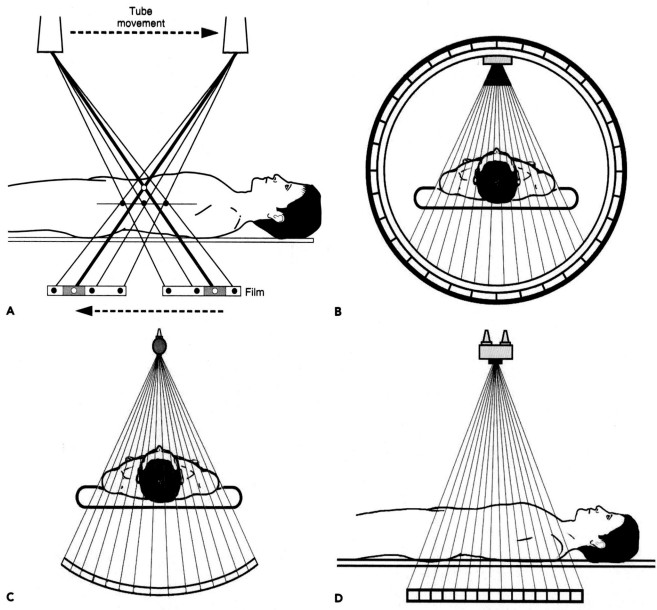

Figure 1.11. Principles of tomography. A. Conventional tomography. The x-ray tube and the film move in opposite directions. The focal point (*open circle*) remains in sharp focus, whereas the other images are blurred. This procedure is no longer performed in the United States. **B.** Computed tomography (CT). In the modern CT scanner, the x-ray tube rotates within the gantry. Instead of film, detectors measure the amount of radiation removed from the x-ray beam. **C and D.** Modern CT scanners use arrays of detectors to shorten the time needed for the scan.

In the United States, conventional tomography has been replaced by CT, which is discussed later in the chapter. Manufacturers no longer make tomographic equipment. However, there are still parts of the world that rely on the technique.

CONTRAST EXAMINATIONS

Plain-film radiography is adequate for situations in which natural radiographic contrast exists between body structures, such as the heart and lungs, or between the bones and adjacent soft tissues. To examine structures that do not have inherent contrast differences from the surrounding tissues, it is necessary to use one of several contrast agents. Contrast examinations were used more extensively in the past to evaluate abdominal or intracranial masses. By putting contrast material in organs that could be opacified, the locations and sizes of the masses could be indirectly determined. CT and MR imaging have made most of these examinations obsolete. The majority of contrast studies are of the gastrointestinal tract, urinary tract, and blood vessels.

The most common contrast material used for gastrointestinal examinations is a preparation of barium sulfate mixed with other agents to produce a uniform suspension. These products are available as premixed powders or liquids. They may be administered alone or, more commonly, in combination with air, water, or an effervescent mixture that produces carbon dioxide. They are administered either by mouth (antegrade) or by rectum (retrograde). Gas-enhanced studies are referred to as air contrast studies (Fig. 1.12).

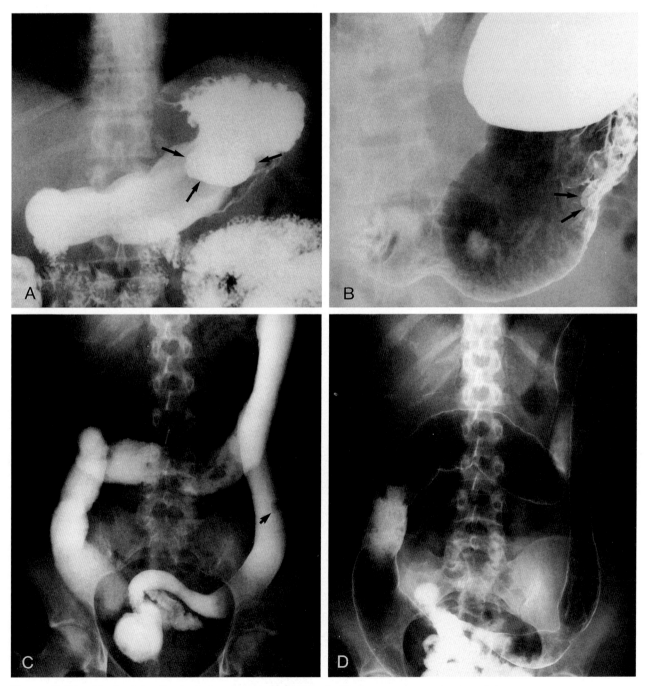

Figure 1.12.   Gastrointestinal contrast examinations. A. Single-contrast examination of the stomach demonstrates a large gastric ulcer (*arrows*). **B.** Double-contrast examination shows a tumor along the greater curvature (*arrows*). **C.** Single-contrast barium enema shows a polyp in the descending colon (*arrow*) in a patient with ulcerative colitis. Notice the loss of haustral markings. **D.** An air contrast barium enema in the same patient.

In addition to barium preparations, water-soluble agents are available for studying the gastrointestinal tract whenever there is a possibility of leakage of the contrast material beyond the bowel wall. Although barium is a chemically inert substance, it produces a severe desmoplastic reaction in tissues. Water-soluble agents, on the other hand, do not produce this type of reaction and are absorbed from the leakage site to be excreted through the kidneys. The water-soluble agents, however, are not without hazard, because they can cause a severe chemical pneumonia if aspirated. Water-soluble agents also cost more and thus are not used on a routine basis.

Urography is the radiographic study of the urinary tract. The contrast agents used for this study are primarily the ionic water-soluble salts diatrizoic or iothalamic acids or the nonionic agents iopamidol or iohexol. The common term for this study is *intravenous urogram;* an older and less appropriate term is *intravenous pyelogram.* The physiology of these agents is discussed in Chapter 2. Intravenous urography largely has been replaced by CT.

Angiography is the study of the vascular system. Water-soluble agents similar to those used for urography are injected either intra-arterially or intravenously, and a rapid sequence exposure is made to follow the course of the contrast material through the blood vessels (Fig. 1.13).

A *sinogram* (or fistulogram) involves the injection of contrast material through an abnormal sinus tract into the body. Water-soluble agents are commonly used for these studies. In evaluating an empyema cavity in the chest, where there is a danger that a bronchopleural fistula may be present, an oil-soluble material such as propyliodone (Dionosil) is used because water-soluble contrast material entering the bronchial tree can produce a severe and often fatal chemical pneumonia.

Diseases encroaching on the vertebral canal may be studied by *myelography.* The main indication is evidence of spinal cord or nerve root compression. The most common lesion is a herniated nucleus pulposus from a lumbar disc. Myelography is performed by inserting a needle between the spinous processes of lumbar vertebrae and entering the subarachnoid space. It may also be performed by puncture of the cisterna magna when there is a complete block within the vertebral canal and it is necessary to inject contrast medium above the lesion. Cerebrospinal fluid may be removed for study at this time. Nonionic, iodinated, water-soluble

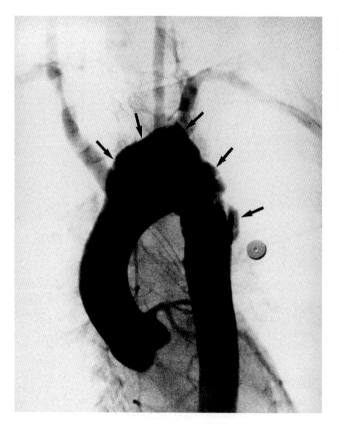

Figure 1.13. Arteriogram in a patient with posttraumatic rupture of the aorta. This is a subtraction film in which black and white are reversed to improve contrast. Notice the irregularity and ballooning of the aortic arch at the site of injury (*arrows*).

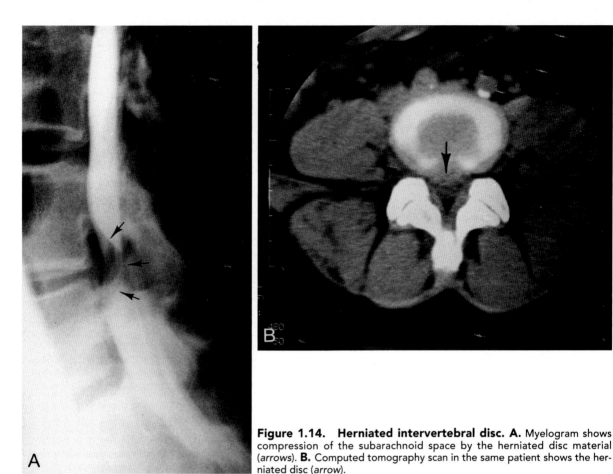

Figure 1.14. Herniated intervertebral disc. A. Myelogram shows compression of the subarachnoid space by the herniated disc material (*arrows*). **B.** Computed tomography scan in the same patient shows the herniated disc (*arrow*).

compounds are injected under fluoroscopic monitoring in varying amounts, and the patient is positioned for the study. Figure 1.14 shows a myelogram of a patient with a herniated lumbar disc. Notice the compression of the thecal sac by the herniated material. Myelography is often performed in conjunction with CT. The development of MR imaging, however, has decreased the number of myelograms performed.

COMPUTED TOMOGRAPHY

Under ordinary circumstances, the fleshy organs of the body, such as the heart, kidneys, liver, spleen, and pancreas, are considered uniform in radiographic density—like water, which produces a gray appearance on conventional radiographs. However, these tissues vary somewhat in their chemical properties, and it is possible, using computer-enhanced techniques, to measure those differences, magnify them, and display them in varying shades of gray or in color. This is the basis of CT. Godfrey Hounsfield was the first to develop the CT scanner in England. For his efforts, he was awarded the 1979 Nobel Prize in medicine.

In CT (Fig. 1.15; see Fig. 1.11B), an x-ray beam and a detector system move through an arc of 360°, irradiating the subject with a highly collimated (restricted) beam. This allows the detector system to measure the intensity of radiation passing through the subject. The data from these measurements are analyzed by a computer system that assigns different shades of gray (CT or Hounsfield numbers) to different structures based on their absorption or attenuation coefficients. The computer reconstructs a picture based on geometric plots of where these measurements were taken. Interestingly, although this system of diagnosis was developed in

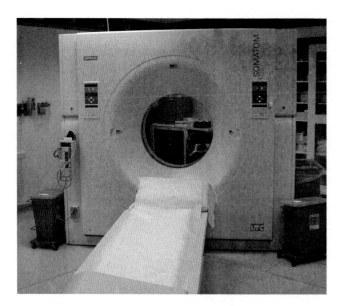

Figure 1.15. Typical computed tomography scanner.

the early 1970s, the mathematical formula for the reconstruction of images based on measurements of their points in space was developed in 1917 by the mathematician Johann Radon.

The latest variation on CT is that it is performed using helical or spiral multislice technology. In the classic CT study, multiple contiguous images are obtained (with or without section overlap) to produce sections resembling the slices of a loaf of bread (Fig. 1.16A). In spiral CT, the data are acquired using technology that produces sections resembling an apple that has been peeled or sliced spirally (Fig. 1.16B). Furthermore, all modern CT systems acquire data using banked rows of 4, 8, 16, 24, 32, or 64 detectors at one time, thus the term *multislice*. The result of using this technology is that images may be obtained rapidly and with overlap of data that provide information on every square millimeter in the area of study. It is now possible to image an entire thorax or an entire abdomen in 20 seconds or less. This speed is important when breath holding is necessary to prevent motion artifacts. Rapid throughput of patients is made possible, as is rapid multiplanar and three-dimensional reconstruction of images (Fig. 1.17). Speed is particularly essential when trauma victims are imaged.

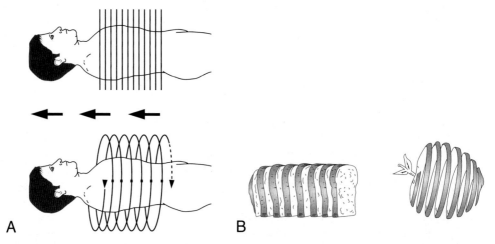

A   B

Figure 1.16. Conventional versus spiral computed tomography (CT). A. Methods of acquisition of the data. In conventional CT (top), individual slices are obtained. In spiral CT (bottom), a continuous band of information is obtained. Horizontal arrows indicate the direction of patient travel through the gantry. **B.** Comparison of data obtained by conventional and spiral CT. Conventional CT obtains individual slices, much like the loaf of bread on the left. Spiral CT produces a continuous band of information, similar to the apple on the right.

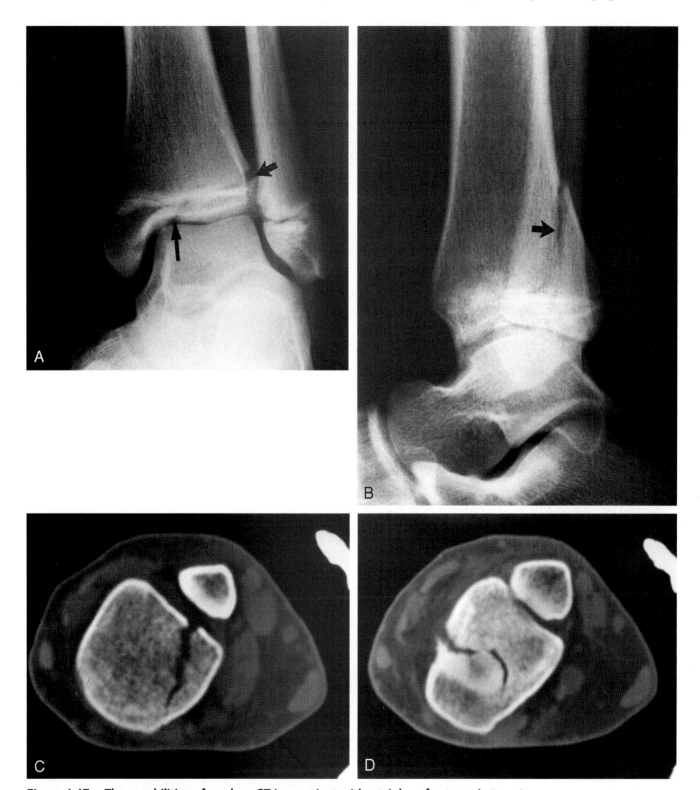

Figure 1.17.   The capabilities of modern CT in a patient with a triplane fracture. A. Frontal radiograph shows a fracture through the distal tibial epiphysis (*long arrow*) as well as separation of the lateral tibial physis (*short arrow*). **B.** Lateral radiograph shows the coronal component of the fracture (*arrow*). **C.** Axial image shows the coronal fracture through the posterior lip of the tibia. **D.** Axial image at the tibial plafond shows the sagittal component. Notice the difference in orientation of the fracture from that demonstrated in C. *(continued on page 18)*

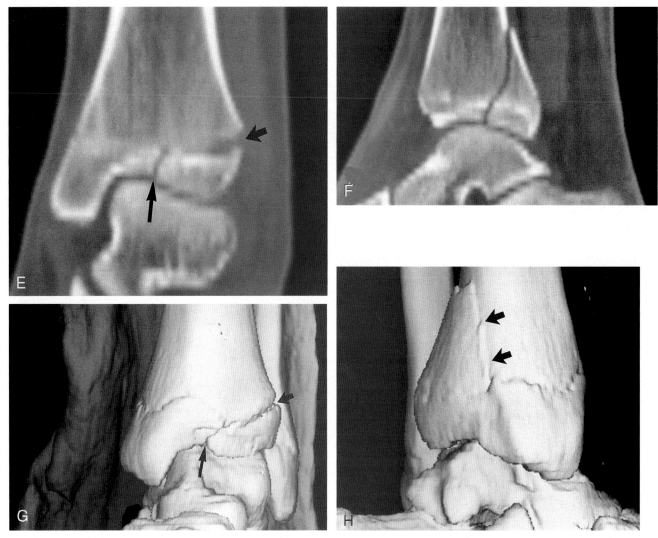

Figure 1.17 *(continued)*   **E.** Coronal tomographic reconstruction shows the sagittal fracture the epiphysis (*long arrow*) as well as the physeal separation laterally (*short arrow*). **F.** Sagittal tomographic reconstruction shows the coronal fracture of the posterior portion of the tibia. **G and H.** Three-dimensional reconstructions show the various components of the fracture (*arrows*)[Unknown font 2: Arial Black];[End Font: Arial Black]ocAU: Two kinds of arrows are used in image G without apparent reason. Should all arrows in G be the same?:.

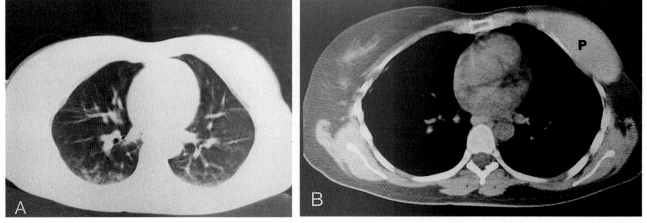

Figure 1.18.   The effects of changes in window settings. A. Image of a patient's thorax made at a window setting to enhance the lungs. **B.** The same section at soft tissue windows. Compare with A. A breast prosthesis (*P*) is evident.

Figure 1.19. Meningioma. Cranial CT shows a mass (*M*) in the right occipital region. Notice the bowing of the septum (*arrow*).

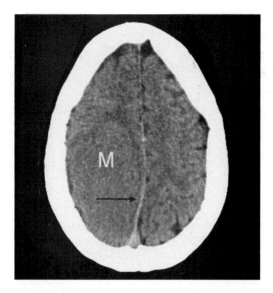

The information obtained with CT systems is displayed on a television (cathode ray tube [CRT]) monitor and recorded on CD or DVD. Once the information has been recorded, it is possible to alter the windows of the various densities to optimally demonstrate the lungs, soft tissues, or bone on the reading console (Fig. 1.18). The data from the CRT are linked to a digital display system such as a PACS or teleradiology or may be transferred to x-ray film using a device known as a multiformat camera. To enhance the appearance of certain viscera or vascular neoplasms, contrast material is injected intravenously. The contrast agents used are identical to those used in angiography or urography.

Cranial scanning is performed to evaluate patients with various neurologic findings. This study is particularly useful in defining and localizing brain tumors (primary or metastatic) and in evaluating patients with neurologic emergencies such as intracerebral hemorrhage or subdural hematoma. Figure 1.19 shows the scan of a patient with a meningioma. Notice how well the tumor is defined against the normal brain tissue. Figure 1.20 shows a patient with a subdural hematoma. Notice the compression of normal brain tissue by the hematoma.

Figure 1.20. Subdural hematoma on the left. Notice the compression of the left side of the brain by the low-density hematoma (*arrows*). There is loss of the sulci on the left as the result of compression. Compare with the right.

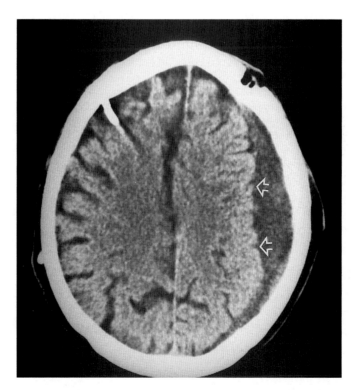

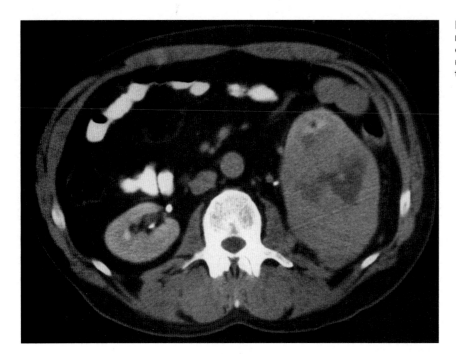

Figure 1.21. Abdominal CT showing a renal carcinoma on the left. Notice the difference in kidney size and loss of the normal parenchymal appearance compared with the right.

Scanning the rest of the body is particularly useful in evaluating visceral neoplasms (Fig. 1.21). Other uses include studies of patients with abdominal trauma (Fig. 1.22), investigation of patients with suspected pancreatic disease, mediastinal studies for defining the extent of tumors, evaluation of patients with Hodgkin disease or lymphoma for staging purposes, diagnosis of intra-abdominal abscess (Fig. 1.23), and scanning the musculoskeletal system for various bone and soft tissue disorders (Fig. 1.24).

NUCLEAR IMAGING

Nuclear medicine traditionally has two divisions: nuclear imaging (radiology) and laboratory analysis. The diagnostic radiologist is concerned with the imaging aspect of the field. The use of isotopes for laboratory purposes and for evaluating physiologic functions are not discussed in this book. However, you should be aware that the laboratory aspect of nuclear medicine is equally as important as the imaging aspect.

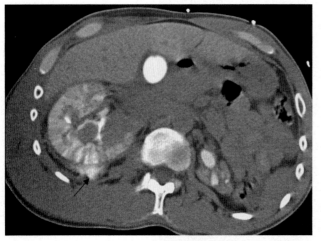

A

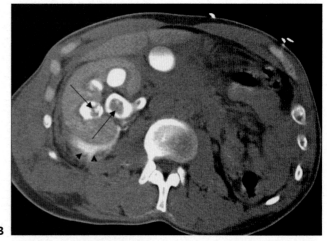

B

Figure 1.22. Renal laceration CT. A. Axial CT image shows enlargement of the right kidney with mottling of its cortex. There is extravasated urine posteriorly in the renal capsule (*arrow*). **B.** Slightly lower image shows blood clots in the collecting system (*arrows*) as well as extravasated contrast posteriorly (*arrowheads*).

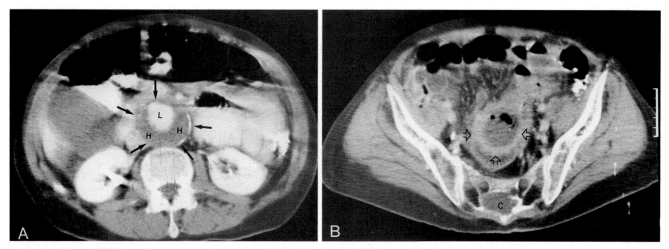

Figure 1.23.   Abdominal aortic aneurysm and perirectal abscess. A. A CT scan through the abdomen shows a large abdominal aortic aneurysm (*arrows*). Notice the central enlarged lumen (*L*), the more peripheral hematoma (*H*), and the calcification of the wall on the left side. **B.** Further down, there is a gas-containing mass (*arrows*) in the perirectal region. Incidental note is also made of a large subarachnoid cyst in the sacrum (*C*).

The principles of nuclear imaging depend on the selective uptake of different compounds by different organs of the body. These compounds may be labeled with a radioactive substance of sufficient energy level to allow detection outside the body. The ideal isotope can be administered in low doses, is nontoxic, has a short half-life, is readily incorporated into "physiologic" compounds, and is relatively inexpensive. Technetium-99m fulfills most of these requirements.

The *half-life* of an element is the time necessary for its degradation to one-half of its original activity. There are actually three types of half-lives: physical, biologic, and effective. The *physical half-life* is the period in which the element would decay on its own. This occurs naturally, whether the element is sitting on the laboratory shelf or has been administered to a patient. *Biologic half-life* concerns the normal physiologic removal of the substance to which the isotope has been attached. For example, the sodium pertechnetate commonly injected for

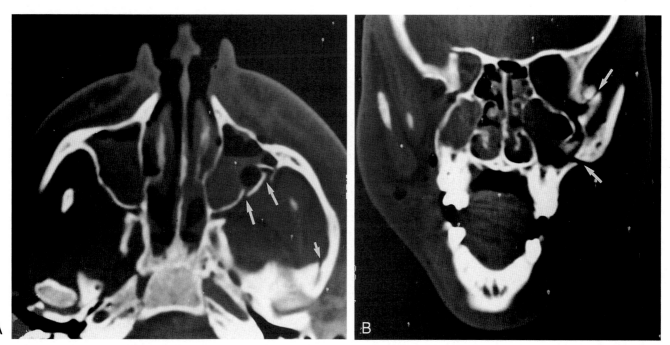

Figure 1.24.   CT evaluation of a patient with facial fractures. A. Axial image shows fractures of the posterior wall of the left maxillary sinus (*long arrows*) as well as a fracture of the posterior portion of the zygomatic arch (*short arrow*). B. Direct coronal image shows fractures of the malar strut (*arrows*) on the left.

TABLE 1.2.
ISOTOPE SCANS AND COMMON USES

Type of Scan	Figure No.[a]	Common Indications
Lung	1.25	Pulmonary embolism, quantification of perfusion
Liver	1.26	Masses (hemangiomas), metastases, cholestasis
Bone	1.27	Metastases, pain, suspected child abuse
Thyroid	1.28	"Goiter" nodules, hyperthyroidism, cancer
Heart	1.29	Myocardial perfusion, function, and viability

[a]Scan illustrated in these figures.

nuclear scanning is excreted into the urine and the gastrointestinal tract. Although the physical half-life of technetium-99m is approximately 6 hours, the biologic half-life is less. The *effective half-life* is a mathematical derivation based on a formula combining the biologic and physical half-lives. It measures the actual time the isotope remains effective within the body.

Nuclear imaging is performed on either a static or dynamic basis. Static studies include the thyroid, liver, and conventional single photon emission computed tomography (SPECT) scans. Dynamic studies additionally include rapid sequence images to assess blood flow to organs such as the skeleton or the kidneys. Common types of scans are listed in Table 1.2 and depicted in Figures 1.25 through 1.29). Equipment for detecting the uptake of isotopes and recording their images includes the γ-camera and the tomographic scanner.

There are basically five mechanisms of isotope concentration within the body:

1. Blood pool or compartmental localization (e.g., cardiac scan)
2. Physiologic incorporation (e.g., thyroid scan, bone scan)
3. Capillary blockage (e.g., lung scan)
4. Phagocytosis (e.g., liver scan)
5. Cell sequestration (e.g., spleen scan)

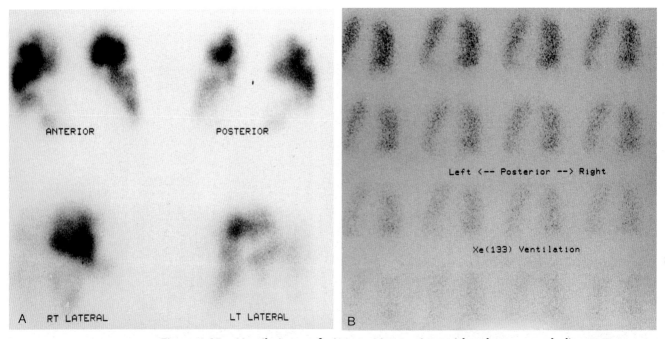

Figure 1.25. Ventilation-perfusion scan in a patient with pulmonary emboli. A. Perfusion scan of the lungs shows many areas devoid of radioisotope (photopenia) bilaterally. B. The ventilation scan is normal. This combination of findings is diagnostic of pulmonary embolism.

Figure 1.26. Liver scan in a patient with multiple metastases to the right lobe of the liver. Notice the large photopenic areas.

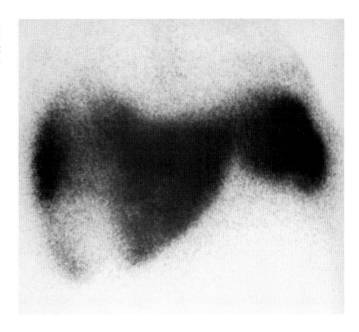

Figure 1.27. Bone scan in a patient with metastatic disease. Notice the areas of the increased tracer concentration (*blackness*) throughout the skeleton.

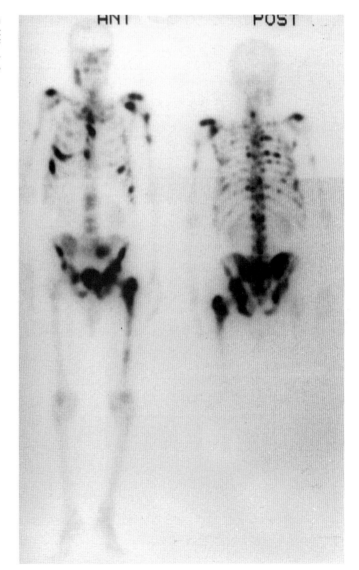

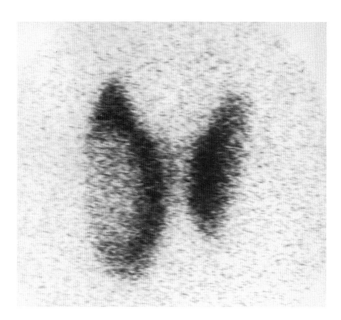

Figure 1.28. Thyroid scan showing a nodule as a photopenic area in the right lobe of the thyroid.

Conventional nuclear scans use isotopes that produce γ- or x-rays. Positron emission tomography (PET) uses cyclotron- or generator-produced isotopes of relatively short half-life that emit positrons, which are significantly higher-energy particles. The initial application of PET scanning was primarily to evaluate brain metabolism by assessing blood flow to a specific part of the brain—for example, measuring focal decrease in epilepsy or differentiating between a tumor and radiation necrosis that might occur after treatment. Areas of increased brain activity show selective uptake of the injected isotope. It has been particularly useful in evaluating patients with senile dementia or Alzheimer disease (Fig. 1.30). PET scanning is more fre-

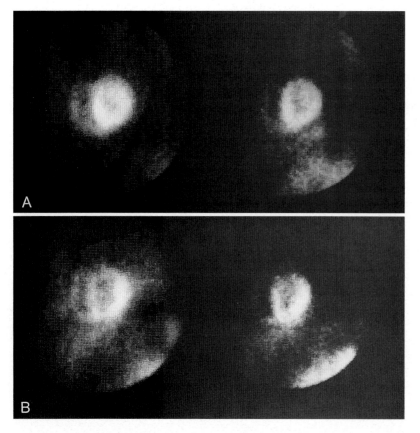

Figure 1.29. Cardiac scan with thallium. A. Resting scan over the apex of the heart is normal. **B.** During exercise, there are photopenic areas within the heart muscle, indicating lack of perfusion.

Figure 1.30. Positron emission tomography (PET) scan for diagnosing Alzheimer disease. A. Focal decrease in perfusion with F-18 fluoro-2-deoxyglucose (F-18 FDG) of parietotemporal lobes along with the frontal and posterior cingulate cortex (*arrows*), with preservation of cortical perfusion in motor cortex and temporal lobes, is characteristic for diagnosis of Alzheimer disease. **B.** Symmetric cortical perfusion in a normal patient.

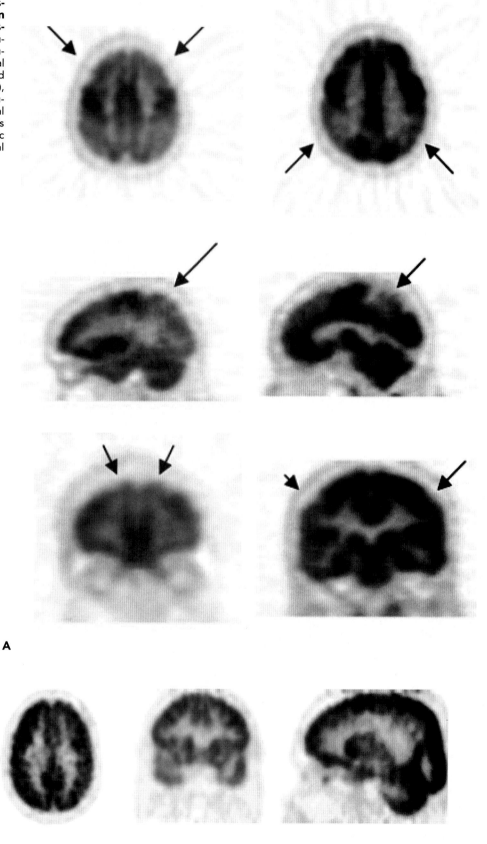

A

B

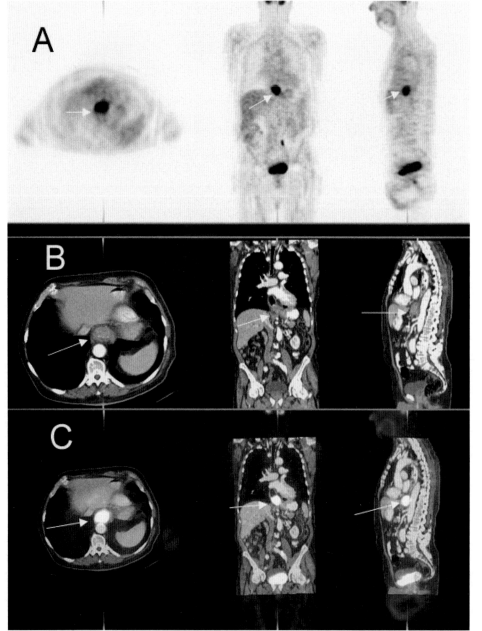

Figure 1.31. PET scan to diagnose metastases. A. Axial, frontal, and lateral images show an area of abnormal tracer activities in the epigastric region (*arrows*). **B.** Corresponding CT scan in axial plane and sagittal and coronal reconstruction show a mass in the retrocardiac area (*arrows*). **C.** Fusing the images of the PET scan with the CT show the exact location of the metastatic lymph nodes (*arrows*). Notice the exact superimposition of the abnormality on the combined study.

quently used for oncologic imaging in diagnosis, staging, and restaging of malignancy after treatment. The reason for this is the ability of the PET scan to show increased use of glucose by the tumor (Fig. 1.31A). With newer technology, the PET image can be combined with a CT image (PET/CT) to allow more accurate localization for either surgery or biopsy of suspected metastases (Fig. 1.31B).

MAGNETIC RESONANCE IMAGING

MR imaging is a noninvasive technique that does not use ionizing radiation. In the parameters used for medical imaging, it is without significant health hazard. MR imaging is based on the principles described by Felix Bloch and Edward Purcell in an experimental procedure they designed to evaluate the chemical characteristics of matter on a molecular level. For their work, Bloch and Purcell were awarded the Nobel Prize in physics in 1962. Raymond Damadian began investigating the possibilities of using MR for imaging in 1971. The development of computer imaging algorithms for CT accelerated the development of MR for medical diagnosis. Paul Lauterbur and Peter Mansfield were able to produce the first successful images using this technique, and for their efforts they received the 2003 Nobel Prize in medicine.

MR imaging uses a pulsed radiofrequency (RF) beam in the presence of a high magnetic field to produce high-quality images of the body in any plane. The nuclei of any atoms with odd numbers of nucleons (protons and neutrons) behave like weak magnets in that they align themselves with a strong magnetic field. If a specific RF signal is used to perturb the nuclei under study, their relationship to the external magnetic field is altered and they will generate a radio signal of their own that has the same frequency as the signal that initially disrupted them (Fig. 1.32). This signal can then be amplified and recorded—the basis for MR imaging. Although many nuclei may be used for MR imaging, the most common is hydrogen because of its abundance in tissue and its sensitivity to the phenomenon of magnetic resonance.

Like CT, MR imaging can display structures in a transverse or axial fashion. However, MR imaging can also produce images in any other planes. The common display parameters used are

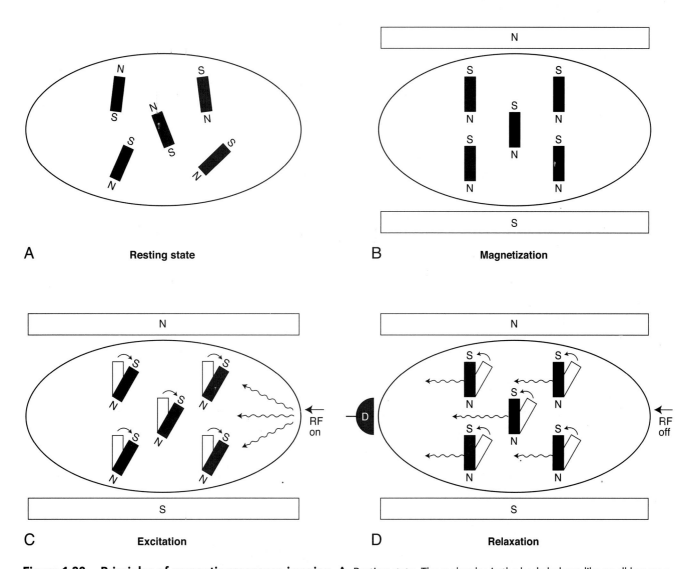

Figure 1.32. Principles of magnetic resonance imaging. A. Resting state. The molecules in the body behave like small bar magnets and are arranged in a random fashion. **B.** Following magnetization. The molecules align themselves along the plane of magnetization. **C.** Excitation. A pulsed radiofrequency (*RF*) beam deflects the molecules as they absorb the energy from that beam. **D.** Relaxation. When the RF beam is switched off, the molecules return to their preexcitation position, giving off the energy they absorbed. This may be measured with a detector (*D*).

the sagittal, coronal, and axial planes. Furthermore, MR imaging has the advantage of being able to highlight the different pathologic changes in different tissues through contrast manipulation. This is accomplished by altering the pattern of RF pulses in a study. The MR image reflects the strength or intensity of the magnetic resonance RF signal received from the sample. Signal intensity depends on several factors, such as hydrogen density and two magnetic relaxation times: T1 and T2. The greater the hydrogen density, the more intense (bright) the MR signal will be. Tissues that contain very little hydrogen, such as cortical bone, flowing blood, and an air-filled lung, generate little or no MR signal and appear black on the images produced. Tissues high in hydrogen, such as fat or cartilage, have high signal intensity and appear white.

Detailed explanation of the physics of MR and of T1 and T2 are beyond the scope of this text. An excellent reference is Stark and Bradley's *Magnetic Resonance Imaging.* However, in simple terms, these two measurements reflect quantitative alterations in MR signal strength owing to interactions of the nuclei being studied and their surrounding chemical and physical milieu. T1 is the rate at which nuclei align themselves with the external magnetic field after RF stimulation. T2 is the rate at which the RF signal emitted by the nuclei decreases after RF perturbation. Following are other terms you will encounter when discussing MR examinations with a radiologist or when reviewing the literature:

- *Tesla* (T): the unit of measure of magnetic flux density, or simply magnet strength; in the International System of Units (SI), 1T equals 10,000 gauss
- *Echo time:* the time between the middle of the RF pulse and the middle of spin echo production
- *Repetition time:* the time between the beginning of one pulse sequence and the beginning of succeeding pulse sequences
- Commonly used imaging parameters: spin echo, short T1 inversion recovery (STIR), and various acronymic gradient echo techniques (FISP, FLASH, etc.)

Again, for a detailed description, see Stark and Bradley's text.

Figure 1.33 shows a typical high-field MR imaging unit, which has a magnet strength of 1.5 to 3.0T. Numerous smaller-strength magnets are also on the market. Machines with magnet strength of 0.1 to 0.5T have the advantage of being open and thus much less likely to produce claustrophobia in patients. However, studies done at lower magnetic strength take longer, raising the possibility of motion artifacts. Furthermore, images from lower-strength magnets tend to be less detailed than those from the high-field units. A third type of magnet is available, designed primarily for office use. This is the extremity magnet, which typically is of 0.1 to 0.2T. These will accommodate knees, ankles, feet, hands, wrists, and elbows. Image quality varies with these units.

MR imaging is used primarily for studying intracranial (Fig. 1.34) and intraspinal (Figs. 1.35 and 1.36) pathology, and for evaluating abnormalities of the musculoskeletal system (Figs. 1.37 and 1.38) and the heart. Additionally, it is used to evaluate abdominal visceral problems (Fig. 1.39). MR angiography is also commonly used for vascular abnormalities (Fig. 1.40).

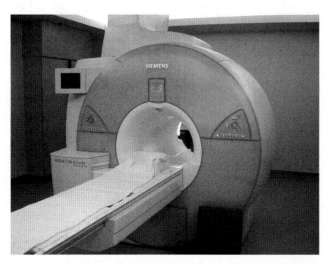

Figure 1.33. A typical magnetic resonance imaging unit. Newer high-field scanners have shorter depth and wider bores, which reduce the patient's sense of claustrophobia.

Figure 1.34. Magnetic resonance imaging of meningioma. (This is the same patient as in Fig. 1.19.) Axial image shows the tumor (*M*) to much better advantage. Notice the internal structure of the tumor compared with Figure 1.19.

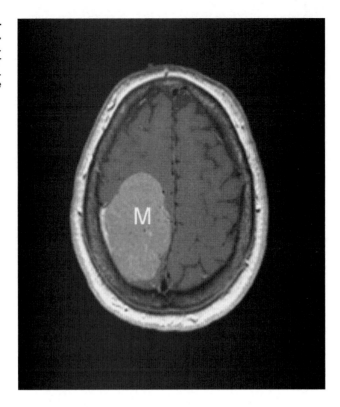

Figure 1.35. Herniated nucleus pulposus. Sagittal magnetic resonance image shows a large posterior herniation (*large arrow*) at the L4 disc space. Notice the posterior displacement of the thecal sac (*small arrows*).

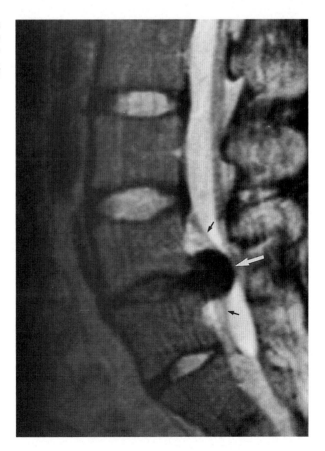

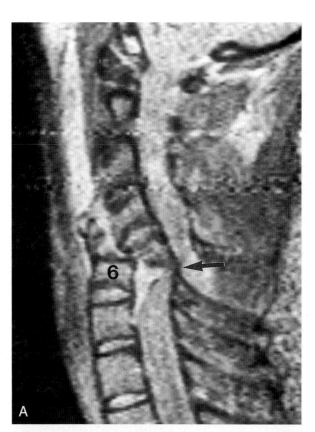

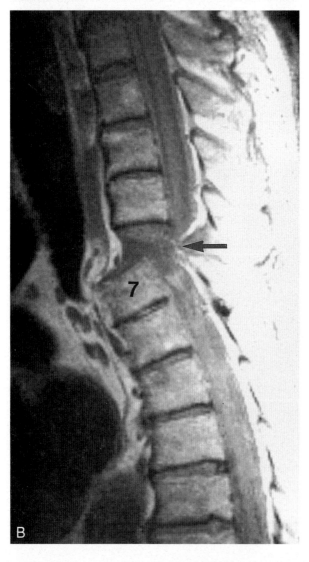

Figure 1.36. Spinal cord transections (*arrows*). **A.** Cervical region. **B.** Thoracic region.

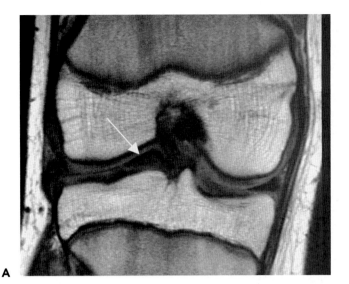

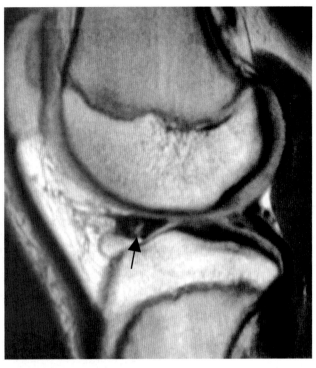

A

B

Figure 1.37. Bucket handle tear of medial meniscus. A. Coronal magnetic resonance image shows flipped fragment of medial meniscus (*arrow*) near the center of the joint. **B.** Sagittal image shows the torn anterior horn of the meniscus (*arrow*). Notice the absence of a normal triangular meniscal image posteriorly.

Figure 1.38. Metastatic disease of the spine. Sagittal magnetic resonance image shows areas of low signal (*dark*) as well as compression in two vertebrae. Other scans showed the tumor to encroach on the subarachnoid space.

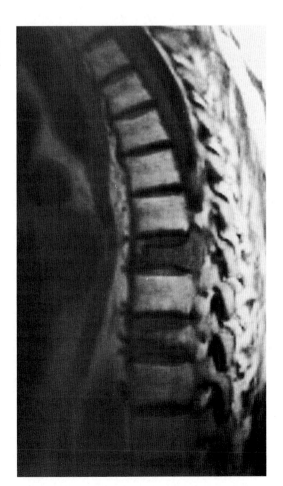

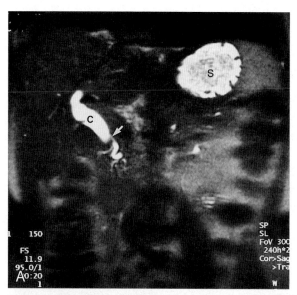

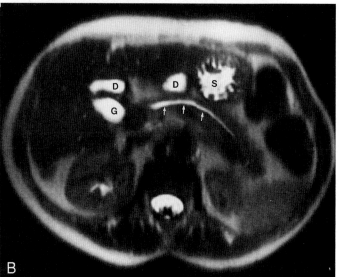

Figure 1.39. Magnetic resonance cholangiopancreatogram. A. Coronal T2 weighted (HASTE) image shows dilatation of the common bile duct (*C*) owing to a stricture (*arrow*). The stomach (*S*) is also indicated. **B.** Axial T2 weighted image shows the normal pancreatic duct (*arrows*). The stomach (*S*), duodenum (*D*), and gallbladder (*G*) are also marked.

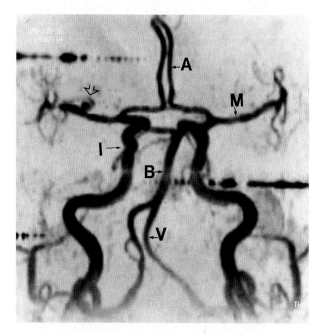

Figure 1.40. Cerebral magnetic resonance arteriogram in a patient with an aneurysm of the middle cerebral artery on the right (*open arrow*). Notice the excellent demonstration of the normal vascular anatomy. The following arteries are demonstrated: anterior cerebral (*A*), middle cerebral (*M*), internal carotid (*I*), basilar (*B*), and vertebral (*V*).

Figure 1.41. An ultrasound machine.

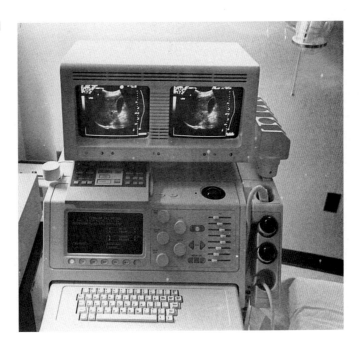

DIAGNOSTIC ULTRASOUND

Diagnostic ultrasound is a noninvasive imaging technique that uses sonic energy in the frequency range of 1 to 10 MHz (1,000,000 to 10,000,000 cps). This is well above the normal human ear response of 20 to 20,000 Hz. Ultrasound is a nonionizing form of energy and, thus, is safe for use on pregnant patients and children. Echoes or reflections of the ultrasound beam from interfaces between tissues with various acoustic properties yield information on the size, shape, and internal structure of organs and masses. Ultrasound waves are greatly reflected by the interface between soft tissue and air or bone, thus limiting its use in the chest and musculoskeletal system. Figure 1.41 shows the components of an ultrasound machine.

Modern ultrasound equipment uses real-time imaging. A continuous stream of ultrasound waves are emitted from the transducer and reflected from the tissues being imaged. The transducer then acts as a receiver, receiving the returning waves and constructing a visual image. Real-time ultrasound allows dynamic scanning of moving objects such as a fetus in utero (Fig. 1.42) or a pulsating aorta. This technique also permits rapid and efficient screening of a body

Figure 1.42. Uterine ultrasound at 22 weeks' gestation. Notice the placenta (*P*), fetal head (*H*), and torso (*T*). Ultrasound has become a primary diagnostic tool in obstetrics.

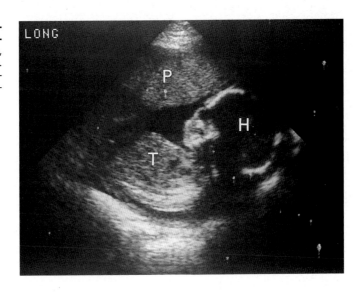

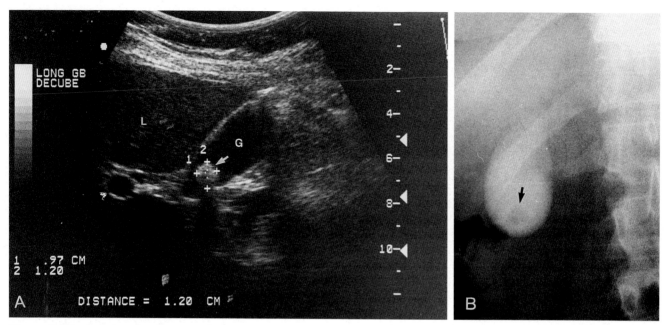

Figure 1.43. **Images of gallstones. A.** Ultrasound examination in the longitudinal plane shows a gallstone measuring 0.97 × 1.20 cm (*arrow*) in the dependent portion of the gallbladder (*G*). The liver (*L*) lies immediately above the gallbladder. **B.** Oral cholecystogram in the same patient shows the lucent gallstone (*arrow*).

region (Fig. 1.43). In the past decade, ultrasound has been used more frequently for evaluating ligaments and tendons, or cystic lesions (Fig. 1.44). Ultrasound is an interactive modality. Observing moving body parts, such as the heart or an aorta, while performing the scan is often more useful than reviewing the static images afterward.

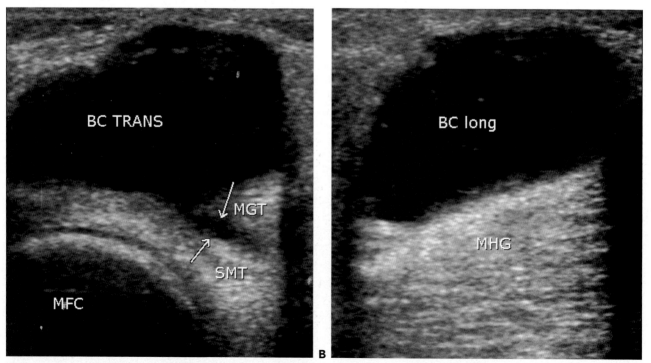

Figure 1.44. **U/S Baker cyst (*BC*) of popliteal area. A.** Transverse section shows the cyst as a sonolucent area above the denser band of the semimembranosus tendon (*SMT*). The arrows point to the neck of the cyst, which leads to the joint. **B.** Longitudinal section shows the cyst above the medial head of the gactrocnemius (*MHG*). MFC, medial femoral condyle; MGT, medial head of gastrocnemius. (Courtesy of Mihra Taljanovic, MD, University of Arizona, Tucson.)

An additional feature of modern ultrasound is Doppler evaluation of blood vessels. With this technique, flow velocities within blood vessels can be measured, and screening for arterial stenosis can be performed. The technique is most commonly done in the carotid arteries (Fig. 1.45). Additionally, Doppler evaluation of venous structures can be performed to rule out occlusion from deep venous thrombosis.

Figure 1.45. Carotid Doppler ultrasound examination. A. Normal left common carotid artery (LCCA). The gray-scale image of a portion of the LCCA shows the vessel to be widely patent. The vessel walls are smooth without visible atheromatous plaques. The rectangle within the vessel lumen (*small arrow*) is the Doppler sample site from which the flow characteristics and velocities generate the Doppler waveform tracing shown to the right of the gray-scale image. There is a normal peak systolic flow velocity of approximately 90 cm/sec (*open arrow*; normal = <125 cm/sec) as well as antegrade blood flow velocity of 40 cm/sec at the end of diastole (*arrowhead*). The Doppler waveform also allows for evaluation of the degree of laminar flow disruption, or turbulence. This is reflected by the range of red blood cell velocities. The greater the velocity range, the greater the turbulence. In this instance, this normal vessel demonstrates a velocity range of 40 to 90 cm/sec. **B.** Significant stenosis in a right internal carotid artery (RICA). The gray-scale image of a portion of a RICA shows gross vessel wall irregularity with significant stenosis near the Doppler sample site (*small arrow*). The Doppler waveform tracing shows an elevated peak systolic flow with velocities of 140 cm/sec (*open arrow*). In addition, there is marked turbulence as a result of the increased red blood cell velocity. Compare these tracings and images with A.

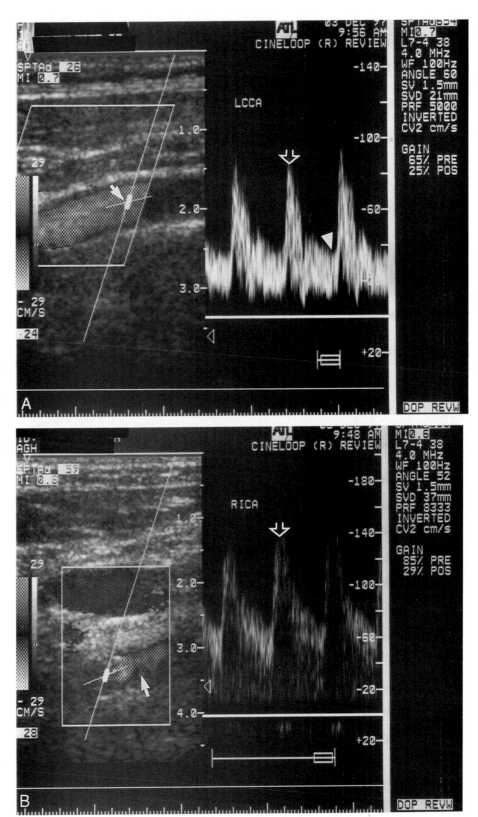

Ultrasound is also a useful tool in performing interventional procedures. Ultrasound-guided fluid aspirations, drainages, and biopsies are routinely performed quickly and safely in skilled hands.

Motion-mode (M-mode) ultrasound is used in echocardiography to study the dynamic changes of cardiac structures. The cardiac structures, including valves, form patterns in the M-mode ultrasound relating to their motion.

An important advantage of ultrasound is the absence of ionizing radiation and the relatively lower cost of the equipment. Most ultrasound units are also portable. Ultrasound, however, is an operator-dependent modality, and a high degree of technical skill is required to perform state-of-the-art examinations.

Because ultrasound is unable to cross a tissue–gas or tissue–bone boundary, it is not useful for evaluating the lung or bones. Furthermore, bony and gas-containing structures can obscure other tissues lying deeper to them.

THE "RADIOLOGIC RESTAURANT"

The impact that medical imaging has on the diagnosis and treatment of disease has changed dramatically in the past six decades. It is also not surprising that the cost of the equipment to perform those imaging studies has also increased dramatically. In 1940, imaging (x-rays) influenced the management of 1 patient in 12. The cost of the most expensive piece of equipment (a fluoroscopic unit) was $9,500. In 1950, the ratio dropped to 1 patient in 6, and the most expensive piece of equipment (usually an image-intensified fluoroscopic unit) was $25,000. By 1960, the ratio was 1 patient in 3, and the cost of the most expensive piece of equipment (again fluoroscopy) was $85,000. In the 1970s, 1 patient in 2 needed imaging, and the cost of the most expensive piece of equipment (usually a CT scanner) topped $1,000,000. Since the 1980s, virtually all patients have been affected by imaging and the costs have risen to the $2,000,000-plus level, usually for MR imaging. However, digital radiography equipment frequently costs nearly $1,000,000. Table 1.3 summarizes these facts.

This chapter has outlined the many studies available to you, the clinician, to solve various clinical problems. You have a large "menu" of studies that can be performed to evaluate your patient. The first choice you must make is the exact approach you wish to take toward this evaluation. Three approaches are currently in use: the "shotgun," the algorithmic, and the directed.

The *shotgun approach* is one that is all too often employed. It takes little thought to order a battery of diagnostic laboratory and imaging studies for each patient in the hope that one or more of those tests will provide important diagnostic information. Primarily based on the principle that if a study is available, it can be done, this approach is often modified toward the specific complaint to give some economy of selected tests.

The *algorithmic approach* follows a more orderly selection of studies based on symptoms and the results of each study (Fig. 1.46). Although this approach requires some thought on the part of the clinician and study selectivity is possible, it is also probable that unnecessary studies will

TABLE 1.3.
IMPACT OF MEDICAL IMAGING AND COSTS

Year	Ratio	Cost	Equipment
1940	1:12	$9,500	Fluoroscopy
1950	1:6	$25,000	Fluoroscopy
1960	1:3	$85,000	Fluoroscopy
1970	1:2	$200,000	CT
1980	1:1	$1,500,000	CT (MR)
1990–2005	1:1	$2,500,000	MR

CT, computed tomography; MR, magnetic resonance.

Figure 1.46. Algorithm for evaluation of low back pain. The clinical, laboratory, or imaging findings will determine the next step. Imaging studies are highlighted.

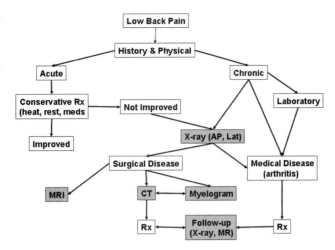

be performed just because they are in the protocol. For example, a patient with an acute back strain usually needs no radiographs and may be treated conservatively with rest, heat, and anti-inflammatory agents. Unfortunately, these patients often receive a complete radiographic evaluation of their lumbar spines and may even undergo MR imaging as well.

The *directed approach* is a carefully thought-out process in which the clinician has performed a thorough history and physical examination and then considers the diagnostic possibilities in that patient. The clinician chooses diagnostic studies based on *probability of diagnostic yield, safety* (invasive versus noninvasive study), *radiation dose, cost,* and *medicolegal aspects.* I prefer this approach and stress it daily to my consulting clinicians as well as to students and residents in all disciplines. Furthermore, in this age of cost containment, third-party payers are demanding that physicians follow this approach in an effort to reduce the soaring costs of medical care.

I have raised two issues in the preceding paragraph: medicolegal concerns and costs. Unfortunately, we live in a litigious society in which it is relatively easy to sue someone. Many patients expect perfect results and, when they are not achieved, feel that somebody must be responsible and therefore somebody must pay. Moreover, the concept of contributory negligence on the part of the patient never enters into the equation. Feeding this is a tort system that has too many lawyers as well as one that operates on the "contingency fee" system, in which plaintiffs owe nothing unless they win. As a result, there is a crisis in health care in which clinicians are closing their doors, denying patients needed medical care. Additionally, the fear of being sued has prompted many physicians to practice "defensive medicine," which has been estimated to cost all U.S. citizens about $70 billion a year.

Not surprisingly, radiologists are being included in lawsuits more frequently, either as primary or, more commonly, as secondary defendants. In radiology, mammography generates the most lawsuits, followed by failure to diagnose other forms of cancer and failure to diagnose fractures. Issues that involve radiology in malpractice cases involve several areas: failure to diagnose, failure to recommend additional (appropriate) studies, failure to communicate, and improper or incomplete informed consent. As a clinician, you can protect yourself by taking the time to listen carefully to a patient, by performing thorough and complete examinations, and by documenting your actions in the patient's chart. When you order diagnostic imaging, you should clearly communicate to the radiologist the reasons for the examination and the diagnosis you suspect. In a recent case involving delayed diagnosis of a fractured hip, in which I was an expert witness for the defense, the only clinical information given to the radiologist was "pain." Had the clinician added that the patient was suspected of having a hip fracture, greater attention might have been paid to the femoral neck, where a subtle fracture was found.

Not only should you communicate with the radiologist, but also you should expect a complete interpretation of the study in a timely manner. The radiologist should communicate any urgent findings back to you and should document the fact that such information was given, as

TABLE 1.4

COMMON IMAGING EXAMINATIONS, COSTS, AND DOSE

Examination	Cost[a]	Dose (mR)
Chest (2 view)	$290	108
Abdomen (2 view)	260	1,460
Femur	250	60
Pelvis	250	545
Wrist	24	04
Cervical (5 view)	410	194
Lumbar (5 view)	420	884
Mammogram (bilateral)	250	300
Upper gastrointestinal	460	1,700[b]
Barium enema	630	4,700[b]
Abdominal aortoiliac angiogram	3,300	151/image
Cranial CT	1,400	4,400
Chest CT	1,400	1,500
Abdominal CT	1,800	3,500
Lumbar CT	1,900	3,000
Abdominal ultrasound	900	0
Pelvic (obstetric) ultrasound	900	0
Cranial MR	2,000	0
Lumbar MR	2,400	0
Pelvic MR	2,200	0
Bone scan (isotope)	1,200	1,000 bone, 260 whole body
Lung scan (isotope)	1,000	900 lung, 61 whole body

[a]2005 figures (includes technical and professional charges).
[b]Includes fluoroscopy time.
CT, computed tomography; MR, magnetic resonance.

well as the method (direct contact, telephone, etc.). You, the clinician, and your patients have the right to rapid consultation.

References to the cost of a study usually bring to mind how much patients are billed for that service. Although it is helpful to consider costs in those terms, it is more useful to consider cost-effectiveness. Furthermore, the actual cost of a study is not what is charged for that examination but rather is based on a formula that takes into account the operating expenses for each machine, the technologist's time in performing the exam, any supplies used, and the efficacy of the diagnosis. For example, CT of the cervical spine has replaced radiography for screening patients suspected of having cervical injury. In addition to being much more sensitive at detecting fractures, CT takes less than half the time needed to do a complete radiographic examination. Radiologists at the trauma center at Massachusetts General Hospital actually showed that CT was more cost-effective than radiography for patients with suspected cervical injury. When considering performing a study, consult your radiologist for the most appropriate method of solving the patient's problem. Table 1.4 lists common imaging procedures, their costs, and their radiation doses.

In 1993, the American College of Radiology (ACR) formed the ACR Task Force on Appropriateness Criteria. The task force consisted of 10 panels of expert radiologists and clinical consultants in each of the 10 subspecialties of diagnostic radiology. Each panel was charged with the task of developing a series of clinical conditions and variations that could serve as the basis for determining the appropriateness of imaging studies. For each clinical condition, the panel performed a literature search with a critical review of the data presented. The panel, after reviewing the data, then made recommendations on the appropriateness of each imaging study using the consensus method. The results were first published by the ACR in 1995. The recommendations, although not perfect, serve as guidelines for radiologists to help their clinical colleagues in making decisions regarding imaging. Additionally, each of the recommendations is subject to periodic review. Figure 1.47 shows a typical appropriateness chart. The full document may be viewed online and downloaded from the ACR Web site at http://www.acr.org/ac.

American College of Radiology
ACR Appropriateness Criteria™

Clinical Condition: Chronic Neck Pain

Variant 1:   Patient of any age, without or with a history of previous trauma, first study.

Radiologic Exam Procedure	Appropriateness Rating	Comments
X-ray, cervical spine, AP, lateral, open mouth	9	
X-ray, cervical spine, AP, lateral, open mouth, oblique, flexion/extension	2	
X-ray, cervical spine, Flexion/extension only	2	
X-ray, cervical spine, AP, lateral, open mouth, oblique	No Consensus	At discretion of clinician
CT, cervical spine	2	
MRI, cervical spine, routine	2	
Myelogram, cervical spine, routine	2	
Myelogram, cervical spine, with CT	2	
NUC, bone scan	2	
Facet injection/arthrography, cervical spine	2	
Appropriateness Criteria Scale 1 2 3 4 5 6 7 8 9 1 = Least appropriate 9 = Most appropriate		

Figure 1.47. Representative American College of Radiology Appropriateness Criteria table for chronic neck pain. (Reprinted with permission from the American College of Radiology Task Force on Appropriateness Criteria. Appropriateness Criteria for Imaging and Treatment Decisions. Reston, VA: American College of Radiology, 2005.)

One final issue to be discussed is that of so-called screening examination. In recent years, a new industry has developed to provide "screening" whole-body CT or MR imaging on otherwise healthy persons. Entrepreneurs have flooded the airwaves, newspapers, and billboards with ads purveying their services. Of course, medical insurance does not cover these studies, but the imaging centers do take credit cards.

Is there a value in such screening? The generic answer is no. Three areas have demonstrated their ability to diagnose malignancies in early stages: mammography, colonoscopy or barium enema, and chest radiography. Screening mammography is effective in identifying small cancers, including ductal carcinoma in situ. Colonoscopy or barium enema is also effective in finding polyps, which have the potential to become malignant. "Remove a polyp, cure a potential cancer," goes the popular mantra. Finally, chest radiography, particularly in patients with certain risk factors such as smoking or occupational exposure to certain substances, has been effective in identifying lung cancers while they are small and potentially curable. No credible evidence exists that whole-body CT or MR screening of the general population is effective at identifying early malignancies or other abnormalities.

THE RADIOLOGIST AS A CONSULTANT

The complexity of today's diagnostic imaging studies makes it imperative that the radiologist be more than an interpreter of imaging studies. As the practice of radiology has become more organ-system oriented in larger hospitals, radiologists have gravitated to subspecialty areas through additional training after residency. Thus, large radiology groups have members who are specialists in neuroimaging, angiography and other invasive procedures, body imaging, musculoskeletal imaging, pulmonary imaging, trauma, gastrointestinal imaging, uroradiology, pediatric radiology, and nuclear imaging. As specialists, these radiologists work closely with specific groups of clinicians to solve their special diagnostic problems. The clinicians, for their part, consult with their radiologic colleagues on a daily basis, either for interpretation of studies or to determine the best method of working up a particular diagnostic problem. Radiologic subspecialists are often on call to perform studies after normal working hours. They make themselves available to consult on request with the clinician. They often participate in multidisciplinary conferences, such as a surgery-radiology-pathology conference, and give lectures to clinicians on topics of mutual interest.

Radiologists have been extensively trained in each of the imaging modalities. They also adhere to the Practice Guidelines and Technical Standards of the ACR. These documents specify indications for studies, qualifications for personnel performing and interpreting them, and the technical specifications for equipment. Like the ACR Appropriateness Criteria, the Practice Guidelines and Technical Standards are subject to periodic review and revision. They, too, may be accessed online at the ACR Web site.

You should learn to make use of this most valuable resource, the radiologist. Keep in mind, however, that he or she can best help you when informed of clinical or laboratory data on a patient. This means that requests for diagnostic studies should contain pertinent clinical information. The radiologist may thus be able to tailor an examination to the exact needs of the patient as well as you, the clinician. This will result in time saved in both the studies obtained as well as the hospital stay. A secondary benefit will be cost containment—a topic of continuing importance. Many studies provide similar information. There is little benefit in ordering expensive studies that will duplicate the diagnostic information. Finally, one of the greatest benefits of using your radiologist is that he or she views the patient and the clinical problem without the "tunnel vision" that medical or surgical specialists often exhibit by focusing solely on the structures within their particular area of expertise. A good example is the patient with back pain. The orthopaedist focuses on the skeletal causes; the urologist concentrates on the kidneys and ureters. However, the radiologist looks at the entire area under study and does not have any ego investment in the diagnosis. Remember, your prime consideration is the welfare of your patient. Consultation with the radiologist is as important for helping that patient as consulting with any other specialist.

SUMMARY AND KEY POINTS

- Diagnostic radiology has emerged over the past one hundred years to become a vital link in the patient care chain. Diagnostic imaging is performed on nearly all patients seen in medical practice.
- Cross-sectional imaging can demonstrate organs and their diseases that previously could be seen only surgically or at the time of necropsy.
- The radiologist has a large variety of studies available for clinicians to use and is in the best position to recommend the appropriate study based on consultation with the clinician.
- This chapter described the various imaging studies offered, reviewed their principles, and made recommendations regarding their appropriate use.
- Blind or protocol-driven ordering of any diagnostic test is to be discouraged. It is best to tailor such examinations to the needs of patients.

SUGGESTED ADDITIONAL READING

American College of Radiology Task Force on Appropriateness Criteria. Appropriateness Criteria for Imaging and Treatment Decisions. Reston, VA: American College of Radiology, 2005. Available at http://www.acr.org/ac. Accessed August 30, 2006.

Brant WE, Helms CA, eds. Fundamentals of Diagnostic Radiology. 3rd Ed. Philadelphia: Lippincott Williams & Wilkins, 2006.

Bushburg JT, Seibert JA, Leidholdt EM Jr., Boone JM. The Essential Physics of Medical Imaging. 2nd Ed. Philadelphia: Lippincott Williams & Wilkins, 2002.

Curry TS III, Dowdy JE, Murry RC. Christensen's Physics of Diagnostic Radiology. 4th Ed. Baltimore: Williams & Wilkins, 1990.

Edelman RR, Hesselink JR, Zlatkin MB, Crues JV. Clinical Magnetic Resonance Imaging. 3rd Ed. Philadelphia: WB Saunders, 2006.

Eisenberg RL. Radiology: An Illustrated History. St. Louis: Mosby-Year Book, 1991.

Fishman EK, Jeffrey RB Jr. Multidetector CT: Principles, Techniques, and Clinical Applications. Philadelphia: Lippincott Williams & Wilkins, 2003

Gagliardi RA, McClennan BL. A History of the Radiological Sciences: Diagnosis. Reston, VA: Radiology Centennial, 1996.

Grainger RG, Allison DJ, Dixon AK, eds. Grainger & Allison's Diagnostic Radiology: A Textbook of Medical Imaging. 4th Ed. New York: Churchill Livingstone, 2002.

Haaga JR, Lanzieri CF, Gilkeson RC. CT and MR Imaging of the Whole Body. 4th Ed. St. Louis: Mosby, 2003.

Rumack CM, Wilson SR, Charboneau JW, Johnson JA. Diagnostic Ultrasound. St. Louis: Mosby, 2005.

Sandler MP, Coleman RE, Patton JA, Wackers FJ, Gottschalk A. Diagnostic Nuclear Medicine. 4th Ed. Philadelphia: Lippincott Williams & Wilkins, 2002.

Stark DD, Bradley WG. Magnetic Resonance Imaging. 2nd Ed. St. Louis: Mosby-Year Book, 1992.[Unknown font 2: Arial Black];[End Font: Arial Black]oc.

Ziessman HA, O'Malley JP, Thrall JH. Nuclear Medicine: The Requisites. 3rd Ed. St. Louis: Mosby, 2006.

Radiographic Contrast Agents

2

Various structures within the body are recognizable on a radiograph either because of their inherent densities (e.g., bone distinguished from muscle) or because they contain one of the basic natural materials (e.g., air). However, because most of the internal viscera are of the radiographic density of water or close to it, it is necessary to introduce into these structures a material that will outline walls, define anatomy, and demonstrate any pathologic conditions. Chapter 1 briefly mentioned these agents and some of the studies for which they are used. This chapter describes their physiology and pharmacology, defines indications and contraindications for their use, and discusses the treatment of reactions to them.

BARIUM PREPARATIONS

Barium sulfate (USP), in one of its many forms, provides the mainstay for radiographic examinations of the gastrointestinal (GI) tract. Barium is of high atomic weight, which results in considerable absorption of the x-ray beam, thus providing excellent radiographic contrast. In the usual preparation, finely pulverized barium mixed with dispersing agents is suspended in water. When administered orally or rectally, it provides adequate coating of the GI tract.

Although barium itself is chemically inert, when it is extravasated outside the GI tract, a severe desmoplastic reaction may develop. This is most likely to occur in a patient with a perforation of the GI tract. In the past, barium mixed with fecal material was deemed to be a rapidly lethal mixture when introduced into the peritoneal cavity. However, studies have shown that the combination of barium and feces is no more lethal than the introduction of feces alone into the peritoneum. Nevertheless, because of the tendency to produce severe granulomas and adhesions, barium should not be used whenever a suspected perforation exists. In these situations, a water-soluble contrast material should be used.

Barium preparations are safe as long as the entire GI tract is patent. Oral barium may be used if an obstruction is present *proximal* to the ileocecal valve, because the contents of the small intestine remain fluid up to that point. If the obstruction is *distal* to the ileocecal valve, the patient is best examined with a retrograde study (barium enema) because once the bowel contents enter the cecum, water is rapidly absorbed. If barium is allowed to remain within the colon for a long time behind an obstruction, it may inspissate and compound the patient's problem.

WATER-SOLUBLE CONTRAST MEDIA

Water-soluble contrast agents are used predominantly for angiography, contrast enhancement of computed tomography (CT) studies, myelography, arthrography, and urography. The most common agents used are the sodium or meglumine salts of diatrizoic or iothalamic acid in concentrations of 60% to 90%.

The common chemical structure of all water-soluble contrast media is a variant of triiodobenzoic acid. These agents are referred to as *ionic* media because of their property in solution to dissociate into the sodium or meglumine cation and their iodine-containing anion.

Ionic agents are very hypertonic (three times that of serum), resulting in a fluid shift from the intracellular or extracellular to the intravascular space or lumen of the GI tract (depending on the route of administration). Although normal persons may not suffer any severe, long-lasting effects from this shift, patients who are dehydrated or in a precarious state of cardiac and fluid balance are at special risk, particularly for renal failure. Secondary effects from the changes in viscosity and tonicity of the blood include platelet aggregation, changes in blood pressure, change in cardiac output, and changes in pulse rate. As the serum osmolality rises, changes in blood coagulation may occur, with a resulting bleeding tendency.

The extent and severity of these changes depend on the volume of the agent injected, the speed of injection, and the tonicity and viscosity of the agent. Rapid injection, high-volume injection, and high tonicity and viscosity of the agent are associated with more-severe reactions. Occasionally, a vagal reaction occurs, marked by vasodilation, systemic hypotension, and bradycardia (rather than tachycardia).

In addition to bradycardia, cardiac changes include a fall in systemic blood pressure, flattening of the T waves, and decreased cardiac output. This occurs especially if the contrast agent is injected directly into the heart. In the kidneys, especially in a dehydrated patient, glomerular and tubular damage may result in temporary impairment of renal function and oliguria.

When ionic agents are injected into a joint for an arthrogram, they tend to draw fluid into that joint. This is the source of the postarthrographic pain many patients experience. Fortunately, the development of magnetic resonance (MR) arthrography has resulted in low dilutions of iodinated contrast being injected into the joints, only for needle localization, nearly eliminating this complication.

The goal of reducing the normal physiologic and abnormal adverse effects of the ionic contrast agents led to the development of a new class of water-soluble media. These agents are of two varieties. The first are *nonionic monomers*—variants of triiodobenzene—in which the sodium or meglumine cation has been replaced by a side chain that will not dissociate from the iodine-containing portion of the molecule. The result is a pronounced lower osmolality than the ionic agents.

The second class of low-osmolar agents is an *ionic dimer* formed by linking two triiodobenzoic acid molecules, one of which contains a sodium or meglumine cation. However, doubling the iodine content in the anionic portion reduces the overall osmolality.

The low-osmolar contrast media are associated with a lower overall incidence of side effects and mortality compared with the older ionic agents and are now used in greater frequency than their ionic counterparts. The main reason for the less-than-universal adoption of the low-osmolar agents is their higher cost (approximately 10 times greater than the ionic agents); this should change in the future.

The low-osmolar contrast media are also used for myelography. In the dilutions used, they provide excellent contrast without excessive density. Thus, they may be used for CT myelography. These agents may produce a headache in up to 30% of patients and transient psychologic disturbances caused by intracranial flow of contrast in less than 5%. The latter complication is reduced by keeping the patient's head elevated after the myelogram.

Additional uses of low-osmolar agents include injection into sinus tracts or, in diluted form, examination of the GI tract when there is a suspected perforation. These agents do not cause any of the undesirable side effects that barium is known to produce when outside the GI tract. However, water-soluble contrast media have one important contraindication: suspected communication between the GI tract and the tracheobronchial tree (tracheoesophageal fistula). As mentioned in Chapter 1, water-soluble materials are extremely irritating to the tracheobronchial mucosa and produce a severe chemical pneumonia that may result in death. A barium or oil-soluble preparation should be used when airway communication is suspected.

Excretion of these agents is by pure glomerular filtration within the kidney. The material is removed intact by the glomeruli. In patients with chronic renal failure, however, the material may be secreted into the bile or small bowel by a process known as *vicarious excretion*. If it is necessary to administer contrast material to a patient with renal failure, the low-osmolar type should be used. In addition, hydration by intravenous infusion with 0.45% sodium chloride at a rate of 100 mL/hour should be performed at least 12 hours before and after contrast injection.

PARAMAGNETIC AGENTS

Despite the variety of pulse sequences available for MR imaging, difficulties still exist for differentiating between neoplasms and chronic cerebral infarctions, tumors and perifocal cerebral edema, or recurrent herniated intervertebral discs and surgical scars. For these reasons, a number of *paramagnetic* contrast agents have been developed for intravenous use during MR imaging. Gadolinium-diethylenetriamine pentaacetic acid (Gd-DTPA) is most commonly used. Gadolinium (Gd) was chosen because of its strong effect on the relaxation time in the scanning sequence. Chelation with DTPA prevents the inherent toxicity of the free Gd ion. In diagnostic doses, Gd-DTPA increases the signal in vascular structures, similar to the effect of conventional water-soluble contrast media. For MR arthrography, a very dilute mixture of Gd (0.4%) is used because of its intense paramagnetic effect. Gadolinium solution may be safely mixed with iodinated contrast materials for needle localization.

Gd compounds carry a slight risk of adverse reactions, particularly in a patient with a history of reaction to iodinated compounds. However, unlike iodinated contrast materials, Gd compounds have no nephrotoxicity, can be used in azotemic patients, and can be removed by dialysis. Interestingly, contrast agents containing gadolinium are slightly radiodense and can be used for opacification in CT and angiography instead of iodinated agents.

CONTRAST AGENTS IN ULTRASONOGRAPHY

Contrast agents for use in ultrasonography have been investigated since 1968. Recently, a family of microbubble-based contrast agents has been developed and offers promise. These agents are used primarily for improving visualization of blood vessels and vascular organs such as the liver and kidneys. Thus, they have been shown to be useful for diagnosing stenotic vessels, identifying areas of ischemia, and in some cases, detecting tumors. This is an area that experts in ultrasound believe has great potential as a relatively noninvasive method to improve diagnoses.

OIL-SOLUBLE AGENTS

Oil-soluble agents such as propyliodone (Dionosil) are occasionally used for esophagography in suspected esophago-airway fistulas. Ethiodized oil (Ethiodol) is an oily agent sometimes used for sialography (study of the salivary ducts) or hysterosalpingography (study of the uterine cavity and fallopian tubes).

ADVERSE REACTIONS TO CONTRAST MATERIALS AND THEIR MANAGEMENT

Incidence of Reactions

Adverse reactions to iodinated contrast material are variable and unpredictable. The Subcommittee on Treatment of Adverse Reactions of the Committee on Contrast Media from the International Society of Radiology reviewed the data from 150,000 case reports. They found that the overall incidence of adverse reactions was 5%. The incidence of serious reactions was reported to vary between 1:1,000 and 1:2,000, with fatalities occurring at a rate of 1:13,000 to 1:40,000. Although many adverse reactions occur in patients with no allergic histories, the study revealed that a patient with a history of allergy has a risk of reaction twice that of the general population. If the patient has experienced a reaction to contrast media, the chances of another reaction are three times greater than that of the general population.

Pretesting with a small injection of the contrast medium was found to have little or no value in identifying patients who would later react. Similarly, pretreatment with antihistamines and steroids in patients with known allergies to contrast materials were shown to be ineffective.

Two studies from Japan and Australia on 337,647 patients reevaluated the incidence of adverse reactions (including death) from ionic and low-osmolar contrast media. The studies revealed that the overall incidence of adverse reactions from ionic contrast materials was 12.7% and from nonionic (low-osmolar) contrasts it was 3.1%. Severe reactions occurred in 0.22% and 0.04% of each group, respectively. One death occurred in each group, but no causal relationship to the contrast medium was found. The conclusions of the studies were that nonionic (low-osmolar) contrast media significantly reduced the incidence of severe and potential life-threatening reactions, and their general use to increase the overall safety for contrast media examinations was recommended.

Types of Reactions

The three basic types of adverse reactions to contrast media are mild, intermediate, and severe. *Mild* or *minor reactions*—including nausea, vomiting, sneezing, flushing, diaphoresis, feeling of warmth, and occasional headache—resolve without therapy. *Intermediate reactions* require therapy to relieve the patient's symptoms but are not life-threatening. These include urticaria, angioneurotic edema, and wheezing. *Severe reactions* include cardiovascular collapse, which may be associated with pulmonary edema, laryngeal edema, and apnea. Central nervous system depression is another possible severe reaction. Death may result if proper treatment of a severe reaction is not instituted immediately.

Table 2.1 lists signs and symptoms of reactions to contrast agents in order of increasing severity.

Treatment of Reactions

Before instituting treatment, the severity of the reaction and the body systems involved should be carefully evaluated. The patient's vital signs should be monitored. Once it has been determined which organ system was involved and the nature and severity of the reaction, proper treatment may be instituted. After successful treatment of a reaction of any kind, the type of reaction, severity, and mode of treatment should be entered in the patient's permanent medical record. In addition, a notation should be made on the patient's x-ray folder or radiology database that an allergic reaction occurred, and the type of reaction should be specified. Furthermore, the patient's referring physician should be notified immediately whenever a reaction occurs.

Mild reactions require that the patient be carefully observed and given reassurance by the radiologist that the symptoms are not serious and will resolve quickly. Most of these symp-

TABLE 2.1
SIGNS AND SYMPTOMS OF REACTIONS TO CONTRAST MATERIALS

Type	Cardiovascular	Respiratory	Cutaneous	Gastrointestinal	Nervous	Urinary
Mild	Pallor	Sneezing	Erythema	Nausea	Anxiety	
	Diaphoresis	Coughing	Feeling of	Vomiting	Headache	
	Tachycardia	Rhinorrhea	warmth	Metallic taste	Dizziness	
Intermediate	Bradycardia	Wheezing	Urticaria	Abdominal	Agitation	Oliguria
	Palpitations	Acute	Pruritus	cramps	Vertigo	
	Hypotension	asthma attack		Diarrhea	Slurred speech	
Severe	Acute pulmonary	Laryngospasm	Angioneurotic	Paralytic	Disorientation	Acute renal
	edema	Cyanosis	edema	ileus	Stupor	failure
	Shock	Laryngeal edema			Coma	
	Congestive heart failure	Apnea			Convulsions	
	Cardiac arrest					

toms will pass within a few minutes. Anxiety is believed to play a key role in the development of minor reactions.

Intermediate reactions are treated by intravenous administration of 25 to 50 mg of diphenhydramine (Benadryl). This may be augmented by 0.3 to 0.5 mL of a 1:1,000 solution of epinephrine subcutaneously. Cimetidine (Tagamet) is a histamine antagonist and may be used as a bolus injection of 300 mg instead of Benadryl or epinephrine. In most cases, the patient will respond favorably within several minutes; hives begin to fade, wheezing subsides, and the patient appears less apprehensive. The use of steroids for intermediate reactions is controversial. Some authorities believe that a 100-mg bolus of prednisolone is useful in treating the more severe type of intermediate reaction.

Severe reactions require immediate recognition and evaluation of the patient's cardiopulmonary status. Cardiopulmonary resuscitation (CPR) equipment should be readily available whenever any contrast medium is used. Furthermore, the radiologist and the technologist staff should be trained in the techniques of CPR. In general, the radiologist is the first physician called to the scene when a reaction occurs. Proper treatment of a severe reaction follows the ABCD system:

- Airway open
- Breathing restored
- Circulation maintained
- Drug and definitive therapy

Following initiation of CPR, a code/crash team should be summoned. The principles and practice of CPR are a subject with which you should be familiar and will not be covered further in this book. You should never inject contrast agents without being familiar with CPR and the management of reactions.

A *vagal type of reaction* has been recognized as a distinct complication of the use of contrast material. This reaction may be recognized by the presence of hypotension and bradycardia rather than tachycardia, the latter occurring in anaphylactoid reactions. Treatment of patients with vagal reactions is administration of 0.5 to 1.0 mg of atropine intravenously.

Adjunctive procedures that should be performed before the patient has a reaction and that may aid in the later treatment of a reaction include recording the patient's pulse and blood pressure and noting the cardiac rhythm. In addition, the use of a cannula type of needle–tubing combination that is taped in place to the forearm will ensure a ready channel of access to the patient's bloodstream in the event of an emergency.

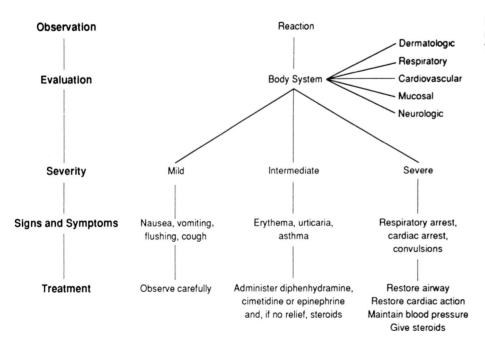

Figure 2.1 Diagram of management of reactions to radiographic contrast materials.

Figure 2.1 is a diagram of steps to follow in managing a patient who has a reaction to a contrast material.

SUMMARY AND KEY POINTS

■ Contrast agents may be categorized as particulate (barium), water-soluble (ionic and non-ionic), paramagnetic, and oily.

■ Barium remains the mainstay for radiographic evaluation of the GI tract. However, barium is toxic outside the lumen of the bowel.

■ Water-soluble agents are among the materials most commonly used for angiography, myelography, enhancement of vessels and organs for CT examinations, arthrography, and urography.

■ Water-soluble agents, when injected intra-arterially or intravenously, may cause life-threatening reactions.

■ Paramagnetic agents are used for the same indications as iodinated agents for MR studies.

■ The types of reactions to contrast media, how to recognize them, and how to treat them were briefly discussed.

■ Thorough familiarity with the technique of CPR is advised.

SUGGESTED ADDITIONAL READING

American College of Radiology. Manual on Contrast Media, Version 5.0. Reston, VA: American College of Radiology, 2004.

Bettman MA, Heeren T, Greenfield A, et al. Adverse events with radiographic contrast agents: results of SCVIR contrast agent registry. Radiology 1997;203:611–620.

Bush WH, Swanson DP. Acute reactions to intravascular contrast media: types, risk factors, recognition, and specific treatment. AJR 1991;157:1153–1161.

Cochran ST, Bomyea K, Sayre JW. Trends in adverse events after IV administration of contrast media. AJR 2001;176:1385–1388.

Cohan RH, Dunnick NR, Bashore TM. Treatment of reactions to radiographic contrast material. AJR 1988;151:263–270.

Goldberg BB, ed. Emergence of contrast ultrasound: a new modality in diagnostic radiology. Appl Radiol 1997;26(suppl):4–7.

Katayama H, Yamaguchi K, Kozuka T, et al. Adverse reactions to ionic and nonionic contrast media. Radiology 1990;175:621–628.

Katzberg RW, Bush WH, Lasser EC. Iodinated contrast media. In: Pollack HM, McClennan BL, eds. Clinical Urography. 2nd Ed. Philadelphia: WB Saunders, 1999:19–66.

Lasser EC, Lyon SG, Berry CC. Reports on contrast media reactions: analysis of data from reports to the U.S. Food and Drug Administration. Radiology 1997;203:605–610.

McClennan BL. Ionic and nonionic iodinated contrast media: evolution and strategies for use. AJR 1990;155:225–233.

Runge VM. Safety of approved MR contrast media for intravenous injection. J Magn Reson Imaging 2000;12:205–213.

Spinosa DJ, Kaufmann JA, Hartwell GD. Gadolinium chelates in angiography and interventional radiology: a useful alternative to iodinated contrast media for angiography. Radiology 2002;223:319–325.

Spring DB, Bettman MA, Barkan HE. Nonfatal adverse reactions to iodinated contrast media: spontaneous reporting to the U.S. Food and Drug Administration 1978–1994. Radiology 1997;204:325–332.

Spring DB, Bettman MA, Barkan HE. Deaths related to iodinated contrast media reported spontaneously to the U.S. Food and Drug Administration, 1978–1994: effect of the availability of low-osmolality contrast media. Radiology 1997;204:333–337.

Interventional and Invasive Radiology

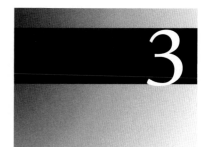

3

Interventional and invasive radiology is the subspecialty of diagnostic radiology that uses imaging guidance to perform many diagnostic and therapeutic procedures. It is also known as surgical radiology. The origins of this subspecialty date to the work of Seldinger, who, in 1953, first reported the technique that allows percutaneous access to many organ systems (Fig. 3.1). In the 1950s and 1960s, interventional radiology was confined primarily to cardiovascular studies. Improvements in imaging, such as the development of high-resolution, image-intensified biplane fluoroscopy, subtraction techniques, and refinements in catheter and guide-wire technology began in the late 1960s. In the early to mid-1970s, the development of ultrasound and computed tomography (CT) and the subsequent development of digital subtraction angiography (DSA) launched the subspecialty into areas previously known only to surgeons. The development of low-osmolar contrast material was an additional benefit.

Interventional radiology is no longer confined to angiography. This exciting and rapidly expanding subspecialty is the most labor-intensive in diagnostic radiology and includes a vast array of vascular and nonvascular procedures, including biopsies, percutaneous puncture, decompression and drainage, balloon dilations (angioplasty), stent placements, shunting, embolization, extraction techniques, vascular chemotherapy, and percutaneous screw placement. In addition, an entirely new field, interventional neuroradiology, has evolved from the techniques derived for the peripheral vascular system.

Invasive radiology has also had a dramatic impact on medical practice. Many procedures previously performed in the operating room, under general anesthesia, are now performed in a special procedures (angiography) suite or in a CT scanner in the radiology department, under conscious sedation, at a lower cost, and with a lower morbidity rate. In addition, high-risk patients who are not surgical candidates may be treated through interventional radiologic techniques. Interventional radiologic procedures are also frequently used preoperatively to improve surgical outcomes—for example, in angioplasty and stenting of iliac vessels before peripheral vascular bypass procedures or in embolization of vascular lesions such as tumors or arteriovenous (A-V) fistulas. Table 3.1 lists the many vascular and nonvascular interventional and invasive radiologic procedures.

This chapter briefly describes some of the techniques and their indications.

ANGIOGRAPHY

Angiography is primarily performed to evaluate the patency and distribution of blood vessels throughout the body. It is used to assess the heart and great vessels, the peripheral circulation, and the cranial circulation. Cardiac angiography is performed almost exclusively by cardiologists. Some neurosurgeons are being trained to perform endovascular procedures on intracranial and vertebral lesions. Most of the remaining procedures are performed by radiologists. Before the development of CT, ultrasound, or magnetic resonance (MR) imaging, angiography

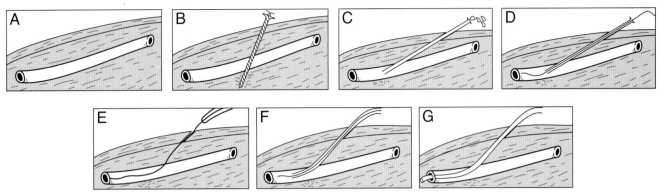

Figure 3.1.   Seldinger technique. This technique is the basis of percutaneous access for most interventional procedures. **A.** The vessel before puncture. **B.** A two-part needle consisting of a central stylet and an outer sheath punctures the vessel through both walls. **C.** The stylet is removed, and the sheath is withdrawn until blood is obtained. **D.** A guide wire is fed through the sheath into the vessel. **E.** The sheath is removed, and a catheter is threaded over the guide wire. **F.** The guide wire and catheter are advanced in the vessel. **G.** The guide wire is removed, leaving the catheter in the vessel ready for injection or infusion of medication.

was much more frequently performed to diagnose suspected neoplasms of the brain as well as of the abdominal viscera and to show the effects of those tumors on the normal vessels. Angiography is less frequently performed for these indications today. Angiograms are now obtained to evaluate vascular malformations, aneurysms (Fig. 3.2), A-V fistulas, thromboembolic phenomena (Fig. 3.3), atherosclerotic vascular disease (Fig. 3.4), and posttraumatic vascular injury (Fig. 3.5). In addition, angiography may serve as a screening examination before any endovascular intervention or therapy, providing the radiographic "road map" needed to complete the procedure. In addition to conventional angiography, magnetic resonance angiography (MRA) and computed tomographic angiography (CTA) offer noninvasive assessments of the vasculature (Fig. 3.6). Conventional angiography in most institutions is now being replaced by MRA or CTA for many diagnostic angiographic procedures. When the intent is to treat the patient with endovascular or surgical techniques, however, conventional angiography is often required.

It is common practice to use *subtraction technique* when performing angiography. Historically, in this process, a "mask" was made of a preliminary radiograph of the area in question by using a special film that reversed the densities (i.e., white becomes black and vice versa). This mask was placed over a radiograph taken after injection of contrast. The whites and blacks canceled each other when additional subtraction was performed, leaving the extra densities—the injected contrast in the vessels. This process is now performed digitally instead of with film, using a technique known as digital subtraction angiography (DSA). On the traditional subtraction angiogram, the vessels are better visualized and little or none of the background structures are visible (see Figs. 3.2 and 3.3). Complications of angiography occur in

TABLE 3.1
INTERVENTIONAL AND INVASIVE RADIOLOGIC PROCEDURES

Vascular Procedures	Nonvascular Procedures
Angioplasty	Biopsy
Vascular stenting	Abscess drainage
Embolization	Biliary drainage
Chemotherapy infusion	Gastrostomy tube placement
Thrombolysis	Nephrostomy
Transjugular intrahepatic portosystemic stents	Stone extraction
Venous access	Foreign body retrieval
Vena cava filter placement	Screw placement

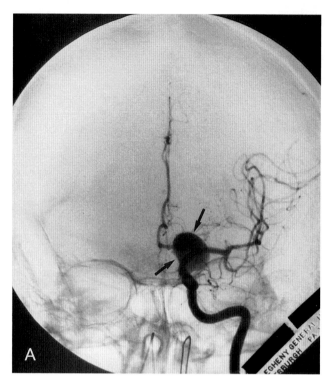

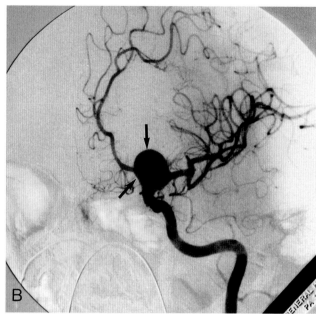

Figure 3.2. Cerebral aneurysm (*arrows*) at the junction of the internal carotid artery and middle cerebral artery. Frontal (**A**) and lateral (**B**) views of subtraction angiogram.

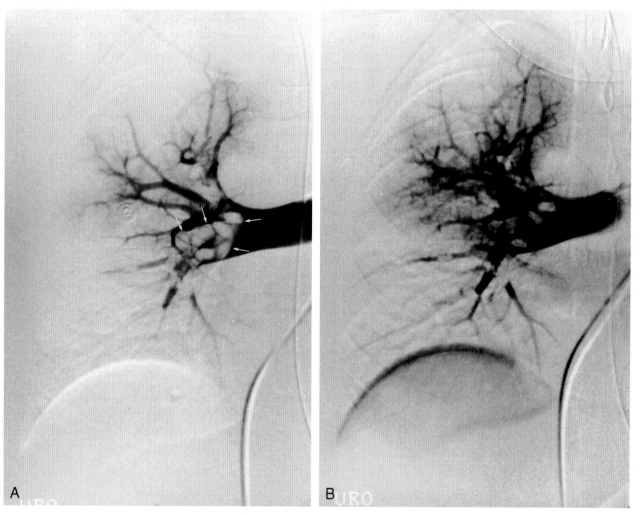

Figure 3.3. Pulmonary thromboembolism. A. Digital subtraction pulmonary angiogram demonstrates multiple lucent filling defects (*arrows*) in the right pulmonary artery. The upper lobe artery looks like a pruned tree. **B.** An image later in the injection shows the paucity of peripheral filling in the middle and lower lobes compared with the upper lobe.

Figure 3.4. Atherosclerotic disease of the abdominal aorta and renal arteries. Notice the irregularity of the abdominal aorta on the left side beneath the renal arteries and the stenosis of both renal arteries near their origin (*arrows*).

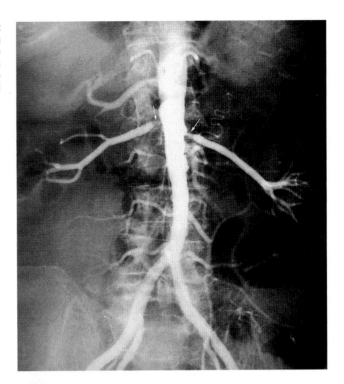

Figure 3.5. Vascular injuries. A. Transection of the distal femoral artery (*arrow*) at the site of a distal femoral fracture. There is partial filling of the remainder of the vessel. **B.** Iatrogenic popliteal pseudoaneurysm (*arrows*) from an arthroscopic examination. Notice the narrowed popliteal artery.

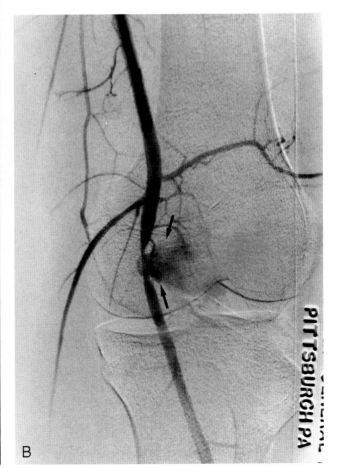

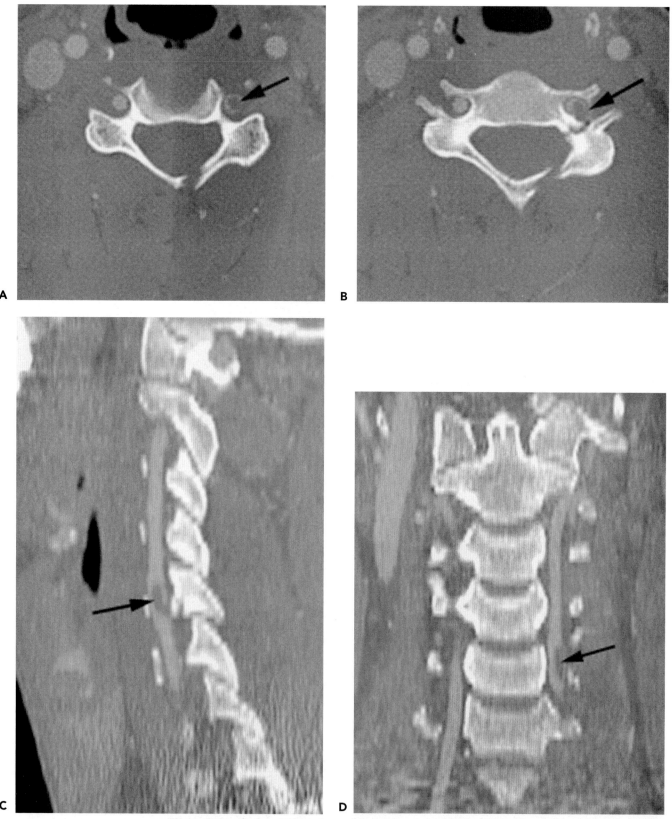

Figure 3.6. Computed tomographic angiogram of the vertebral arteries in a patient with a cervical fracture. A and B. Axial images show the contrast-filled vertebral arteries in the transverse foramina. On the right, the vessel is normal; on the left, there is a filling defect (*arrows*). Sagittal **(C)** and coronal **(D)** reconstructed computed tomography images show the filling defect (*arrows*) in the left vertebral artery.

fewer than 1% of patients and include contrast reaction, hematoma, pseudoaneurysm formation, A-V fistulas, arterial occlusion, spasm, and stroke.

VASCULAR INTERVENTION—ANGIOPLASTY

Angioplasty is a technique that uses special dilating catheters (Fig. 3.7) to open occluded or
stenotic blood vessels (Fig. 3.8). This procedure was originally introduced by Dotter and
Judkins in 1964 using fairly rigid sequential dilators. Grüntzig subsequently developed the
balloon angioplasty catheter. However, it was not until the 1980s that catheter technology
became refined enough to allow the widespread use of angioplasty. Today angioplasty is used
routinely for treatment of coronary, renal, peripheral vascular, and carotid stenoses. The more
recent development of the vascular stent, as described in the next section, has expanded the
indications of a treatable lesion and has greatly improved the results.

STENTS

One of the more innovative endovascular procedures developed within the last few years has
been the use of stents. These meshlike metallic tubes are inserted through a catheter into
a stenotic vessel in an attempt to prevent further stenosis and restore adequate blood flow

Figure 3.7. Catheters used for angioplasty.
A. Entire catheter. **B.** Close-up of tip (inflated).

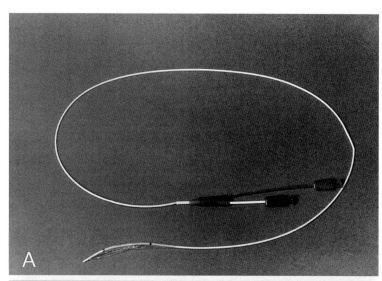

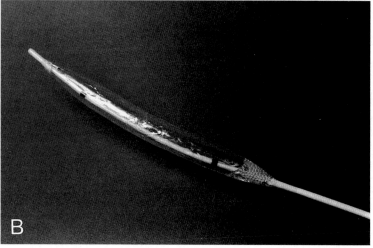

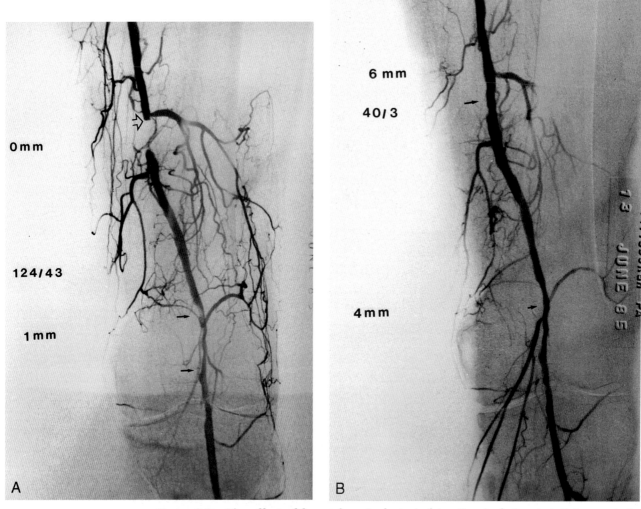

Figure 3.8.   The effect of femoral angioplasty (subtraction technique). A. Before angioplasty, a segment of the femoral artery is completely occluded (*open arrow*). The distal vessels fill through collaterals. There is an area of stenosis of the popliteal artery (*solid arrows*). Before angioplasty, no lumen is at the occluded area, and a 1-mm lumen is at the distal lesion. The gradient is 124/43. **B.** Following angioplasty, flow is reestablished through the occluded area (*long arrow*). Flow through the distal stenotic area (*short arrow*) is also improved. The proximal lumen now measures 6 mm and the lower measures 4 mm. The gradient is now 40/3. Notice the less prominent appearance of the collateral circulation.

(Fig. 3.9). They are being used for a variety of vessels, including the coronary arteries. Covered stents are metallic with a fabric covering without fenestrations, allowing coverage within aneurysms, perforated vessels, or A-V fistulas. Interventional radiologists, in conjunction with vascular surgeons, now routinely repair abdominal aortic aneurysms with a less invasive approach using covered stents (stent grafts). These stents are also called endografts.

IMAGE-GUIDED VASCULAR INTERVENTIONS AND EMBOLIZATION

Therapeutic embolization involves the deliberate occlusion of arteries, veins, or abnormal vascular spaces by introducing various materials through a selectively positioned catheter. Occlusive materials used include gelfoam, polyvinyl alcohol particles, metallic coils, glue (cyanoacrylate), and detachable balloons. The procedure is particularly advantageous to high-risk patients who otherwise might have to undergo surgery to occlude these vessels. The usual indications are acute bleeding (Figs. 3.10 and 3.11) occluding the vascular supply of neoplasms,

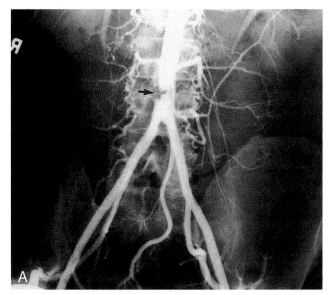

Figure 3.9. Stenting of the abdominal aorta in a patient with claudication. A. Abdominal aortogram demonstrates focal atherosclerotic narrowing of the distal aorta (*arrow*). **B.** Subtraction angiogram after repair using a single stent. Notice the meshlike appearance of the stent. The stenosis is no longer present.

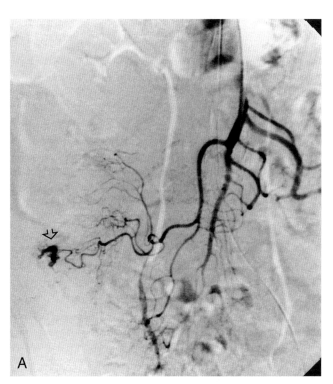

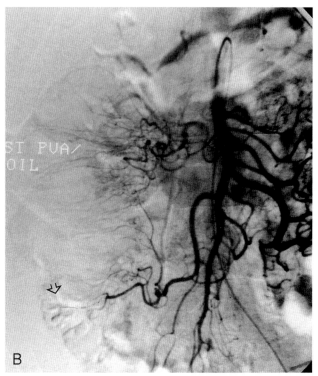

Figure 3.10. Embolization for lower intestinal bleeding. A. Injection into the superior mesenteric artery demonstrates an area of active bleeding from a small branch of the ileocolic artery (*arrow*). **B.** A postembolization injection made after insertion of an occlusive coil (*arrow*) shows the bleeding has stopped.

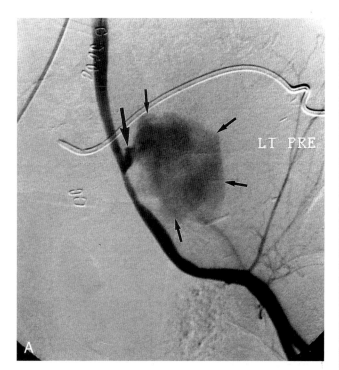

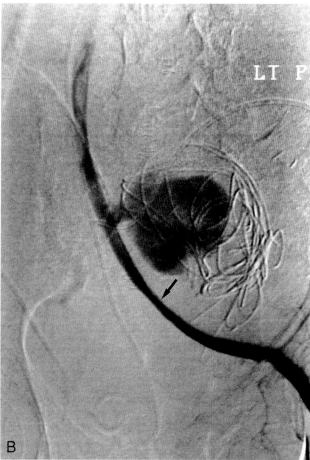

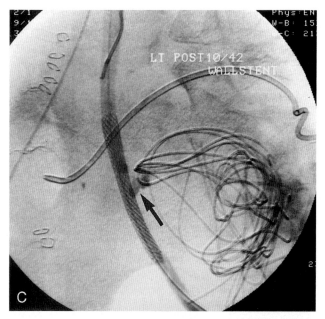

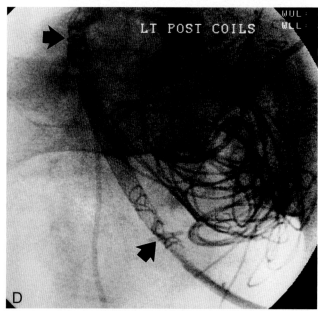

Figure 3.11.   Occlusion of posttraumatic tear of the left external iliac artery. A. Iliac artery injection shows active extravasation of contrast (*large arrow*) and pseudoaneurysm formation (*small arrows*). **B.** Injection made immediately after placement of occlusive wires shows persistent bleeding. Notice the compression of the iliac artery distal to the tear (*arrow*). Compare with A. **C.** A mesh stent has been placed to open the iliac artery. There still is some bleeding (*arrow*). **D.** Occlusive coils (*arrows*) were placed above and below the stent because of persistent bleeding that was considered life threatening.

Figure 3.11. *(continued)* **E.** Following the procedure, an abdominal radiograph shows the many interventional devices inserted, including urinary stents (*arrowheads*), occlusive coils (*small arrows*), vascular stent (*large arrow*), and the large occlusion wires on the left. The safety pins are on a dressing.

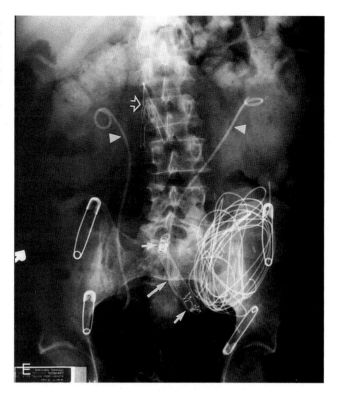

A-V malformations (Figs. 3.12 and 3.13), and intracranial aneurysms (Fig. 3.14). Embolization procedures require the utmost care to ensure that the embolized materials do not end up in vessels other than those intended.

Catheter-directed drug delivery can be used for various indications. Chemotherapeutic agents alone or in combination with an embolic agent are used with selective arterial catheterization to deliver a high concentration of the drugs into the feeding vessels of a tumor. The procedure is most commonly used to treat certain types of hepatic neoplasms. The procedure can also be used as a prelude to the surgical removal of a tumor to reduce blood loss, especially with vascular tumors (i.e., renal cell carcinoma metastases). In addition to embolization, vasoconstrictor agents such as vasopressin are sometimes infused into feeding vessels that are responsible for gastrointestinal bleeding. Finally, thrombolytic agents such as tissue plasminogen activator may be introduced for such conditions as pulmonary embolism, deep venous thrombosis, or coronary or peripheral arterial thrombosis to reestablish blood flow through clotted vessels.

In certain situations, such as in hemodialysis access grafts or fistulas or when thrombolytics are contraindicated, mechanical thrombectomy can be performed. Various devices, such as rotating brushes and baskets and suction-type devices, are available to macerate or remove the thrombus.

VENOUS ACCESS

Interventional radiologists are frequently asked to establish venous access routes in patients needing hemodialysis or chemotherapy or in patients with difficult venous access. The use of ultrasound and fluoroscopic guidance and knowledge of vascular anatomy greatly improve success with fewer complications. Commonly placed devices include peripherally inserted central catheters (PICC), subcutaneous ports, dialysis catheters, and nontunneled triple- or quad-lumen catheters.

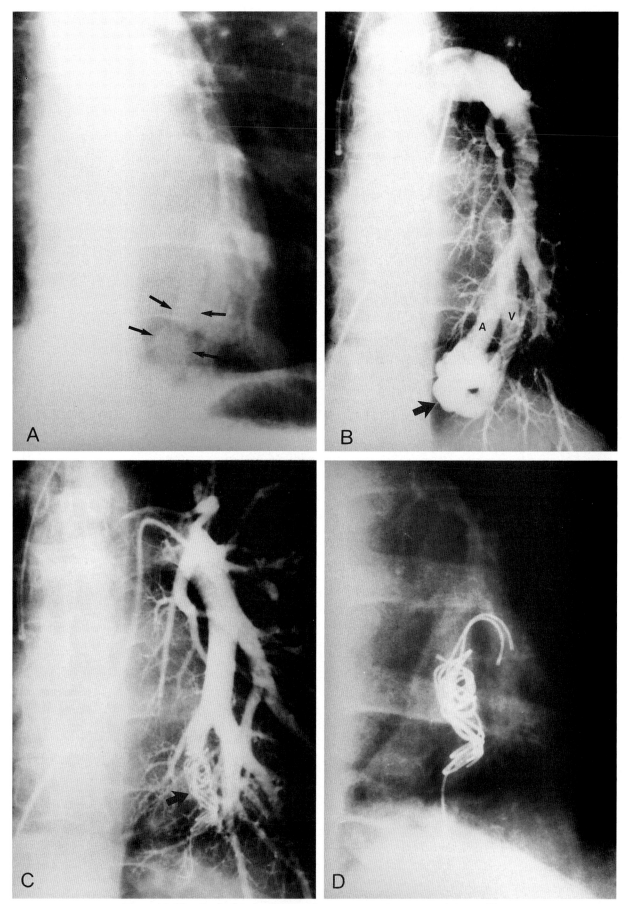

Figure 3.12.   Embolization of a pulmonary arteriovenous (A-V) malformation. A. Cone-down view of the left lower lobe shows the masslike A-V malformation (*arrows*). **B.** Pulmonary arteriogram shows the arterial (*A*) and the venous (*V*) branches of the malformation (*arrow*). **C.** Arteriogram following embolism of the vessel with an occluding coil (*arrow*) shows no flow of contrast into the malformation. **D.** Radiograph of the left lower lobe after embolization shows the coil in place.

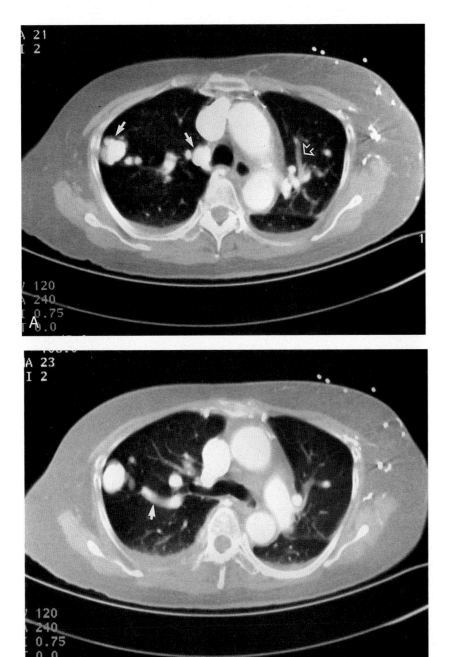

Figure 3.13. Embolization of multiple pulmonary A-V malformations in a patient with Rendu-Osler-Weber syndrome. A. Contrast-enhanced spiral computed tomography (CT) image shows two large malformations in the right lung (*solid arrows*) and serpentine vessels on the left (*open arrow*). **B.** CT image slightly more distal shows a large vein (*arrow*) draining the peripheral lesion on the right. **C.** Right selective pulmonary arteriogram shows the two large malformations (*arrows*). Notice the large feeding artery (*A*) and draining vein (*V*). **D.** Left selective pulmonary arteriogram shows the large malformation (*arrow*) and the feeding and draining artery (*A*) and vein (*V*). **E.** Selective right pulmonary injection after placement of occluding coils (*arrows*) shows successful occlusion of the malformations. **F.** Selective left pulmonary injection after placement of occluding coils (*arrows*) shows successful occlusion of the malformations.

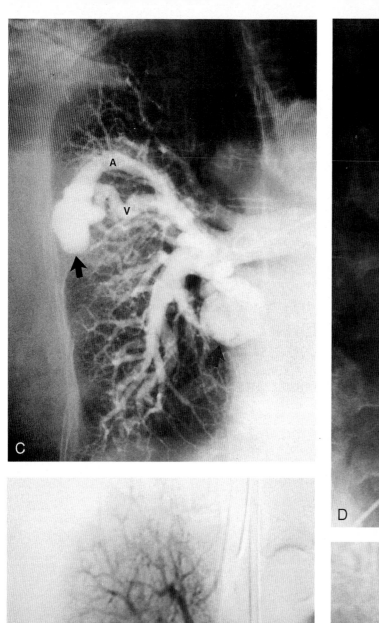

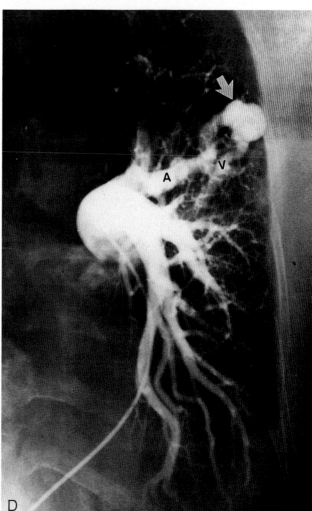

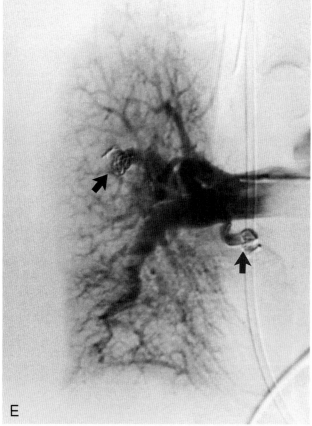

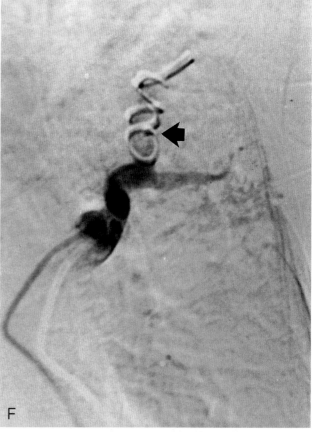

Figure 3.13. *(continued).*

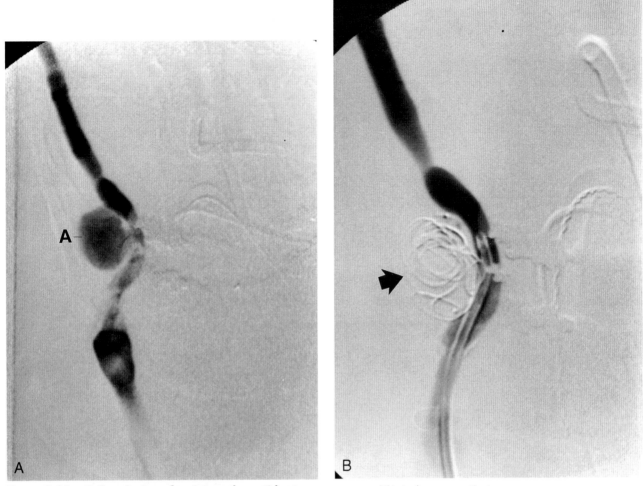

Figure 3.14.   Coil occlusion of an internal carotid artery aneurysm. (This is the same patient as in Fig. 3.13.) **A.** Digital subtraction angiogram of the right internal carotid artery shows the large aneurysm (*A*). **B.** Digital subtraction angiogram following coil occlusion of the aneurysm. Notice the coil just lateral to the artery (*arrow*).

VENA CAVA FILTERS

An inferior vena cava filter may be placed in patients who have lower extremity deep venous thromboses (DVT) or pulmonary embolism (PE) with a contraindication for anticoagulation, or in patients who have developed a worsening PE or DVT despite anticoagulation. Sometimes a filter is placed prophylactically in high-risk patients with expected long-term immobility. First, access is gained into the femoral, jugular, or antecubital veins. After a venogram is performed to determine the size of the inferior vena cava and the location of branch vessels, the self-expanding filter is deployed through a 3- to 4-mm-diameter catheter and placed just below the level of the renal veins. Various permanent and removable filters are available (Fig. 3.15).

TRANSJUGULAR INTRAHEPATIC PORTOSYSTEMIC SHUNTS

Patients with portal hypertension who present with variceal hemorrhage or intractable ascites may benefit from creation of a transjugular intrahepatic portosystemic shunt (TIPS). Variceal hemorrhage is treated first pharmacologically and endoscopically. If these measures fail, a TIPS procedure is often needed. These shunts can now be placed through a right internal jugular vein. Using a long, curved needle, a communication is made from the right hepatic vein to the right portal vein (Fig. 3.16), allowing placement of a stent between the two vessels and decom-

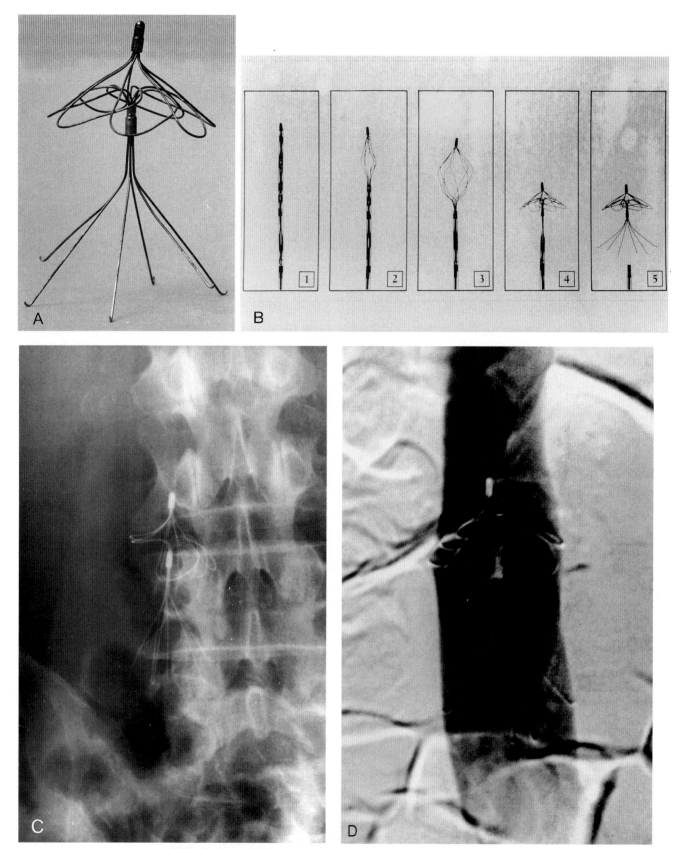

Figure 3.15. Simon-Nitinol inferior vena cava filter. A. Photograph of the filter. **B.** Photographs showing deployment of the filter from its catheter. (Courtesy of Cardiomedics, Inc.) **C.** Radiograph showing the filter in place. **D.** Subtraction inferior vena cavagram shows a filter in place. The filter does not obstruct the flow of blood through the cava but will trap any emboli.

Figure 3.16. Transjugular intrahepatic portosystemic shunts (TIPS) procedure. A. Drawing showing the shunt in place (*open arrow*). **B.** Radiograph made following a TIPS procedure shows the shunt in place in the liver and occlusive coils (*arrows*) in gastric varices.

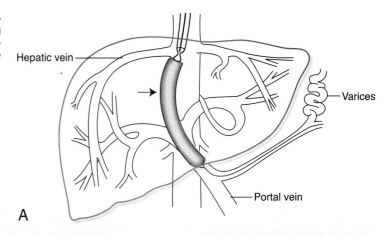

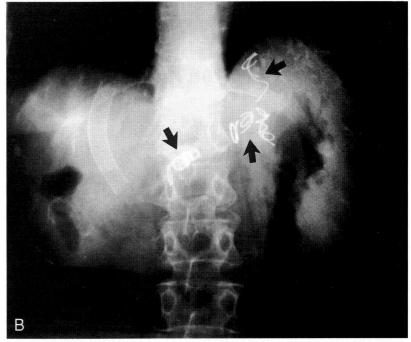

pressing the portal venous system. Before this procedure was developed, these high-risk patients had to undergo surgery for which the morbidity and mortality was high.

PERCUTANEOUS BIOPSY

Biopsy procedures are performed using various needles (Fig. 3.17) throughout the body. Percutaneous biopsy has prevented countless surgical operations for which the sole purpose was to obtain tissue. Biopsies should be performed using whatever imaging modality shows the lesion to best advantage. In most instances, CT guidance is used because it gives the best overall depth control (Fig. 3.18). Large skeletal lesions that are apparent on radiographs may undergo biopsy under fluoroscopic control. Ultrasound is helpful for most thyroid and liver biopsies or for aspiration of cystic lesions. Breast lesions may be biopsied under ultrasound or stereotactic guidance (see Chapter 6).

In our department, we have an older CT scanner that is used solely for interventional procedures (biopsies, drainages, and screw placements). In addition, we have provided space for our cytopathologist to have a small "wet lab" to provide immediate assessment of the tissues removed during biopsies. We have found that both of these innovations have hastened the process of obtaining information and eliminated delays in routine diagnostic studies by freeing up our main CT scanners.

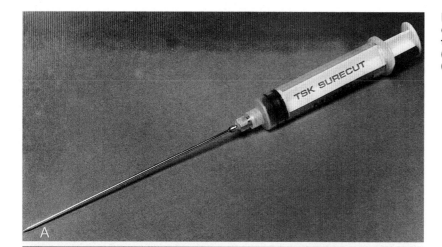

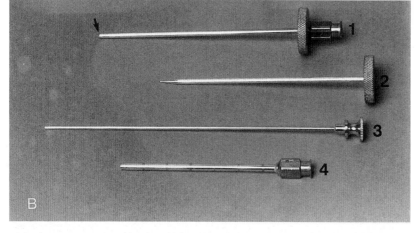

Figure 3.17. Representative biopsy needles. A. Surecut Menghini needle used for soft tissue lesions. **B.** Ackerman bone biopsy set: (*1*) Toothed (*arrow*) biopsy needle. (*2*) Trocar. (*3*) Clearing rod. (*4*) Outer, depth-marked sheath.

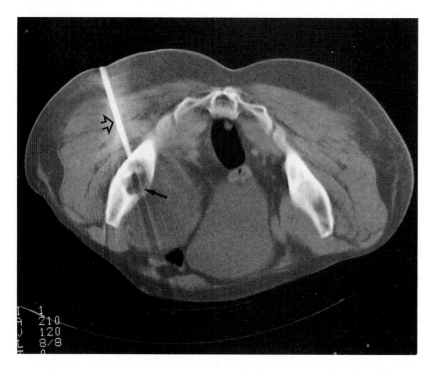

Figure 3.18. CT-guided biopsy of a pelvic chondrosarcoma on the left. The patient is prone. The biopsy needle (*open arrow*) is directly over the lesion (*thin arrow*).

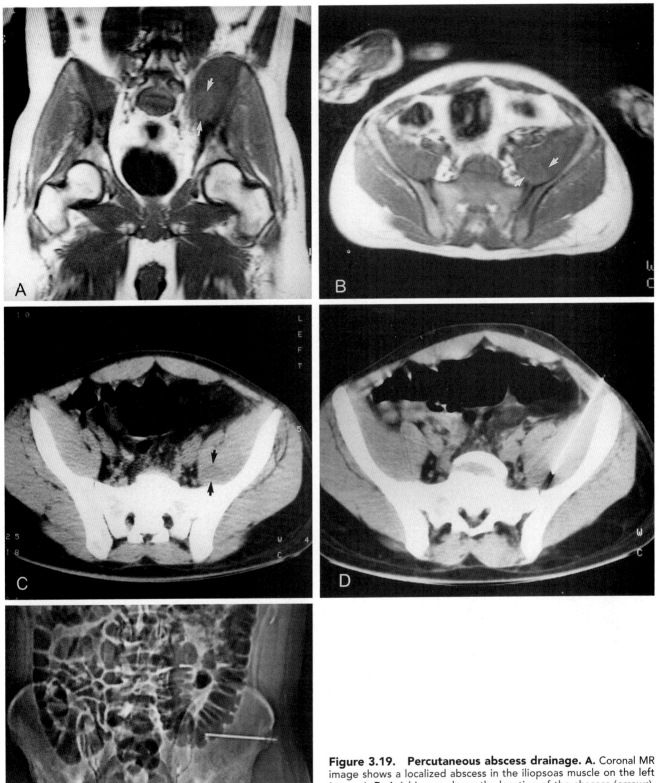

Figure 3.19. Percutaneous abscess drainage. A. Coronal MR image shows a localized abscess in the iliopsoas muscle on the left (*arrows*). **B.** Axial image shows the location of the abscess (*arrows*). **C.** CT image also shows the abscess (*arrows*). **D.** CT image shows the placement of the drainage needle in the abscess. **E.** Scout view shows the position of the needle. Compare this location with the abscess as shown in A.

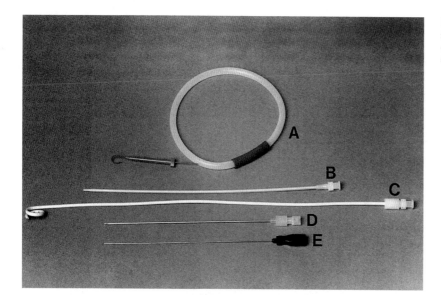

Figure 3.20. Percutaneous nephrostomy set. A. Guide wire. **B.** Dilator. **C.** Pigtail drainage catheter. **D.** Needle and stylet. **E.** Thin-walled needle.

DECOMPRESSION AND DRAINAGE

Decompression and drainage is performed as a variation of the Seldinger technique. A needle is placed into the fluid collection using imaging (usually ultrasound or CT) guidance (Fig. 3.19). A guide wire is then advanced through the needle, the needle is removed, and a drainage catheter is introduced into the fluid-filled space. The catheter is either taped or sutured in place and then attached to a vacuum bottle for further drainage. Variations of this technique may be used to drain obstructed renal collecting systems (nephrostomy) (Fig. 3.20), obstructed biliary ducts (biliary drainages), and gastric outlet obstruction (percutaneous gastrostomy). Once access to the obstructed system is achieved, invasive radiologic procedures may be used to correct the obstruction by placing temporary catheters or permanent metallic stents or by performing angioplasty in the biliary duct (Fig. 3.21). Benign strictures can be dilated, and malignant obstructions can be stented open (see Fig. 3.21B).

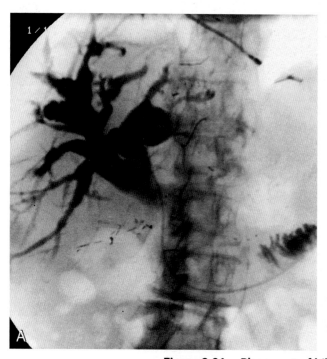
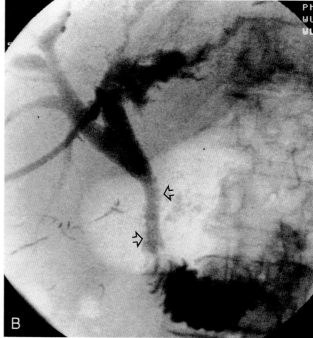

Figure 3.21. Placement of biliary stent in an obstruction of the common bile duct. A. Injection of contrast through a catheter following percutaneous transhepatic cholangiography shows complete obstruction of the common bile duct near the catheter tip. Notice the dilation of the biliary tree. **B.** After placement of a stent (*arrows*), there is decompression of the biliary tree.

With improvements in catheter technology and imaging systems, radiologists can now perform extraction procedures for biliary and renal stones as well as foreign bodies. The procedure is a variant of that used for decompression, with the exception being the use of an extraction instrument through the catheter within the lumen of the occluded duct.

PERCUTANEOUS SCREW PLACEMENT

In recent years, musculoskeletal radiologists have been called on to assist orthopaedic surgeons in the placement of screws across unstable sacroiliac joints or across acetabular fractures. These procedures have been performed traditionally under fluoroscopic guidance by the orthopaedist in the operating room. For some obese patients who could not undergo fluoroscopic-guided placement, radiologists have been asked to perform the procedure using CT guidance. CT has the advantages of permitting precise localization, accurate determination of angles, and exact depth measurements for screw placement (Fig. 3.22).

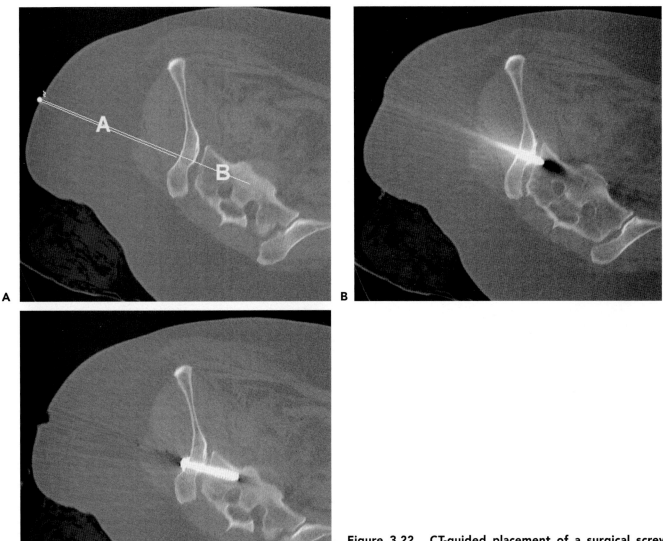

Figure 3.22. CT-guided placement of a surgical screw across an unstable sacroiliac joint. A. CT image shows a wide right sacroiliac joint. Lines are for measurement of depth from the skin to the iliac bone (A) and for length of screw (B). **B.** CT image shows the screw being placed. **C.** CT image showing final position of the screw. Notice that the sacroiliac joint is now narrower.

SUMMARY AND KEY POINTS

- Interventional and invasive radiology is an exciting subspecialty that uses various diagnostic and therapeutic techniques.
- Percutaneous puncture using the Seldinger technique forms the backbone of this subspecialty..
- Interventional and invasive radiologic procedures use imaging technologies such as fluoroscopy, digital subtraction, CT, and ultrasound.
- Invasive radiologic procedures may be performed instead of a surgical procedure in the operating room, saving the patient the risk of general anesthesia as well as that of the surgical procedure itself.

SUGGESTED ADDITIONAL READING

Baum SA, Pentecost MJ, eds. Abrams' Angiography: Interventional Radiology. 2nd Ed. Philadelphia: Lippincott William & Wilkins, 2005.

Fenton DS, Czervionke LF. Image-Guided Spine Intervention. Philadelphia: WB Saunders, 2003.

Kaufman JA, Lee MJ. Vascular and Interventional Radiology: The Requisites. St. Louis: Mosby, 2004.

LaBerge JM, Gordon RL, Kerlan RK Jr., Wilson MW. Interventional Radiology Essentials. Philadelphia: Lippincott Williams & Wilkins, 2000.

Pulmonary Imaging

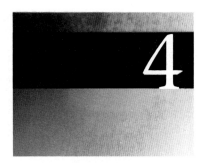

The chest radiograph is the examination you will be requesting and observing with the greatest frequency. In addition, it is the examination that you will most likely be reviewing alone. Chest radiographs account for more than half of all the examinations performed in any radiology practice. One of the reasons for this is that the chest is the "mirror of health or disease." Besides giving information about the patient's heart and lungs, the chest radiograph provides valuable information about adjacent structures such as the gastrointestinal (GI) tract, the thyroid gland, or the bony structures of the thorax. Furthermore, metastatic disease from the abdominal viscera, head and neck, or skeleton frequently manifests itself in the lungs. Thus the "routine" chest radiograph should not be considered quite so "routine." Figures 4.1 through 4.4 illustrate some of these entities.

TECHNICAL CONSIDERATIONS

The Patient

The first technical consideration for any imaging study is to be certain that the examination is of the *correct* patient (Fig. 4.5). It is important to check the patient's name, gender, age, and medical identification number on the study with that given on the requisition slip. Mismatches do occur. Furthermore, because many critically ill patients have multiple studies performed the same day, it is important to check the time of each examination (Fig. 4.6). Actual patient identification is checked by looking for congruent bony structures, soft tissue characteristics such as breast shadows (or their absence), and the presence of surgical hardware (see Fig. 4.5). *Always use old studies (films) for comparison, whenever they are available.* Old studies are your best friends in radiology!

Analysis

Once you have assured yourself that the radiograph presented is that of the correct patient, the film should be analyzed for *density, motion,* and *rotation.* A determination should be made as to whether the entire thorax is displayed. Be sure that the technologist has not cut the costophrenic angles off the film. On a properly exposed radiograph, the thoracic vertebrae should be barely discernible through the image of the heart. The medial ends of the clavicles should be equidistant from the patient's midline, indicating no rotation.

The next step is to decide what *type of examination* has been performed. The ordinary chest radiograph is made with the patient in the erect position with the anterior portion of the chest against the film cassette. The x-ray tube is positioned 6 feet behind the patient, and the

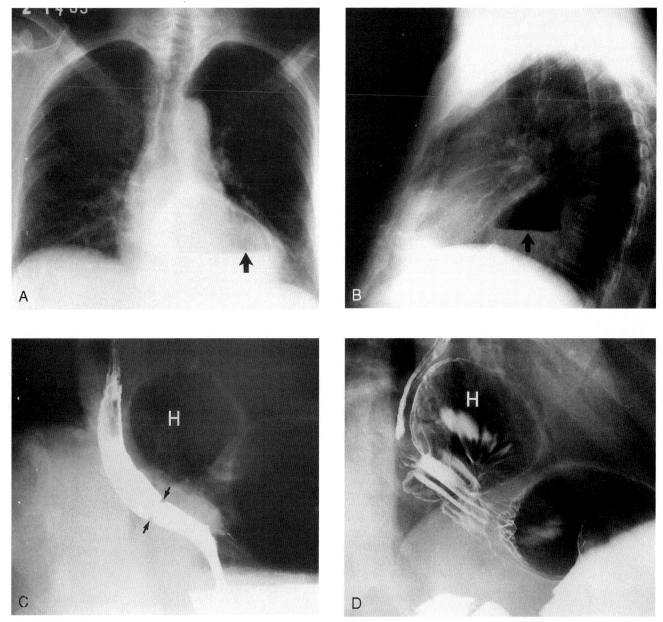

Figure 4.1.   Large paraesophageal hiatal hernia detected on a "routine" chest examination. A, frontal and **B,** lateral radiographs demonstrate a mass behind the heart with a large air-fluid level (*arrows*). **C,** detail view of an upper gastrointestinal examination shows the esophageal hiatus (*arrows*). The large hernia sac is seen above (*H*). **D,** detail film taken slightly later shows barium and air within the hernia sac (*H*).

horizontal beam enters from the back (posterior) and exits through the front (anterior): the PA radiograph. If the patient turns completely around and the beam enters from the front, the film is termed an AP film. Figure 4.7**A** is a PA erect film of a young patient; Figure 4.7**B** is an AP erect film of the same patient. Figures 4.7**C** and **D** illustrate the differences between an erect film and a supine film.

In general, the following are features that commonly identify PA chest radiographs: identification markings, if present, are oriented so that the observer may read them without reversing the film; the clavicles are superimposed over the upper lungs and are slanted with the medial aspect lower than the lateral; and the posterior portions of the cervical and thoracic vertebrae (neural arch, articular processes, apophyseal joints, and laminae) are more

Figure 4.2. **"Routine" chest radiograph showing a thyroid mass (goiter) on the left displacing the trachea to the right** (*arrow*).

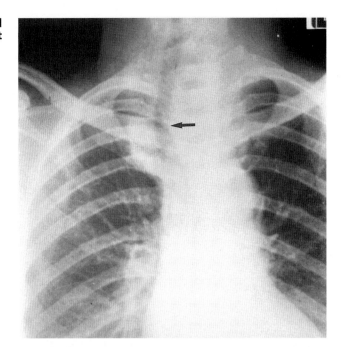

Figure 4.3. **Cleidocranial dysplasia.** Note the absence of the clavicles.

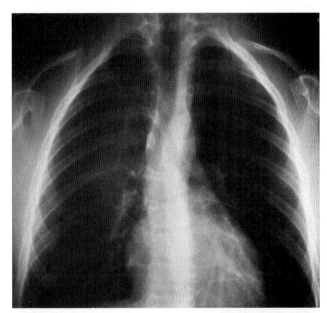

Figure 4.4. **Multiple pulmonary and mediastinal metastases in the right hemithorax detected on a "routine" chest radiograph.**

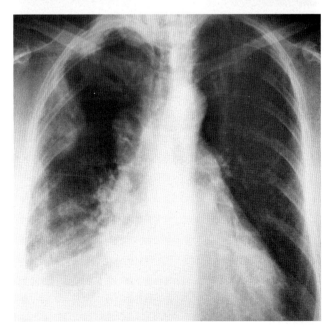

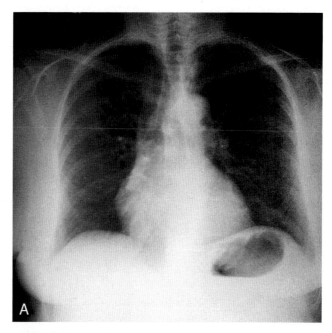

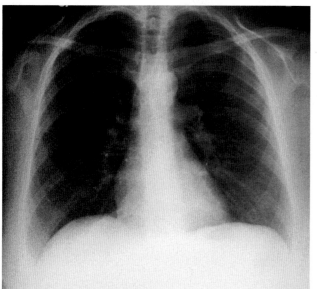

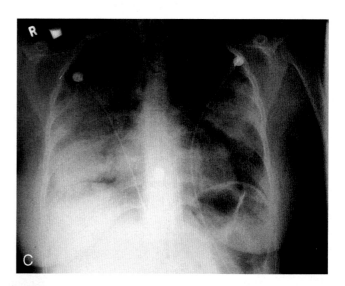

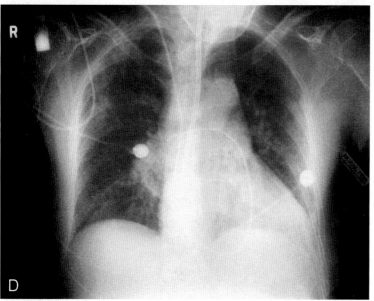

Figure 4.5. Mislabeled chest radiographs. A and **B,** consecutive films from the outpatient imaging center were both labeled with the same patient identification. Note the differences between each patient with regard to heart and aortic configuration, clavicle shape, and breast size. **C** and **D,** portable chest radiographs from patients in adjacent beds in an intensive care unit. Both films were obtained at the same time. In addition to the pulmonary pathology, note the differences in heart size, aortic configuration, clavicle position, breast size, and bone structure, particularly in the shoulders. *Always compare radiographs with old studies and check pertinent patient information on the requisition slip!*

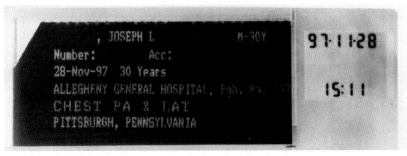

Figure 4.6. Film identification label. The information on the dark part of the label is printed on the film at the time it is processed. The top line contains the patient's name and to the right, gender and age. The next line has the patient's hospital identification number and immediately adjacent the film accession number (Acc) that refers only to the current examination. The next line contains the date of the examination, and the patient's age, once again. The fourth and sixth lines give the identification of the hospital. The fifth line tells what type of examination was performed. The numbers in the light portion of the label include the date on top and the time of the examination on the bottom. This is important if a patient has multiple examinations in one day. Digital images contain the same information. (Name and other patient ID data intentionally blacked out for HIPAA compliance.)

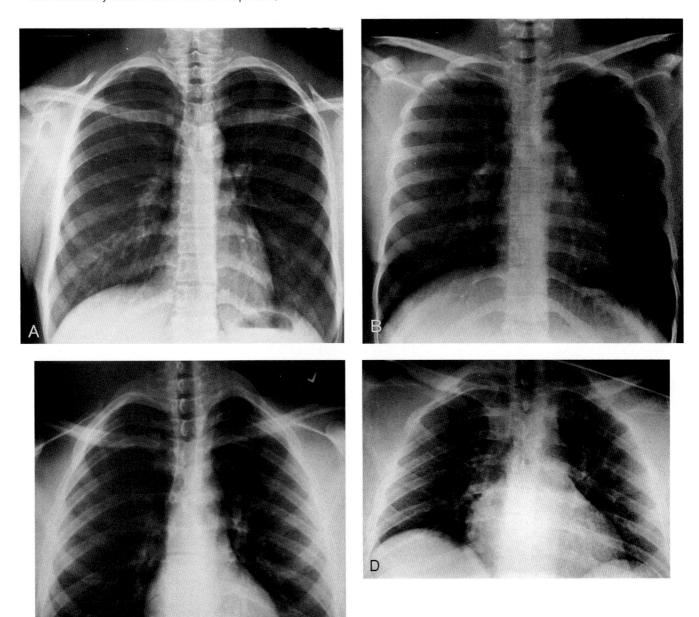

Figure 4.7. Normal chest radiographs. A, PA view. **B,** AP view. (See text for description). **C,** upright PA and **D,** supine AP views on another patient. Note the differences in the appearance of the heart and skeletal structures caused by the changes in position.

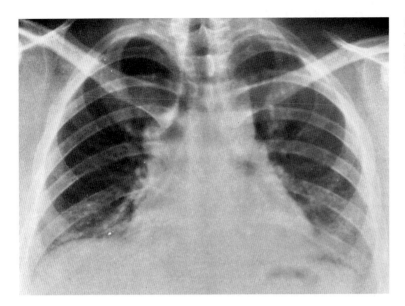

Figure 4.8. Expiratory chest radiograph. This film was made in deliberate expiration..There is elevation of the diaphragm, crowding of the lower lung markings, and apparent heart enlargement. (Compare with Figure 4.9.)

clearly visible. These findings suggest an AP radiograph: identification marks and writing are reversed; the heart appears slightly large; the clavicles are usually higher; and there is demonstration of the bodies and Luschka joints of the lower cervical vertebrae.

One of the most important technical considerations in evaluating the chest radiograph is determining whether or not the film is in optimal *inspiration*. Figure 4.8, a film of a healthy man, was deliberately made in forced expiration. Failure to observe that the film was a poor inspiratory *result* could easily lead to a mistaken diagnosis of congestive heart failure (CHF). After all, the heart appears large and rather poorly defined, the pulmonary vessels appear slightly prominent, and there is apparent blunting of both lung bases, suggesting fluid. Figure 4.9 is a maximal inspiratory film of the same individual; it is perfectly normal.

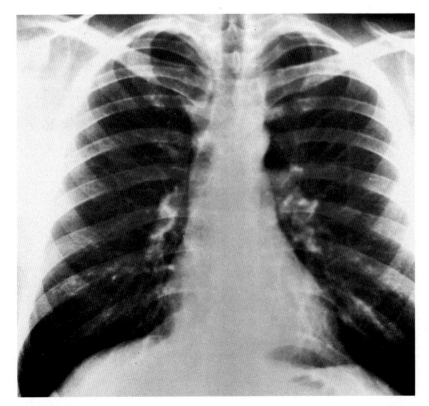

Figure 4.9. Normal inspiratory chest radiograph. (This is the same patient as in Fig. 4.8.) Note the differences in full inspiration.

There are many reasons why a film may not be obtained in full inspiration. Massive obesity is a mechanical cause; pain in a patient postoperatively results in voluntary restriction; the cardiac patient with CHF is unable to displace the edema fluid in the "waterlogged" lungs; and the patient with chronic restrictive lung disease cannot expand his/her chest to expected maximum because of scarring and loss of compliance in the lung tissues. For all these reasons, the term *"poor inspiratory result"* is used rather than *"poor inspiratory effort."* In most instances, these patients will have made a good inspiratory *effort,* but the *result* is poor.

A film is considered to be in optimal inspiratory result when we are able to see the diaphragm crossing the tenth rib or interspace posteriorly or the eighth rib anteriorly. The reader is cautioned not to fall into the pitfall of diagnosing "nondisease" in a patient with a poor inspiratory film.

Interestingly enough, there are certain circumstances in which it is desirable to have a film deliberately taken in *expiration.* These include evaluation of the patient with a suspected foreign body in a bronchus, a "ball-valve" type of bronchial obstruction, or a suspected pneumothorax. In the first instance (Fig. 4.10), the PA inspiratory film is normal; the expiratory film demonstrates no change in the volume of the lung on the obstructed side. The normal lung decreases in volume, and the mediastinum swings toward the normal side. In the second instance, the pneumothorax is enhanced by the decrease in lung volume (Fig. 4.11).

Rotation of the patient or angulation may result in distortion of normal anatomic images. As mentioned previously, you should be able to detect rotation by observing the position of the medial ends of the clavicles.

Lordotic views have been advocated as a means of examining lesions in the lung apices. The examination is made by having the patient lean backward toward the film while a horizontal beam is used to make the exposure. We do not use this view frequently because anterior lesions are often not demonstrated by this technique. An alternative to a lordotic view, a coned-down view of the apex of the lung, is more useful for suspected upper lobe lesions.

Another technical consideration is the analysis of radiographs made by *portable technique.* Studies of this kind are performed on severely debilitated or gravely ill patients who are unable to come to the radiology department. In reviewing these studies, it is important to recognize the circumstances under which they were made. There may be slight motion on the film (the

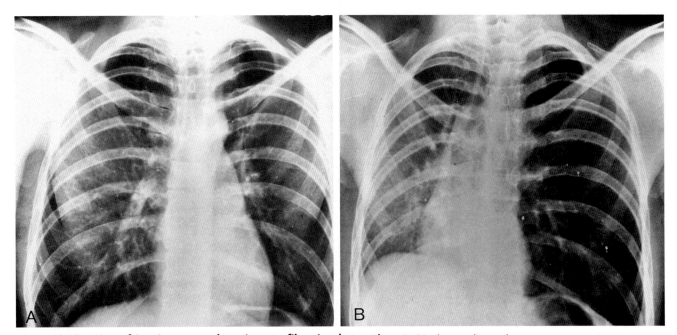

Figure 4.10. Use of inspiratory and expiratory films in obstruction. A, PA chest radiograph made in full inspiration is normal. **B,** radiograph made in expiration shows the mediastinum and heart to shift to the right. There is no volume change on the left. These findings indicate an obstructing lesion in the mainstem bronchus on the left, found to be a bronchial adenoma on subsequent bronchoscopy.

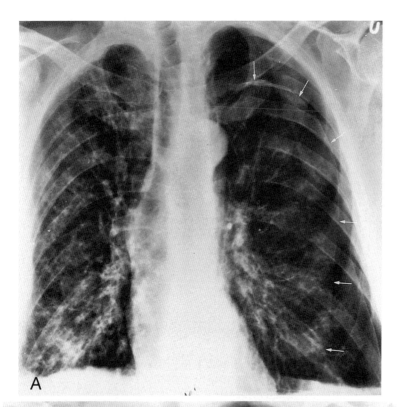

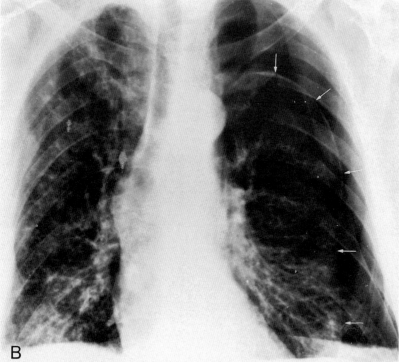

Figure 4.11. Use of inspiratory and expiratory film in pneumothorax. A, inspiratory film shows a pneumothorax on the left (*arrows*). **B,** expiratory film shows enlargement of the pneumothorax (*arrows*).

patient cannot hold his/her breath), the patient may be rotated, or the patient may sag down against the pillow; the result is a lordotic view of the chest. This is easy enough to detect because the heart assumes an egg-shaped configuration, the ribs appear tapered, and the clavicles are seen above the ribs (Fig. 4.12).

Many portable studies are obtained with the patient supine. This can result in a redistribution of blood to the upper lobes of the lung, a finding that is an early sign of CHF. The

Figure 4.12. Lordotic positioning. A, supine lordotic film shows the clavicles to be positioned high. The mediastinum appears widened, and the heart is egg-shaped. **B,** upright radiograph on the same patient shows striking differences.

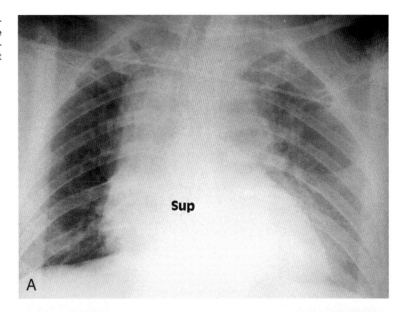

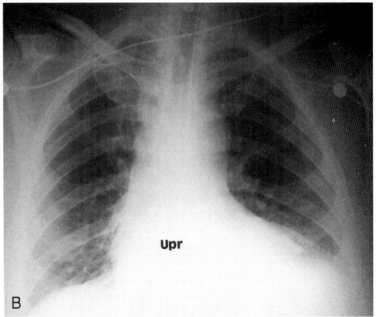

reader is again cautioned to observe whether the study was performed with the patient in the upright position or in the supine position. The presence or absence of an air-fluid level in the gastric air bubble may aid in determining upright versus supine positioning. Our technologists routinely use a vial of radiographic contrast material to indicate the degree of erectness. An upright film will have a sharp fluid meniscus; a recumbent film will not (Fig. 4.13).

Occasionally it may be useful to make a film with the patient lying on one side (*decubitus position*). This study is primarily used for patients suspected of having pleural effusions to determine if the effusion will layer out. The technique may also be used to "clear" a portion of the lung base that is obscured by fluid. Unfortunately, loculated effusions often do not shift with changes in patient position.

Chest radiographs made using computed radiography offers the operator the additional feature of dual-energy subtraction. This allows one to selectively subtract the bones to see just the lungs and the heart, or conversely, to subtract the heart and lungs to see the bones (See Fig. 1.6). The advantages of this technique are to enable finding subtle lung lesions; to

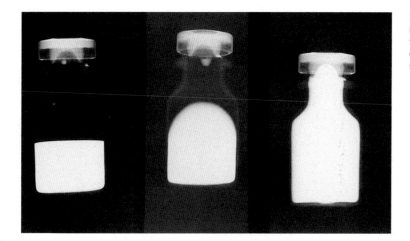

Figure 4.13. Film position marker. Radiographic appearance of a vial of dilute radiographic contrast in the erect (left), 45° recumbent (center), and supine (right) positions.

be able to differentiate between lung and bone lesions; and to assess pneumothorax or inserted lines. There are disadvantages, however, including longer examination times and higher radiation dose.

A final technical consideration is, once again, the use of *old films* to compare with the current study. Many individuals have abnormal chest radiographs from inactive or old diseases. The most common conditions encountered are old, healed granulomas; scarring; and chronic obstructive pulmonary disease. Without the old radiographs for comparison, the patient may have to undergo extensive (and expensive) evaluation that may include a biopsy. Every effort should be made to obtain old studies. *Every* current study should be compared with a previous one if it is available. If old studies are not available, you should place a note to that effect in the medical record.

Other Imaging Modalities

Although chest radiography is the mainstay for diagnosing thoracic disease, other imaging modalities are also used. Chest fluoroscopy is a valuable, but unfortunately infrequently used, technique for confirmation and localization of suspected lung nodules (Fig. 4.14). This procedure is simple to perform, takes little time, is inexpensive, and has relatively low radiation exposure. Fluoroscopy is also useful for evaluating cardiac and diaphragmatic motion. In most instances, however, it is easier to obtain a CT examination of the chest. The rationale for doing this is that if the fluoroscopic study was positive, CT would be performed anyway.

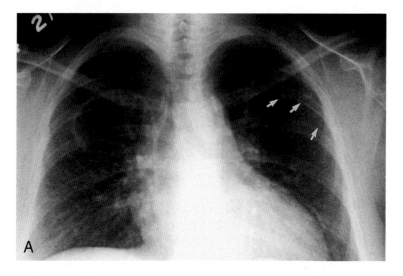

Figure 4.14. Use of chest fluoroscopy. A, chest radiograph shows "lung nodules" in the left upper lobe (*arrows*). *(continued on page 79)*

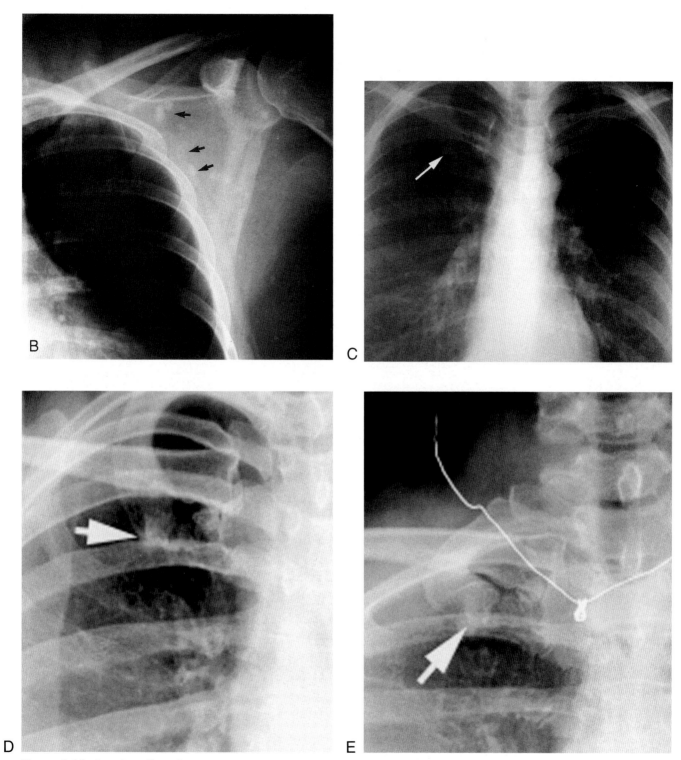

Figure 4.14. *(continued)*   **B,** fluoroscopic spot film shows the "nodules" are, in fact, multiple calcified axillary lymph nodes (*arrows*). **C,** chest radiograph in another patient shows a "nodule" in the right upper lobe. **D, E,** fluoroscopic spot films shows the "nodule" to be prominent costochondral cartilage.

Computed tomography (CT), particularly with spiral technology, is an extremely valuable technique for assessing lung nodules as well as lung and mediastinal masses (Fig. 4.15). It is also useful for evaluating chronic pleural effusions, chronic infiltrates, and pulmonary emboli. By far, the most common use will be for suspected primary or metastatic neoplasms. CT is much more sensitive in detecting the calcification in nodules that would suggest a benign postinflammatory condition. CT is also now routinely used in trauma victims to detect mediastinal hemorrhage from injury to the aorta or other great vessels (Fig. 4.16).

Magnetic resonance (MR) imaging is now used primarily to evaluate hilar and other mediastinal masses, more peripheral nodules, and vascular lesions (including superior vena cava

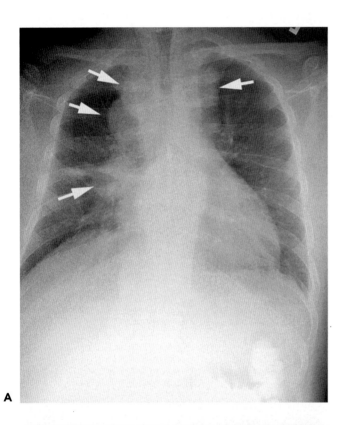

A

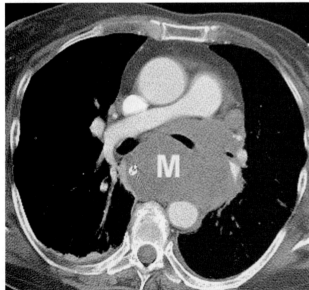

B

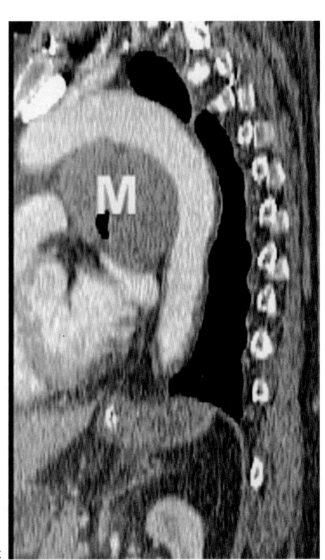

C

Figure 4.15.   Mediastinal mass. A, frontal radiograph shows bilateral mediastinal masses (*arrows*). The paraspinal stripe is widened as well. This is a case of "too many bumps". **B,** axial CT image shows a large mass (*M*) in the infracarinal area. **C,** sagittal reconstructed CT image shows the mass (*M*) beneath the aorta.

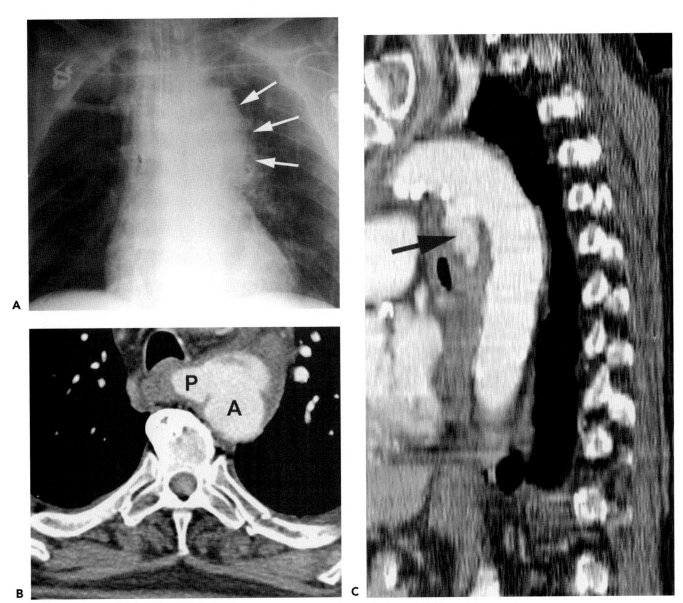

Figure 4.16.   Posttraumatic aortic tear. A, frontal chest radiograph shows widening of the superior mediastinum and straightening and irregularity of the aortic knob (*arrows*). **B,** axial contrast-enhanced CT image just below the aortic arch (*A*) shows extravasation of contrast anteriorly, and a pseudoaneurysm (*P*) medially. **C,** sagittal reconstructed CT image shows the hemorrhage and pseudoaneurysm (*arrow*).

syndrome). This technique is particularly advantageous over CT because flowing blood has no signal on MR and appears black. Thus, it is possible to differentiate a hilar mass from a dilated pulmonary vessel (Fig. 4.17). MR is also used to determine the extent of chest wall involvement in pulmonary lesions and to evaluate the brachial plexus. The ability of MR to image in sagittal and coronal planes is another distinct advantage over CT, as is the fact that it requires no intravenous contrast to identify vessels.

Diagnostic ultrasound is used to diagnose suspected pleural fluid collections, particularly on the right side, where imaging is performed in the transhepatic plane. Ultrasound is not useful for lung lesions because it cannot cross tissue-air borders.

Finally, *nuclear imaging* is performed to assess pulmonary blood flow and ventilation. It is most commonly used to diagnose suspected pulmonary emboli. The typical ventilation-perfusion (V/Q) scan uses inhaled xenon-133 or technetium-99-m-labeled DTPA for ventilation imaging followed by technetium-99-m-labeled macroaggregated albumin (MAA) particles injected intravenously for perfusion imaging (Fig. 4.18).

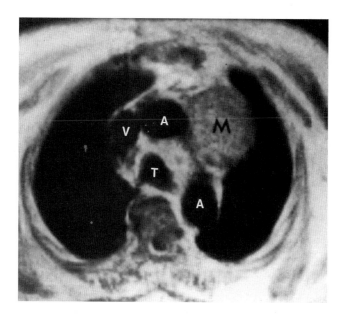

Figure 4.17. MR image differentiation of a hilar vessel from a mass. The mass (*M*) is of higher signal than either of the adjacent vessels. *A*, aorta; *V*, vena cava; *T*, trachea.

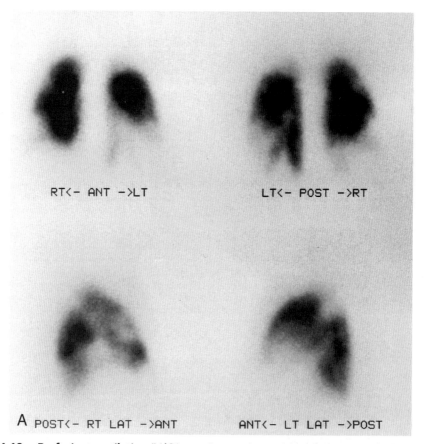

Figure 4.18. Perfusion-ventilation (V/Q) scan in a patient with pulmonary emboli. A, perfusion scan of the lungs demonstrates many areas devoid of radioisotope (photopenia) bilaterally. *(continued on page 83)*

Figure 4.18. *(continued)* **B,** ventillation scan is normal. This combination of findings is diagnostic of pulmonary emboli, particularly when the chest radiograph is normal or near normal.

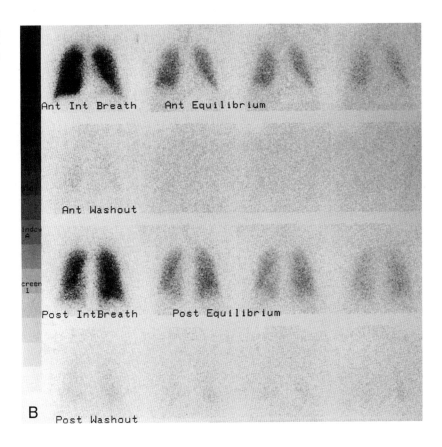

ANATOMIC CONSIDERATIONS

A logical approach to the interpretation of chest radiographs is predicated on the observer developing an orderly system for scanning each image. It matters not whether the review begins from the outside and proceeds inward or vice versa. What is important is that the system is followed each and every time that particular type of study is reviewed. Working from the inside outward, the method I use, observe the following:

1. Trachea and mediastinum
2. Heart and great vessels
3. Lungs
4. Pleura
5. Costophrenic angles
6. Diaphragm
7. Bones and soft tissues

The order of visual scan is illustrated in Figure 4.19, which shows a patient who has had a right radical mastectomy and has a congenital anomaly of the left shoulder. The analysis of this study and its reporting is as follows: "The heart and mediastinal structures are normal. The pulmonary vessels and aorta are normal. The lungs, costophrenic angles, pleura, and diaphragm are normal. The patient has had a right radical mastectomy as indicated by the absence of the right breast shadow and increased lucency (radiability) from the missing pectoralis muscle. A bony anomaly is present in the left shoulder: elevation of the scapula, the presence of an omovertebral bone, and a cleft vertebra at C-6. This particular type of anomaly is called Sprengel deformity."

The lateral chest radiograph should receive the same attention as the PA film and is analyzed similarly. Consider the report on the lateral chest radiograph in a patient with known esophageal carcinoma (Fig. 4.20): ". . . on the lateral chest film, the trachea is deviated anteriorly by a soft tissue mass that contains an air-fluid level (*arrow*). This is most consistent with the

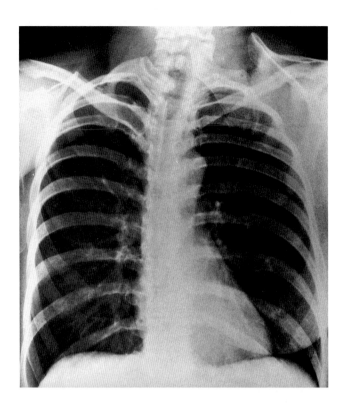

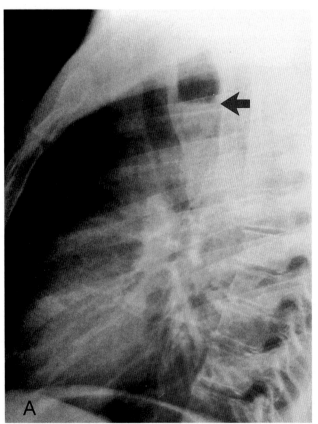

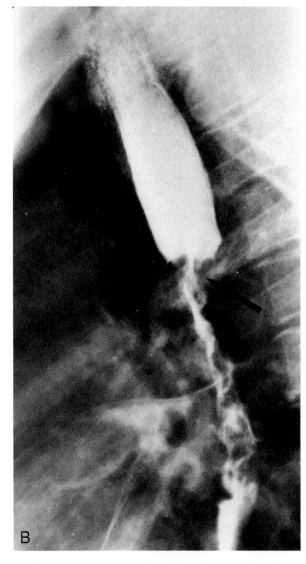

Figure 4.20. Carcinoma of the esophagus. A, lateral chest radiograph shows an air-fluid level (*arrow*) immediately behind the trachea. There is thickening of the retrotracheal line. Compare with Figure 4.21. B, esophagogram shows nearly complete obstruction to the passage of barium (*arrow*).

diagnosis of an obstructing esophageal lesion. The cardiac silhouette is normal. The lungs, costophrenic angle, posterior recesses, and diaphragm are normal. There are no significant vertebral abnormalities."

Let us now review the normal anatomic structures found on the chest radiograph in the same order as the film analysis.

The *trachea* is a midline structure whose air-filled image stands out in bold contrast to the surrounding soft tissues of the neck and mediastinum. On a well-penetrated frontal film, the carina (tracheal bifurcation) may be found at the level of the T4-T5 interspace. On the lateral film, the tracheal air column may be seen slowly angling down from the thoracic inlet. The soft tissue line (retrotracheal line) along its posterior wall should not be bowed and should not exceed 3 mm in thickness (Fig. 4.21). In young children, it is not uncommon for the tracheal air column to bow to the right. A trachea deviated to the left should be considered abnormal and CT of the neck should be performed to determine the cause, if not otherwise apparent (such as an associated cervical fracture).

The *mediastinum*, the extrapleural space between the lungs, is the midregion of the thorax. Contained within it are the heart, pericardium, great vessels, trachea, thoracic duct, thymus, fat, numerous small blood vessels, nerves, lymph nodes, and lymphatic vessels. Traditionally, the mediastinum has been divided into four regions—one superior and three inferior components (anterior, middle, and posterior). We may make this division by drawing a horizontal line from the sternal angle (of Louis) back to the T4-T5 intervertebral disc (Fig. 4.22). In the living patient, this line traverses the midportion of the aortic arch. Any structures above this line lie in the superior mediastinum, and any below are in the inferior mediastinum. The anatomic anterior mediastinum is bounded by the sternum anteriorly and by the pericardium posteriorly. The middle mediastinum is located between the anterior and posterior pericardium. The posterior medi-

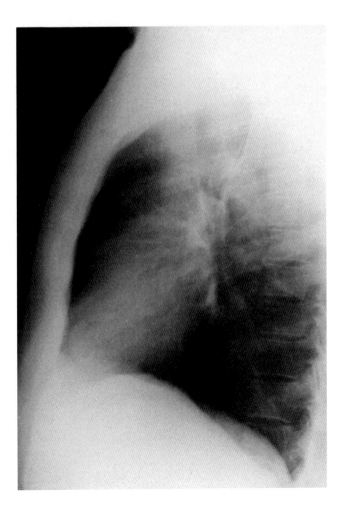

Figure 4.21. Normal lateral chest radiograph.

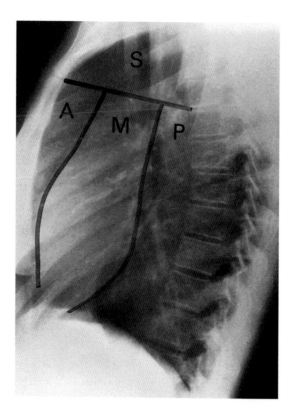

Figure 4.22. Anatomic mediastinum. Anatomically, the mediastinum is divided into anterior (*A*), middle (*M*), posterior (*P*), and superior (*S*), segments.

astinum is bounded anteriorly by the posterior pericardium and posteriorly by the vertebral column. All three subdivisions of the anatomic inferior mediastinum are bounded inferiorly by the diaphragm.

Although this classification may be satisfactory for the anatomist, radiologists and surgeons prefer to use the *radiologic mediastinum,* a concept proposed by Felson that is far more useful in clinical practice than the anatomic mediastinum, especially when dealing with neoplasms, because tumors of the mediastinum tend to spread in a craniocaudal manner rather than anteroposteriorly.

To delineate the three parts of the radiologic mediastinum, the following lines may be imagined on a lateral radiograph (Fig. 4.23). Line A–A′ begins at the diaphragm just behind the image of the inferior vena cava and extends upward along the back of the heart and in front of the trachea to the neck. The second line, B–B′, runs across the body of each thoracic vertebra 1 cm from its anterior margin and extends upward. The area anterior to line A–A′ is the anterior mediastinum; the area between lines A–A′ and B–B′ is the middle mediastinum; and the area posterior to line B–B′ is the posterior mediastinum. Pathologic aspects of these compartments will be discussed in the following section.

The anatomy of the *heart and great vessels* will be described in the next chapter. It is sufficient to say at this point, however, that all lung markings found on the normal chest radiograph are made by pulmonary arteries and veins and not by bronchi. After all, the blood-filled vessels are of water density; air-filled bronchi, which normally have thin walls, provide no significant contrast to the aerated lungs.

There are three lobes in the right *lung* and two in the left. Each lobe is divided into anatomic segments supplied by its own bronchus and blood vessels (Fig. 4.24). In the right upper lobe are the apical, anterior, and posterior segments; the middle lobe has medial and lateral segments. The right lower lobe contains a superior segment and, in clockwise fashion, posterior, medial, anterior, and lateral basal segments.

The left upper lobe consists of a fused apical-posterior segment, an anterior segment, and superior and inferior lingular segments. The left lower lobe is similar to the right lower lobe except that the anterior and medial basal segments are fused. A knowledge of the location of these segments is important in localizing disease. The reader is advised to note that there is a

Figure 4.23. The radiologic mediastinum. (See text for description.) *A*N, anterior mediastinum; *M*, mediastinum; *P*, posterior mediastinum.

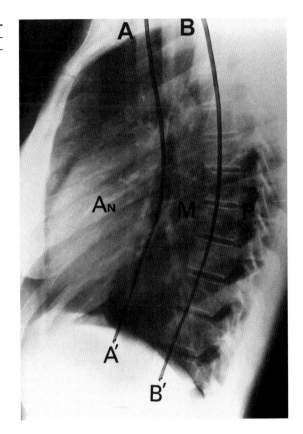

Figure 4.24. Segmental bronchial anatomy. Right upper lobe: *A*, apical; *P*, posterior; *An*, anterior. Right middle lobe: *L*, lateral; *M*, medial. Right lower lobe: *S*, superior; *Ab*, anterior basal; *Lb*, lateral basal; *Pb*, posterior basal; *Mb*, medial basal. Left upper lobe: *AP*, apical-posterior; *A*, apical; *P*, posterior; *An*, anterior; *Sl*, superior lingular; *I*, inferior lingular. Left lower lobe: *S*, superior; *AMb*, anterior-medial basal; *Lb*, lateral basal; *Pb*, posterior basal.

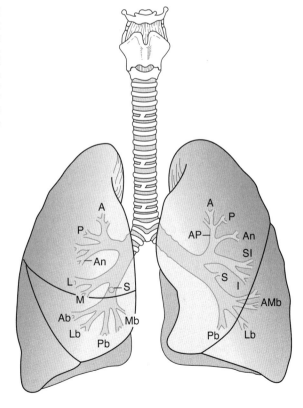

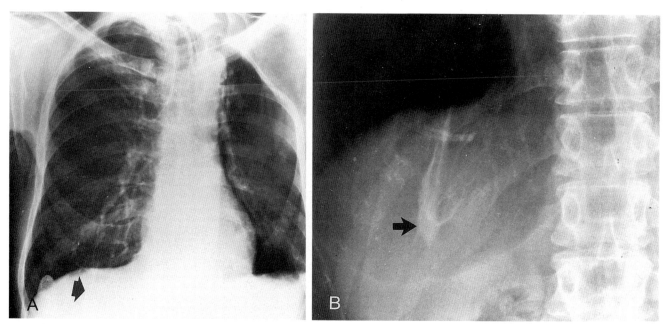

Figure 4.25.   Carcinoma of the right lower lobe in an extreme basal segment. A, PA chest radiograph barely shows a lesion beneath the diaphragm on the right (*arrow*). **B,** detail view from an abdominal radiograph shows an irregular mass (*arrow*) in an extreme basal segment of the right lower lobe.

significant portion of lung contained in the costophrenic recesses posteriorly. These recesses extend as far down as the level of L-2. Occasionally, tumors occur within the lung in this location. These lesions often will not be seen on chest radiographs but may be detected on an abdominal radiograph (Fig. 4.25) or on CT.

The basic anatomic and functional pulmonary unit is the *acinus*, the portion of lung distal to the terminal bronchiole where gas exchange takes place. It contains respiratory bronchioles, alveolar ducts, alveolar sacs, and alveoli. Anatomically and radiographically, a consistently rec-

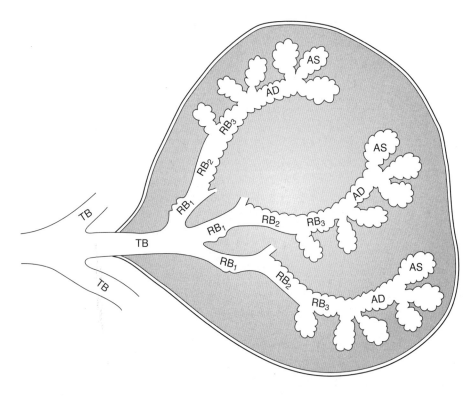

Figure 4.26.   The pulmonary lobule. This consists of a terminal bronchiole (*TB*), several levels of respiratory bronchioles (*RB*), alveolar ducts (*AD*), and alveolar sacs (*AS*). Each acinus is surrounded by its own interstitial structures and interlobular septum.

ognizable structure results from the grouping of three to five acini together to form the *pulmonary lobule.* The usual lobule is approximately 1 cm in diameter in the adult. Each of these lobules is surrounded by its own interlobular septa and interstitial structures (Fig. 4.26). Diseases that affect the air spaces are referred to as having an *acinar- or alveolar-type* pattern; diseases that affect the interstitial tissues are referred to as having an *interstitial* pattern.

The interlobular septa are not seen normally. However, when they become edematous or thickened by other pathologic processes, they become visible as faint linear lines known as septal (*Kerley*) lines (Fig. 4.27).

There are microscopic communications between the distal portions of the bronchiolar tree and surrounding alveoli known as the *canals of Lambert.* They provide an accessory route for air

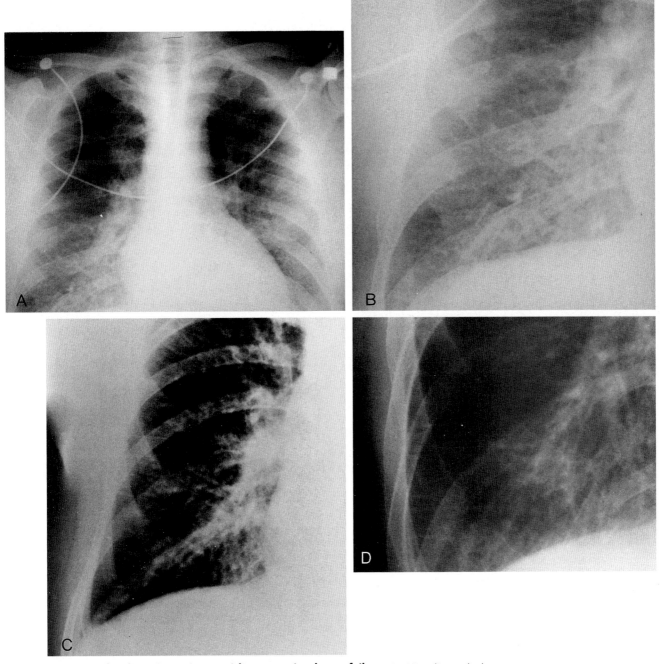

Figure 4.27. Kerley lines in patients with congestive heart failure. A, AP radiograph shows prominent interstitial markings in both bases with a fine interlacing pattern. **B,** detail view shows the linear horizontal Kerley B-lines in the periphery. **C** and **D,** detail views of two other patients show similar findings.

passage from the bronchioles to the alveoli. Another connection, the *pores of Kohn*, are small openings in the alveolar wall 10 to 15 microns in diameter. These permit the lung distal to an obstructed bronchus or bronchiole to be ventilated by a process known as collateral air drift. They also allow infection to spread.

The *pleura* consists of two layers, the visceral pleural and the parietal pleura. The visceral pleura encases the lungs. Under normal circumstances the pleura is not visualized with the exception of the normal interlobar fissures (Fig. 4.28). On the right there are two fissures, the oblique (major) and the horizontal (minor). The left lung contains an oblique fissure only. The oblique fissure begins at the level of the fourth thoracic vertebra, extending obliquely downward and forward and ending approximately at the level of the sixth rib anteriorly. The horizontal fissure begins roughly at the level of the sixth rib laterally and extends anteriorly and slightly downward to end near the medial portion of the fourth rib. Occasionally, an accessory fissure may be found bordering a segment of lung that has become partially or completely separated from its adjacent segments. The best known of these is the azygos fissure, which is created by the downward migration of the azygos vein through the apical pleura of the right upper lobe. In doing so, the vein invaginates a portion of pleura and results in a comma-shaped structure seen in the vicinity of the right upper lobe (Fig. 4.29). It is a normal variant.

The pleura is frequently involved in inflammatory and traumatic insults to the chest. These may result in areas of thickening or distortion along the pleural surface or in the *costophrenic or cardiophrenic angles.* Pleural calcification (Fig.4.30) may also occur.

The *diaphragm*, which separates the thoracic from the abdominal cavities, appears most often seen as a smooth, dome-shaped structure on either side. There may be scalloping or irregularities along the diaphragmatic surface, a frequent finding considered to be of little significance. The right hemidiaphragm is slightly higher than the left. Occasionally, gaseous distension of the stomach or colon produces elevation of the left hemidiaphragm above the right. The reason for the lower left hemidiaphragm is the contiguity of the left ventricle of the heart with it and not the bulk of the liver elevating the right hemidiaphragm.

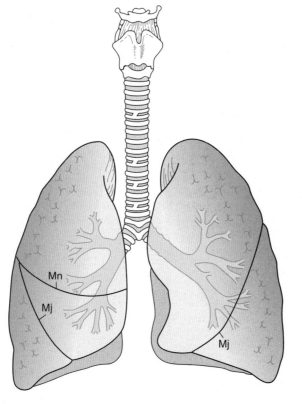

Figure 4.28.   Division of the lungs by fissures. *Mn*, minor fissure; *Mj*, major fissure.

Figure 4.29. **Azygous fissure** (*open arrows*) **and azygous vein** (*solid arrow*). This is a normal variant. **B, C,** CT images show the azygous vein (*A*) traversing the thorax. The azygous fissure, which represents pleural invagination around the vein as it descends, is seen just posterior to the vein in **B**.

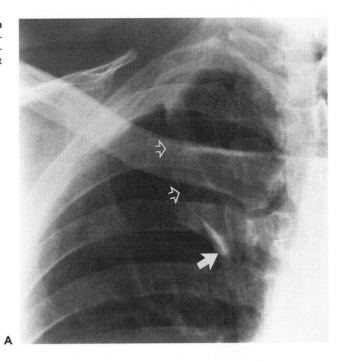

A

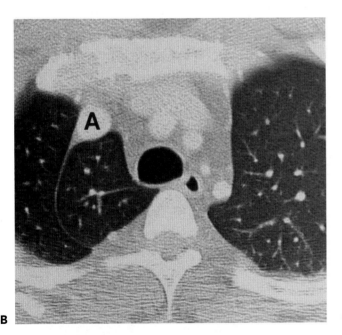

B

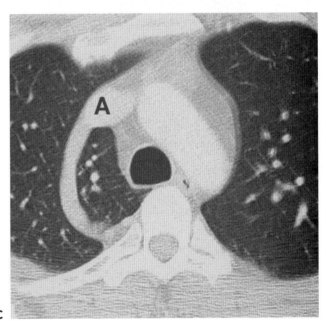

C

Soft tissue images commonly visible on the routine chest radiograph are the anterior axillary fold produced by the bulk of the pectoral muscles, soft tissue images along the upper surfaces of the clavicles, images of the sternocleidomastoid muscles in the neck, and breast images. In addition, nipple images are frequently seen over the lower chest radiographs in men. They may be mistaken for lung nodules, particularly when they are bilateral. When this poses a problem, a repeat radiograph with markers on the nipples is indicated (Fig 4.31).

Bony structures visible on the chest radiograph include the ribs, thoracic vertebrae, lower cervical vertebrae, clavicles, scapulae, and occasionally the heads of the humeri. In addition, the sternum is clearly visible on the lateral chest film. Occasionally, the manubrium projects as a prominence just to the right of the midline. It should not be mistaken for a pulmonary mass. Not uncommonly, cervical ribs are encountered. An abnormal-appearing rib in the cervicothoracic region can be considered a cervical rib if the transverse process to which it is

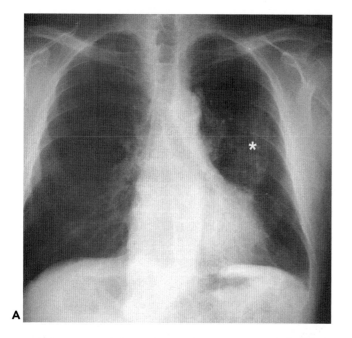

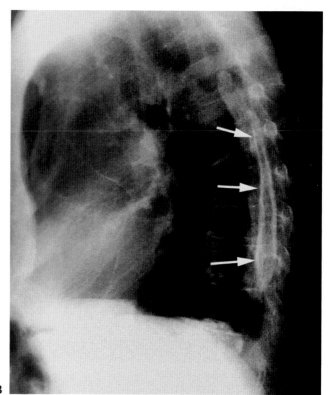

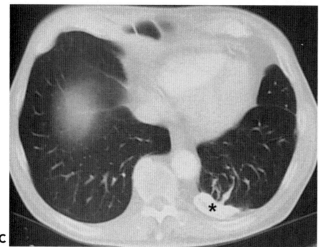

Figure 4.30.   Pleural calcification. A, Frontal radiograph shows a "mass" in the left mid lung field (*). **B,** Lateral radiograph shows the "mass" to be an area of thick pleural calcification posteriorly (arrows). **C,** CT image shows the dense pleural calcification posteriorly (*).

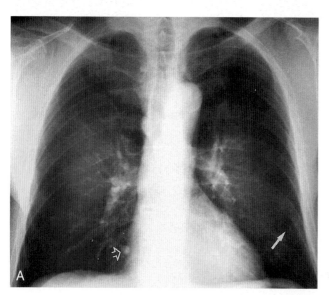

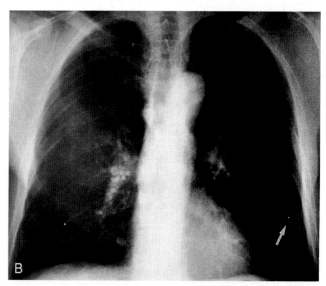

Figure 4.31.   Use of nipple markers. A, Frontal radiograph shows a rounded density in the left mid-lung field (*solid arrow*). There is a granuloma in the right lower lobe (*open arrow*). **B,** Repeat radiograph made with markers on both nipples. Notice how the rounded density on the left corresponds to the nipple shadow (*arrow*).

Figure 4.32. Bilateral cervical ribs (*open arrows*). The cervical transverse processes (*C*) point downward; the thoracic (*T*) point upward.

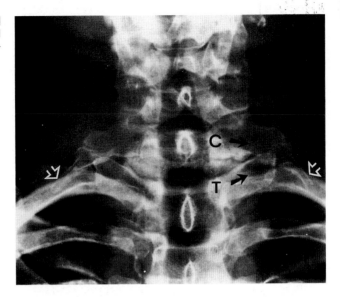

articulating points inferiorly. *Cervical transverse processes point down; thoracic transverse processes point up* (Fig. 4.32).

PATHOLOGIC CONSIDERATIONS

Six basic pathologic patterns may alter the normal appearance of the lungs. The reader should be aware that any or all of these may be present at one time in the same patient. Furthermore, any of these entities may be combined with abnormalities of the heart and pulmonary vessels. The six abnormalities are as follows:

1. Air space disease - consolidation
2. Atelectasis - collapse
3. Pleural fluid accumulation - effusion
4. Masses – tumors and tumor-like abnormalities
5. Emphysema - overinflation
6. Interstitial changes – fibrosis and/or edema

Figure 4.33 illustrates the effect of these abnormalities on the pulmonary lobule.

Air Space Disease—Consolidation

When the air spaces become filled with fluid (inflammatory exudate, blood, edema, or aspirated fluid), they lose their normal lucency and become opaque. In pneumonia, the inflammatory infiltrate usually follows normal anatomic planes and has a *segmental* distribution. By knowing the location of the lung segments and their relationship to the mediastinum and diaphragm, it is possible to accurately localize an area of consolidation by noting the loss of these normal anatomic landmarks.

The basis for visualization of the border of a structure depends on its contiguity with another structure of *different radiographic density.* Hence, we normally see the *silhouette* of the mediastinal structures and the diaphragm because they are of water density and are outlined by the adjacent air density in the lung. Consolidations adjacent to these borders result in the loss of the normal-appearing borders or silhouettes. This concept was first described by Fleischner and popularized by Felson as the *silhouette sign.*

Fleischner's famous experiment demonstrating the silhouette sign is illustrated as follows (Fig. 4.34): An empty film box was tilted on end; liquid paraffin was poured into it and allowed to congeal into a triangular density. A second empty film box was taped behind the first box, and both were radiographed (see Fig. 4.34A). The gray image of the solid paraffin represents a "cardiac border," and the blackness of the air within both boxes represents "aerated lung," creating a model for demonstrating the effects of consolidation on the

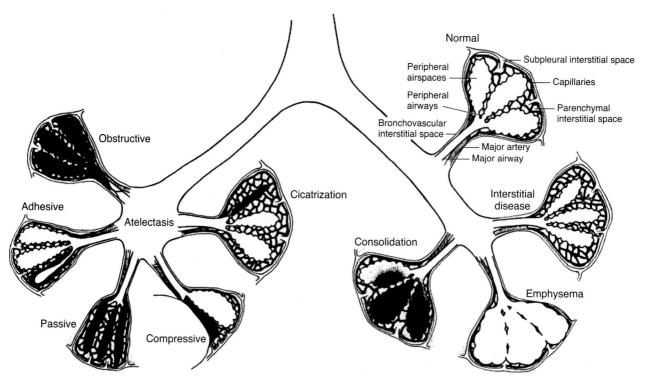

Figure 4.33. Schematic drawing of the four basic pathologic patterns affecting the lungs, atelectasis (five variations), consolidation, emphysema, and interstitial disease, compared with a normal pulmonary lobule.

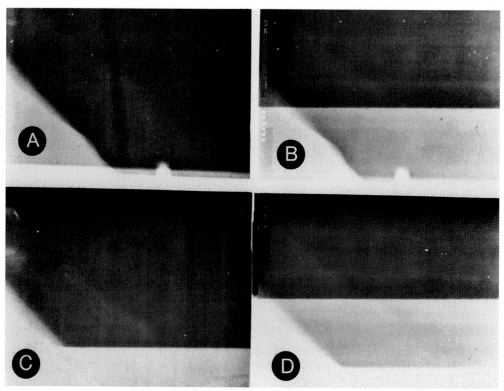

Figure 4.34. Reproduction of Fleischner's classic experiment to demonstrate the silhouette sign. **A,** radiograph shows the paraffin in one box with air in the second. **B,** radiograph shows paraffin in one box with mineral oil in the second box. The border of the paraffin is still visible. **C,** radiograph shows mineral oil added to the box with paraffin. The silhouette of the lower portion of the paraffin now disappears. **D,** radiograph shows mineral oil in both boxes. The only portion of the paraffin obscured is that covered by mineral oil sitting immediately adjacent to it (lower air-fluid level).

silhouette of the "heart". The boxes were again radiographed in the upright position after mineral oil (of approximately the same radiographic density as solid paraffin) was poured into the empty box behind the one containing the paraffin (see Fig. 4.34B). Note the air-fluid level at the border between the mineral oil and the air in the second box. More importantly, the image of the "heart" is still clearly visible because of the air adjacent to its border. Thus, an area of consolidation behind the cardiac silhouette does not obliterate its border.

The mineral oil was then poured out of the back box and into the box containing the paraffin. A radiograph of this (see Fig. 4.34C) shows obliteration of a portion of the border of the "heart" image because of the contiguity of the two structures of similar radiographic density. This is analogous to pneumonia in the right middle lobe or in the lingula obliterating the cardiac border (Fig. 4.35).

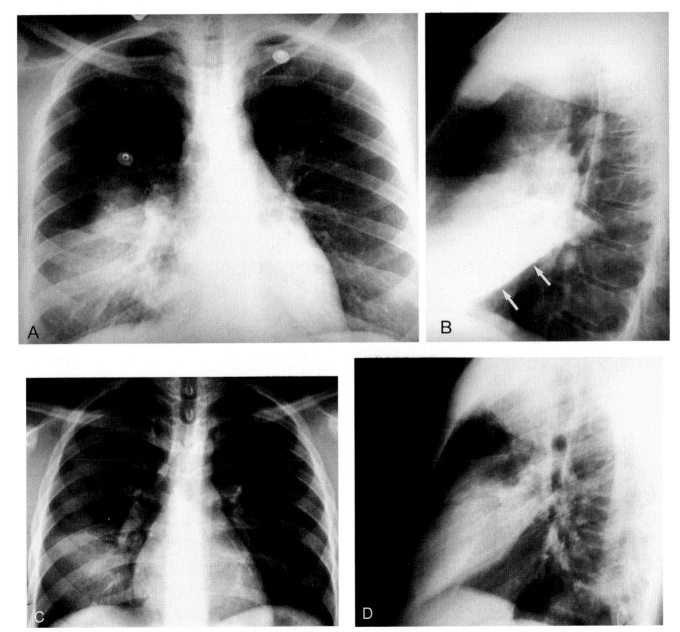

Figure 4.35.   Right middle lobe pneumonia. A, PA radiograph shows the right cardiac silhouette to be obliterated. **B,** lateral radiograph shows the consolidation to involve the middle lobe. Note the sharp definition of the major fissure (*arrows*) on the right side. **C,** frontal radiograph in another patient shows consolidation in the right lower lung field. The cardiac silhouette and the diaphragmatic margin are normal. **D,** lateral radiograph shows the consolidation to be located in the right middle lobe. In this instance, the lateral segment of the right middle lobe is involved, accounting for preservation of the silhouette of the right cardiac border.

Finally, mineral oil was poured into the second box, with the resultant radiograph (shown in Figure 4.34D). Note the obliteration of the lower "cardiac" border by the "consolidated" area adjacent to it. However, the upper "cardiac" border is clearly visible along with an air–fluid level behind it because this upper border is still surrounded by air.

In summary, an intrathoracic lesion that is contiguous with the border of the heart, aorta, or diaphragm will result in the loss of that border on the radiograph. This border will not be obliterated unless the lesion is anatomically contiguous with it. These principles apply not only to the PA or AP chest radiograph but also to the lateral view and, in addition, to certain abdominal radiographs that show loss of the psoas margin with retroperitoneal inflammation or hemorrhage.

The following consolidations are illustrated: right middle lobe (see Fig. 4.35), right upper lobe (Fig. 4.36), right lower and middle lobe (Fig. 4.37), left upper lobe (and lingula) [Fig. 4.38], lingula (Fig. 4.39), and left lower lobe (Fig. 4.40).

On the lateral film, we can identify each hemidiaphragm because of a normal-appearing silhouette sign. The anterior portion of the cardiac border lies in contiguity with the left hemidiaphragm. Therefore, the anterior one-third of the left diaphragmatic image is obliterated by the cardiac border. This is the most reliable way to identify the hemidiaphragms (Fig. 4.41). A summary of localization using the silhouette sign is in Table 4.1. Although the localizing signs are extremely useful, the reader is cautioned that they are not always infallible. For example, an area of consolidation in the lateral segment of the right middle lobe will not always obliterate the right cardiac border. It is therefore important to use two views at all times when evaluating patients with lung disease.

The *cervicothoracic sign*, a variant of the silhouette sign, is useful in determining whether a mass that is seen above the level of the clavicles is wholly intrathoracic or mediastinal. If this lesion is seen in its entirety, it must lie *posteriorly* because it is surrounded by air and therefore must be entirely within the thorax. If it is located *anteriorly*, its border will be obliterated by the

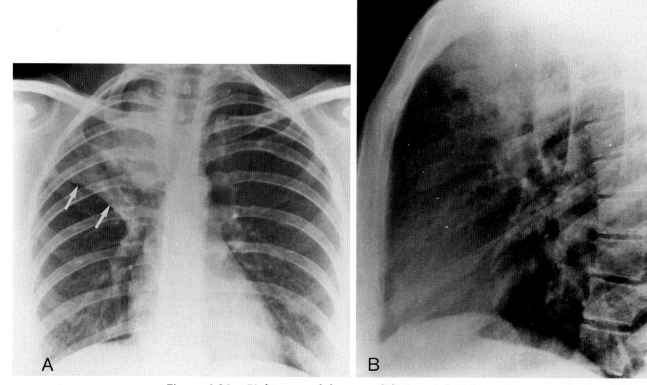

Figure 4.36. Right upper lobe consolidation and atelectasis. A, Frontal radiograph shows obliteration of the superior mediastinal silhouette on the right. Volume loss is present as evidenced by elevation of the minor fissure, which is well demarcated (*arrows*). **B,** Lateral radiograph shows the upper lobe consolidation.

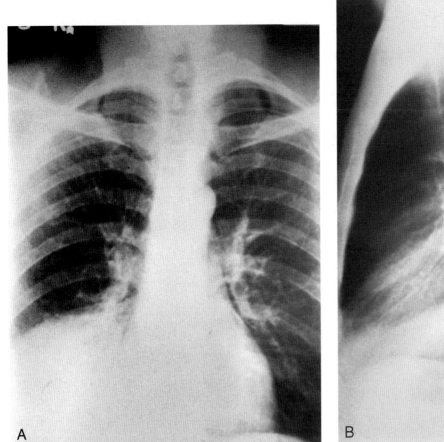
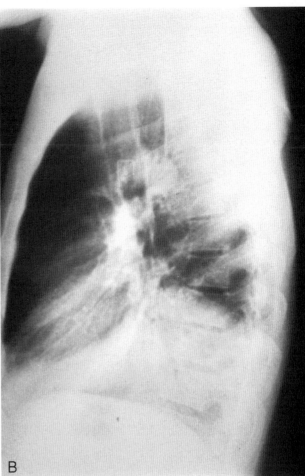

Figure 4.37. Right lower and middle lobe infiltration. A, frontal radiograph shows increased density in the right lower lung field that obscures the right hemidiaphragm and also a portion of the right heart border. **B,** lateral view shows the right hemidiaphragm to be obscured by the right lower lobe infiltrate. The lower portion of the cardiac silhouette shows increased density as a result of the involvement of a portion of the right middle lobe as well.

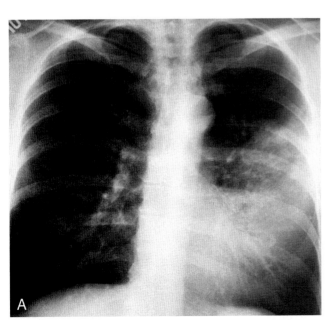
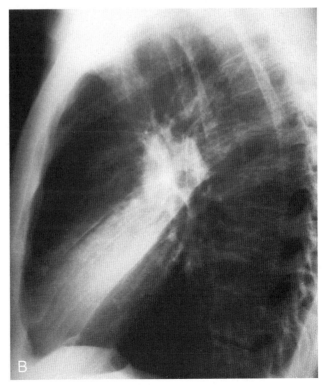

Figure 4.38. Combined left upper lobe and lingular consolidation. A, Frontal radiograph shows the left cardiac border obscured. Consolidation extends above the cardiac shadow into the anterior segment of the left upper lobe. **B,** Lateral radiograph shows consolidation to mostly overlap the heart.

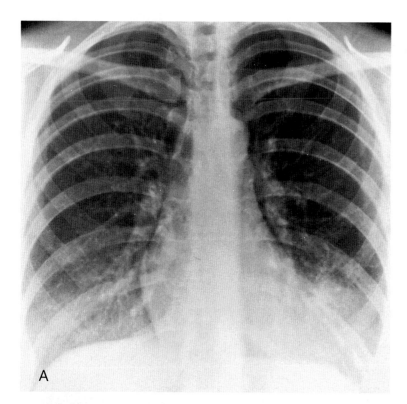

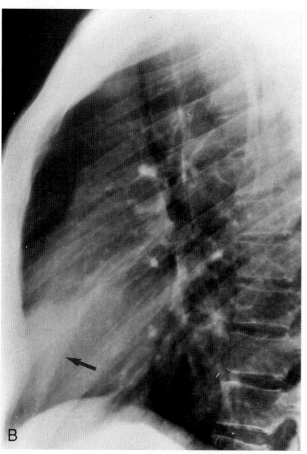

Figure 4.39. Consolidation in the lingula.
A, Frontal radiograph shows the silhouette of the apex of the heart to be obscured by the overlying consolidation. **B,** Lateral radiograph shows the consolidation anteriorly (*arrow*).

Figure 4.40. Left lower lobe pneumonia.
A, Frontal radiograph shows the silhouette of the diaphragm on the left to be obliterated. **B,** Lateral radiograph shows the posterior consolidation.

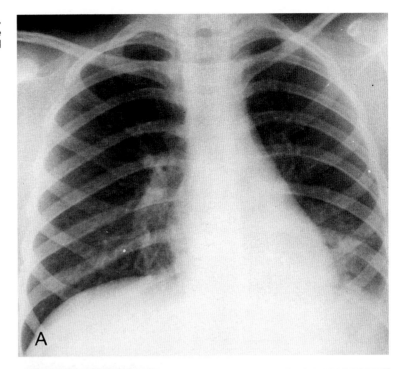

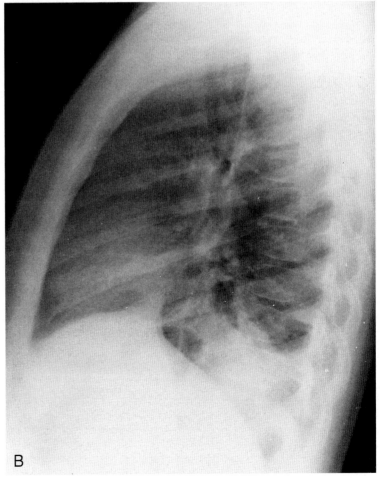

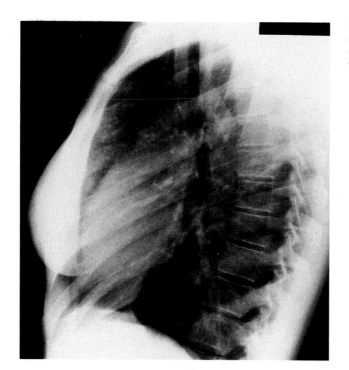

Figure 4.41. Normal lateral radiograph showing the diaphragm. (See text for description.)

TABLE 4.1
LOCALIZATION USING THE SILHOUETTE SIGN

Structure	Obliteration/Overlap of Border	General Location	Anatomic Location
Heart	Obliteration	Anterior	Middle lobe Lingula Anterior mediastinum Anterior segment of an upper lobe Lower end of oblique fissure Anterior portion of pleural cavity
	Overlap	Posterior	Lower lobe Posterior mediastinum Posterior portion of pleural cavity
Ascending aorta (right border)	Obliteration	Anterior	Anterior segment, right upper lobe Right middle lobe Right anterior mediastinum Anterior portion, right pleural cavity
	Overlap	Posterior	Superior segment, right lower lobe Posterior segment, right upper lobe Posterior mediastinum Posterior pleural cavity
Aortic knob (left border)	Obliteration	Posterior	Apical-posterior segment, left upper lobe Posterior mediastinum Posterior pleural cavity
	Overlap	Anterior	Anterior segment, left upper lobe Far posterior portion mediastinum or pleural cavity
Descending aorta	Obliteration	Posterior	Superior and posterior basal segments, left lower lobe

images of the neck structures and will seem to disappear into the neck. Therefore, it is cervicothoracic, lying partially in the anterior part of the mediastinum and partially in the neck. Figure 4.42 illustrates this in a patient with a prominent brachiocephalic artery, the most common cause of this finding.

Another useful sign that indicates consolidation within the lung is the *air bronchogram.* As previously mentioned, normal bronchi are not visible on the chest radiograph. This is because they have thin walls, they contain air, and they are surrounded by air within the lung parenchyma. However, parenchymal consolidation that results in a water density in the alveolar spaces in the lung may demonstrate adjacent bronchi because the air within their lumens

Figure 4.42.   Cervicothoracic sign. A, there is a right paratracheal density (*arrows*). Notice that the image of this density disappears as it crosses the clavicle. This indicates that the structure in question is located anteriorly and has entered the neck. This density is, in fact, the tortuous right brachiocephalic artery. If this structure were located posteriorly, it would be seen in its entirety above as well as below the clavicle, as in **B. B,** a right paratracheal density (*arrows*) extends above as well as below the clavicle. *(continued on page 102)*

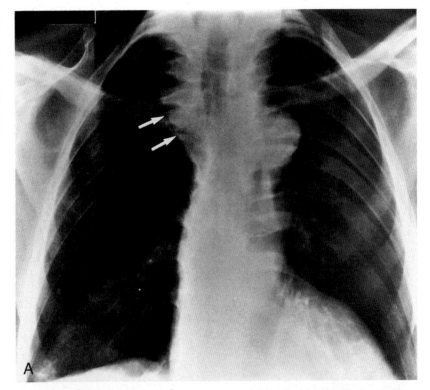

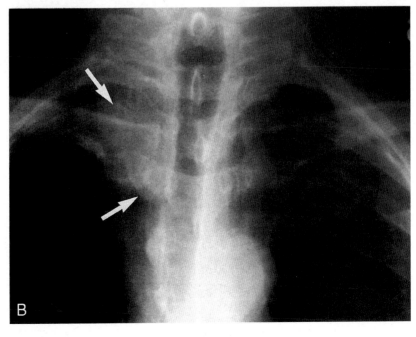

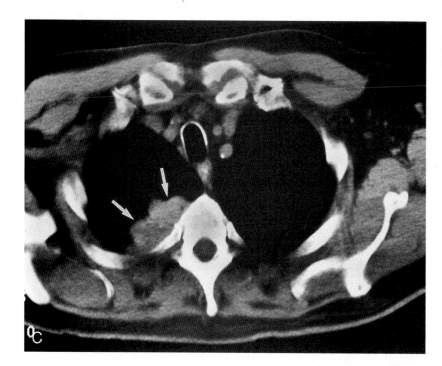

Figure 4.42. *(continued)* **C,** CT scan shows the density to be located in the posterior aspect of the apical segment of the right upper lobe (*arrows*).

will stand out in stark contrast to the dense lung (Fig. 4.43). The formation of the air bronchogram sign is illustrated in Figure 4.44. Plastic tubing sealed at each end was placed in an empty plastic container and radiographed (Fig. 4.44A). The walls are barely discernible, because the tubing contains air and there is air surrounding it. Water was then added to the container to cover the tubing (Fig. 4.44B). The wall is barely visible. However, the air within

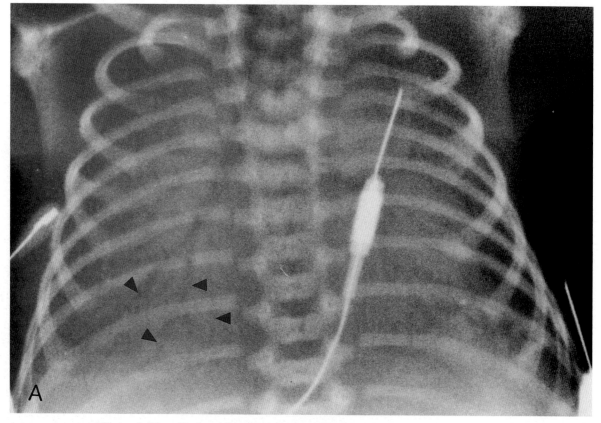

Figure 4.43.   Air bronchograms. A, air bronchograms in the right lung (*arrowheads*) in an infant with hyaline membrane disease. *(continued on page 103)*

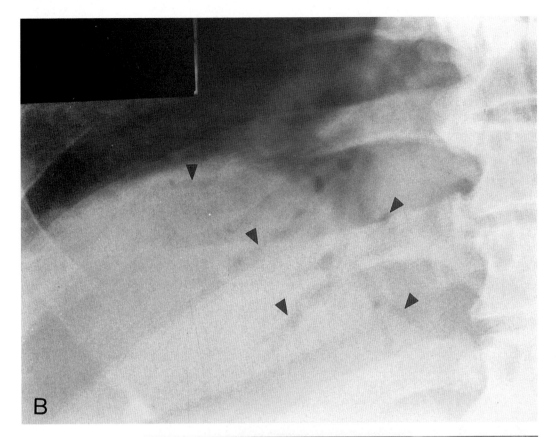

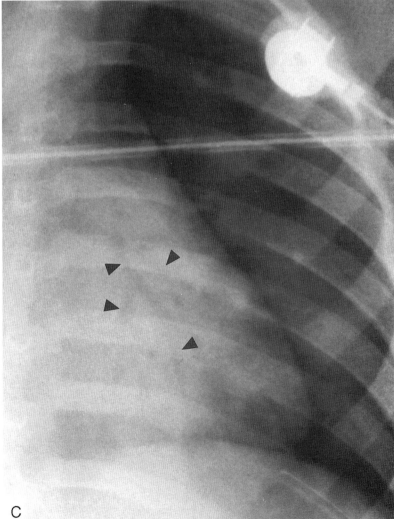

Figure 4.43. *(continued)* **B** and **C,** detail views of the lower lobes in two other patients with pneumonia show multiple air bronchograms *(arrowheads).*

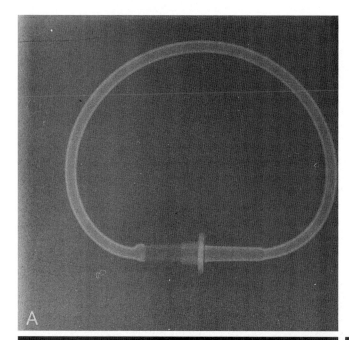

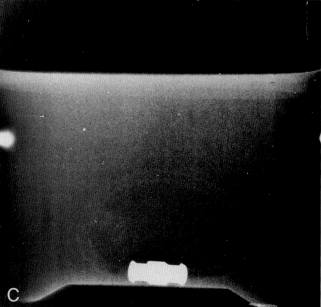

Figure 4.44.   Air bronchogram formation. A, radiograph of a plastic tube shows its walls. **B,** when the tube is submerged in water, the lumen and walls are still visible as would be seen in an air bronchogram. **C,** when water fills the tubing, the lumen is obscured.

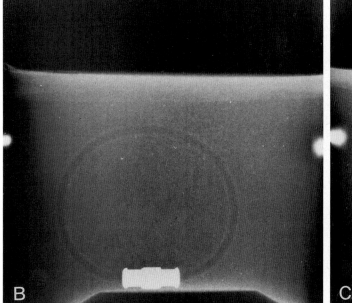

the tubing defines its lumen (air bronchogram). Water was then poured into the tubing with the resultant radiographic appearance (shown in Figure 4.44C). As illustrated here, there is no difference between the water inside the tube and the outside (no air bronchogram).

The air bronchogram is a valuable sign that, when present, is virtually diagnostic of air–space (acinar) disease. A pleural or mediastinal lesion may be excluded because there are no bronchi traversing these lesions. Similarly, a mass in the lung should engulf, occlude, or displace bronchi, and therefore the air bronchogram would not occur. If an air bronchogram is seen within a round pulmonary density, the lesion is most likely an inflammatory process, an infarct, a contusion, or, more rarely, an alveolar cell carcinoma or lymphoma. All of these are acinar lesions. Rare exceptions to this rule are bronchiectasis and chronic bronchitis, in which thickening of the bronchial walls may result in tubular air profiles (Fig. 4.45).

Figure 4.45. Bronchiectasis.
Thickened bronchial walls produce a tubular pattern in a patient with bronchiectasis.

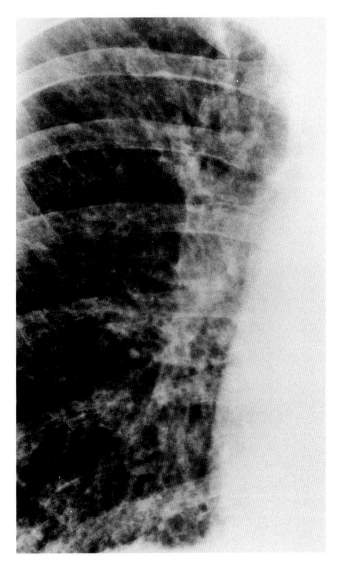

Atelectasis - Collapse

Atelectasis is a condition of volume loss of some portion of the lung. It may be massive, with complete collapse of an entire lung or, more commonly, less extensive and involve a lobe, segment, or subsegment. Atelectasis results from a number of causes, which are illustrated in Figure 4.33.

Obstructive atelectasis, the most common type, results when a bronchus is obstructed by a neoplasm, foreign body, mucous plug, or inflammatory debris (Fig. 4.46). Quite often, there is associated pneumonia distal to the site of obstruction.

Compressive atelectasis is a purely physical phenomenon in which the normal lung is compressed by a tumor, emphysematous bulla, pleural effusion, or an enlarged heart (Fig. 4.47).

Cicatrization atelectasis is produced by organizing scar tissue (Fig. 4.48). This occurs most often in healing tuberculosis and other granulomatous diseases, as well as in entities such as pulmonary infarct and pulmonary trauma.

Adhesive atelectasis is a unique type of volume loss that occurs in the presence of patent airways. The mechanism involved is believed to be the inactivation of surfactant. A common example of this is hyaline membrane disease (Fig. 4.49).

Passive atelectasis results from the normal compliance of the lung in the presence of either pneumothorax or hydrothorax. The airways remain patent (Fig. 4.50).

The radiographic signs of lobar and segmental collapse are of two types: *direct* and *indirect*. Of the direct signs, displacement or deviation of a fissure is the most reliable, indicating not

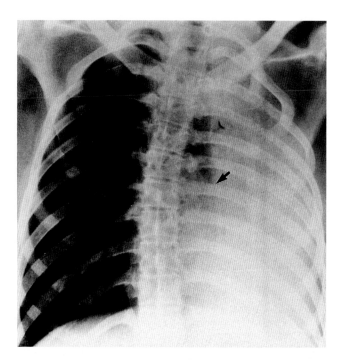

Figure 4.46. Obstructive atelectasis on the left. There is complete collapse of the left lung caused by a central obstructing lesion in the left mainstem bronchus (*arrow*). The heart and mediastinum have shifted to the left.

only volume loss in the collapsed segment(s), but also compensatory hyperinflation in an adjacent lobe to take the place of some of the collapsed lung. Other direct signs of collapse are increased opacity, crowding of vessels, and the presence of a silhouette sign. In any patient, one or all of these signs may be present (Figs. 4.51 and 4.52).

Of the indirect signs, the most reliable is displacement of the hilar vessels, which shift in the direction of the collapse. Other indirect signs include a shift of the mediastinum (see Fig. 4.51), elevation of the hemidiaphragm, compensatory emphysema, herniation of the lung across the midline, and approximation of the ribs. This last sign generally indicates that the collapse has been long-standing. As with the direct signs, any or all of these may occur in a particular patient.

In general, the upper lobes collapse medially, upward, and anteriorly. On the right side, the most reliable signs are an increase in density with obliteration of the upper mediastinal images

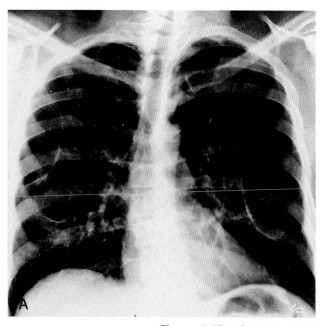
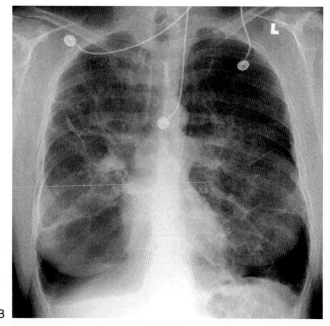

Figure 4.47. Compressive atelectasis in two patients with bullous emphysema. The large bullae in each lung compress and displace the remaining lung markings.

Figure 4.48. Cicatrization atelectasis. Scarring in the left lung has produced atelectatic changes in the left upper lobe. Note the hyperinflation of the lower lobe.

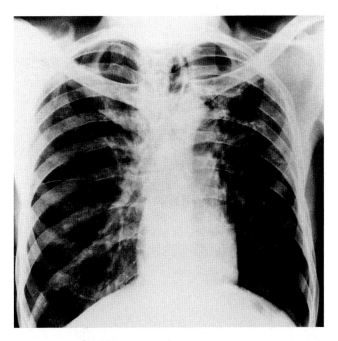

Figure 4.49. Adhesive atelectasis in a premature newborn with hyaline membrane disease. There is a "ground glass" opacification to both lungs.

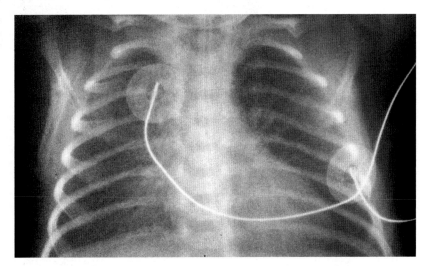

Figure 4.50. Passive atelectasis. There is collapse of the right lung in a patient with large pneumothorax on the right.

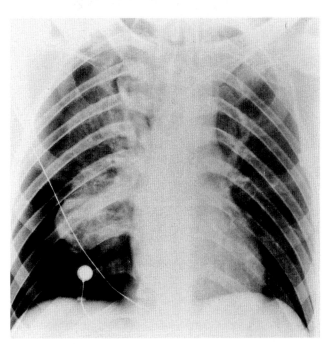

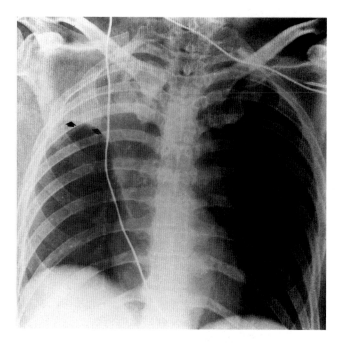

Figure 4.51.   Right upper lobe collapse in a patient with a central lung carcinoma. There is consolidation in the atelectatic right upper lobe. The minor fissure is elevated (*arrows*). There is a mass in the right hilar region. The mediastinum is shifted to the right.

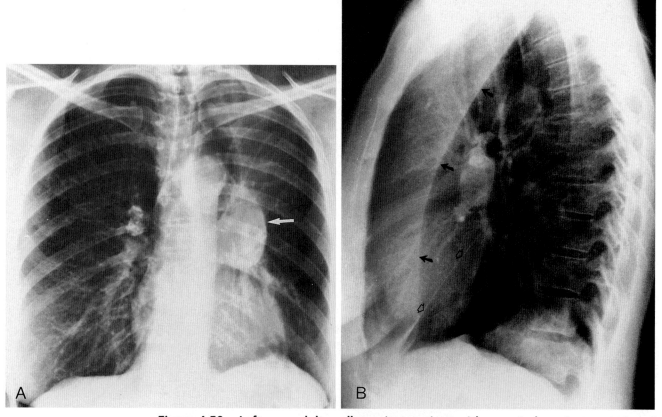

Figure 4.52.   Left upper lobe collapse in a patient with a central carcinoma. A, frontal radiograph shows a mass in the left hilar region (*arrow*). Note the shift of the left-sided pulmonary vessels upward. **B,** lateral radiograph shows anterior bowing of the major fissure on the left (*solid arrows*). The normal right-sided major fissure is also shown (*open arrows*).

on the right and shift of the minor fissure obliquely upward (see Fig. 4.51). On the left, the most reliable sign is the presence of increased density near the midline, with preservation of the aortic knob. In both instances, the ipsilateral diaphragm is usually elevated. On the lateral view, the major fissure is displaced anteriorly and superiorly (see Fig. 4.52).

The right middle lobe and lingula collapse downward and medially, producing haziness adjacent to the cardiac border on the frontal film. A lordotic view orients the atelectatic segment of lung more perpendicular to the direction of the x-ray beam and allows better visualization. On the lateral film, a triangular-shaped density is seen overlying the cardiac silhouette (Fig. 4.53).

Figure 4.53. Lingular collapse. A, frontal radiograph shows obliteration of the silhouette of the apex of the heart. **B,** lateral radiograph shows consolidation in the lingula. The major fissure on the left is sharply defined and bowed slightly anteriorly (*arrows*).

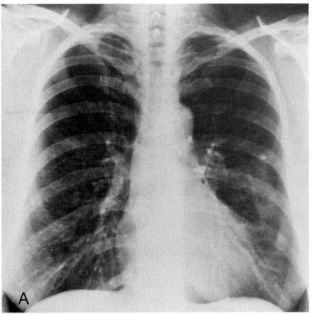

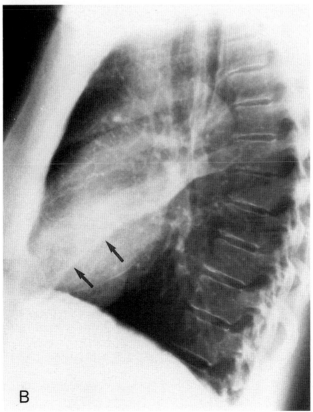

The lower lobes collapse posteriorly, medially, and downward. On a frontal radiograph, the classic lower lobe collapse is a triangular-shaped density behind the cardiac shadow. On the lateral film, a fissure shift may also be appreciated. In total collapse, a wedge-shaped density occurs posteriorly and inferiorly, extending down to the diaphragm (Fig. 4.54). In some instances, lower lobe collapse is difficult to detect on the frontal radiograph. Oblique films or CT are quite useful in making this diagnosis. Because of the orientation of the bronchi, left lower lobe atelectasis is most common, and is frequently found on the chest radiographs of patients in the immediate postoperative period.

Linear or *"plate-like"* atelectasis, a less severe form of partial collapse, may occur throughout the lungs, and appears as a dense line in one or more lobes (Fig. 4.55). It is most often found in a lower lobe where it will obscure a portion of the subjacent diaphragm (Fig. 4.56).

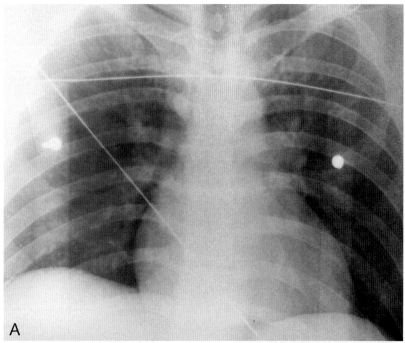

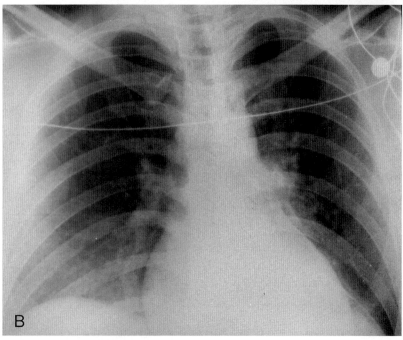

Figure 4.54. Left lower lobe atelectasis. A, admission radiograph shows both lungs expanded and clear. Note the images of both sides of the diaphragm. **B,** 2 days later, the patient has experienced left lower lobe atelectasis. There is increased density behind the heart on the left. The left hemidiaphragm is no longer visible and there is a shift of the hilar vessels downward. Compare with **A.**

Figure 4.55.   Linear atelectasis in the left lower lobe (*large arrow*) **in a patient with a tension pneumothorax on the right** (*small arrows*).

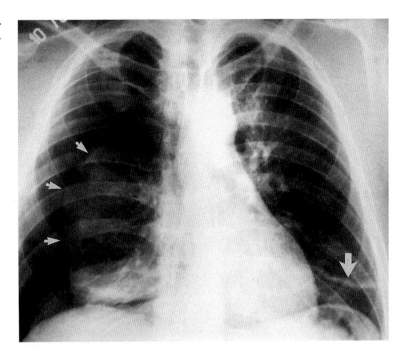

Pleural Fluid Accumulation - Effusion

Pleural effusion is a sign rather than a disease and occurs in a variety of pathologic conditions, including infection, embolism, neoplasm, CHF, and trauma. Pleural fluid may be either free or loculated within the pleural space. Free pleural fluid occupies the most dependent portion of the pleural cavity and can occur as a meniscus and elevation of the "diaphragm" on an upright film (Fig. 4.57**A**) or as an increase in the overall opacity of one hemithorax on a recumbent film. It also may be demonstrated on the decubitus film (Fig. 4.57**B**).

Loculation of pleural fluid occurs when fibrous adhesions form. Occasionally, the fluid will collect in a fissure to form a "*pseudotumor*" or "*phantom tumor*" (Figs. 4.58 and 4.59). This usually occurs in patients with CHF and clears when that condition resolves. A pseudotumor may be recognized by its tapered margins at a fissure as well as the fact that it changes shape with positioning.

Figure 4.56.   Left basilar atelectasis. There are linear densities in the left lung base that obscure the diaphragm. Compare with the right.

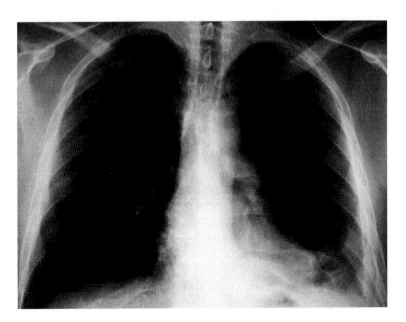

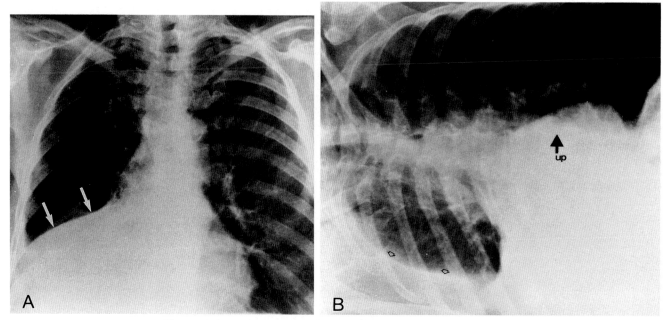

Figure 4.57.   Large right pleural effusion. A, frontal radiograph shows a subpulmonic collection of fluid with a straight border (*arrows*). **B,** right lateral decubitus film shows most of the fluid layers out (*open arrows*).

Other signs of pleural effusion include widening of the pleural space, blunting of the costophrenic angle, and mediastinal shift in massive effusion. It is estimated that up to 300 mL of pleural fluid may be accumulated in the costophrenic sulcus posteriorly before an effusion is apparent on the frontal radiograph!

Patients with unexplained pleural effusions should be carefully studied for neoplasm. In addition to cytologic studies of the fluid itself, it is desirous to clear those portions of the lung that would be obscured by the fluid. To do this, a lateral decubitus or *Trendelenberg* position (head down) is used to make the fluid flow away from the lung bases. A more useful technique is to use CT, in which the fluid layers in the horizontal position (Fig. 4.60).

Masses – Tumors and Tumor-Like Abnormalities

Lung and mediastinal masses are a very important group of diseases. In general, a variety of clinical, historic, and radiologic findings are used to predict the nature of the lesion. Ultimately, the diagnosis rests in the hands of the pathologist. The most common etiologies of the solitary pulmonary nodule are either tumors or granulomas. Table 4.2 lists the differential diagnoses of common and uncommon pulmonary nodules.

Some nodules may cavitate (Fig. 4.61). The most common lesions to undergo cavitation are lung carcinoma (Figs. 4.61**A** and **B**), granulomas (tuberculosis or fungal) [Fig. 4.61**C**], and metastatic lesions (usually squamous cell). Abscesses, hematomas, and pneumatoceles are other cavitary lesions that may be encountered. Much has been made of the thickness of the wall of a cavitary lesion regarding its pathogenesis. As a rule, this is not as reliable a diagnostic parameter as CT-guided needle aspiration of the cavity or its parent nodule. In some instances, such as trauma, it may be possible to observe cavitation develop as in a pneumatocele (Fig. 4.62). In most instances, the lesion will be detected on the initial chest radiograph. Fluid levels in a nodule are pathognomonic of cavitation.

In evaluating the solitary pulmonary nodules, the following studies are useful: an old chest film, chest fluoroscopy, CT, MR, and PET imaging. As mentioned previously, the most valuable study a radiologist can have for evaluating a solitary nodule is the patient's old chest film. The reader should be cautioned, however, that in reviewing serial chest films, it is necessary to examine not only the most recent old chest film, but also one that dates back a considerable period of time. A very slowly growing lesion may not appear to have grown from one study to

Figure 4.58.   Pseudotumor caused by pleural effusion. A, radiograph taken on admission (*ADM*) shows a mass-like collection of fluid along the minor fissure (*P*). There is loculated fluid (*L*) in the right costophrenic angle in this patient with congestive heart failure. **B,** radiograph made 4 days later shows a decrease in the cardiac size. The pleural effusion is also diminished. The pseudotumor is no longer present.

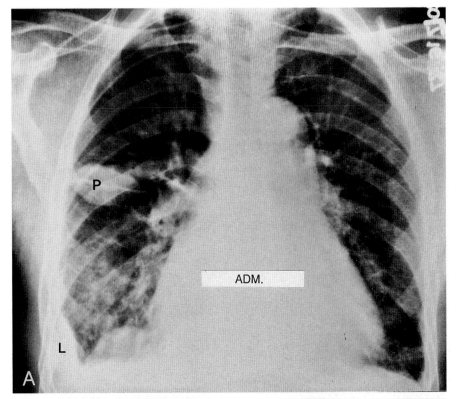

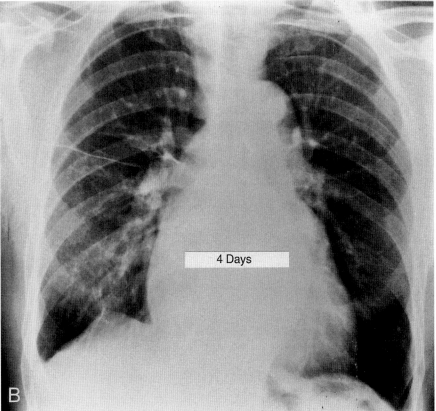

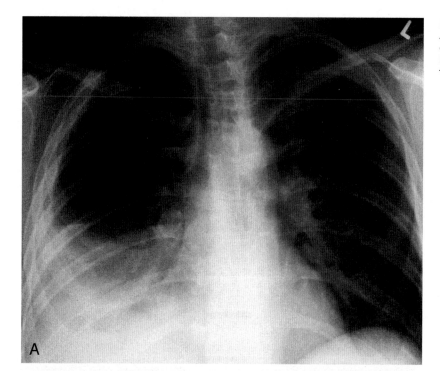

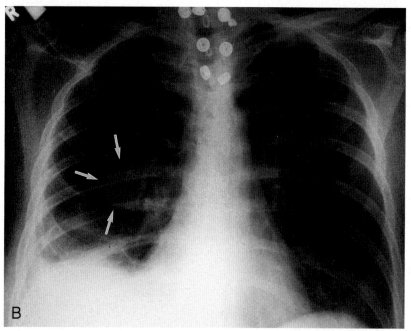

Figure 4.59. Pulmonary pseudotumor. **A,** initial radiograph shows a large right pleural effusion. **B,** 1 day later, the overall effusion is less. However, loculated pleural fluid in the major fissure produces a pseudotumor (*arrows*).

Figure 4.60. Right-sided pleural effusion (*E*) **as demonstrated on a CT scan.**

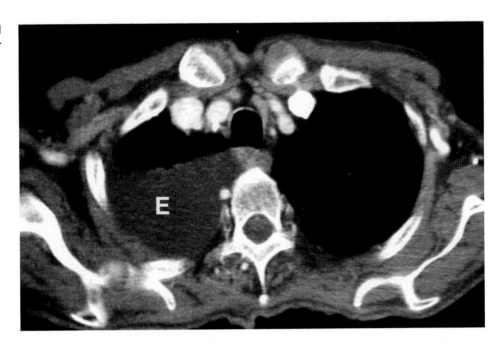

TABLE 4.2
DIFFERENTIAL DIAGNOSES OF PULMONARY NODULES

Diagnosis	Solitary	Multiple	Growth*
Common			
Bronchial adenoma	X		I
Carcinoma, primary	X	X	I
Granuloma—tuberculosis, fungus	X	X	0
Hamartoma	X	X	0
Metastases	X	X	I
Simulated nodule-nipple, bone lesion, skin tumor, foreign body, artifact	X	X	0
Uncommon			
Abscess	X	X	D
Hematoma	X	X	D
Infarct	X	X	D
Loculated pleural fluid	X	X	D
Pneumonia, organized	X	X	D
Pneumoconiosis, conglomerate mass	X	X	0
Sarcoidosis		X	0
Sequestration (fluid-filled cyst)	X		0
Vascular lesion	X	X	0

*I, increase in time; D, decrease in time; 0, no growth.

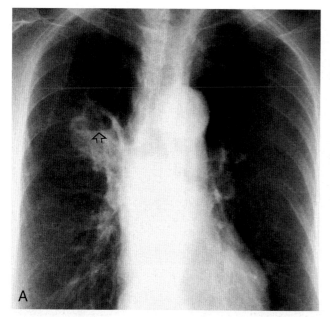

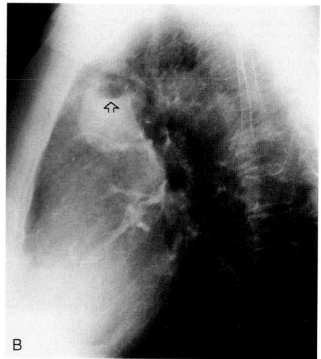

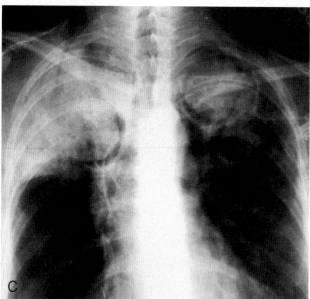

Figure 4.61.   Cavitating lung lesions. A, frontal and **B,** lateral views show cavitation in a right upper lobe carcinoma. Note the air-fluid level within the cavity (*arrows*). **C,** aspergillosis with bilateral upper lobe cavities containing large mycetomas ("fungus balls").

the next. However, in comparing films *out of sequence*, the difference may be quite dramatic. Figure 4.63 shows a series of circles, each differing in diameter by 1 mm. It is difficult to tell the difference between consecutive circles. However, by comparing drawings out of sequence a significant difference is apparent. A change in size also represents a change in volume, which increases by the cube power of its radius. Thus, a lesion that doubles in its diameter has actually increased eightfold in volume!

Chest fluoroscopy is an important examination for a patient with lung nodules. It is rapid, easy to perform, and inexpensive. The fluoroscopist should first make sure that the nodule is not an artifact such as hair braids, a button or snap on a gown, or a skin lesion. The next step is to determine the location of the lesion, especially whether it is in the lung or is a bony abnormality such as an osteochondroma, a healing rib fracture or vertebral osteophytes (Fig. 4.64), or in an adjacent anatomic region such as the axilla (see Fig. 4.14) or the abdomen.

Spiculation of the margin of a lesion (Fig. 4.65) is a sign of malignancy. It indicates that the mass is invading the surrounding tissue. This finding is similar to that seen at the border of a

Figure 4.62. **Left upper lobe pneumato-cele in an area of pulmonary hematoma secondary to trauma. A,** frontal radiograph shows the cavity (pneumatocele) in the area of consolidation (*arrow*). **B,** detail view. If you look closely you will see the overlying rib fracture.

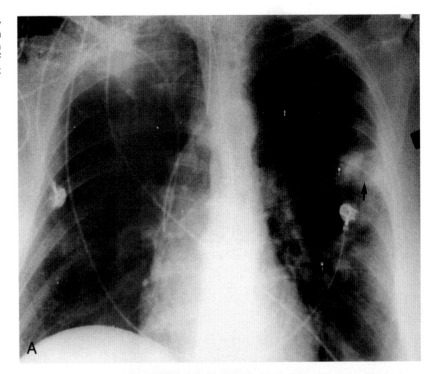

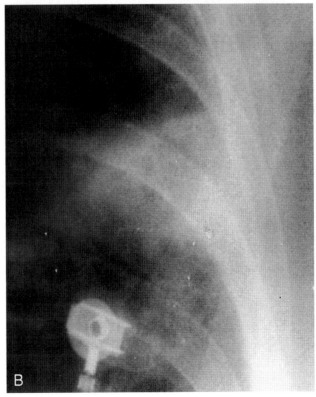

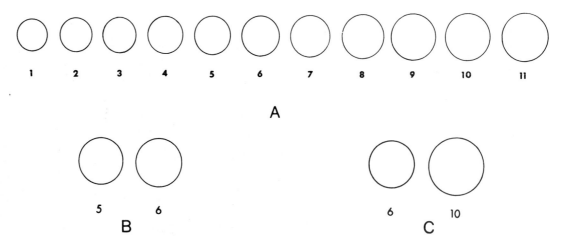

Figure 4.63. Importance of viewing serial radiographs out of sequence. A, each of these circles varies in diameter by 1 mm. **B,** comparing circles 5 and 6 shows the difference to be minimal, if any. **C,** comparing circle 6 and 10 shows a significant change. Often the human eye cannot detect the small changes in the size of nodules.

breast carcinoma (Fig. 4.66). Calcification in a lesion is considered almost pathognomonic of a benign entity, especially when it is centrally located or "popcorn-shaped" (Fig. 4.67). The reader is cautioned, however, in using calcification as the sole criterion of the nature of the lesion, because a scar carcinoma may engulf a calcified granuloma. In these instances, the calcification may be eccentric.

CT is most useful in evaluating patients with pulmonary and mediastinal masses (Fig. 4.68). The information gained includes evidence of mediastinal invasion (Fig. 4.69), chest wall invasion (Fig. 4.70), presence of peripheral or multiple nodules (Fig. 4.71), and calcification (Fig.4.72). Contrast-enhanced or dynamic CT may be used to differentiate hilar masses from dilated or enlarged pulmonary vessels. The latter will enhance with contrast, while a tumor will not. CT is also useful for detecting multiple metastases (Fig. 4.73) and is also the mainstay for guided percutaneous biopsy (Fig. 4.74).

As previously mentioned, MR imaging of the chest is useful for evaluating suspected mediastinal masses (see Fig. 4.17). The flow void easily allows vessels to be distinguished from neoplasm.

Finally, with the emergence of PET scanning in oncological diagnosis, a patient with a solitary pulmonary nodule that is worrisome for malignancy can undergo PET imaging. The advantage may be best for a patient who is a poor candidate for biopsy. Furthermore, the fact that a "whole body" PET scan is usually performed allows simultaneous initial staging evaluation in the case of finding a malignant nodule. This has had a significant impact on management.

Patients with solitary pulmonary nodules are often submitted to a battery of diagnostic studies, including chest and abdominal CT, and metastatic bone surveys. These are performed before histologic confirmation of the lesion in the hope that a primary lesion will be found, thus indicating that the pulmonary lesion is metastatic. The yield from this process is extremely low and results in longer hospitalization and more expense for the patient. The final diagnosis rests on tissue examination. It is now routine to perform a biopsy of these lesions percutaneously or transbronchially under fluoroscopic or CT control (see Fig. 4.74). We have a cytology "minilab" in our department where a cytopathologist examines aspirated material and "touch" preparations to determine whether, 1) the biopsy or aspiration is adequate; 2) the sample is neoplastic or inflammatory; and 3) malignant cells are present. If either of these studies fails to provide an adequate answer, thoracotomy with excision of the lesion in toto is the next step.

Mediastinal masses are sometimes difficult to separate from pulmonary parenchymal masses. However, most show extraparenchymal signs such as sharp margins, tapered borders,

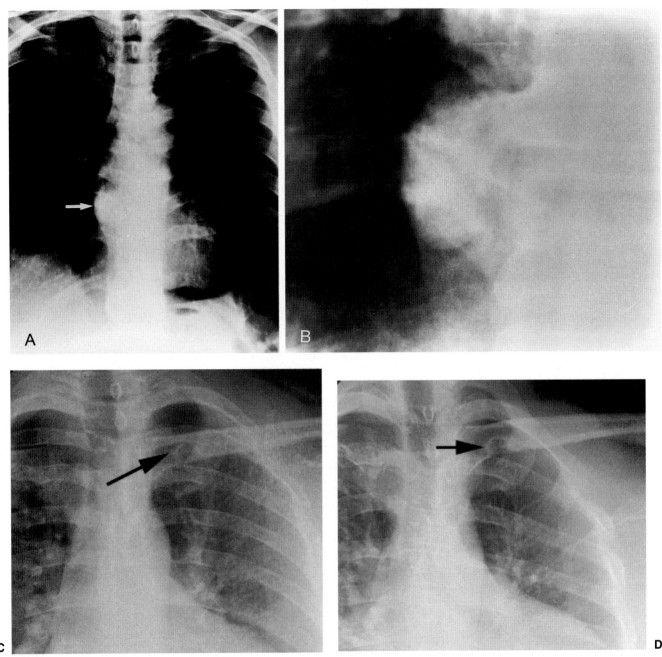

Figure 4.64.   Use of chest fluoroscopy. A, frontal radiograph shows a "mass" behind the heart (*arrow*). **B,** fluoroscopic spot film shows the mass to be osteophytes bridging two thoracic vertebrae. **C,** detail of chest radiograph in another patient shows a "cavity" (*arrow*) in the left upper lobe. **D,** fluoroscopic spot film shows the "cavity" to be a rhomboid fossa (*arrow*), a normal variant in the distal clavicle.

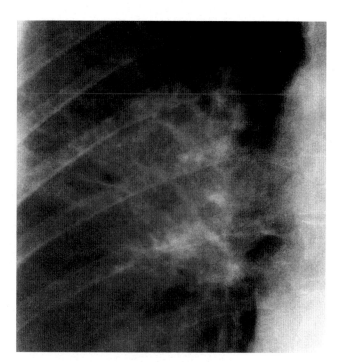

Figure 4.65. Spiculation in a lung carcinoma. Close-up view shows the irregular spiculated margins of this large perihilar carcinoma.

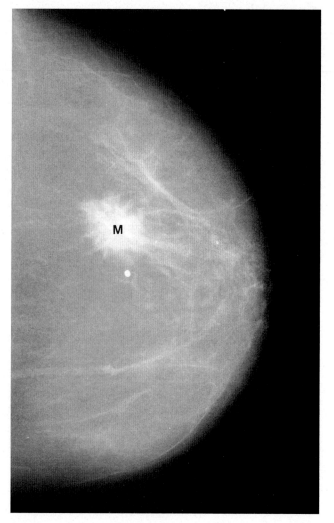

Figure 4.66. Carcinoma of the breast (*M*) showing irregular spiculated margins. Spiculation indicates invasion. Note the similarity to Figure 4.64.

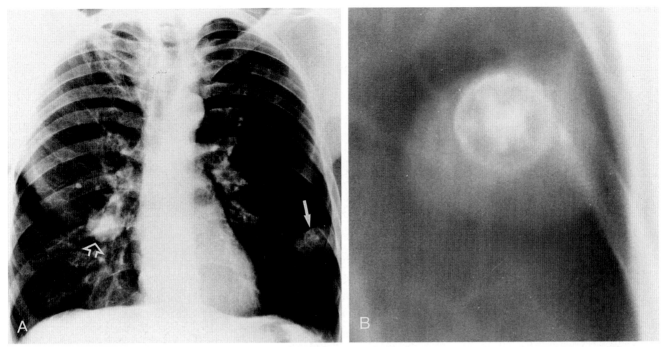

Figure 4.67.   Calcification in a lung lesion. A, frontal radiograph shows bilateral lung masses. The mass on the right (*open arrow*) contains no calcification. There is calcification on the left (*solid arrow*). **B,** tomogram of the left-sided mass shows the calcification. This lesion was a granuloma that was later engulfed by a carcinoma.

Figure 4.68.   Lung carcinoma, right upper lobe.
A, frontal radiograph shows a mass (*arrow*) just above the right hilum. The mass does not obscure the image of the ascending aorta (*arrowheads*), indicating a location either anterior or posterior to that structure. **B,** CT section shows the mass to be located in the anterior segment of the right upper lobe (*arrow*) adjacent to the pleura.

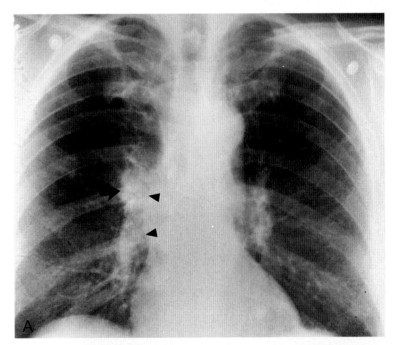

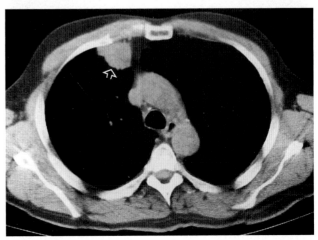

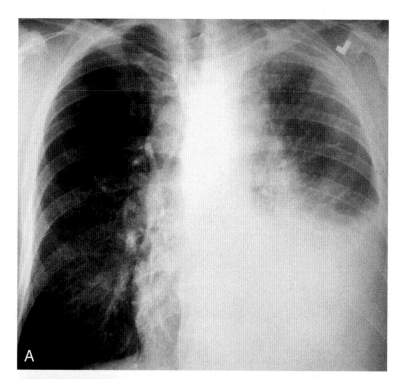

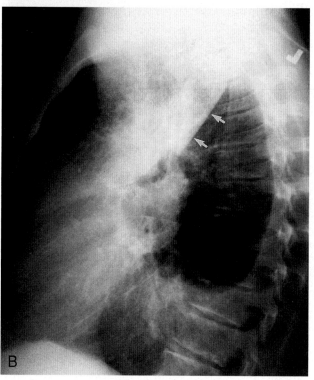

Figure 4.69. Mediastinal invasion from metastatic carcinoma. A, frontal radiograph shows consolidation in the lingula and left lower lobe. There is a large left pleural effusion. The upper mediastinum is widened, particularly on the left, where the aortic arch is indistinct. **B,** lateral radiograph shows increased density along the upper major fissure on the left (*arrows*) as well as over the area of the aortic arch. *(continued on page 123)*

Figure 4.69. *(continued)* **C,** CT section shows a broad area of consolidation in the left upper lobe as well as necrotic (gray) foci of tumor in mediastinal lymph nodes (*arrows*). **D,** CT section adjacent to the aortic arch shows the mediastinal invasion (*arrow*). Note the pleural effusions in **C** and **D.**

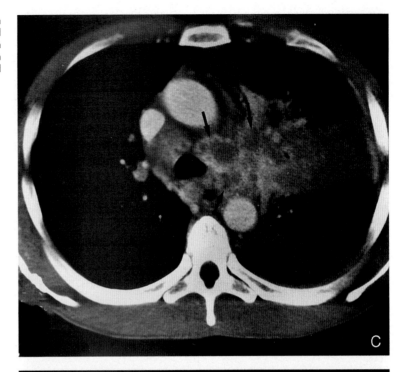

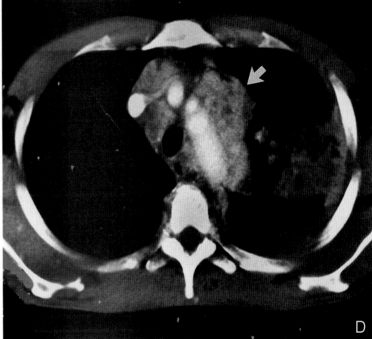

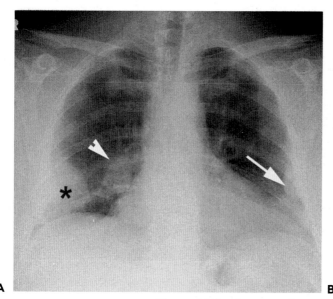
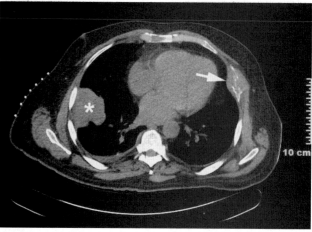

Figure 4.70. Lung carcinoma with chest wall invasion. A, Frontal radiograph shows a large peripheral mass in the right lower lung field (*), a smaller adjacent mass (arrowhead), and another mass along the chest wall on the left (arrow). **B,** CT image shows the large right peripheral mass (*). The left sided mass is invading the chest wall (arrow).

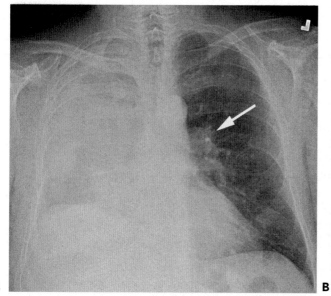
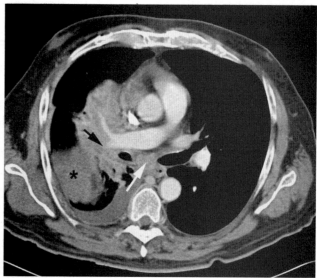

Figure 4.71. Lung carcinoma with multiple pulmonary nodules. A, chest radiograph shows opacification of the right hemithorax from a central obstructing carcinoma of the right bronchus. There is a metastatic nodule (*arrow*) on the left. **B,** CT image shows the mass on the right pinching the bronchus closed (*black arrow*). Note the collapsed right lower lobe (*) and metastatic deposit in a subcarinal lymph node (*white arrow*).

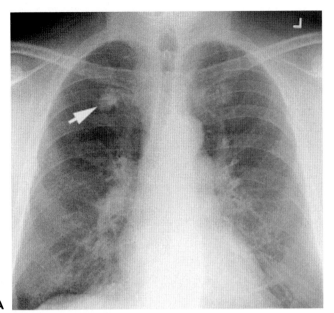

A

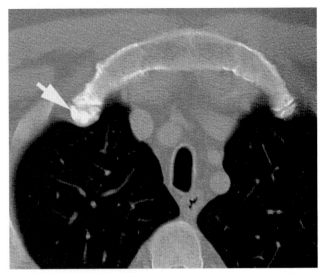

B

Figure 4.72. Calcified granuloma. A, chest radiograph shows a "nodule" in the right upper lobe (*arrow*). **B,** CT image shows the "nodule" to be a hypertrophied and calcified granuloma (*arrow*) immediately beneath the first costochondral junction.

Figure 4.73. Multiple pulmonary metastases (*arrows*) **demonstrated by CT.** These nodules are too large to be considered vessels.

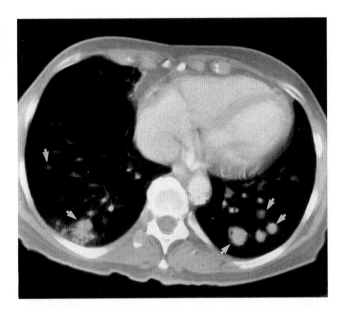

Figure 4.74. Use of CT guidance for biopsy of a lung mass. (This is the same patient as in Fig. 4.70). A needle (*arrow*) has been placed into the right sided mass. Note the left sided mass invading the chest wall (*).

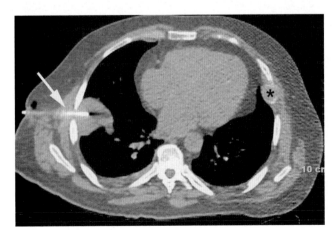

and convexity toward the lung. The majority of all primary mediastinal masses occur in the anterior compartment, one-third occur in the middle compartment, and the remainder occur in the posterior compartment. Most patients with mediastinal masses are asymptomatic. Table 4.3 lists abnormalities found in each compartment of the radiologic mediastinum.

The most common lesions of the anterior mediastinum are lymphomas (Fig. 4.75), thymic lesions (Fig. 4.76), and teratomas. Other anterior lesions that may occur include foramen of Morgagni hernias (Fig. 4.77) and pericardial cysts (Fig. 4.78).

The majority of masses arising in the middle mediastinum are lymph nodes representing lymphoma, metastatic disease, sarcoidosis (Fig. 4.79), or response to infection. Hiatal or paraesophageal hernias are the most common masses immediately behind the heart. If they contain an air–fluid level, the diagnosis is confirmed (Fig. 4.80). In some instances, it may be necessary to administer oral barium to establish the diagnosis.

The most likely cause of a posterior mediastinal mass is a neurogenic tumor (Fig. 4.81). These generally appear as a paraspinous mass and are often associated with changes in the vertebrae or of the posterior ribs. Neurofibromas frequently enlarge the neural foramina. Calcification may occur in neuroblastomas in children.

Bronchogenic carcinoma may occur as a mediastinal mass in *any* compartment. This should always be considered in any adult with a mediastinal mass.

Multiple pulmonary nodules may be granulomas or metastases. If the lesions contain calcium and are widely disseminated (Fig. 4.82), the diagnosis is most likely a granulomatous disease. Multiple large nodules, particularly of varying sizes and with fuzzy borders

---

TABLE 4.3

CONDITIONS FOUND IN EACH COMPARTMENT OF THE RADIOLOGIC MEDIASTINUM

Condition	Compartment		
	Anterior	**Middle**	**Posterior**
Neoplasms	Lymphoma Thymic lesion Thyroid lesion Parathyroid Teratoma Carcinoma (lung)	Lymphoma Carcinoma (lung, esophagus) Metastases	Neurogenic tumor Lymphoma Carcinoma (lung) Pheochromocytoma Myeloma
Cystic lesions	Thymic cyst Pericardial cyst	Bronchogenic cyst Esophageal duplication cyst	Neurenteric cyst Thoracic duct cyst Lateral meningocele
Vascular abnormalities	Buckled brachiocephalic artery Anomalous or dilated superior vena cava Aortic aneurysm Cardiac aneurysm (including sinus of Valsalva)	Aneurysm of aorta or great vessels Right aortic arch Aortic ring Azygos vein enlargement	Aortic aneurysm
Other	Foramen of Morgagni hernia Hematoma Mediastinitis Abscess Postoperative esophageal bypass	Hiatal hernia Enlarge lymph node (other than lymphoma) Mediastinitis Abscess Hematoma	Bochdalek hernia Extramedullary hematopoiesis Hematoma Abscess

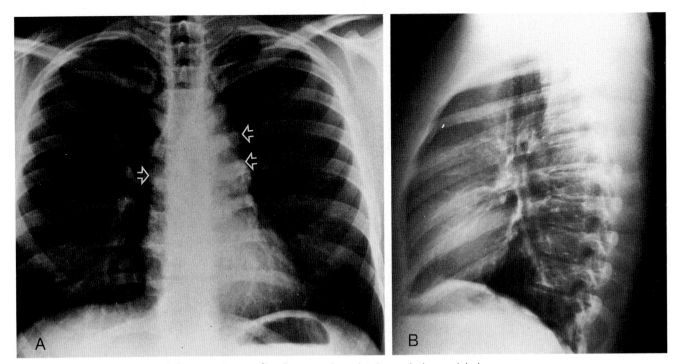

Figure 4.75. Lymphoma of the anterior mediastinum. A, frontal radiograph shows a lobular mass in the mediastinum (*arrows*). **B,** lateral radiograph shows the mass to be anteriorly located.

(Fig. 4.83), usually are metastases. Metastases may also occur in a "lymphangitic" form as a result of lymph node infiltration and lymphedema producing a prominent interstitial pattern (Fig. 4.84).

Emphysema - Overinflation

One does not need a chest radiograph to make a diagnosis of emphysema. There are adequate physical findings for that. However, there are certain radiographic findings that corroborate those of the physical examination. A better use of the chest film in the emphysematous patient is to detect localized bullae, peribronchial infiltrates, and pneumothorax or pneumomediastinum.

The radiographic findings of classic emphysema reflect the overinflation, loss of compliance, and parenchymal destruction that denote the pathophysiology of the disease. The most reliable radiographic sign is decreased ("pruned") vascularity. Other signs are hyperlucency; increased retrosternal clear space; increased lung volume; depression, flattening, or reversal of the curvature of the diaphragm; decreased diaphragmatic excursion; presence of prominent central pulmonary arteries with rapid tapering ("marker") vessels; bowing of the sharply defined trachea ("saber trachea"); and vertical cardiac configuration. Bullae may be present to a greater or lesser extent (Figs. 4.85 and 4.86).

Patients with chronic pulmonary disease may not have all the classic findings of emphysema. Some may have prominent interstitial markings, the so-called "dirty lung" seen particularly in smokers. In some younger individuals, the only finding may be hyperlucency, representing early overinflation (Fig. 4.87). Emphysematous changes are often combined with other abnormalities.

Interstitial vs. Acinar Disease

Diseases that primarily involve the interlobular connective tissue with or without secondary involvement of the air spaces are called interstitial diseases. They constitute a group of diseases

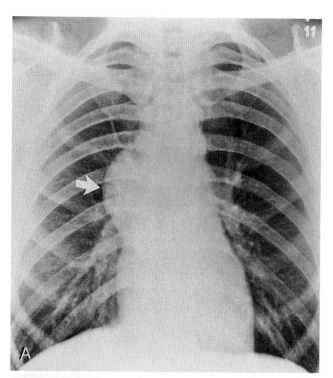

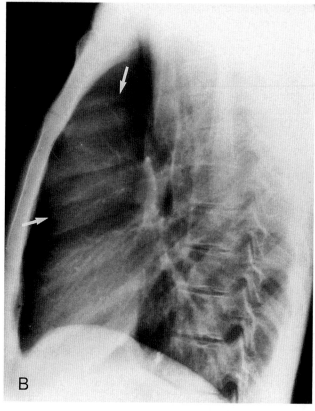

Figure 4.76. **Thymoma** (*arrows*). **A**, frontal radiograph. **B**, lateral radiograph.

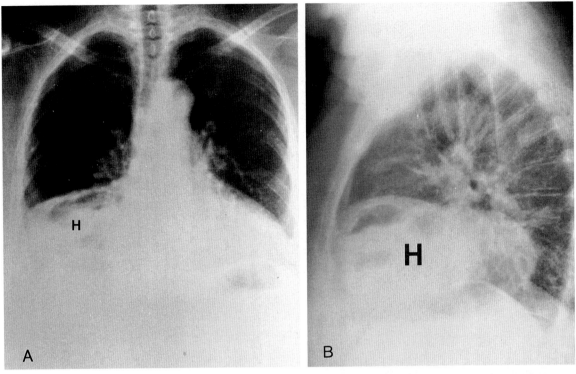

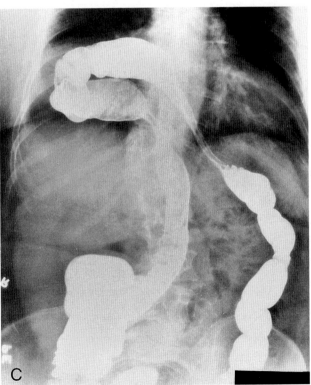

Figure 4.77.   Foramen of Morgagni hernia.
A, frontal radiograph shows apparent consolidation in the right lower lobe containing gaseous shadows. This is the hernia sac (*H*). **B,** lateral radiograph shows the gas-containing hernia (*H*). **C,** barium enema shows the herniated colon in the right hemithorax.

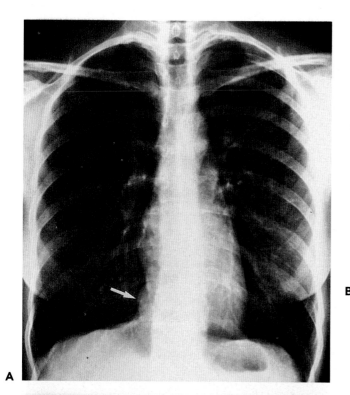

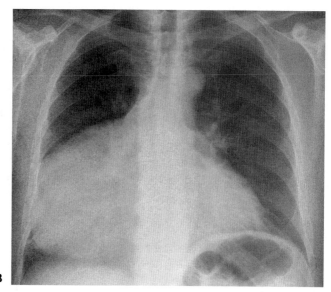

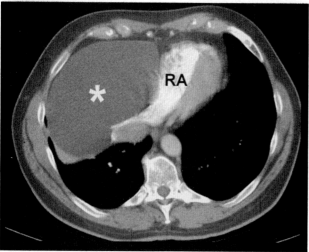

Figure 4.78.   Pericardial cysts. A, frontal radiograph shows a small bump along the right cardiophrenic angle (arrow). **B,** frontal radiograph shows a large mass adjacent to the heart on the right. **C,** CT image shows the mass (*) compressing the contrast-filled right atrium (RA). (*Courtesy Carl Fuhrman, M.D.*)

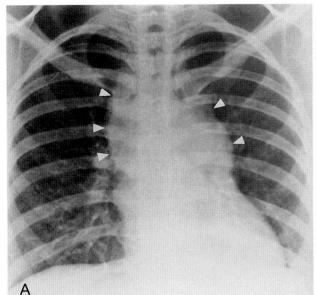

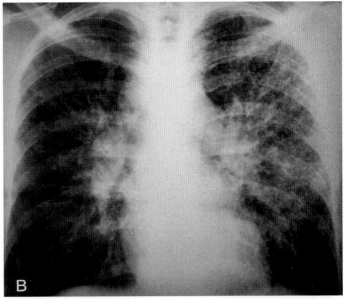

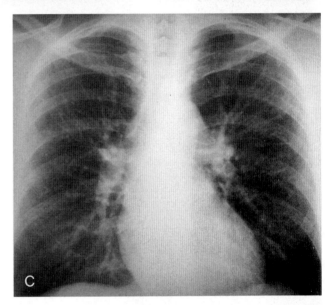

Figure 4.79.   Sarcoidosis. A, nodal pattern. There are too many "bumps" (*arrowheads*). **B,** mixed parenchymal and nodal pattern in another patient. Note the enlargement of mediastinal and hilar lymph nodes as well as diffuse interstitial disease, particularly on the left. **C,** the same patient 2 months after treatment. The nodes are smaller and the peripheral lungs are normal.

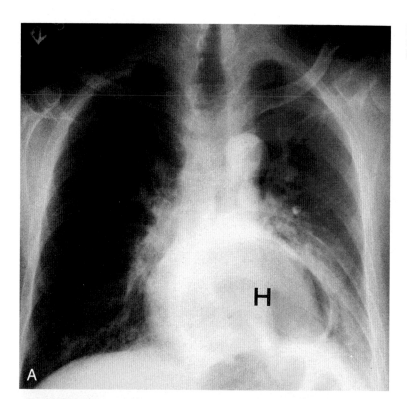

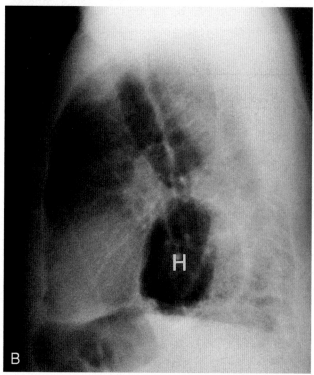

Figure 4.80.   Hiatal hernia. A, frontal and **B,** lateral radiograph shows the large hernia sac (*H*) behind the heart.

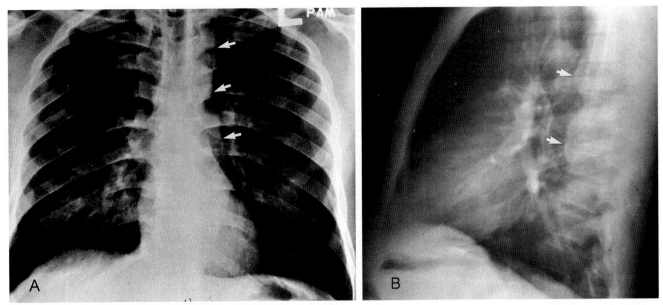

Figure 4.81.   Posterior mediastinal widening in a patient with neurofibromatosis. A, frontal radiograph shows lobulation in the left paraspinal region (*arrows*). **B,** lateral radiograph confirms the posterior location of the masses (*arrows*).

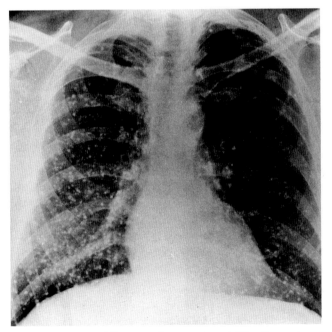

Figure 4.82. Diffuse pulmonary calcifications in a patient with histoplasmosis.

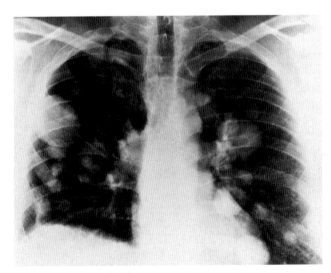

Figure 4.83.   Multiple metastases.

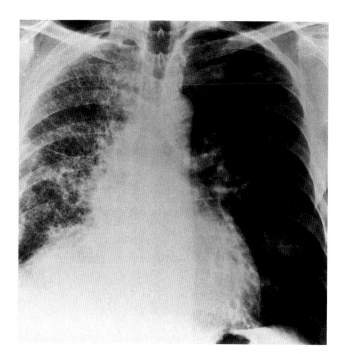

Figure 4.84. Lymphangitic spread of carcinoma. There is enlargement of the right hilum and a prominent interstitial pattern on the right that indicates lymphedema and lymphangitic spread of tumor.

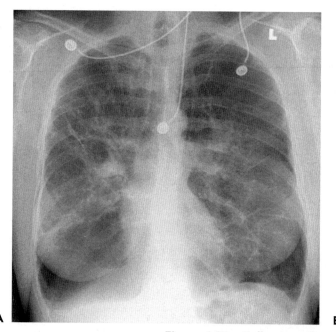

A

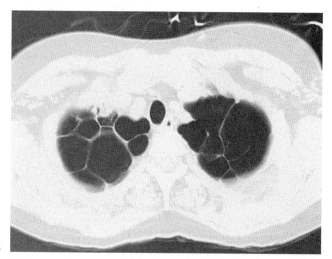

B

Figure 4.85. Bullous emphysema. Note the large bilateral blebs. **A,** radiograph, **B-D,** CT images. Note the large areas devoid of lung markings. *(continued on page 135)*

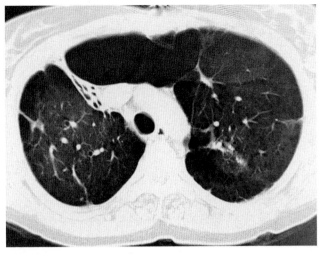

C

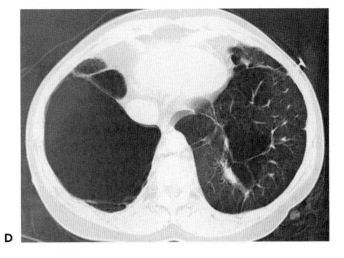

D

Figure 4.85. *(continued)*

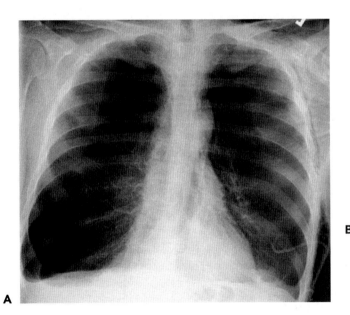

A

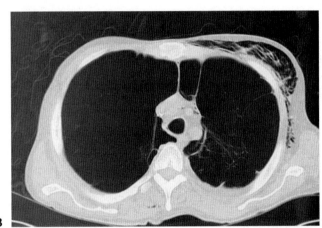

B

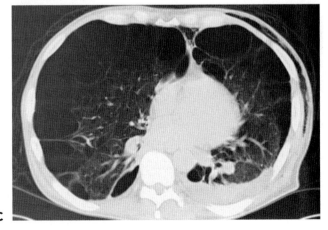

C

Figure 4.86. Bullous emphysema. A, Frontal radiograph shows large bullae in both upper lobes in the periphery of the lower lobes. Note the absence of lung markings in these areas. **B, C,** CT images show the large cystic bullae. Note the crowding of the normal lung by the bullae.

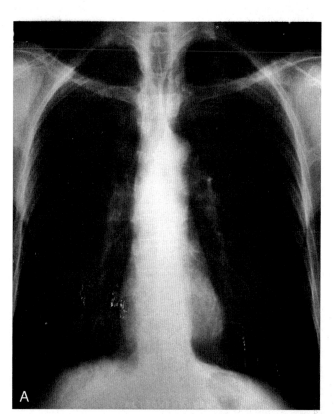
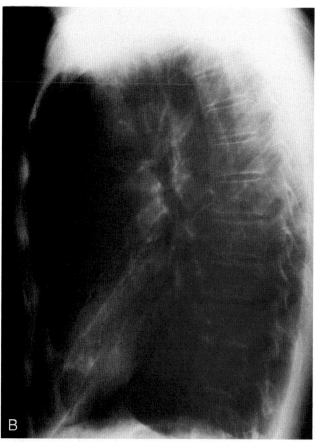

Figure 4.87. Chronic obstructive pulmonary disease (COPD). A, frontal and **B,** lateral radiographs show hyperinflation with flattening of the diaphragm. In **A,** note the vertical appearance of the heart, which is compressed by the overinflated lungs.

that have recognizable radiographic patterns: linear, nodular, combined lineonodular, and reticular (web-like, "honeycombing"). The etiologies vary and include early CHF (edema), pneumoconiosis, collagen disease (fibrosis), metastatic neoplastic (lymphangitic) permeation, and primary inflammatory conditions (early viral pneumonia, interstitial pneumonia). Many of these diseases produce some degree of air space or acinar pattern as they progress.

Pure acinar lesions produce a pattern characterized by fluffy margins, coalescence, a segmental or lobar distribution, a "butterfly" appearance (radiating out from the hila), air bronchograms, and a rapid sequence of onset and clearing. Conditions that produce acinar patterns include acute alveolar edema (pneumonia, CHF with pulmonary edema, toxic or chemical reaction), bleeding (idiopathic pulmonary hemorrhage), aspiration of any fluid, and alveolar cell carcinoma. A rare condition that produces this pattern is alveolar proteinosis.

It is possible to differentiate many of the more common acinar diseases on the basis of pattern, distribution, and resolution. Pulmonary edema is one of the most common acinar diseases encountered. The causes include CHF, fluid overload (iatrogenic), narcotic poisoning, central nervous system depression, aspiration, inhalation of noxious gases, uremia, pulmonary thromboembolism, and trauma. Pulmonary edema in the presence of cardiac enlargement is usually of cardiac origin (Fig. 4.88). Edema in the presence of a normal heart is generally from some other cause. Upper lobe distribution occurs more with neurologic abnormalities. The pattern changes rapidly, often on a daily basis. In more severe cases, usually of cardiac origin, interstitial edema may also be present.

Pneumonia, on the other hand, may involve any lobe, an entire lung, or be unilateral or bilateral. There are few distinguishing features of the acute bacterial pneumonias. However, those caused by an unusual organism tend to produce a more widespread acinar pattern. *Klebsiella* pneumonia often produces bulging of a fissure away from the consolidated lobe;

Figure 4.88. Pulmonary edema. There are fluffy alveolar densities throughout both lungs. The cardiac silhouette is obscured in this patient with congestive heart failure.

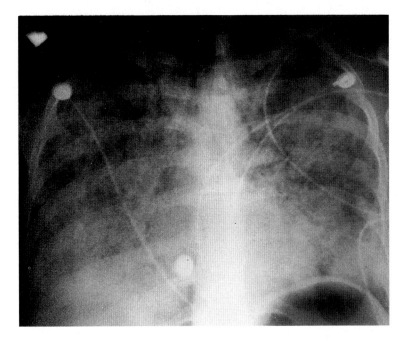

Staphylococcus aureus may produce multiple cavities and pneumatoceles. Pneumonic consolidations, as a rule, clear by slowly fading. The acinar consolidation often remains visible on the chest radiograph after the patient has become clinically better. You should be careful to treat your patient and not the radiograph.

Other acinar processes have the same appearance as pneumonia or pulmonary edema. The pattern and timing of the clearing often may provide clues to their cause. Consolidation from a lung infarct clears slowly with a gradual reduction in size of the lesion, keeping the same basic shape ("melting ice cube" pattern). Lung contusions from trauma (Fig. 4.89) generally clear within 24 to 48 hours. Persistent consolidation (with or without interstitial disease) in these patients may mean the onset of adult respiratory distress syndrome (ARDS, see below).

Pure acinar disease may frequently be distinguished from pure interstitial disease by pattern recognition. For demonstration purposes, consider the lung to be analogous to a piece of

Figure 4.89. Pulmonary contusions in a trauma victim. Radiograph made 2 hours after the accident shows multiple areas of consolidation throughout the right lung. A right pleural effusion is present.

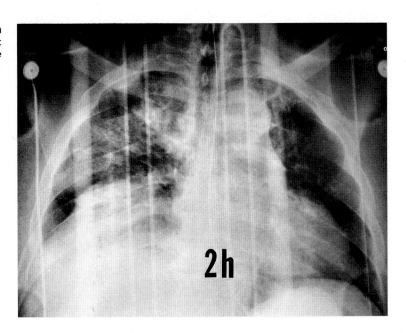

chicken wire, where the wire hexagons represent the interstitial tissues and the spaces represent the air spaces. Under normal circumstances, there is a uniform black background with thin interlacing strands of gray (Fig. 4.90A). In acinar disease, the air spaces are filled in. Unless there is total consolidation of a lobe or a lung, an alveolar process will appear as *white dots* (representing the so-called acinar shadows) *on a black background* of aerated lung (Fig. 4.90B). If, however, the disease is primarily interstitial, there is thickening of the borders around the acini and the resulting pattern is that of *black dots* (representing aerated acini) *surrounded by a white background* of the thickened interstitial tissue (Fig. 4.90C). Combined airway and interstitial disease produce a combined pattern. The following outline lists some of the more common interstitial diseases:

> *Primary Pulmonary Interstitial Diseases*
>   I. Infections
>   A. Tuberculosis
>   B. Histoplasmosis
>   C. Coccidioidomycosis
>   II. Inhalation disorders
>   A. Inorganic dust
>   1. Silicosis
>   2. Asbestosis
>   3. Pneumoconiosis (mixed dust)
>   4. Siderosis
>   5. Other inorganic dust diseases
>   B. Organic dust
>   1. Farmer's lung
>   2. Mushroom worker's disease
>   3. Bagassosis
>   4. Other organic dust diseases
>   III. Miscellaneous
>   A. Sarcoidosis
>   B. Drug-induced disease
>   C. Rheumatoid arthritis
>   D. Scleroderma

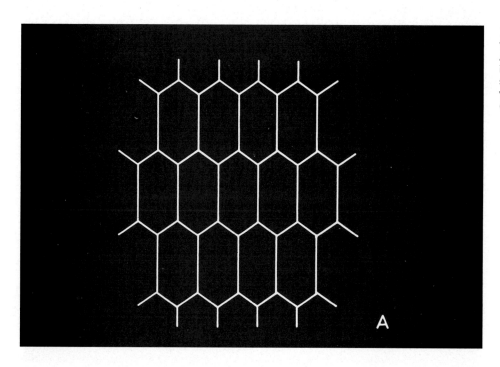

Figure 4.90. Acinar pattern versus interstitial pattern. A, the normal parenchymal pattern is a uniform black background ("air spaces") with thin interlacing white strands ("interstitial tissues"). *(continued on page 139)*

Figure 4.90. *(continued)* **B,** in acinar disease, the air spaces are filled in, producing a pattern of white dots on a black background. **C,** in interstitial disease, there is thickening of the interstitial tissues resulting in a pattern of black dots on a white background.

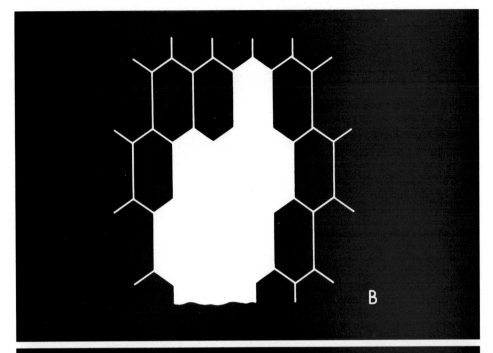

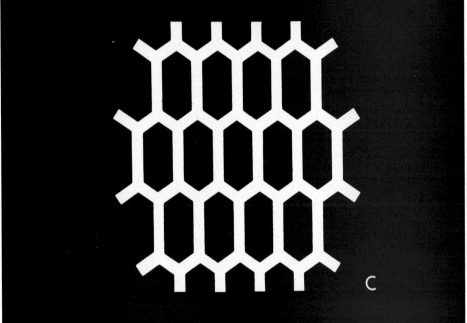

E. Hemosiderosis
F. Chronic thromboembolism
G. Histiocytosis
H. Desquamative interstitial pneumonia
I. Idiopathic interstitial fibrosis (Hamman-Rich syndrome)

Often the presence of ancillary radiologic and clinical findings will be needed to make the correct diagnosis. A good clinical history is also essential, especially if we are entertaining a diagnosis of pneumoconiosis or other industrial exposure. Figures 4.91 through 4.93 show representative examples of pure interstitial disease.

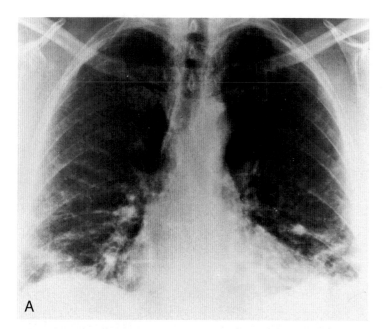

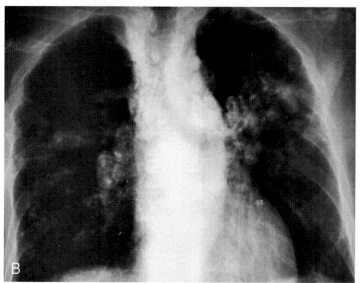

Figure 4.91.   Silicosis. A, there is prominence of the interstitial markings, worse in the lung bases. **B,** there are confluent parenchymal densities and "egg shell" calcifications of hilar and peritracheal lymph nodes.

Pneumothorax

Pneumothorax may result from a variety of causes, including trauma (laceration by fractured rib, stab, or bullet wound) and iatrogenic factors (following thoracentesis, lung biopsy, or placement of subclavian catheter) or may occur spontaneously. The most common radiographic findings are absence of pulmonary vessels extending to the chest wall, a visible pleural line displaced from the chest wall, and increased lucency of one hemithorax. If the patient has a tension-type pneumothorax, air continuously enters the pleural space and builds up pressure, which compresses the mediastinum toward the opposite lung. This may result in severe respiratory distress unless immediately recognized. The most common sign of tension pneumothorax is a shift of the mediastinum away from the abnormal side (Fig. 4.94). This is a true emergency and requires immediate tube decompression. An ancillary sign in tension pneumothorax is depression of the affected hemidiaphragm. A pneumothorax may be made more visible by an expiratory film (Fig. 4.95).

Some pneumothoraces are not as obvious. Free air will be found over the apex of a lung on erect radiographs (Fig. 4.96). CT is very sensitive for identifying pneumothorax. In supine patients, free air collects anteriorly and superiorly (Fig. 4.97).

Figure 4.92. Diffuse interstitial disease in a chronic smoker. Note the prominent interstitial markings. This is the so-called "dirty lungs" pattern.

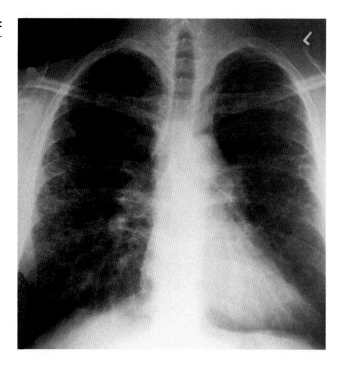

Pulmonary Embolus

It is estimated that pulmonary embolus is the most common abnormality found in hospitalized patients who die and are examined by autopsy. Fortunately, in most cases, embolism occurs without infarction because of the double blood supply to the lung. Pulmonary emboli are most likely to occur in severely ill patients who are bedridden, in those with venous disease, and in those with chronic CHF.

Interestingly, there may be few radiographic findings of pulmonary embolus in any particular patient. Clinicians and radiologists should have a high index of suspicion to make

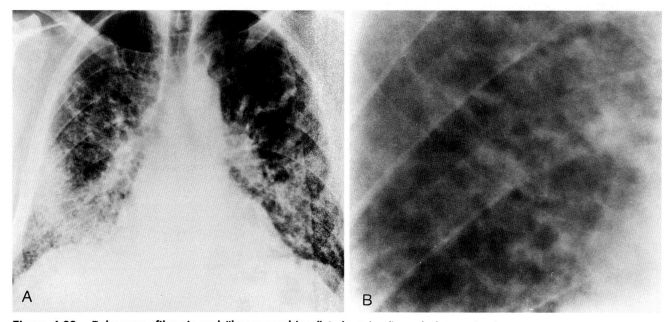

Figure 4.93. Pulmonary fibrosis and "honeycombing." A, frontal radiograph shows extensive interstitial disease with confluent margins (massive pulmonary fibrosis). **B,** detail view shows the honeycombing pattern.

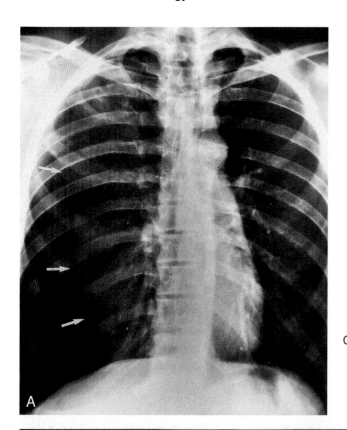

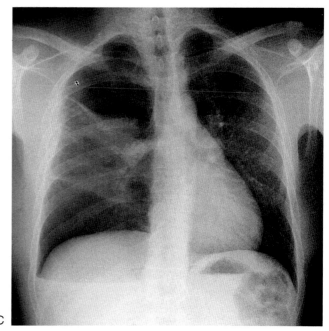

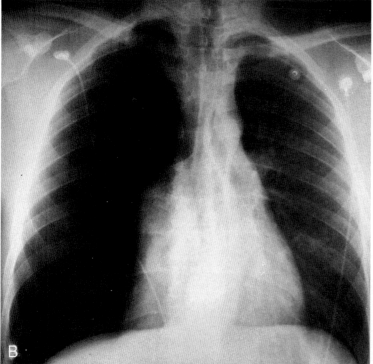

Figure 4.94. Tension pneumothorax in three patients. There is displacement of the mediastinum (*arrows*) toward the left in **A.** The density on the right in **B** is the collapsed lung. In **C** there is incomplete collapse of the right lung due to pleural scarring. The mediastinum is shifted to the left, however.

Figure 4.95. Right-sided pneumothorax (*arrows*) **demonstrating the use of inspiratory (A) and expiratory (B) radiographs.** Note how the pneumothorax is "enlarged" on the expiratory film (**B**).

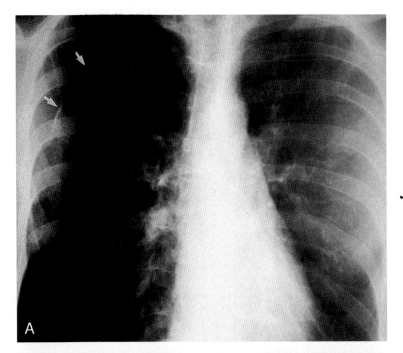

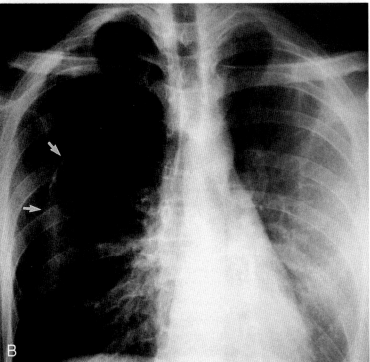

Figure 4.96. Left apical pneumothorax (*arrows*).

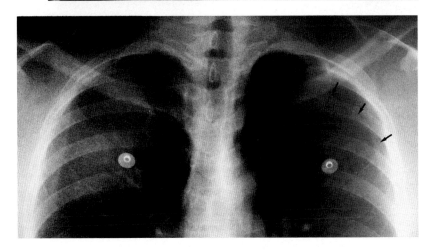

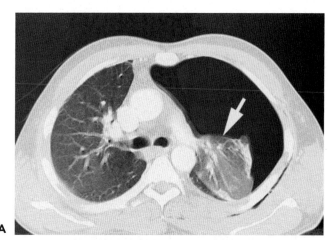

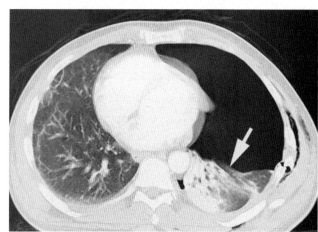

Figure 4.97. Tension pneumothorax as demonstrated on CT. Two CT images show the large collection of free air on the left. The mediastinum is shifted to the right. Note the collapsed lung posteriorly (arrows).

this diagnosis because the most common radiographic finding is that of a "normal" chest, which is incompatible with a patient in acute cardiopulmonary distress. Radiographic signs that may be seen, however, include pleural effusion, pulmonary infiltrates, focal atelectasis, elevation of the diaphragm, and hypovascular peripheral lung segments. Infiltration and formation of a "mass" may occur with infarction. With healing, these areas of consolidation shrink in the same pattern as a melting ice cube, retaining its original outline, only becoming smaller.

Ventilation-perfusion (V/Q) lung scintigraphy is a useful diagnostic procedure in patients suspected of having pulmonary emboli. Injected particles are trapped in the capillary bed, and thus give an index of pulmonary arterial perfusion. Inhaled particles demonstrate the ventilation pattern of the lungs. Patients with emphysema, pneumonia, pulmonary fibrosis, or pleural effusions may demonstrate displacement of vessels, physiologic shunting of blood flow, or poorly ventilated areas. However, a "mismatched" decrease in perfusion of a lung zone that is receiving ventilation is a very reliable sign of an intrinsic vascular defect, i.e. a pulmonary embolus obstructing blood flow (Fig. 4.98). It is critical to assess the VQ scan with simultaneous chest radiographs to reduce the likelihood of false positive outcomes. Furthermore, if a patient is shown to have normal perfusion to part of the lung despite an abnormal radiographic appearance, you can exclude embolus as a cause of that abnormality. The V/Q scan has the advantage of less radiation exposure than CT (see below). Furthermore, it may still be used as a first line imaging modality in otherwise healthy patients with normal chest radiographs who are suspected of having pulmonary emboli.

Chest CT has largely replaced the V/Q scan for diagnosing pulmonary emboli. The main reasons for this are the "indeterminate" outcome of V/Q scans in patients with known lung diseases, mentioned above and the ready availability of CT, particularly at night and on week-

Figure 4.98. Pulmonary embolism.
A, perfusion scan shows photopenic areas throughout both lungs, representing regions of lack of perfusion. **B,** ventilation scan shows that these areas are normally ventilated.

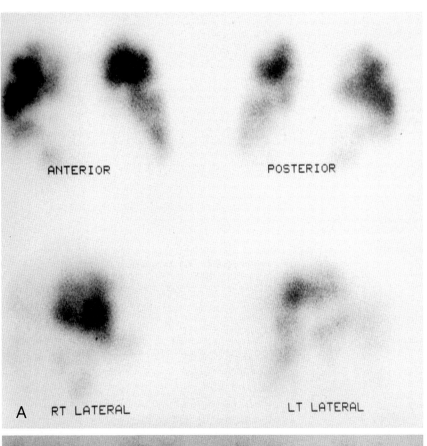

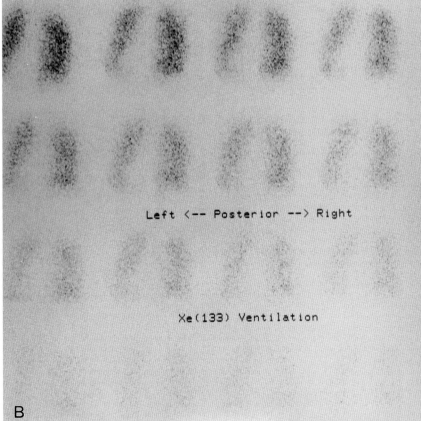

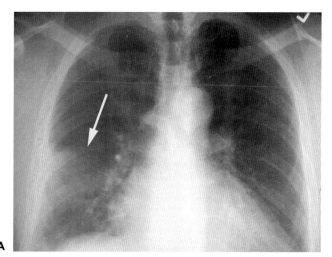

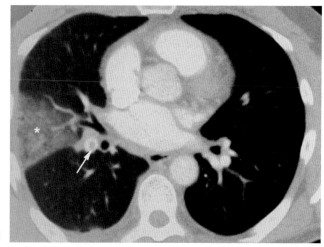

Figure 4.99.   CT of small pulmonary embolism. A, Radiograph shows a wedge-shaped area of increased density in the right middle lobe (arrow). **B,** CT image shows the wedge-shaped area in the right middle lobe (*) representing an infarct. Note the small filling defect in the adjacent pulmonary artery (arrow).

ends when nuclear medicine divisions are normally closed. In most instances, the CT can be obtained in a significantly shorter period of time than that required to call in a nuclear medicine technologist, and have the technologist prepare the isotope for injection. Modern CT is fast and more importantly, more effective in demonstrating small peripheral emboli, as well as the larger more central ones (Figs. 4.99, 4.100). With modern multidetector CT scanners, the thorax may be studied in as little as 15 to 20 seconds. Most patients are able to breath-hold in that short time period. Thus the advantages of CT lie in its availability, high sensitivity for central and clinically significant emboli, as well as its ability to provide more information about the lungs and thoracic organs in the absence of pulmonary emboli. There are, however, some limitations in the use of CT. In approximately 10% of patients the study is suboptimal. This may be the result of patient obesity or respiratory motion. The sensitivity is only about 86%, although the specificity is 96%.

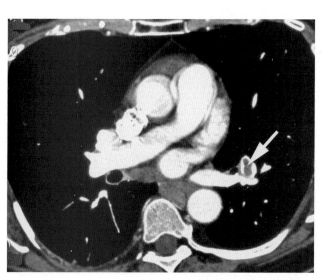

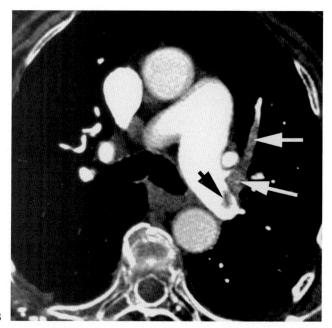

Figure 4.100.   CT of large pulmonary embolisms in two patients. A, CT image shows the defect in a central pulmonary artery (arrow). **B,** CT image shows a long thrombus on the left (white arrows). Note the smaller clot in the main pulmonary artery (short black arrow).

Figure 4.101. Pulmonary embolism. Pulmonary arteriogram shows a large saddle embolus (*arrow*). Note the poor perfusion of the right middle and lower lobes as opposed to the upper lobe.

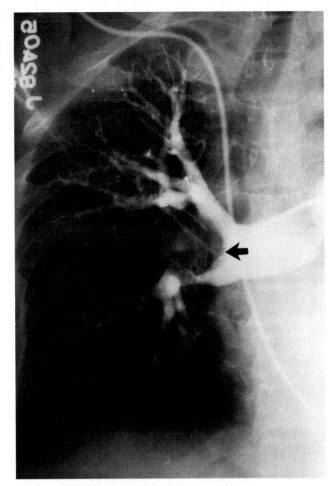

Pulmonary arteriography was considered the "gold standard" for diagnosing pulmonary emboli (Fig. 4.101) prior to the emergence of CT for that purpose. In many places outside the US, however, arteriography is still used, particularly when the isotope study is equivocal. However, in the US, CT has replaced it.

Appearance of the Chest After Surgery

Monumental advances have been made in thoracic surgery in the past 40 years: development of new techniques for cardiopulmonary bypass, lung surgery, and coronary revascularization procedures; stents; development of new prosthetic heart valves; advancements in heart transplantation; and perfection of new techniques for esophageal bypass surgery. These changes have reduced the morbidity and mortality in patients who were formerly subjected to cardiothoracic surgery.

Although the appearance of the chest radiograph in a patient who has undergone cardiac, thoracic, or esophageal surgery may be quite characteristic of the procedure following recovery from surgery, in the immediate postoperative period there are many generic findings common to all procedures. Operative manipulation of the lung may result in areas of patchy consolidation. Pleural effusion is a common finding following both cardiac and pulmonary surgery. Patients who have undergone cardiac surgery often show enlargement of the cardiac silhouette. CHF, pneumonia, atelectasis (particularly the left lower lobe), and pneumothorax are frequent findings in the immediate postoperative period (Fig 4.102).

Following heart or lung surgery, a variety of foreign objects may be seen within the thorax. These include chest tubes placed anteriorly in the supine patient for drainage of air and posteriorly for drainage of fluid, wire staples representing lines of resection of lung, metal clips placed across vessels or at the site of dissection around vessels, wire sutures in the sternum, mediastinal drains, a variety of intravascular catheters, and prosthetic heart valves.

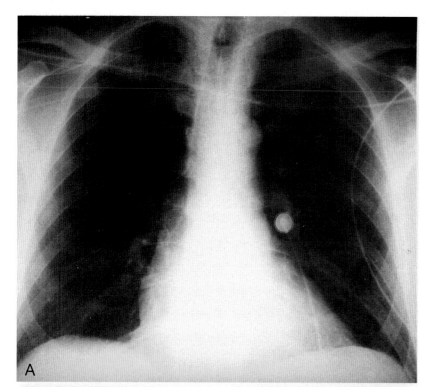

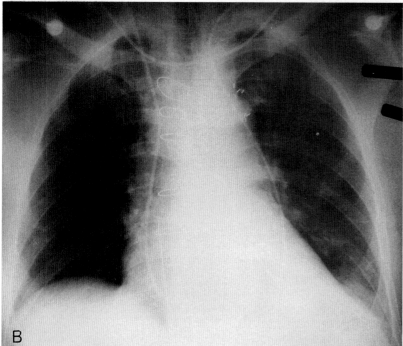

Figure 4.102. Changes of thoracic surgery. A, preoperative portable frontal radiograph is normal. **B,** following cardiac surgery, there are multiple sternal wires present. There are surgical clips adjacent to the aorta. An endotracheal tube, Swann-Ganz catheter, and mediastinal drains are also present.

Furthermore, pacemaker leads may be seen either intraventricularly or epicardially. Electrocardiographic leads may also be seen on the chest wall. Some of these "foreign bodies" are illustrated in Figure 4.102.

We can divide the discussion of the chest during the postoperative period into four categories:

1. Primary lung surgery
2. Primary cardiac surgery
3. Primary esophageal surgery
4. Mastectomy

PRIMARY LUNG SURGERY

Patients undergo *lung surgery* in basically three types of procedures: excisions, pneumonectomy, and lobectomy.

The most common radiographic manifestation of excisional biopsy or wedge resection of a lesion is a line of wire staples across the lung (Fig. 4.103). Often this is accompanied by the absence of a portion of a rib, generally the fifth or sixth posteriorly.

Following pneumonectomy, the affected hemithorax fills with fluid (Fig 4.104A). Air within the affected side gradually resorbs, leaving an opaque hemithorax. As fibrosis ensues, the heart and mediastinum are drawn toward the side of surgery. Often the cardiac silhouette will not be seen. The remaining lung hyperinflates to fill the space vacated by the shifted heart and mediastinum, as illustrated in Figure 4.104B.

In patients who have undergone a lobectomy, wire staples representing the line of resection across the bronchus are seen. Metal clips may be present across the vessels. There is a shift of fissures as with atelectasis, the directions being the same as in atelectasis of the affected lobe. Hyperinflation of the remaining lobes on the side of a lobectomy is also seen. These findings are illustrated in Figure 4.105.

Thoracoplasty and plombage are procedures that were once performed to eliminate dead space within the chest. A patient who has undergone thoracoplasty exhibits deformity of the upper chest wall on the affected side (Fig. 4.106A). Patients who have undergone plombage will exhibit foreign material, as in Figure 4.106B.

PRIMARY CARDIAC SURGERY

Cardiac surgery is performed most often to replace damaged heart valves, to bypass stenotic coronary arteries, to palliate congenital heart disease, and for transplantation. The majority of the patients who have had operations for acquired disease will demonstrate wire sutures in the sternum, the common exposure of the surgical field. Small wire sutures seen in an adult indicate that the surgery was performed when the patient was a child.

Prosthetic valves are of several varieties. When observing these valves, one can easily appreciate the location on plain film of the mitral and aortic rings (Figs. 4.107 and 4.108).

Patients who undergo bypass surgery of the coronary arteries often show multiple metal clips in the epicardial portions of the heart. On occasion, small metal rings may represent the aortic root origin of the coronary bypass grafts. These findings are illustrated in Figure 4.109. Coronary arterial stents may also be seen on a well-penetrated radiograph.

Figure 4.103. Changes following lung resection in the left lower lobe. There are multiple surgical staples present in the left lower lobe.

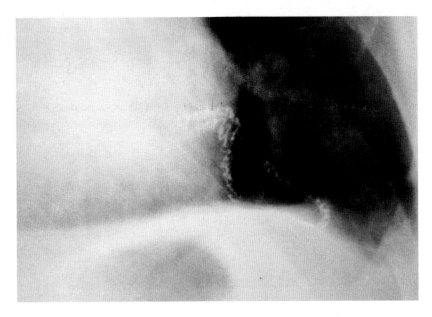

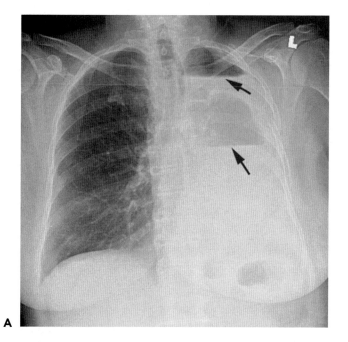

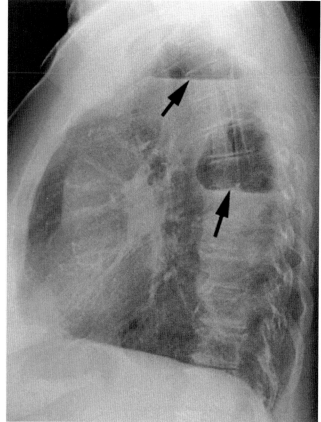

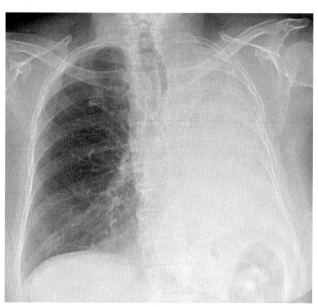

Figure 4.104. Changes following left-sided pneumonectomy. A, B, frontal and lateral radiographs respectively taken two days following surgery, show a multilocular hydropneumothorax on the left side. Note the multiple air-fluid levels (arrows). **C,** follow-up radiograph several months later shows complete opacification of the left hemithorax. The heart and mediastinum are shifted to the left and the trachea is bowed to the left.

Patients who have had palliative surgery for congenital heart disease may exhibit a variety of changes, depending on the surgical procedure. In some instances, as with palliation of a septal defect or ligation of a patent ductus arteriosus, the findings may be perfectly normal if the surgery has been successful.

Pacemakers are of two varieties, intravascular and epicardial. The intravascular leads are generally placed into the right atrium and right ventricle. When seen on the routine PA and lateral chest films, there should be a gentle curve to the catheter (see Fig. 4.110). Any kinking or odd course of the lead should suggest that the catheter is not in the right position. The pacer box is in the subclavicular area. Epicardial leads are placed along the outside of the heart in the vicinity of the interventricular septum. Generally, these wires go through the diaphragm to the power box, which is in the abdominal wall (Fig. 4.111).

Cardiologists are now using an automatic implantable cardiac defibrillator (AICD). When ventricular tachycardia or fibrillation occurs, the device automatically discharges a cardioverting shock. One device is implanted either directly on the heart surface or subcutaneously in the ante-

Figure 4.105.   Changes following partial right upper lobectomy. Note the shift of the minor fissure upward (*open arrow*). A suture line is visible medially (*solid arrows*).

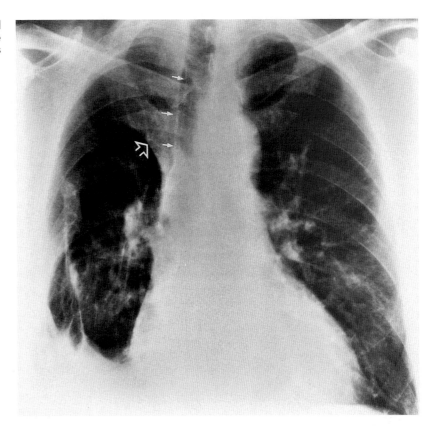

rior chest wall. The leads are attached to the transmitter box that is contained subcutaneously in the abdomen. Internal defibrillators have been proven effective in preventing sudden death from arrhythmias. The device may be recognized on a chest radiograph by the fly swatter-like pad over the heart (Fig. 4.112). A more commonly used device is the intracardiac defibrillator. This is inserted the same way as a pacemaker, from one of the subclavian veins (usually on the left). The

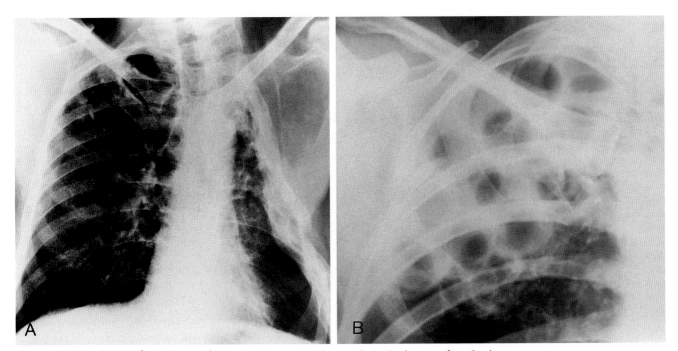

Figure 4.106.   Unusual postoperative appearances. A, thoracoplasty. **B,** changes after plombage in which plastic balls were placed in the right hemithorax.

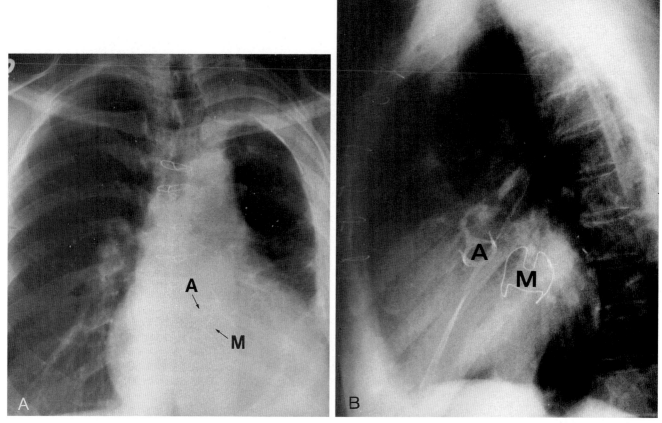

Figure 4.107. **Prosthetic mitral** (*M*) **and aortic** (*A*) **valves. A,** frontal view. **B,** lateral view shows the valves to better advantage.

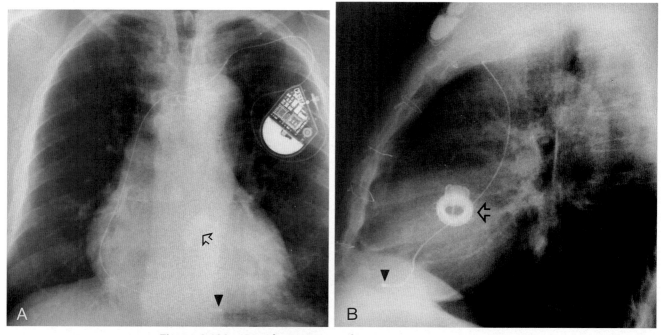

Figure 4.108. **Prosthetic aortic valve** (*arrows*) **and transvenous pacemaker.** The tip of the pacing lead (*arrowheads*) is in the right ventricle. **A,** frontal view. **B,** lateral view.

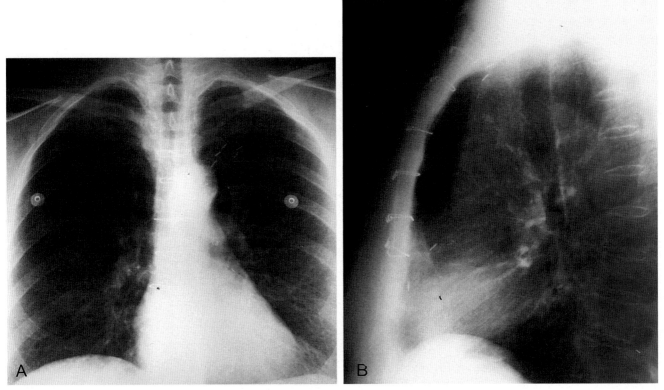

Figure 4.109.   Changes following cardiac surgery. Note the presence of sternal wires and mediastinal vascular clips. **A,** frontal view. **B,** lateral view.

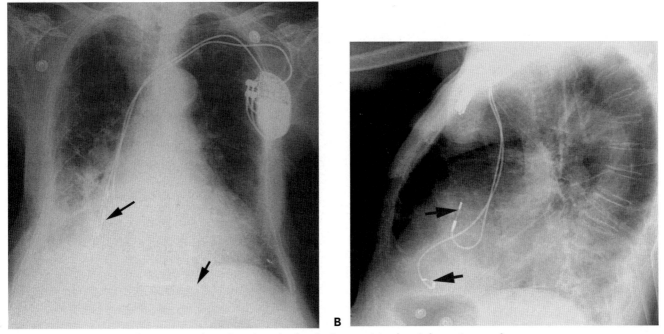

Figure 4.110.   Intracardiac pacemaker showing the leads *(arrows)* **in the right atrium and right ventricle. A,** frontal view. **B,** lateral view.

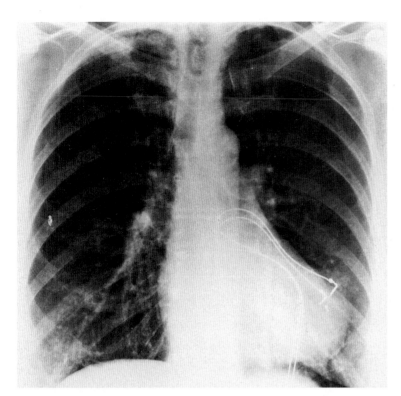

Figure 4.111.   Epicardial pacemaker leads on the left side.

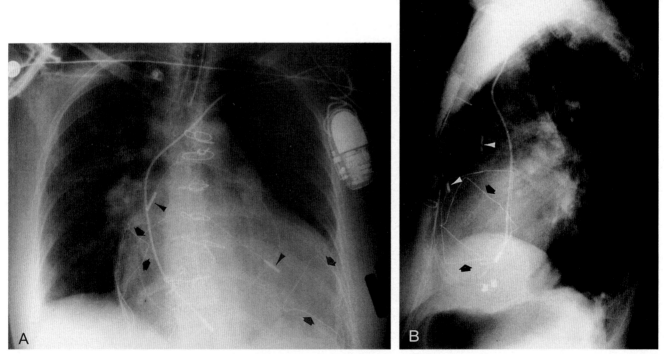

Figure 4.112.   Automated internal cardiac defibrillator. Frontal **(A)** and lateral **(B)** views show the defibrillator pads (*arrows*) over the right atrium and left ventricle. The leads (*arrowheads*) previously connected to the power box in the abdominal wall. Note the pacemaker in place.

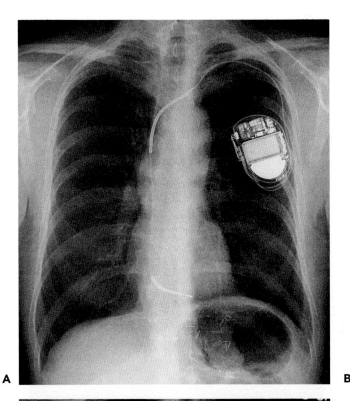

A

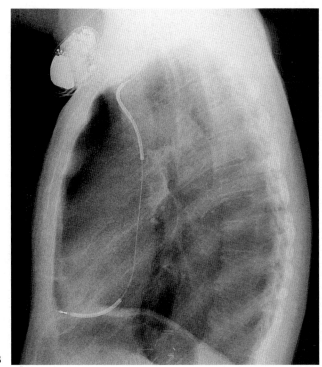

B

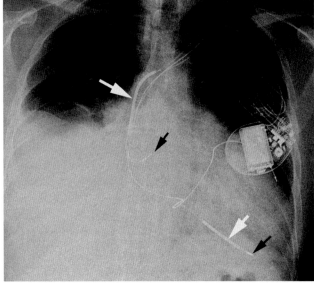

C

Figure 4.113.   Automated internal cardiac defibrillator.
A, PA and **B,** lateral views show the power box over the left chest wall. The defibrillating leads are in the superior vena cava and the right ventricle. **C,** another patient with a combined pacemaker and defibrillator. The coiled defibrillating leads are in the superior vena cava and the right ventricle (large arrows). The pacing leads are in the right atrium and right ventricle (small arrows).

defibrillator is often combined with a pacemaker or may be implanted alone. The intracardiac defibrillator may be recognized by the coiled spring appearance of the defibrillating leads in the superior vena cava or right atrium and the right ventricle (Fig 4.113).

PRIMARY ESOPHAGEAL SURGERY

Numerous procedures have been devised for palliation of esophageal disease. There are basically two types, bypass surgery and hiatal hernia repair. In a *bypass procedure,* the stomach or a segment of colon may be used to bypass a stenotic segment of esophagus or a neoplasm. The bypassing conduit is often visible on the chest radiograph, as illustrated in Figure 4.114. *Hiatal hernia repair* may on occasion show a mass in the immediate postcardiac region. This

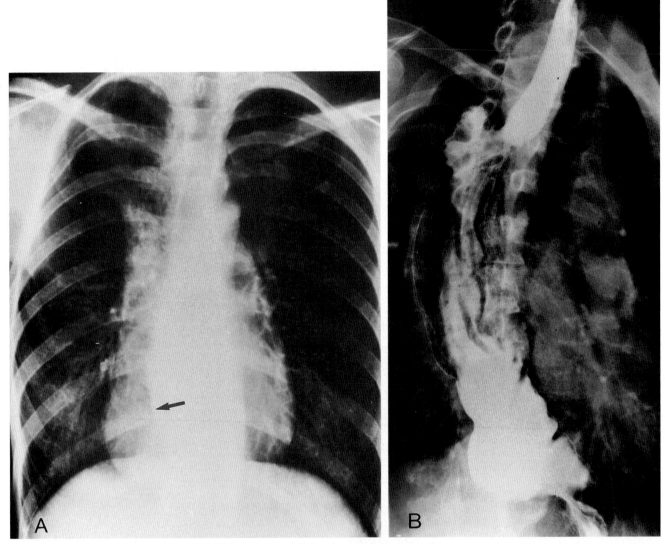

Figure 4.114. Changes following esophagogastrectomy. A, frontal radiograph shows apparent enlargement of the cardiac silhouette. The real cardiac border is seen just to the right of midline (*arrow*). **B,** contrast examination shows the stomach in the right hemithorax.

represents the fundus of the stomach, which has been plicated around the distal esophagus to create a competent esophageal sphincter. Metal clips may also be seen in this region. Various types of stents may also be used to bypass the obstructed esophageal segment.

MASTECTOMY

You should also be familiar with postoperative appearance of the patient following radical mastectomy for carcinoma of the breast. Following mastectomy, the affected side appears more lucent. This is because of the absence of the breast shadow and pectoralis major muscle. If we follow the soft tissue lines of the axilla on the normal side, we can see that the axillary fold merges imperceptibly with that of the breast shadow. However, on the affected side, the axillary fold extends up to and crosses over onto the thorax. These findings are illustrated in Figure 4.115. Occasionally, we may see metal clips that were left at the site of nodal resection within the axilla in patients who have undergone radical mastectomy. These changes are now

Figure 4.115.   Changes following left radical mastectomy. There is hyperlucency in the left hemithorax from the absence of pectoral tissues. Note the differences in soft tissues between right and left.

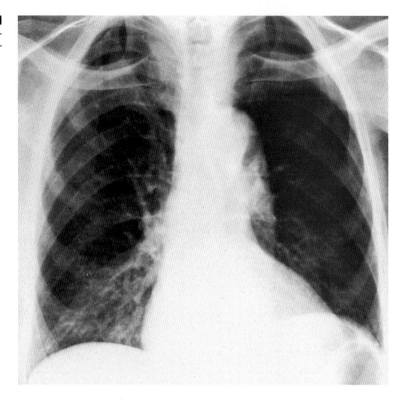

less common since the introduction of breast conservation therapy (lumpectomy combined with radiation and chemotherapy).

You should familiarize yourself with the various appearances of the chest postoperatively. Remember, once the patient has recovered and is free of symptoms of the previous disease, we can consider this chest "normal" for that individual.

Finally, when dealing with postoperative patients or any other patient in an intensive care unit, one should always be cognizant of the placement and location of the various life-support devices used. Many times endotracheal or nasogastric tubes are inadvertently inserted into a bronchus (Fig. 4.116) or the esophagus. Similarly, intravenous or arterial catheters occasionally end up in a position not intended. Chest tubes may be kinked or have their tips of side holes in the axilla. Wayward support devices may have disastrous results.

Figure 4.116.   Nasogastric tube in right main-stem bronchus (*arrow*).

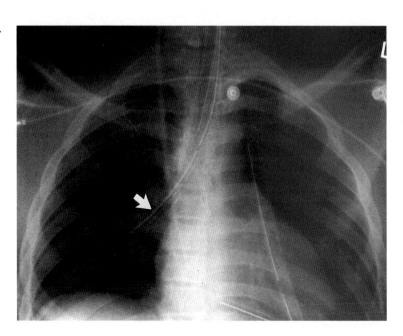

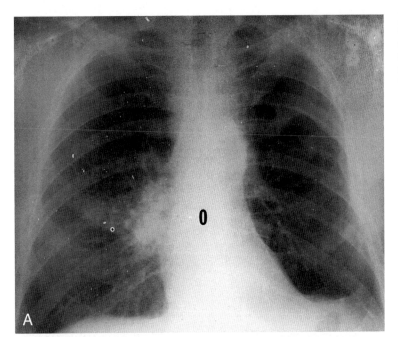

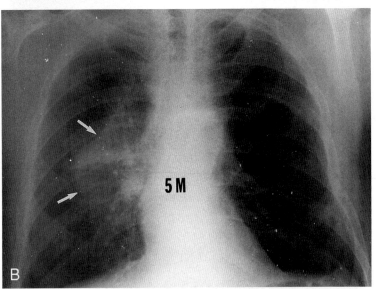

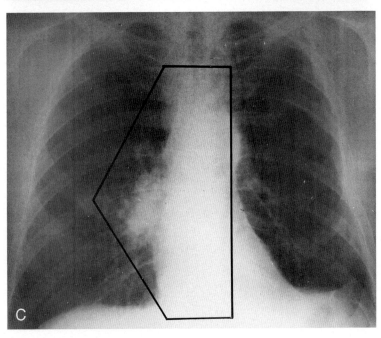

Figure 4.117. Radiation pneumonitis. A, pre-treatment film shows a large mass in the right hilum. **B,** 5 months after radiation therapy, there is a sail-like sharply outlined density in the right lung (*arrows*). **C,** pretreatment film with radiation port superimposed. Note the similarity of the density in **B** to the treatment port.

Other Considerations

Radiation Pneumonitis

Radiation pneumonitis is a form of interstitial lung disease that produces pulmonary scarring and volume loss. It is found whenever the lung is exposed to radiation of a dose of 20 Gy or greater. Typically, the dose is 60 Gy or more administered over a period of 5 to 6 weeks. In the acute stage there is consolidation, similar to that from other etiologies. However, the radiographic clue to the diagnosis is that the distribution of the abnormalities is nonanatomic and follows the borders of the radiation therapy portal that was used. These borders are usually well defined (Fig. 4.117). In the late stages, fibrosis occurs. This usually produces hilar and/or fissure displacement, depending on the portals. Obtaining a history of previous radiation therapy is key to making the diagnosis. On occasion, there may be skeletal changes from radiation therapy as well.

AIDS-Related Abnormalities

Acquired immunodeficiency syndrome (AIDS) is the result of infection with the human immunodeficiency virus (HIV). Patients with this disease suffer a variety of pulmonary infections and neoplasms. Of the infections, *Pneumocystis carinii* pneumonia (PCP) is reported to occur in approximately 75% of these patients. In the early stage of the disease there are subtle fine reticular or nodular deposits found in a predominantly upper lobe distribution. A more fulminant pattern may be encountered in which there are rapidly developing coalescent opacities (Fig. 4.118). Another pattern is that of symmetric perihilar opacification that resembles pulmonary edema. The heart, however, is normal sized, as are the pulmonary vessels (Fig. 4.119).

Pneumocystis infection is not the only pathogen to infect HIV patients. Pyogenic organisms, most commonly *Haemophilus influenzae* and *Streptococcus pneumoniae* also cause pneumonia. In addition, fungal, nocardial, and mycobacterial infections (*Mycobacterium tuberculosis, Mycobacterium avium-intracellulare*) are not uncommon. The pulmonary patterns produced by these organisms are similar to those seen in other immunocompromised patients, such as those who have hematologic malignancies (leukemia, lymphoma), patients on chemotherapy for malignancies, organ transplant patients, and those receiving high-maintenance doses of steroids for chronic systemic diseases such as rheumatoid arthritis or systemic lupus erythematosus.

Figure 4.118. *Pneumocystis carinii* **pneumonia (PCP) in a patient with AIDS.** There are bilateral patchy pneumonic densities.

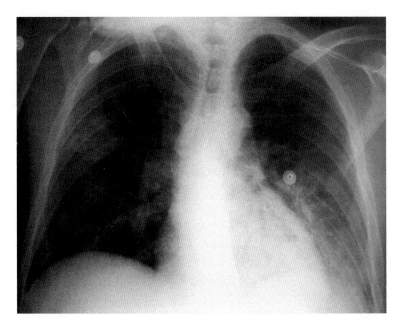

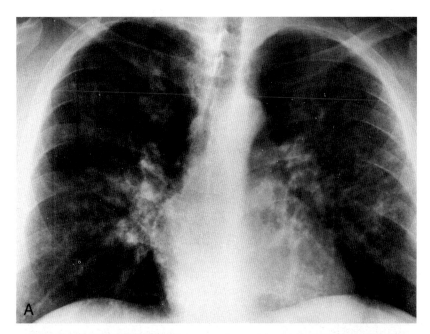

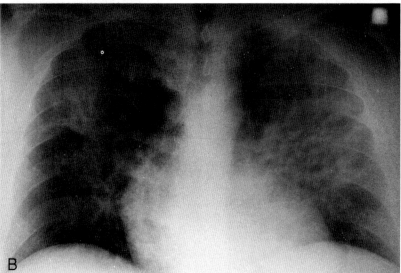

Figure 4.119. PCP—edema pattern in an AIDS patient. A, radiograph shows bilateral interstitial pneumonic densities. **B,** 1 day later, there is an edema pattern, that is particularly noticeable on the left.

Kaposi sarcoma occurs in approximately one-third of patients with AIDS. Radiographically, this usually presents as asymmetric bilateral pulmonary nodules, coarse reticulonodular parenchymal pattern, mediastinal or hilar adenopathy, and pleural effusion. Air space densities represent areas of pulmonary hemorrhage. Figure 4.120 illustrates some of these findings.

Tuberculosis

Tuberculosis (TB) has been one of the scourges of humankind. This disease, which had been in decline in the United States, began to make a dramatic comeback in the early 1980s. The reasons for this included a number of medical and social factors, such as an increasing incidence of drug abuse, increasing numbers of homeless people, and the rise in the number of patients infected with HIV. TB has always been known as "the great imitator" because of its propensity to mimic other diseases.

Pulmonary TB may occur in primary or secondary forms. Primary TB begins with a pulmonary parenchymal pattern that is radiographically mostly interstitial. The upper lobes are the

Figure 4.120.   Pulmonary Kaposi sarcoma in a patient with AIDS. Note the bilateral parenchymal and intersititial pulmonary densities. (*Courtesy David Epstein, M.D., from Radiology 1982;183:7–10. Reproduced with permission.*)

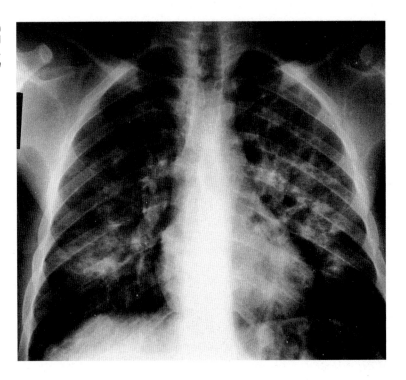

areas most commonly infected (Fig. 4.121). There is usually enlargement of ipsilateral hilar lymph nodes. Upon treatment and healing, it is not unusual for the parenchymal lesion to calcify along with the hilar nodes. When this occurs, it leaves a characteristic radiographic pattern known as the *"primary inflammatory complex."* A second, more massive form of tubercular infection occurs, in which there is diffuse involvement of both lungs. The radiographic appearance is that of a "snow storm" that, again, is interstitial. This is termed *miliary TB* (Fig. 4.122).

The secondary form of TB involves reactivation of dormant foci of infection. In these patients, new interstitial densities may occur with or without cavitation. In end stage of reactivation TB there is fibrosis and scarring with volume loss, shift of fissures and/or vessels and calcification (Fig. 4.123).

Adult Respiratory Distress Syndrome

Critically ill patients frequently undergo a serious pulmonary complication known as *adult respiratory distress syndrome (ARDS)*. These patients undergo prolonged anoxia, receive large amounts of blood products for resuscitation, or are on extended ventilatory assistance, and develop an evanescent pulmonary pattern that combines features of pneumonia, pulmonary edema, and atelectasis. The pattern changes on a daily basis, with improvements and relapses. Trauma patients who suffer initial pulmonary contusions generally experience a worsening of their pulmonary function, coinciding with a chest radiograph that indicates the same (Fig 4.124). Generally, it is not difficult to make the diagnosis when confronted with the radiographic pattern described above in an at-risk patient.

Special Pediatric Considerations

Chest radiographs make up at least one-third of all radiologic examinations performed at most children's hospitals. Although many of the diseases, such as pneumonia and atelectasis, produce changes that are identical in children and adults, there are a number of entities that are unique to newborns, infants, and children. Congenital cardiac abnormalities and their radiologic manifestations will be described in the next chapter.

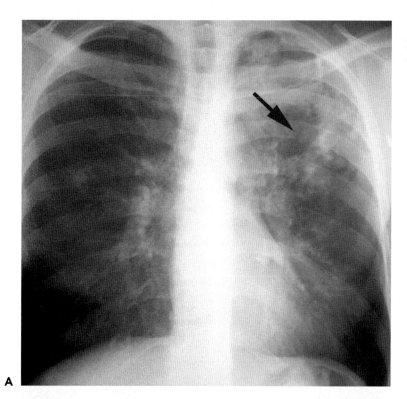

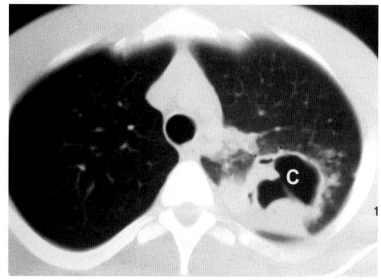

Figure 4.121. Tuberculosis left upper lobe. A, frontal radiograph shows interstitial densities of a fibronodular nature. This is the typical picture for reinfection tuberculosis. Note the cavity (*arrow*). **B,** CT image shows the cavity (*C*) within the area of consolidated lung.

Upper Airway Obstruction

Choanal atresia is an obstruction to the posterior wall of the nasopharynx. It is a threat to newborns who are obligate nasal breathers, particularly during feeding. In approximately 90% of patients the obstruction is bony. Thirty-three percent are bilateral. CT is the best modality for making the diagnosis.

Tonsillar and adenoidal enlargement may be found in asymptomatic healthy children. A radiograph showing such enlargement (Fig. 4.125) usually does not provide any more information than a good clinical examination.

Epiglottitis and *croup* are upper airway diseases that produce respiratory stridor, cough, fever, and irritability. True epiglottitis is less common but more dangerous than croup. The peak incidence is around age 3 1/2. It is usually caused by infection with *H. influenzae*. A lateral radiograph of the neck typically shows increase in the size of the epiglottis and thickening of the aryepiglottic folds (Fig. 4.126). It is this thickening of these folds that obstructs the airway.

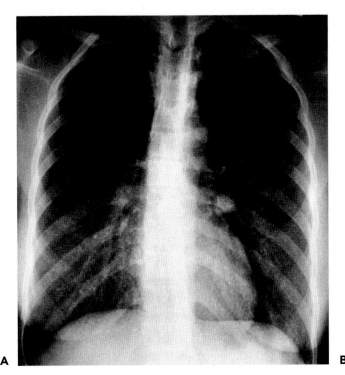

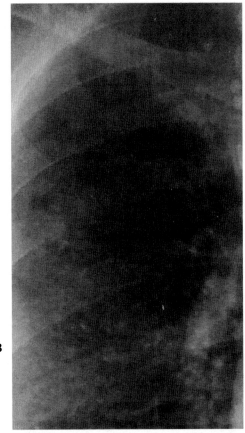

Figure 4.122.   Miliary tuberculosis in a patient with AIDS. Note the fine diffuse nodular pattern throughout both lower lobes. **A,** overview radiograph, **B,** detail view.

Figure 4.123.   Old tuberculous infection. There is a dense irregular granuloma in the left upper lobe (*arrow*). Note the cephalad shift of the hilar vessels on the left side. Compare with the right.

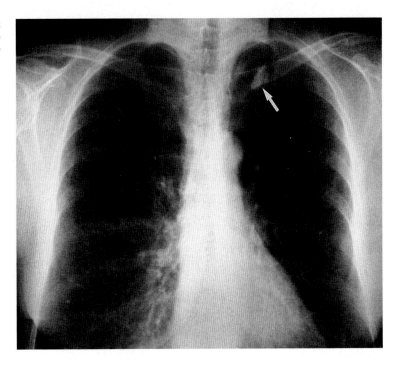

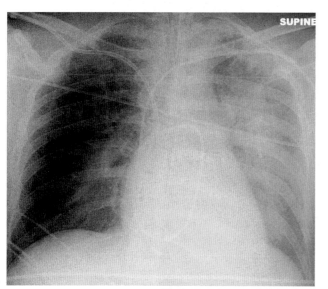

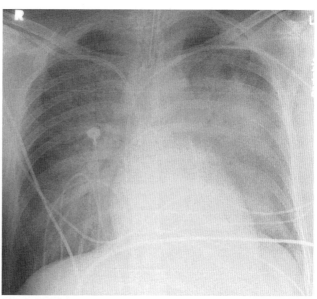

Figure 4.124. Adult Respiratory Distress Syndrome (ARDS). A, portable chest radiograph on a trauma victim shows bibasal pulmonary densities. Note the presence of an endotracheal tube and Swann-Ganz central venous catheter. **B,** 12 hours later the portable radiograph shows a dramatic increase in consolidation throughout both lungs. The cardiac size remains normal.

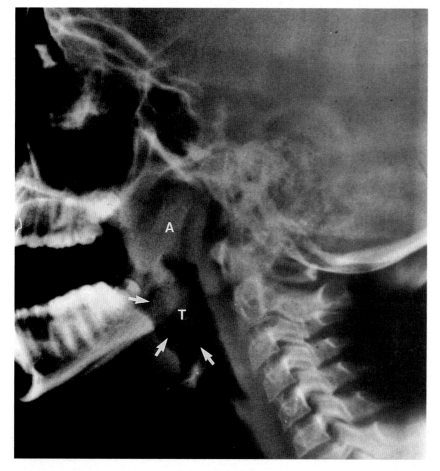

Figure 4.125. Enlarged tonsils (*T*) (*arrows*) **and adenoids** (*A*) **in an 8-year-old.** The adenoidal enlargement has virtually occluded the nasopharynx.

Figure 4.126. Epiglottitis. There is blunting and thickening of the epiglottis (*arrows*). This has severely narrowed the airway immediately below. Note the dilated hypopharynx.

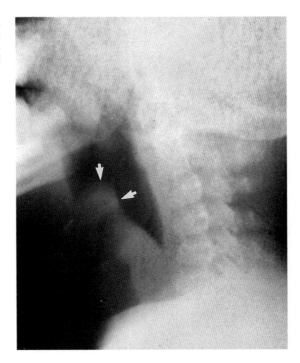

Most cases of croup are caused by viral pathogens. Frontal radiographs of the neck show loss of the lateral contours of the subglottic trachea. On the frontal view, there is narrowing of the airway to produce an inverted "V" that has been called the "steeple sign" (Fig. 4.127).

Disorders Of Newborns

There are a number of conditions that affect newborn infants, especially those who are premature or of extremely low birth weight. These entities are immature lung disease, respiratory distress syndrome (RDS), bronchopulmonary dysplasia, wet lung disease, and meconium aspiration.

Immature lung disease occurs in newborns of birth weight under 1500 g. These patients usually do not become symptomatic until they are 4 to 7 days old. Radiographically, there is a diffuse granularity to both lungs *without* air bronchograms (which differentiates this entity from RDS). Smaller newborns weighing less than 1000 g may have their respiratory illness complicated by intracranial hemorrhage, necrotizing enterocolitis, and bronchopulmonary dysplasia. In uncomplicated cases, over 80% of patients survive.

RDS, also known as *hyaline membrane disease* (*HMD*), is a disorder of hypoventilation and pulmonary immaturity. It occurs predominantly in newborns under 36 to 38 weeks' gestation, who typically weigh less than 2500 g. It is a leading cause of death in newborns. Radiologically, the disease produces a diffuse coarse granular alveolar pattern that has a distinct "ground glass" appearance (Fig. 4.128). Air bronchograms are common and serve to differentiate RDS from immature lung disease, as mentioned above. Complications of RDS include pneumothorax, pneumomediastinum, and interstitial emphysema. In many instances, the patient develops bronchopulmonary dysplasia (BPD).

BPD, also known as chronic lung disease of premature infants, is a complication of prolonged ventilator therapy. Four distinct clinical and radiographic stages have been described. Stage I is identical to RDS both clinically and radiographically. Stage II occurs between 4 and 10 days of age and is manifest by marked opacity of both lungs ("white-out"). Stage III occurs at 10 to 20 days of age and is characterized by a bubbly radiographic appearance to the lungs, with many "lung cavities." Stage IV occurs after 1 month of age and is characterized by hyperaeration, particularly of the lung bases, and by fibrosis (Fig. 4.129). Many authorities consider *Wilson-Mikity syndrome* to be identical to BPD.

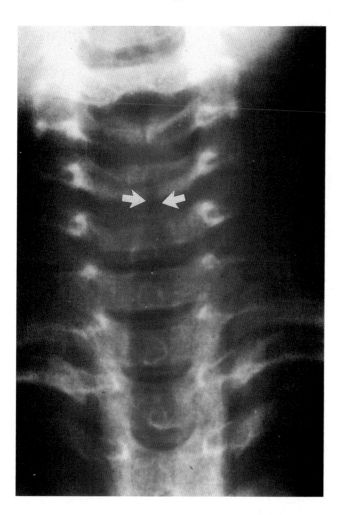

Figure 4.127. Croup. Frontal radiograph of the neck shows a "steeple sign" of the subglottic region (*arrows*).

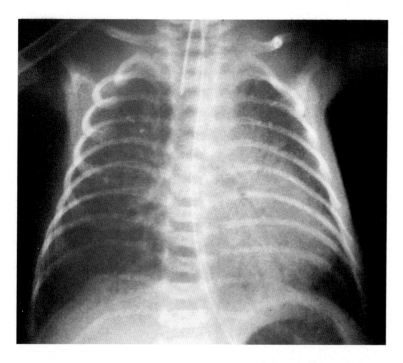

Figure 4.128. Hyaline membrane disease. There is a "ground glass" appearance to both lungs. Note the air bronchograms in the left lung base.

Figure 4.129. Bronchopulmonary dysplasia (BPD). There is marked hyperinflation and interstitial prominence. The bubbly appearance of the left lung is caused by interstitial emphysema, a complication of BPD.

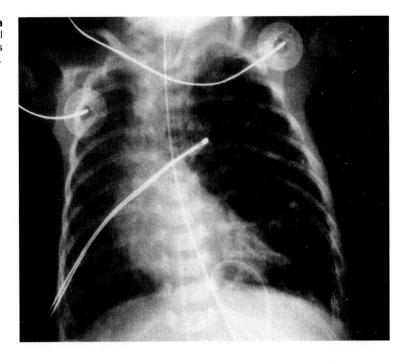

Wet lung disease (*transient tachypnea of the newborn*) is caused by delayed resorption and clearing of fetal lung fluid. It is a common cause of respiratory distress in the newborn. Radiographically, there is a pattern of fluid in the lungs, somewhat "ground glass," resembling that of RDS that develops within 2 to 6 hours of life (Fig. 4.130). At 10 to 12 hours it begins to clear. The chest radiograph is usually normal by 48 hours of age. One important clue to the diagnosis is that the findings occur in a newborn of normal size and birth weight.

Meconium aspiration syndrome occurs as the result of meconium aspiration at the time of birth. This produces a chemical pneumonitis that has the appearance of patchy bilateral asymmetric pulmonary opacities. Pneumothorax or pneumomediastinum may occur in as many as 25% of patients. Because of the chemical nature of the inflammation, radiologic clearing is slower than other pneumonias. The diagnosis is usually assured when the clinical picture includes a history of meconium staining at birth.

Pneumonias from other sources have a radiographic pattern similar to those seen in older children and adults. The reader is cautioned not to "overcall" a pneumonia on a crying child,

Figure 4.130. Wet lung. There is a fine haze to both lungs on this radiograph made several hours after birth. A follow-up radiograph the next day was normal.

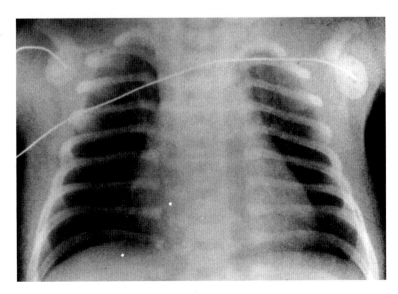

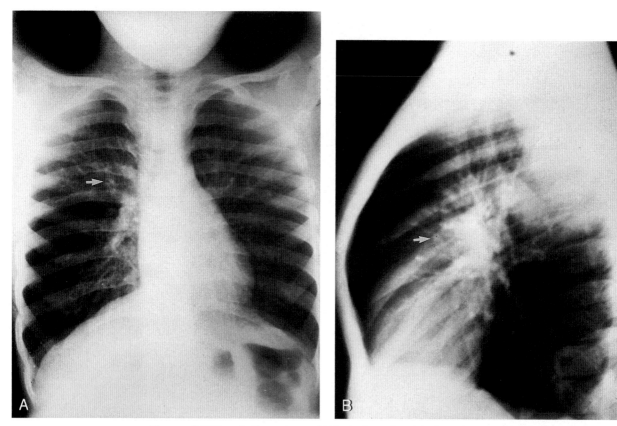

Figure 4.131. Asthma in a child. A, frontal and **B,** lateral views show hyperinflation. There is peribronchial cuffing (*arrows*). Note the flat diaphragm in **B.**

in whom the radiograph is obtained in *expiration*. In these instances, crowding of markings, particularly in the right lower lobe, may be misinterpreted as an infiltrate. Always look for the presence of a silhouette sign as well as for air bronchograms. One other note of caution. Viral pneumonias frequently produce an interstitial pattern *with* enlarged hilar lymph nodes, a pattern not unlike that found with TB. Remember that viral pneumonia is much more common than TB!

Bronchiolitis and Asthma

Bronchiolitis is a clinical condition caused by a virus (usually respiratory syncytial virus) that typically occurs in patients over 1 year of age. These infants typically have a syndrome of wheezing, tachypnea, and low-grade fever. Radiographically, the condition is characterized by hyperinflation, peribronchial cuffing, with or without perihilar linear opacities (Fig. 4.131). The chest radiograph becomes normal once the disease resolves.

Asthma typically occurs in older patients. The radiographic findings are typically hyperinflation and peribronchial cuffing. These findings are similar to those found in bronchiolitis. Pneumonic consolidation may be superimposed on these changes.

SUMMARY AND KEY POINTS

- Chest radiography is the most common imaging examination performed today.
- Chest CT is an integral technique in finding lung lesions and in delineating the extent of their involvement. It is particularly important in the diagnosis of pulmonary emboli, as well as in detecting intrathoracic tumors.
- The unit of structure and function in the lung is the pulmonary lobule. This serves on a macroscopic and microscopic level to explain lung pathology.

- Pathologic alterations seen in the lung include consolidation, atelectasis, pleural fluid, masses, emphysema, pneumothorax, and pulmonary embolus. Each of these abnormalities produces clearly recognizable patterns.
- The concepts of the silhouette sign and the air bronchogram were described as was their importance in localizing pulmonary consolidations.
- Acinar (air space) disease produces distinctive radiographic changes of "white dots on a black background" that allows its differentiation from interstitial disease which produces "black dots on a white background."
- Specific entities discussed included postoperative appearances, the effects of radiation, the changes that may occur in patients with AIDS, and the findings in pulmonary tuberculosis.
- Conditions specific to newborns and older children include immature lung disease, hyaline membrane disease, bronchopulmonary dysplasia, wet lung disease, meconium aspiration, and bronchiolitis.
- "Garden variety" pneumonias and asthma appear similar in the pediatric age group as well as in adults.

SUGGESTED ADDITIONAL READING

Fraser RS, Colman N, Muller N, Paré PD. Synopsis of diseases of the chest. 3rd ed. Philadelphia: WB Saunders, 2005.

Hansell D, Armstrong P, Lynch, McAdams HP. Imaging of diseases of the chest. 4th ed. St. Louis: Mosby, 2005.

Hedlund GL, Griscom NT, Cleveland RH, Kirks DR. Respiratory system. In: Kirks DR, Griscom NT, eds. Practical pediatric imaging. Diagnostic radiology of infants and children, 3rd ed. Philadelphia: Lippincott-Raven, 1998.

Ketai L, Meholic A, Lofgren R. Fundamentals of chest radiology. 2nd ed. Philadelphia: W.B. Saunders, 2006.

McLoud T. Thoracic radiology. The requisites. St. Louis: Mosby, 1999.

Reed JC. Chest radiography: plain film patterns and differential diagnoses. 5th ed. St. Louis: Mosby, 2003.

Cardiac Imaging

5

Cardiovascular radiology is a subspecialty shared by radiologists and cardiologists. Although most cardiac imaging is performed by cardiologists, radiologists still play an important role in the diagnosis of heart disease. Too often, the clinician is content merely to have made a diagnosis of "large heart," "congestive heart failure," or "congenital heart disease." It is possible, however, for you, as the clinician, to recognize certain patterns of disease based on the alterations those diseases produce in the pulmonary vascularity and in specific chambers of the heart on routine radiographs. The evaluation of the patient with suspected cardiac disease should be directed along two distinct lines—imaging of anatomic changes and demonstration of physiologic function—often simultaneously. Although the former goal can be attained through radiographs, radionuclide studies, and echocardiography, the latter may be achieved only through cardiac catheterization, which permits hemodynamic measurements and injection of contrast material. As discussed in the following section, developments in imaging technology have made it possible to make accurate diagnoses using noninvasive techniques.

This chapter discusses the criteria for certain *categories* of diseases rather than describing specific entities. For a complete discussion of those entities, you should consult a comprehensive text on cardiology.

TECHNICAL CONSIDERATIONS

The advances in diagnostic imaging techniques in the past three decades have revolutionized cardiac imaging. Radiography, cardiac series, cardiac fluoroscopy, and cardiac catheterization were the mainstays of cardiac imaging before 1975. However, real-time ultrasound imaging, radionuclide cardiac perfusion studies, computed tomography (CT), and magnetic resonance (MR) imaging have become standard evaluation tools in the hands of the cardiovascular radiologist and the cardiologist. High-detail CT cardiac images, using intravenous contrast, allow the demonstration of coronary arteries with a high degree of accuracy, approaching that for coronary angiography. MR coronary arteriography has also achieved significant success as a noninvasive method of studying cardiac circulation. The clinician has a great number of options available to evaluate patients. As with any other organ system, your choice of diagnostic studies will depend on getting the most information in the safest way at the lowest cost. Therefore, consulting with your radiologist or referring cardiologist is mandatory.

The same technical considerations for chest radiography that were discussed in Chapter 4 for pulmonary disease apply when evaluating the heart radiographically. You should first decide if the film is a posterior-anterior (PA) or anterior-posterior (AP) view, if the patient is lordotic, and if rotation is present. The degree of penetration on the film (darkness or lightness), the presence of motion, and the degree of inspiration are important factors to consider. A radiograph made with the patient in a slightly lordotic position will falsely distort and magnify the cardiac size. A film that is too light will accentuate the pulmonary vessels. A film with

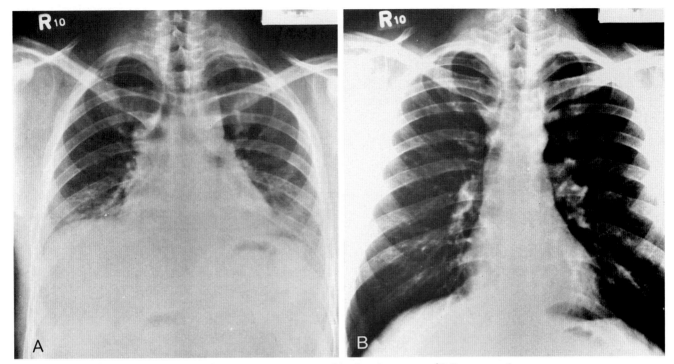

Figure 5.1.   Difference in radiographic appearance caused by inspiratory result in a normal individual. A. PA radiograph made in forced expiration. There is poor inspiratory result. The diaphragm is flat and the heart appears enlarged. Prominence of the pulmonary vessels can be seen. **B.** The same individual in full inspiration. Notice the differences in appearance.

the patient not in maximum inspiration may result in further accentuation of pulmonary vessels and cause an appearance of cardiac enlargement and/or an erroneous diagnosis of congestive heart failure (Fig. 5.1).

It is also necessary to pay close attention to the patient's body habitus. A narrow AP diameter of the chest or a pectus excavatum deformity may result in anterior compression of the heart and a spurious appearance of cardiac enlargement (Fig. 5.2).

In the bony thorax, particular attention should be given to the undersurfaces of the ribs for any evidence of rib notching. Although the most common cause of rib notching is coarctation of the aorta, many other conditions, such as tetralogy of Fallot, truncus arteriosus, status following a Blalock-Taussig operation, or neurofibromatosis, produce this abnormality.

The basic imaging techniques used for evaluating the heart are (1) chest radiography, (2) cardiac fluoroscopy, (3) cardiac catheterization and coronary arteriography (angiocardiography), (4) echocardiography, (5) radioisotope studies, (6) CT, and (7) MR imaging. Echocardiography is the most commonly used diagnostic imaging tool for evaluating patients with suspected heart disease. This procedure is performed almost exclusively by cardiologists and, in the United States, has largely replaced the cardiac series and cardiac fluoroscopy. The other imaging modalities are used in various combinations, as discussed in the following sections.

Chest Radiography

Chest radiography is the standard imaging examination in patients with suspected cardiac disease. By knowing the normal anatomy portrayed on the PA and lateral films and by analyzing the sizes of pulmonary arteries and veins, you may be able to make correct diagnoses in many patients. The four-view "cardiac series" was used to determine heart chamber enlargement. It has been largely replaced by echocardiography.

A popular method used to determine cardiac size is the *cardiothoracic ratio:* the maximum width of the cardiac shadow on the PA chest film divided by the maximum width of the thorax. This method has received criticism because a true determination of cardiac enlargement requires evaluating the cardiac silhouette on *both* the PA and lateral views. Generally, however, the cardiac width should never exceed half the width of the thorax on the PA film.

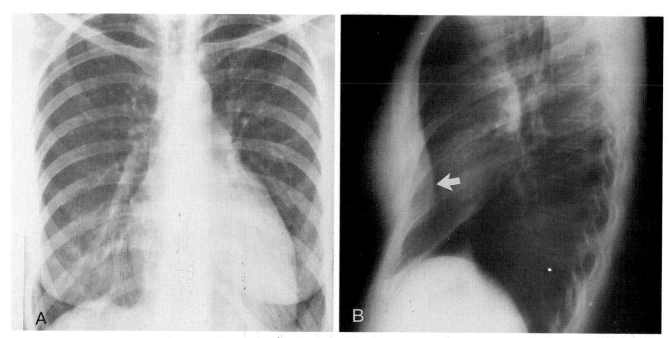

Figure 5.2. Pectus excavatum deformity. A. Frontal radiograph shows apparent enlargement of the heart. The ribs are slightly more horizontal posteriorly and steeper anteriorly. **B.** Lateral radiograph shows a prominent pectus excavatum deformity (*arrow*). The sternal deformity compressed the heart and gave the spurious appearance of enlargement.

Cardiac Fluoroscopy

Fluoroscopic examination of the heart and pulmonary vessels is only occasionally used for assessing cardiac motion, contour, and dynamics (useful for evaluation of cardiac aneurysms); investigating intracardiac calcifications (valvular, coronary artery, or pericardial); and evaluating patients with suspected pericardial effusion (dampened pulsations and displaced subepicardial fat line). It has largely been replaced in the United States by echocardiography.

Cardiac Catheterization and Coronary Arteriography

Cardiac catheterization and coronary arteriography are invasive procedures performed almost exclusively by cardiologists or cardiovascular radiologists. These procedures allow accurate evaluation of the size and configuration of the cardiac chambers, the great vessels, and the coronary arteries. The most common use is in patients with known or suspected vascular occlusive disease. The tests are also performed to evaluate patients with suspected shunt lesions. Real-time echocardiography has decreased the number of catheterizations used to determine cardiac chamber size and configuration. Coronary artery CT may further decrease the number of catheterizations performed for patients with chest pain.

Echocardiography

Echocardiography is an ultrasound examination of the heart and great vessels primarily using one of three techniques: motion-mode (M-mode), cross-sectional (two-dimensional) imaging, or Doppler technique. Two other methods, exercise echocardiography and transesophageal echocardiography, are used for special circumstances. Cardiac ultrasound is the principle diagnostic tool for investigating cardiac abnormalities in both children and adults.

Conventional ultrasound of the solid viscera relies on the principle of the velocity of sound traveling through a medium, reflecting off a tissue interface, and returning to the transducer. An internal computer calculates the distance of that interface from the transducer and displays the image on a monitor. Moving interfaces, such as would be encountered in the beating heart, produce echographs that change as a result of variations in the distance to the transducer. For

Figure 5.3. Ultrasound display modes.
The transducer passing over objects of varying size portrays those objects in a different fashion depending on the display mode. In brightness mode (B-mode), the objects appear as dots; in motion mode (M-mode), they appear as a series of wavy lines.

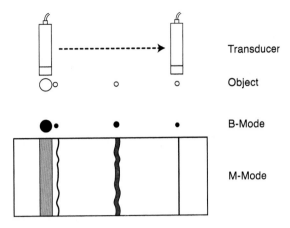

this reason, cardiac and vascular (Doppler) ultrasound studies are significantly different from those of static organs.

All forms of cardiac ultrasound evolved from M-mode echocardiography. M-mode ultrasound displays cardiac motion as a one-dimensional recording over a period that can be displayed either on a cathode ray tube (CRT) monitor or on a paper strip tracing (Fig. 5.3). This allows for measuring the depth of each structure as well as displaying its motion (Fig. 5.4). Two-dimensional cross-sectional echocardiography provides real-time images of the moving heart chambers. By shifting the transducer and altering the depth of penetration of the ultrasound beam, a tomographic image of the heart and its chambers can be obtained.

Doppler echocardiography, with or without color-flow technology, makes possible the study of interruptions or obstruction of flowing blood and thus is used primarily to assess the direction and velocity of blood flow within the heart and great vessels. It is particularly useful in evaluating the carotid vessels in patients with transient ischemic attacks (Fig. 5.5) as well as the integrity and motion of the cardiac valves. Color-flow Doppler superimposes a color-coded, real-time depiction of velocity and direction of blood flow on a two-dimensional image. The added color helps in the interpretation of the study.

Echocardiography is performed by placing the transducer on the neck, chest, and abdomen to obtain parasternal long- and short-axis, apical, subcostal, and suprasternal images (Figs. 5.6 and 5.7). Figure 5.8 illustrates some of the normal anatomic structures demonstrated by this technique. For greater detail, consult either of the excellent texts by Feigenbaum or Higgins listed at the end of this chapter.

Overall, the most common indications for echocardiography are suspected chamber enlargement, congenital heart disease, abnormalities of heart valves, abnormalities of contractility, and suspected pericardial effusions. This examination is performed primarily by cardiologists.

Figure 5.4. M-mode echocardiogram showing a pericardial effusion (*eff*). A. Pericardium. **B.** Left ventricular wall. **C.** Chorda tendinea. **D.** Mitral valve. **E.** Septal wall. **F.** Electrocardiogram. **G.** Right ventricular wall. **H.** Chest wall.

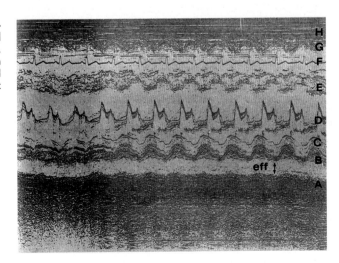

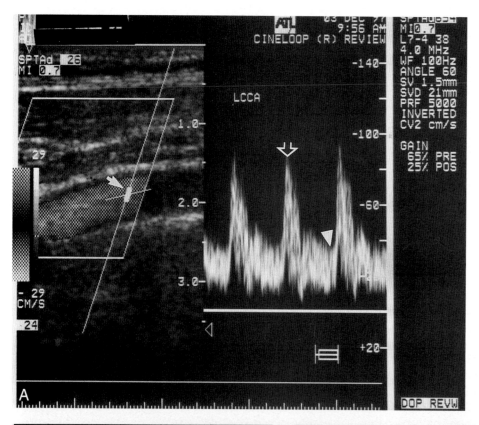

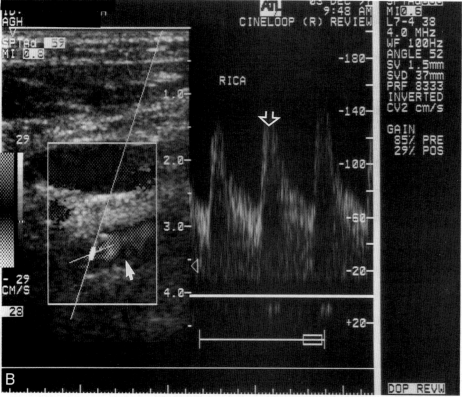

Figure 5.5. Carotid Doppler ultrasound examination. A. Normal left common carotid artery (LCCA). The gray-scale image of a portion of the LCCA shows the vessel to be widely patent. The vessel walls are smooth, without visible atheromatous plaques. The rectangle within the vessel lumen (*small arrow on left*) is the Doppler sample site from which the flow characteristics and velocities generate the Doppler waveform tracing shown to the right of the gray-scale image. There is a normal peak systolic flow velocity of approximately 90 cm/sec (*open arrow; normal = <125 cm/sec*) as well as antegrade blood flow velocity of 40 cm/sec at the end of diastole (*arrowhead*). The Doppler waveform also allows for evaluation of the degree of laminar flow disruption or "turbulence." This is reflected by the range of red blood cell velocities. The greater the velocity range, the greater the turbulence. This normal vessel demonstrates a velocity range of 40 to 90 cm/sec. **B.** Significant stenosis in a right internal carotid artery (RICA). The gray-scale image of a portion of the RICA shows gross vessel wall irregularity with significant stenosis near the Doppler sample site (*small arrow on left*). The Doppler waveform tracing shows an elevated peak systolic flow with velocities of 140 cm/sec (*open arrow*). In addition, there is marked turbulence as a result of the increased red blood cell velocity. Compare these tracings and images with A.

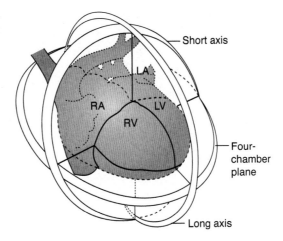

Figure 5.6. Normal planes of echocardiographic scans. LA, left atrium; LV, left ventricle; RA, right atrium; RV, right ventricle.

Radioisotope Studies

Radioisotope studies are performed primarily to evaluate cardiac perfusion and function. Radioisotopes such as thallium-201 and technetium-99m sestamibi are injected intravenously, and myocardial perfusion is recorded. A myocardial imaging study can be performed with a combination of both radioisotopes or with sestamibi alone for both rest and stress imaging (Fig. 5.9). This technique is most useful for evaluating significant cardiac disease in the setting of risk factors and for determining subsequent risk stratification for significant future myocardial events in the setting of abnormal findings (Fig. 5.10).

Positron emission tomography (PET) studies with F-18 fluoro-2-deoxyglucose (F-18 FDG) are used to assess the viability of myocardial tissue, especially when coronary artery bypass

Parasternal Long-Axis View

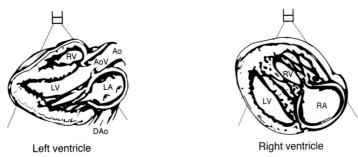

Left ventricle   Right ventricle

Parasternal Short-Axis View

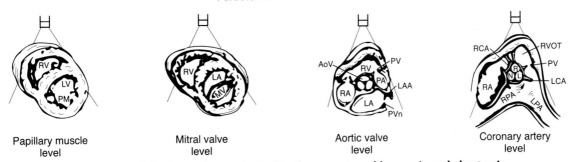

Papillary muscle   Mitral valve   Aortic valve   Coronary artery
level   level   level   level

Figure 5.7. Anatomy of the heart demonstrated in the parasternal long-axis and short-axis views. Ao, aorta; AoV, aortic valve (with right, left, and neutral cusps); DAo, descending aorta; LA, left atrium; LAA, left atrial appendage; LCA, left coronary artery; LPA, left pulmonary artery; LV, left ventricle; MV, mitral valve; PA, pulmonary artery; PM, papillary muscle; PV, pulmonic valve; PVn, pulmonary vein; RA, right atrium; RCA, right coronary artery; RPA, right pulmonary artery; RV, right ventricle; RVOT, right ventricular outflow tract.

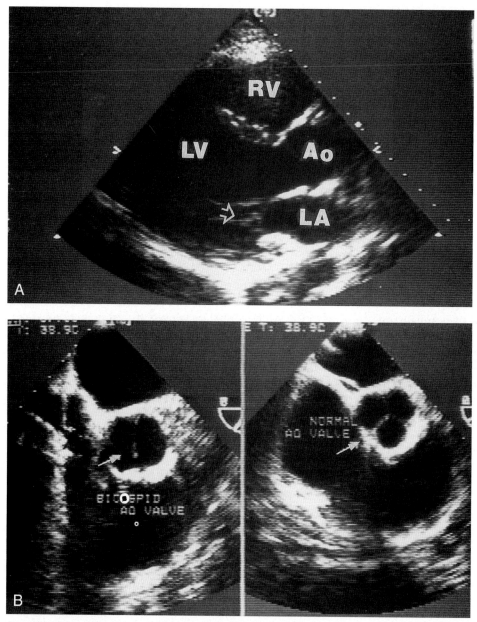

Figure 5.8. Normal echocardiographic anatomy. A. Two-dimensional parasternal view showing the normal right ventricle (*RV*), left ventricle (*LV*), ascending aorta (*Ao*), and left atrium (*LA*). The aortic valve is open in this view made in systole. The mitral valve is closed (*arrow*). **B.** Aortic valve variations showing a bicuspid valve in the left panel and a normal tricuspid valve in the right panel (*arrows*).

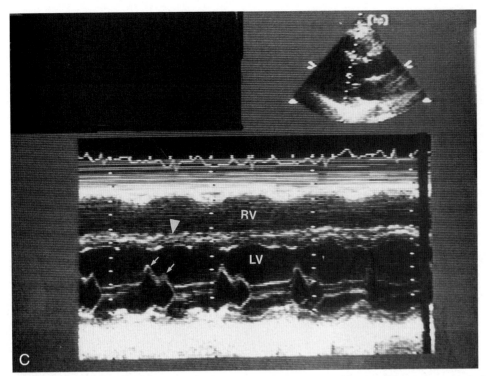

Figure 5.8. *(continued)* **C.** M-mode parasternal view shows a normal right ventricle (*RV*), interventricular septum (*arrowhead*), mitral valve (*small arrows*), and left ventricle (*LV*).

surgery is being considered. Acquiring this data in concordance with gating of the cardiac cycle allows functional assessment of the left ventricular ejection fraction as well.

Although the new advances in PET and CT angiography are significantly improving the diagnosis and management of cardiac disease, the previously mentioned conventional techniques are still quite viable because of their widespread availability and lower cost.

Lastly, radioisotope ventriculography studies with technetium-99m–tagged red blood cells is also used to analyze the right and left ventricular ejection fractions in patients who are scheduled to undergo cardiothoracic surgery or are going to receive chemotherapy that may affect cardiac function.

Computed Tomography

CT, performed with electrocardiographic CT gating, is used with contrast enhancement for various cardiac conditions. In this technique, dynamic scanning—multiple images of one section—is performed to evaluate flow through a particular chamber or vessel. In addition, CT is used to evaluate the patency of coronary artery bypass grafts, to assess the extent of myocardial infarcts, to depict the size and location of left ventricular aneurysms, to detect aneurysms of the thoracic aorta, to diagnose aortic dissections (Fig. 5.11), to define certain congenital

Figure 5.9. Normal thallium cardiac scan during stress testing. Distribution of blood flow is uniform over the left ventricle, as evidenced by the uniform distribution of the isotope.

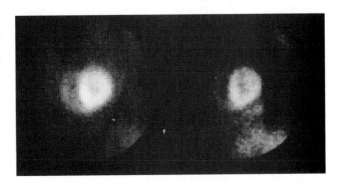

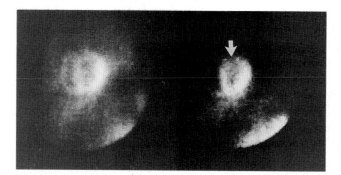

Figure 5.10. Cardiac ischemia. Ischemic disease of the anterior left ventricular wall, as demonstrated by a photopenic area (*arrow*) during a stress test. Compare with Figure 5.9.

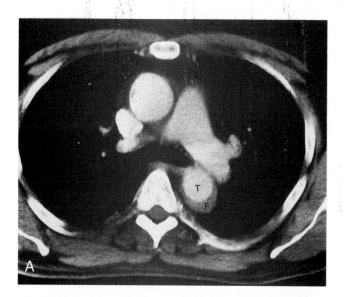

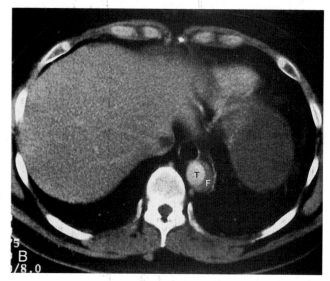

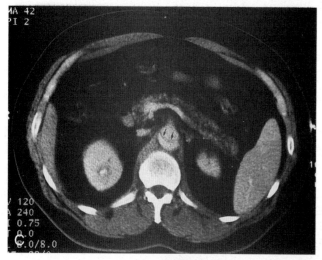

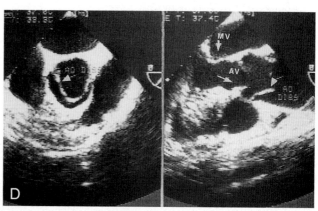

Figure 5.11. Aortic dissection demonstrated by computed tomography (CT) and echocardiography. A and B. CT sections at the levels of the carina and liver, respectively, demonstrate the true (*T*) and false (*F*) lumens. Notice the contrast-opacified blood in the true lumen. **C.** Section near the top of the kidneys shows contrast in both the true and false lumens. Notice the intimal flap (*arrows*). **D.** Echocardiogram. Left panel is a short-axis image of the aortic root and shows the intimal flap (*arrowhead*) of the dissection with the crescent false lumen beyond. Right panel shows a long-axis image of the aortic root with the intimal flap of the dissection (*arrowhead*). The mitral valve (*MV, short arrow*) is closed and the aortic valve (*AV, long arrow*) is open.

Figure 5.12.   Volume-rendering technique image from a cardiac CT angiogram performed on a 64-row multidetector CT scanner. This 62-year-old man had a strong family history of coronary artery disease and hypercholesterolemia. The left main coronary artery arises from the root of the aorta beneath the left atrial appendage. The left anterior descending coronary artery (LAD) is in the interventricular groove. A large diagonal branch (DB) arises from the LAD. No significant plaque formation or stenosis is evident. (Courtesy of H. Scott Beasley, MD, Department of Radiology, Western Pennsylvania Hospital.)

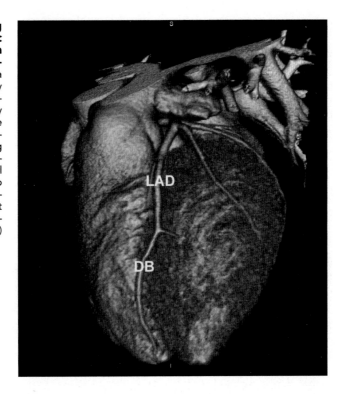

abnormalities such as coarctation of the aorta and anomalous venous connections, and to assess the pericardium for effusions. Dynamic CT is also used to determine myocardial wall thickness and dynamics, although echocardiography is used much more commonly. *Helical CT* is especially useful because of its speed and its ability to overlap areas of interest. *Electron beam CT*, a variation of conventional CT, is used to detect and quantify coronary artery calcifications. It is primarily a screening type of examination for determining the risk of ischemic heart disease.

The introduction of multidetector CT scans (with 16, 32, or 64 rows) has expanded the application of CT scanning for evaluation of coronary artery disease. The fast scan times and the ability to gate the CT images to certain portions of the cardiac cycle has made possible CT reconstruction of the relatively small coronary arteries with excellent anatomic detail and without any motion artifact resulting from the beating heart (Fig. 5.12). CT can often detect soft plaque (Fig. 5.13), which cannot be visualized on cardiac catheterization studies. This imaging technology also allows the reconstruction of three-dimensional images displaying the anatomic relationships of the coronary arteries (Figs. 5.14 and 5.15). Multidetector CT is very useful for the evaluation of congenital anomalies of the coronary artery (Fig. 5.16). The radiation dose from a cardiac CT is similar to a nuclear medicine thallium scan.

In summary, 64-slice CT cardiac angiography offers several advantages over invasive angiography:

- It is noninvasive and thus without the complications of traditional angiography.
- A CT scan of the entire heart may be performed in less than 15 seconds.
- There is no need for a hospital stay.
- It is cost-effective.
- It gives better depiction of coronary anomalies.
- It provides clear demonstration of calcium deposits and plaque morphology.
- It better delineates stenoses at the origins of the coronary arteries.
- It allows "one-stop shop" analysis of the coronary arteries, heart valves, myocardial mass, ventricles, plaque morphology, and lung parenchyma.
- It allows three-dimensional volume-rendered images.

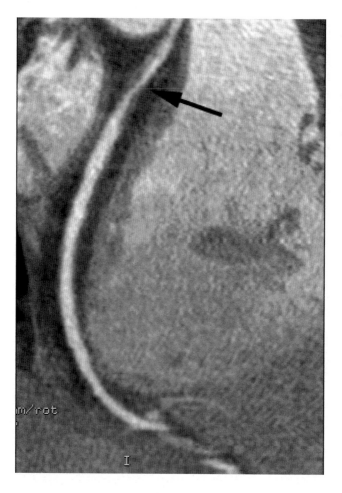

Figure 5.13. CT scan shows the right coronary artery arising from the left cusp. The right coronary artery (*arrow*) must pass between the aorta (*A*) and the pulmonary artery. This anatomic variant can lead to fatal arrhythmias. (Courtesy of Carl Fuhrman, MD, Department of Radiology, University of Pittsburgh School of Medicine.)

Magnetic Resonance Imaging

MR imaging is used to diagnose many of the same abnormalities that can be seen with CT. Electrocardiographic gating is used for "stop-action" images of the heart and great vessels. MR imaging has the advantage of portraying flowing blood as a signal void (black) so that it is easy to distinguish blood from solid structures. MR imaging is very useful for evaluating patients with aortic dissections and aortic coarctation (Fig. 5.17), although multidetector CT is increasingly used for evaluation of aortic disease in patients who do not have a contraindication to

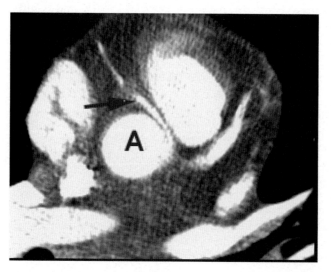

Figure 5.14. CT reconstruction of right coronary artery shows atheromatous (*arrow*) plaque narrowing the proximal portion of the artery in a young man with atypical chest pain and a normal stress test. A stress test is usually not positive until a vessel is 75% narrowed. This abnormality would not be detected on electron beam CT because there are no calcifications. (Courtesy of Carl Fuhrman, MD, Department of Radiology, University of Pittsburgh School of Medicine.)

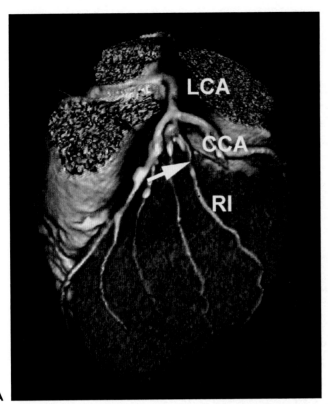
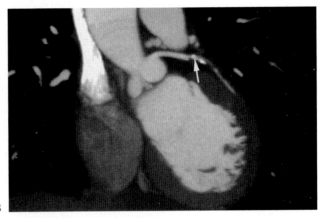

A

B

Figure 5.15.   A 63-year-old female with atypical chest pain and a negative nuclear stress test. A. Volume-rendered image from a 64-slice cardiac CT angiogram shows the left main coronary artery (*LCA*) arising from the aortic root (cut away). The circumflex coronary artery (*CCA*) in the atrioventricular groove and a large ramus intermedius branch (*RI*) have been outlined in gray in this image. A mixed calcified and soft plaque is present in the proximal portion of the ramus intermedius, causing significant stenosis (*arrow*). **B.** Coronal maximal intensity projection image of the left main coronary artery shows the lesion in the proximal segment of the ramus intermedius (*arrow*). (Courtesy of H. Scott Beasley, MD, Department of Radiology, Western Pennsylvania Hospital.)

Figure 5.16.   Volume rendered three-dimensional image of the origin of the left coronary artery from the aorta. The left main coronary artery (*arrow*) is very short before dividing into the left anterior descending (LAD) and circumflex (CIR) coronary arteries. The first and second diagonal branches are clearly defined. (Courtesy of Carl Fuhrman, MD, Department of Radiology, University of Pittsburgh School of Medicine.)

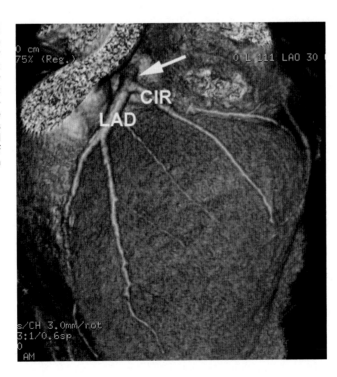

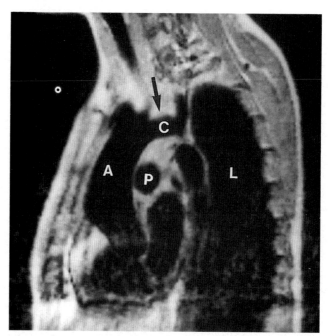

Figure 5.17.   Cardiac application of magnetic resonance (MR) imaging. Parasagittal MR image showing coarctation of the aorta (arrow). Notice the following landmarks: A, ascending aorta; C, coarctation; P, pulmonary artery; L, lung.

the use of contrast. In addition, *magnetic resonance angiography (MRA)* is used as a noninvasive method of evaluating vascular problems (Fig. 5.18).

Other uses for MR imaging are routinely evaluating cardiac anatomy and morphology, evaluating global and regional myocardial function and assessing heart valves (including calculating pressure gradients and quantifying valvular regurgitation), and calculating any shunt fractions. MR imaging is also very useful for evaluating pericardial disease and differentiating restrictive pericardial disease from restrictive myocardial disease, which is not easily done with echocardiography. Research is continuing into the use of MR for coronary artery imaging, although it is not available for routine clinical use at the present time.

MR imaging is also used for evaluating myocardial perfusion, or detecting nonperfused portions of myocardium (Fig. 5.19), after the intravenous injection of MR contrast (gadolinium). The nonperfused portions of the myocardium remain dark, and the perfused portions of myocardium become brighter as a result of the delivery of gadolinium to the myocardium. Tissue viability can then be determined by imaging a short time later. A special pulsing sequence is chosen to make normal myocardium very dark, and the nonviable myocardium becomes bright (Figs. 5.20 and 5.21). The distinction between viable and nonviable myocardium can be very important in the decision to perform coronary artery bypass surgery, and MR imaging is useful in distinguishing between "stunned" and "hibernating" myocardium and nonviable myocardium.

MR imaging is very useful in the evaluation of cardiac masses and tumors and can often be useful in separating thrombus from tumor in the heart chambers (Fig. 5.22). The ability of MR to distinguish different signal characteristics among different tissues is very useful for evaluating infiltrative diseases of the myocardium. MR can detect fatty and fibrous infiltration of the right ventricle and is useful in the evaluation of patients with suspected arrhythmogenic right ventricular dysplasia and other cardiomyopathies.

Remember that the presence of a cardiac pacemaker is a contraindication to MR, and MR images must be obtained before placement of pacemakers and intracardiac defibrillating devices. MR imaging requires a relatively normal electrocardiogram (ECG), and arrhythmias (including atrial fibrillation and frequent premature ventricular contractions) may not permit adequate imaging.

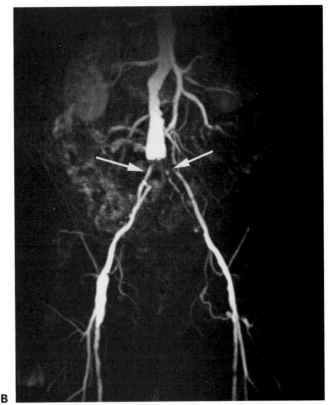

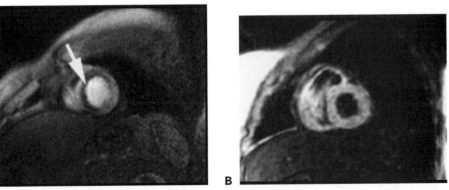

Figure 5.18. Magnetic resonance angiograms (MRA). A. MRA of the great vessels in a patient with subclavian steal syndrome. Notice the stenosis of the right subclavian artery (*arrow*) and poststenotic dilatation. Compare with the left. **B.** MRA of aortoiliac runoff. There is stenosis of both common iliac arteries (*arrows*). Notice the plaque in the distal aorta.

Figure 5.19. Short-axis image of right and left ventricles. A. The septum (*arrow*) and portions of the anterior wall remain dark after administration of intravenous gadolinium, indicating ischemic or nonviable myocardium. **B.** A different patient with normal uniform perfusion of the myocardium. (Courtesy of Carl Fuhrman, MD, Department of Radiology, University of Pittsburgh School of Medicine.)

Figure 5.20. Normal myocardial viability. The left ventricular myocardium (*) remains very dark on this pulsing sequence. Intravenous gadolinium was administered approximately 15 minutes earlier for perfusion imaging. (Courtesy of Carl Fuhrman, MD, Department of Radiology, University of Pittsburgh School of Medicine.)

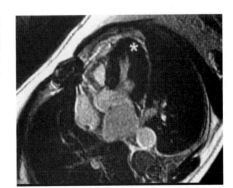

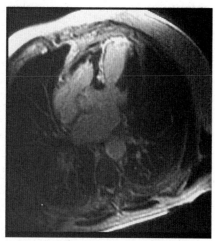

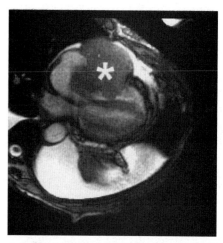

Figure 5.21.   Abnormal myocardial viability. (This is the same patient as in Fig. 5.19A.) The septum and portions of the anterior wall are bright on this pulsing sequence, indicating nonviable myocardium. Compare with Figure 5.20. Coronary artery revascularization would not be beneficial for this patient. (Courtesy of Carl Fuhrman, MD, Department of Radiology, University of Pittsburgh School of Medicine.)

Figure 5.22.   Cardiac plasmacytoma (*) involving the right atrium and right ventricle. (Courtesy of Carl Fuhrman, MD, Department of Radiology, University of Pittsburgh School of Medicine.)

ANATOMIC CONSIDERATIONS

To appreciate the anatomic relationships of the heart and its chambers, you need to think in three-dimensional terms. The following sections examine the position of the cardiac chambers, the great vessels, and the aortic and mitral valves, as seen in the four radiographic views in Figure 5.23.

Cardiac Chambers

On the *PA view* (see Fig. 5.23A), most of the cardiac silhouette is made up almost exclusively of the right side of the heart; the left ventricle forms the left cardiac border. The position of the anterior interventricular sulcus may be determined on an angiocardiogram by following the course of the anterior descending branch of the left coronary artery. The right atrium forms the right border of the heart, merging imperceptibly into the image of the superior vena cava. The left atrium is not seen in this view under normal circumstances. However, a small portion of the left border of the heart just beneath the pulmonary trunk is represented by the left atrial appendage. In this view, the aortic valve is positioned obliquely, with its lower end oriented to the right approximately in the midline just below the waist of the cardiovascular silhouette. The mitral valve, which is oriented on a similar plane in this view, lies just below the aortic valve area and to the left. Occasionally, calcification of these valves or their annuli will be seen on this view (Fig. 5.24).

In the *normal lateral view* (see Fig. 5.23B), the anterior border of the cardiac silhouette consists of the right ventricle. The posterior and inferior cardiac border is that of the left ventricle. The image of the inferior vena cava superimposes on the posteroinferior border of the left ventricle, occasionally extending just posterior to the left ventricular outline. The left atrium forms the superoposterior border of the heart. The esophagus, when filled with barium, courses almost immediately posterior to the cardiac silhouette. Normally, it should not be indented by the heart. Occasionally, the image of the pulmonary artery is observed arching up from the right ventricle and passing inferiorly to the arch of the aorta, which is also visible on the lateral film. In this view, the aortic valve lies almost horizontally just below the narrow waist of the cardiovascular pedicle. As indicated in Figure 5.23B, the mitral valve ring lies in an oblique plane, inferior and posterior to that of the aortic valve. Valvar calcification can also be seen in this view.

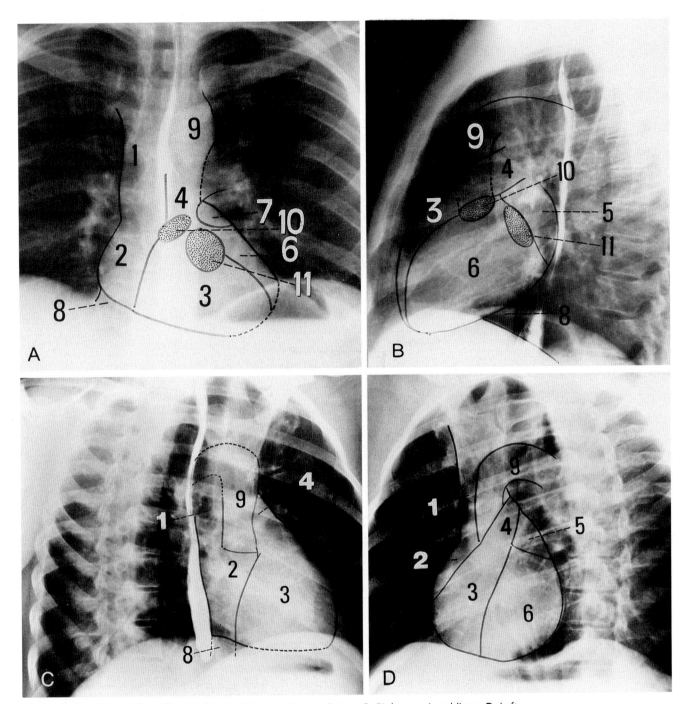

Figure 5.23.   Normal cardiac series. A. PA view. **B.** Lateral view. **C.** Right anterior oblique. **D.** Left anterior oblique. 1, superior vena cava; 2, right atrium; 3, right ventricle; 4, pulmonary outflow tract; 5, left atrium; 6, left ventricle; 7, left atrial appendage; 8, inferior vena cava; 9, ascending aorta and aortic arch; 10, aortic valve; 11, mitral valve.

In the *right anterior oblique view* (see Fig. 5.23C), the bulk of the cardiac silhouette consists of the right ventricle. The left ventricle contributes a small portion to the cardiac silhouette over the apex anteriorly. The right cardiac border consists of the right atrium inferiorly and the left atrium superiorly. In this position, a barium-filled esophagus should not be indented in any way; if this occurs, it indicates an enlarged left atrium.

In the *left anterior oblique position* (see Fig. 5.23D), all the cardiac chambers contribute to the cardiac silhouette. Only a small segment of the upper portion of the right heart border is

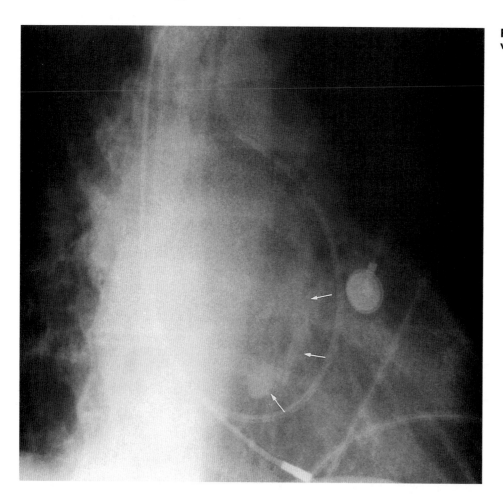

Figure 5.24. Calcified mitral valve annulus (*arrows*).

formed by the right atrial appendage; the rest is delineated by the right ventricle. On the left side, the lower border is exclusively the left ventricle. The left atrium forms the upper portion of the left silhouette. In a normal heart, the image of the left ventricle should not overlap that of the thoracic vertebrae by more than 1 cm. An overlap larger than this indicates left ventricular enlargement. A small, "clear," aerated area is present just above the border of the left atrium. In patients with left atrial enlargement (LAE), this area "fills in."

One additional useful anatomic relationship to note is that of the *mainstem bronchi* to the heart. The trachea bifurcates below the aortic arch. The bronchi continue downward and branch from this point. The left mainstem bronchus, however, has a close relationship with the left atrium. Consequently, enlargement of the left atrium may result in elevation of the left mainstem bronchus and widening of the normal carinal angle to greater than 75° in adults; greater angulation is allowed for infants and children.

On an echocardiogram, the normal anatomy is as depicted in Figures 5.7 and 5.8.

Pulmonary Vasculature

The pulmonary arteries and veins constitute the lung markings seen on a chest radiograph. It is sometimes difficult to differentiate between arteries and veins on a radiograph. However, a useful method is by analyzing the *direction* of the vessels to determine whether they are arterial or venous. Normally, the pulmonary arteries radiate from the hilar region in a fairly uniform, fanlike appearance (Fig. 5.25A). The veins, on the other hand, follow a different course because of the lower location of the left atrium, into which they must terminate. The upper lobe veins assume an obliquely downward course, in some instances almost vertical, as they "dive" for the left atrium; the lower lobe veins assume a more horizontal course, located

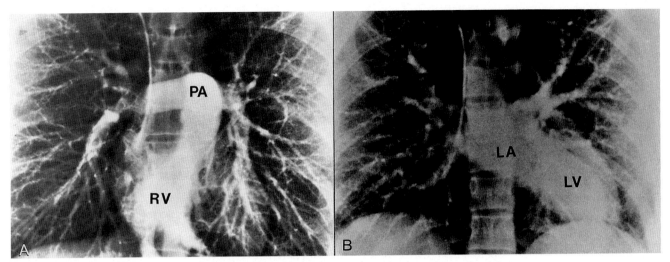

Figure 5.25.   Normal pulmonary arteriogram. A. Arterial phase. Injection was made into the right ventricle (*RV*). Contrast material passes through the pulmonary outflow tract into the pulmonary arteries (*PA*). **B.** Venous phase. Contrast material passes from the pulmonary veins into the left atrium (*LA*) and then into the left ventricle (*LV*). Notice the difference in orientation between the pulmonary arteries and pulmonary veins.

almost directly opposite the level of the left atrium (see Fig. 5.25B). It is important to be able to differentiate arteries from veins because the proposed approach for diagnosis is based on analysis of the pulmonary vasculature.

In a normal heart, the vascularity of the lower lobes is more prominent than that of the upper lobes. This relationship is altered in a normal person in the recumbent position, where gravity results in greater flow to the cephalic regions.

Aortic Arch

Finally, it is important to observe the side on which the aortic arch is located and the position of the gastric air bubble. Under normal circumstances, the aortic arch is on the left. However, there are anomalies of this vessel in which the arch is on the right (Fig. 5.26). The gastric air bubble is ordinarily on the left. However, in patients with certain forms of *situs inversus* and *dextrocardia* (Fig. 5.27), the gastric bubble is on the right. Always check the film orientation and markings carefully to avoid the pitfall this condition engenders.

Figure 5.26.   Right aortic arch (*AA*) in an elderly patient with no evidence of heart disease.

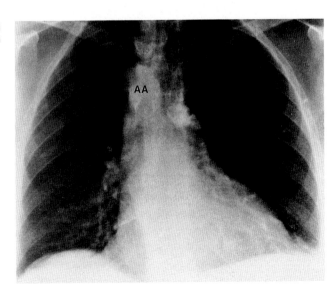

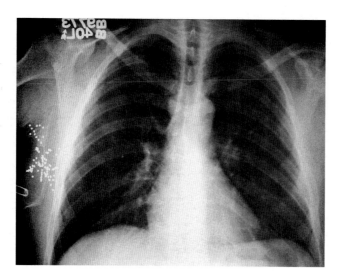

Figure 5.27. Situs inversus and dextrocardia in a patient who suffered a gunshot wound to the left axilla. The radiograph is oriented in the customary viewing position. If one were in doubt about the laterality, the easiest way to solve the dilemma would be to examine the patient!

PATHOLOGIC CONSIDERATIONS

There are many ways to classify cardiac disease. A popular classification uses two large categories—*congenital* and *acquired*. Congenital cardiac disease is further subdivided into *cyanotic* and *acyanotic* types. Most books on cardiology prefer this method. For the noncardiologist, a *physiologic* approach affords an understandable and useful basis for dealing with congenital and acquired heart disease. In addition, it is preferable to evaluate patients with cardiac disease on the basis of their age. This discussion focuses on the radiographic evaluation of these patients, because that is the type of imaging examination you will order first and with which you will be most familiar. Once you have an idea of the kind of cardiac disease you are dealing with, you can order more-sophisticated imaging procedures, such as echocardiography, angiography, or MR imaging, to make a definitive diagnosis.

Adult Patients

From a physiologic standpoint, all types of cardiac disease may be categorized into the following:
  I. Obstruction
 II. Volume overload
    A. Shunt (right-to-left, left-to-right)
    B. Admixture
    C. Valvular insufficiency
III. Disorders of contraction or relaxation
    A. Myocardial disease
    B. Conduction disorders (arrhythmias)
 IV. Combination of the preceding
No matter what the cause, all cardiac diseases will show evidence of one or more of these patterns.

Evaluation of the *pulmonary vascularity* is an important step that allows one to exclude many diseases. The *physiologic* type of disease may be inferred from the pattern of pulmonary blood flow. Pulmonary vascularity may be normal, decreased, or increased. Figure 5.28 illustrates the varying forms of pulmonary blood flow and lists some important disease processes that accompany those patterns. Normal pulmonary vessels should be about the same size as those of an accompanying airway. Any significant disparity in size is abnormal (Fig. 5.29).

Surprising as it may seem, patients with *normal pulmonary vascularity* may have significant cardiac disease. In these patients, the heart has compensated for the abnormality by becoming enlarged. The pulmonary vascularity remains normal until the heart decompensates. Diseases that enlarge cardiac chambers without appreciably changing the pulmonary vascularity until decompensation occurs include cardiomyopathy, coronary artery disease, hypertensive

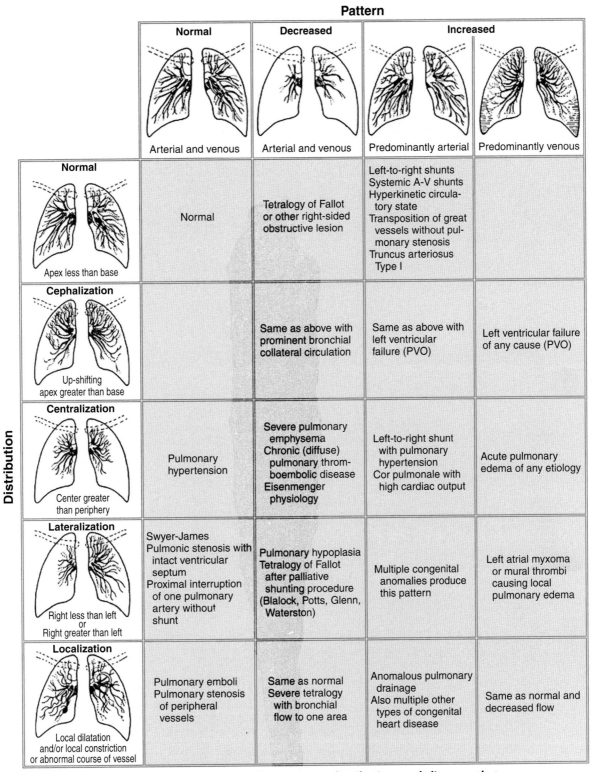

Figure 5.28. Correlation of pulmonary vascular patterns, distribution, and diseases that produce the patterns. A-V, arteriovenous; PVO, pulmonary venous obstruction.

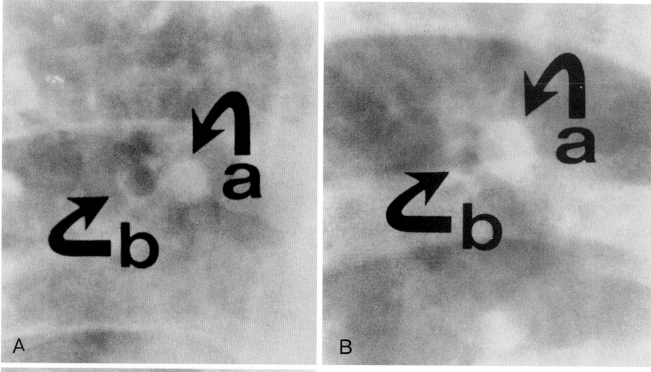

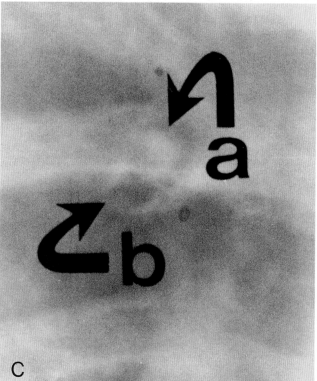

Figure 5.29.   Comparison of pulmonary artery (a) with companion bronchus (b). A. Normal blood flow. The artery and the bronchus are approximately equal in size. **B.** Shunt vascularity (increased arterial flow). The artery is larger than the bronchus in this patient with an atrial septal defect. **C.** Diminished pulmonary arterial flow. The artery is smaller than the bronchus in this patient with tetralogy of Fallot.

cardiovascular disease, aortic stenosis, and coarctation of the aorta. All these conditions, except coarctation and a form of aortic stenosis, are acquired.

Decreased vascularity indicates a severe obstruction to the outflow of blood from the right ventricle, usually at the pulmonic valve or subvalvular level. Patients exhibiting this pattern are often visibly cyanotic. If the decreased vascularity is of a diffuse nature, a congenital anomaly is most likely. This pattern is seldom found in adults because the abnormalities that produce this pattern will have resulted in the patient's death unless corrective surgery was performed during childhood.

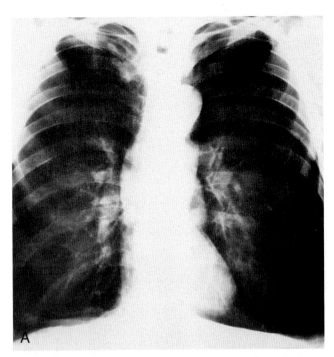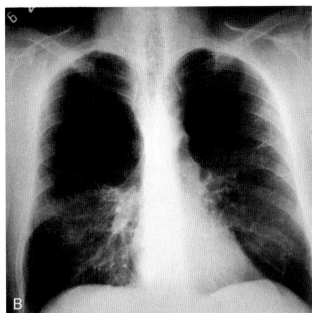

Figure 5.30.   Decrease in pulmonary vascularity in two patients with emphysema. Notice the crowding of vessels centrally and the paucity of peripheral vessels.

Decreased vascularity may be apparent locally or unilaterally. A local decrease in vascularity may be the result of pulmonary embolism (Westermark sign), emphysema (Fig. 5.30), or scarring with rearrangement of vessels in a lung. A unilateral decrease in vascularity without changes in the cardiac size may result from either hypoplasia of a lung or the Swyer-James syndrome—a rare condition caused by diffuse, unilateral bronchitis (Fig. 5.31).

Increased vascularity is of four types: (1) shunts, (2) pulmonary venous obstruction (PVO), (3) precapillary hypertension, and (4) high-output state.

Figure 5.31.   Unilateral decrease in pulmonary vasculature in a patient with left-side unilateral hyperlucent lung (Swyer-James syndrome). Compare the vessels in this patient's normal right side with those in the abnormal left side.

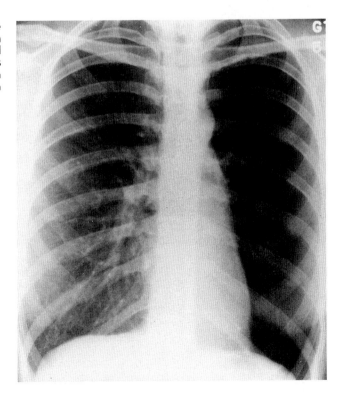

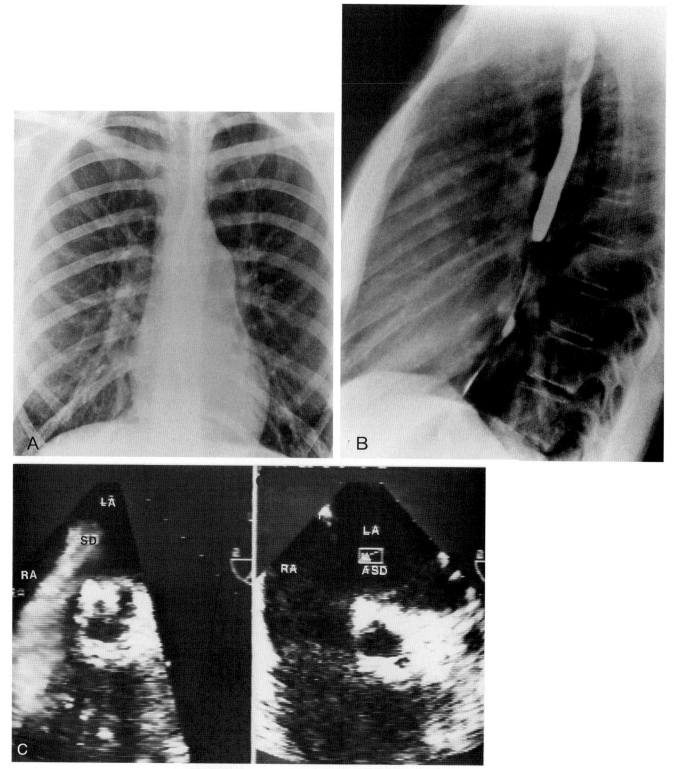

Figure 5.32.   Increased pulmonary vascularity in a patient with an atrial septal defect. A. Frontal radiograph shows prominent vessels. **B.** Lateral radiograph shows right ventricular prominence in the substernal region. **C.** Echocardiogram. The left panel, a color-flow Doppler image, shows the turbulence of flow through the defect (*SD*). The right panel shows the septal defect (*ASD, arrowhead*) between the right atrium (*RA*) and the left atrium (*LA*).

Shunts represent an increased flow through the pulmonary bed. They are characterized by large vessels in the upper and lower lobes. A similar pattern may occur in high-output states. In a patient who has a shunt and is not in congestive heart failure, the redistribution of blood will be in the same proportion as that occurring normally: greater to the lung bases than to the upper lobes. This vascular pattern occurs most commonly in a left-to-right shunt at the cardiac or great vessel level (septal defect or patent ductus arteriosus). This pattern is uncommon in adults because the condition is usually diagnosed and treated in childhood (Fig. 5.32).

A patient with a *PVO* demonstrates large veins in the upper lobe as a reflection of reversal of the normal flow pattern. This indicates increased left atrial pressure. A severe PVO is manifested by pulmonary edema and prominent interlobular septal (Kerley) lines (Figs. 5.33 and 5.34).

Patients with *precapillary hypertension* (pulmonary arterial hypertension) have large central vessels that taper rapidly into small vessels peripherally. This is referred to as centralized flow

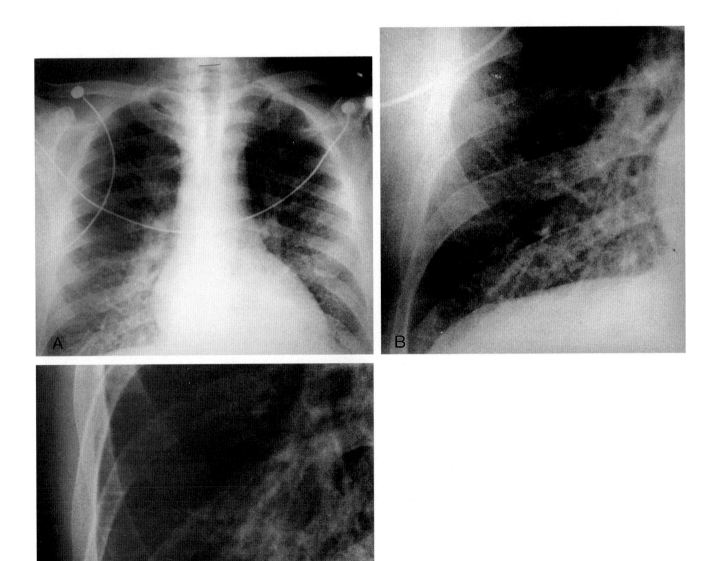

Figure 5.33.   Congestive heart failure and pulmonary edema. A. Frontal view shows mild pulmonary edema and pulmonary venous engorgement. **B.** Detail view shows the edema and prominent septal (Kerley) lines. **C.** Detail view in another patient shows the prominent horizontal Kerley lines.

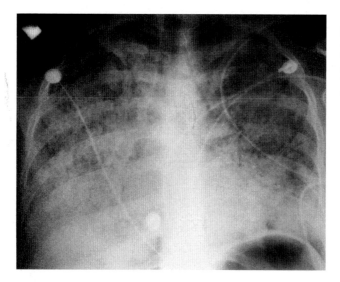

Figure 5.34. Alveolar and interstitial pulmonary edema. Notice the fluffiness of the densities, the indistinctness of the cardiac border, and the combination of findings that indicate alveolar and interstitial abnormalities.

and occurs in patients with severe pulmonary disease, recurrent pulmonary embolism (Fig. 5.35), and Eisenmenger physiology.

Once you have determined the pulmonary vascular pattern, look at the heart to ascertain if specific chamber enlargements are present. If there is evidence of an LAE (with or without a PVO), rheumatic heart disease (mitral stenosis) or an obstruction at or proximal to the mitral valve is present (Fig. 5.36). If there is evidence of left ventricular enlargement with a "concavity" in the area of the main pulmonary artery, the disease is one of left ventricular stress, such as hypertensive cardiovascular disease (Fig. 5.37), coronary artery disease, aortic stenosis, or coarctation of the aorta.

A PVO plus a left ventricular configuration (LVC) equals left ventricular stress with failure. All the preceding conditions occur with this pattern. It is possible to further narrow the list of causes in this situation by scanning the film for evidence of rib notching and/or decreased size

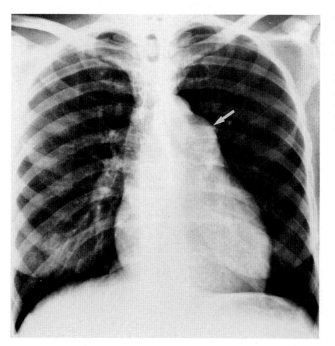

Figure 5.35. Pulmonary arterial hypertension in a patient with recurrent pulmonary emboli. Prominence of the main pulmonary artery is evident near the outflow tract on the left (*arrow*). The right mainstem pulmonary artery is enlarged and tapers rapidly peripherally. This is a sign of pulmonary arterial hypertension.

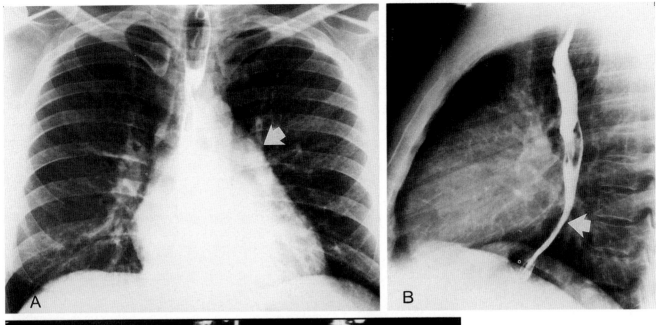

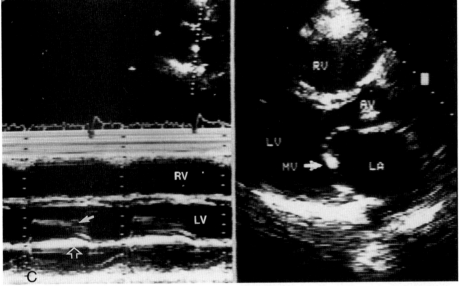

Figure 5.36. Mitral stenosis. A. Frontal radiograph shows a prominent bulge in the vicinity of the left atrium (*arrow*). **B.** Lateral radiograph shows impingement of the barium-filled esophagus (*arrow*) by the enlarged left atrium. **C.** Echocardiogram. The left panel is an M-mode image and shows a reduced opening slope of the mitral valve (*solid arrow*). The bright and continuous echodensity at the base of the valve (*open arrow*) is a calcified mitral annulus. The right panel is a parasternal view of the mitral valve area (*MV*) and shows "doming" in systole as the valve closes (*arrow*). AV, aortic valve; LA, left atrium; LV, left ventricle; RV, right ventricle.

of the aortic knob, as in aortic coarctation (Fig. 5.38), or for calcification in or about the aortic valve (Fig. 5.39), as in calcific aortic stenosis.

A *high-output state,* such as severe anemia or thyrotoxicosis, may produce increased vascularity with a normal distribution as a result of the increased volume being pumped through the heart. The heart itself may be normal or slightly enlarged as a result of this increased activity.

Pediatric Patients

Cardiac disease in pediatric patients is usually congenital. However, rheumatic heart disease is an important form of acquired disease that may occur in this age group.

Before beginning an analysis of the pulmonary vascularity in pediatric patients, it is important to know whether or not they are visibly cyanotic. The presence of visible cyanosis changes the physiologic state of the patient and the category of disease. It is also important to know whether the cyanosis was present at birth (as in transposition of great vessels) or developed later (as in tetralogy of Fallot). Radiographic analyses of the acyanotic patient and the cyanotic patient are presented in the following sections.

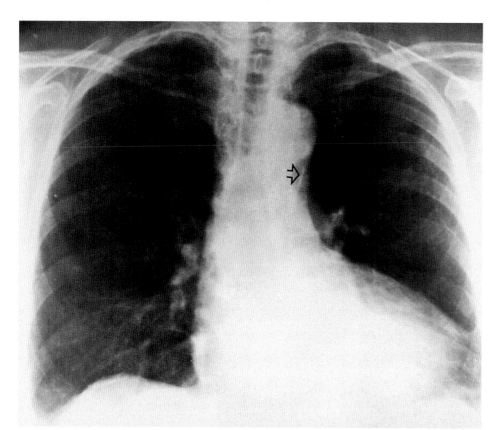

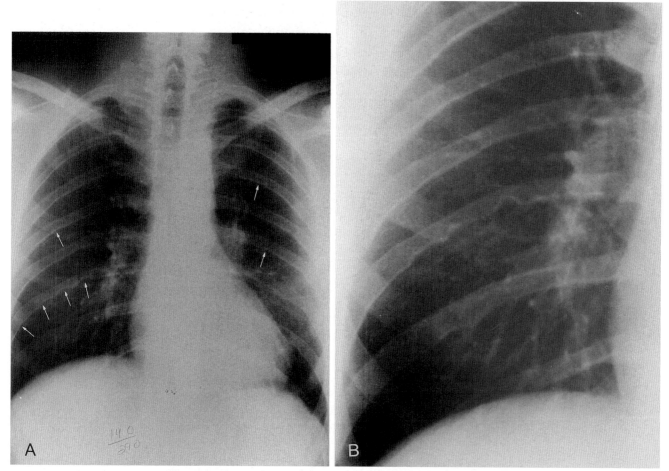

Figure 5.38. Coarctation (A–C) and pseudocoarctation (D–G) of the aorta. A. Frontal radiograph at first glance appears normal. However, slight left ventricular prominence can be seen. The aortic knob is small. Notice the rib notching bilaterally (*arrows*). **B.** Detail view shows the rib notching to better advantage. *(continues)*

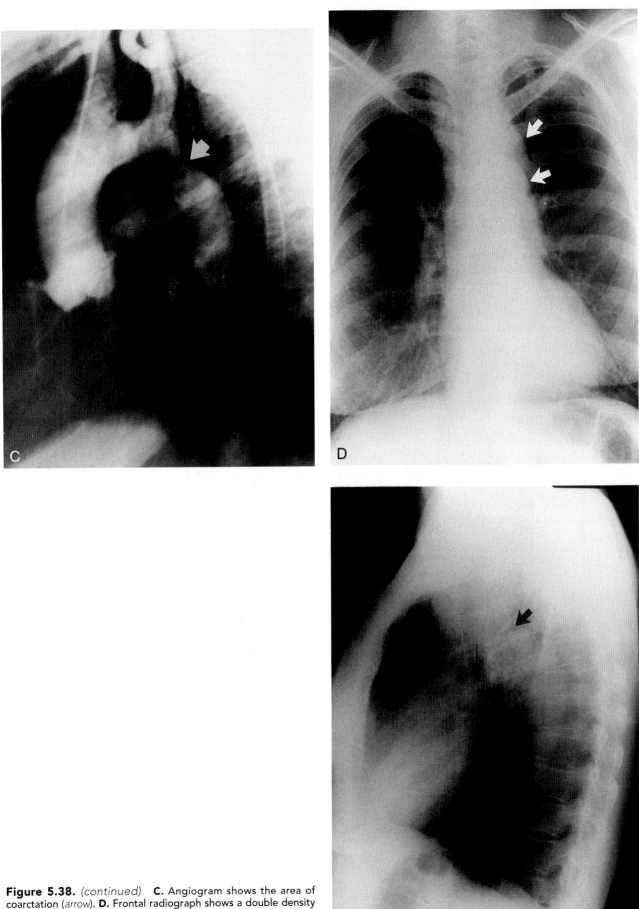

Figure 5.38. *(continued)* **C.** Angiogram shows the area of coarctation (*arrow*). **D.** Frontal radiograph shows a double density of the aortic arch (*arrows*) owing to its tortuosity. There is no rib notching. **E.** Lateral radiograph shows a kink in the aortic arch (*arrow*). *(continues)*

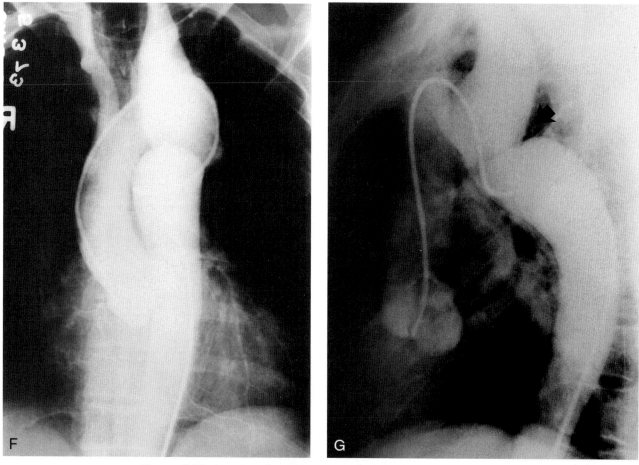

F

G

Figure 5.38. *(continued)* **F and G.** Frontal and lateral angiographic images show the kinking of the aorta *(arrow)*. Notice the course of the catheter.

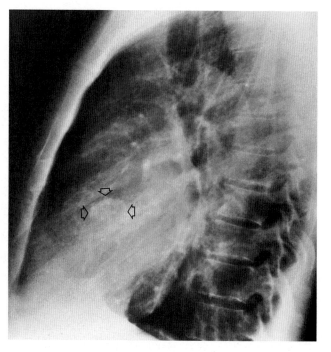

Figure 5.39. Aortic valve calcification *(arrows)*. Compare with the mitral valve calcification shown in Figure 5.24.

Figure 5.40 is a diagram summarizing the analyses necessary in the diagnosis of congenital cardiac disease.

Acyanotic Patients

Normal Vascularity

If the vascularity is normal, it is necessary to rely on the heart size and configuration and the appearance of the great vessels to provide clues to the cause of the suspected cardiac disease. A normal heart size does not rule out a heart lesion. A mild or compensated lesion may be accompanied by a normal-appearing heart on radiographs. Furthermore, an obstructive lesion may cause hypertrophy but may not enlarge the heart enough to be detectable on the chest

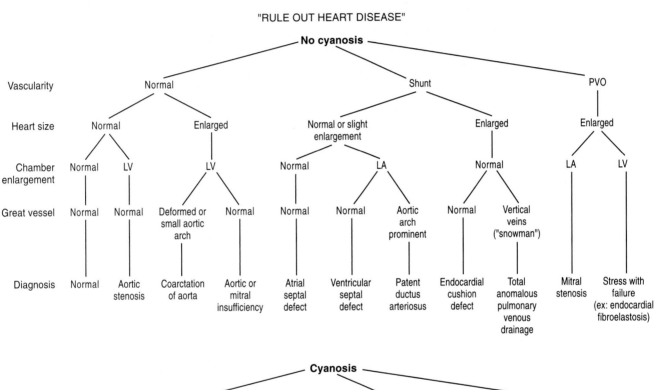

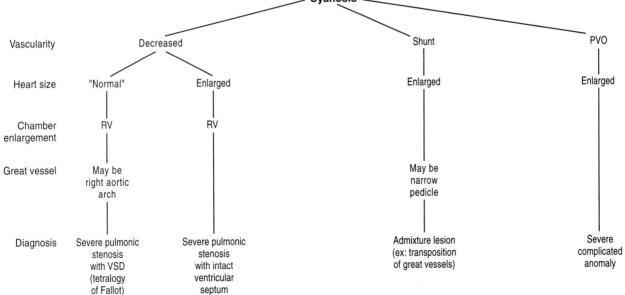

Figure 5.40.   Diagram of a plain-film radiographic diagnosis of congenital cardiac diseases.

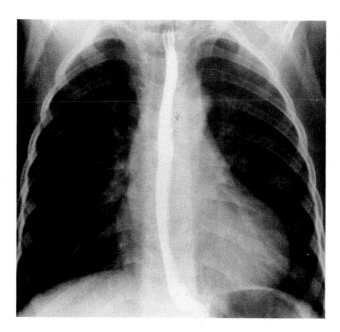

Figure 5.41.   Aortic stenosis in a child. Notice the left ventricular configuration.

radiograph. A diagnosis of left or right ventricular *hypertrophy* is an electrocardiographic or ultrasonic, not radiographic, diagnosis. Radiography identifies chamber *enlargements*, not hypertrophy.

An LVC in a child indicates a left-sided obstructive lesion, such as aortic stenosis (Fig. 5.41) or coarctation of the aorta. Although usually normal in adults, an LVC is always abnormal in children.

A prominent main pulmonary artery or proximal left pulmonary artery segment suggests a right-sided obstructive lesion, pulmonic valvular stenosis with poststenotic dilatation (Fig. 5.42). If the peripheral vascularity is normal, the degree of stenosis is not severe.

In patients with enlarged hearts but normal vascularity, volume overload most likely caused by valvular insufficiency may be inferred. Volume overload dilates the involved cardiac chambers without causing increased pressure until cardiac failure occurs. An LVC (indicating left ventricular stress) with an enlarged heart suggests aortic or mitral insufficiency (Fig. 5.43). In mitral insufficiency, volume overload occurs in the left atrium as well. This may be detected on plain films or on the cardiac series as a bulge along the left cardiac border (indicating displacement of the left atrial appendage); a double density seen on the PA film, representing the

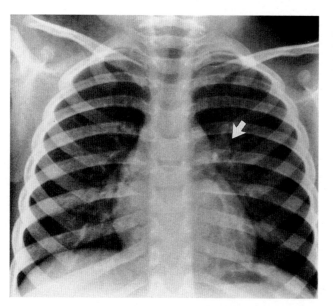

Figure 5.42.   Pulmonic stenosis in a child. There is prominence of the left main pulmonary artery (*arrow*) near the outflow tract caused by the "jet phenomenon."

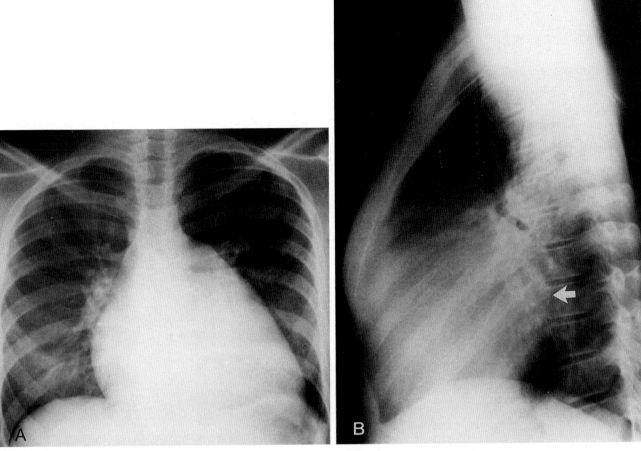

Figure 5.43.   Mitral insufficiency. A. Frontal radiograph shows prominence and straightening of the left cardiac border from left atrial enlargement. Notice the left ventricular prominence. **B.** Lateral radiograph shows left ventricular enlargement (*arrow*).

enlarged left atrium itself; splaying of the carinal angle greater than 75°; and impingement on the barium-filled esophagus. These findings are illustrated in Figure 5.44 in a patient with mitral stenosis and insufficiency.

The findings for normal vascularity are summarized as follows:

- Normal vascularity + Normal heart size = Normal or "mild anything"
- Normal vascularity + LVC (overall heart size normal) =
  Left ventricular obstructive lesion without heart failure
- Normal vascularity + Prominent main pulmonary artery =
  Right ventricular obstructive lesion
- Normal vascularity + Big heart = Volume overload lesion, valvular insufficiency type

Shunt Vascularity

As mentioned previously, a general increase in the size of the pulmonary arteries throughout the lungs indicates either a left-to-right shunt or a hyperdynamic state, such as thyrotoxicosis or large systemic arteriovenous (A-V) fistula. In the pediatric age group, the most common congenital lesion to produce this pattern is a shunt.

Once shunt vascularity is identified, the size of the left atrium is used to determine the level of the shunt. An LAE indicates that the atrial septum is intact (LAE results from the increased pulmonary venous return). In this situation, the shunt must be distal to the A-V valves, as in a ventricular septal defect (VSD; Fig. 5.45) or patent ductus arteriosus.

Shunt vascularity without atrial enlargement indicates an atrial septal defect (ASD; see Fig. 5.32). The excess blood flows immediately into the lower-pressure right atrium, resulting in no

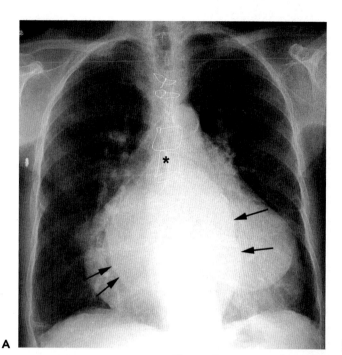

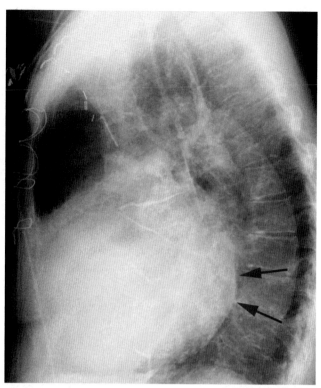

Figure 5.44. Mitral insufficiency and mitral stenosis. When these two lesions are combined, there is greater cardiomegaly than in an isolated lesion. **A.** Frontal radiograph shows a double density over the heart, representing the enlarged left atrium (*arrows*). The carina is splayed (*). **B.** Lateral radiograph shows posterior bulging of the enlarged left atrium (*arrows*). The patient has had previous heart surgery.

net volume overload of the left atrium. In a patient with an isolated ASD, the heart is either normal in size or mildly enlarged. Shunt vascularity coupled with marked cardiomegaly indicates a complicated ASD.

The findings of shunt vascularity are summarized as follows:

- Shunt vascularity + LAE = Shunt distal to AV valves
- Shunt vascularity + Normal-sized left atrium = ASD
- Shunt vascularity + Normal-sized left atrium + Big heart = Complicated ASD

Pulmonary Venous Obstruction

A severe PVO in a newborn usually occurs in conjunction with cyanotic congenital heart disease. However, cardiac failure may occur in very young children in the presence of large systemic A-V fistulae. Interestingly, because infants spend most of their hours in a recumbent position, the pulmonary blood flow is equally distributed throughout the lungs, and the adult pattern of PVO—a redistribution to the upper lobes—is therefore not observed. The older a child becomes, however, the closer the appearance is to the adult pattern of PVO.

As in the adult, once a pattern of PVO is recognized in a child, attention should be directed to the cardiac configuration to determine the level of the obstruction. If the heart is triangular in shape—that is, having a prominent bulge along the left cardiac border—and there is evidence of an LAE, the obstruction is at or proximal to the mitral valve. The most common source of this situation is rheumatic heart disease. Remember, however, that the failure pattern may also occur in patients with mitral insufficiency or aortic valve disease. Such a patient will have an LVC. If the heart shows a pure LVC with no evidence of an LAE, primary left ventricular stress is present. This is similar to the case of the adult patient and results from a variety of causes.

The findings of a PVO are summarized as follows:

PVO + LAE = Obstruction at or proximal to the mitral valve (usually rheumatic)
PVO + LVC = Primary left ventricular stress (of any cause) with failure

Figure 5.45.   Ventricular septal defect. A. Radiograph shows shunt vascularity. **B.** Echocardiogram. Left panel is a color-flow Doppler image through the septal defect and shows the turbulent flow from the left ventricle to the right ventricle. Arrow indicates the direction of flow. Right panel is a four-chamber image and shows the defect (*VSD*). MV, mitral valve; RA, right atrium; RV, right ventricle; TV, tricuspid valve; VSD, ventricular septal defect.

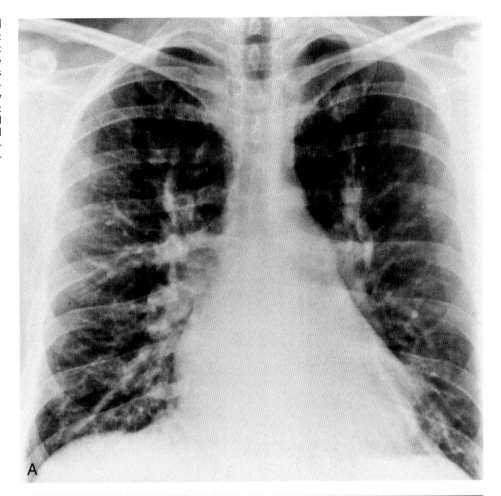

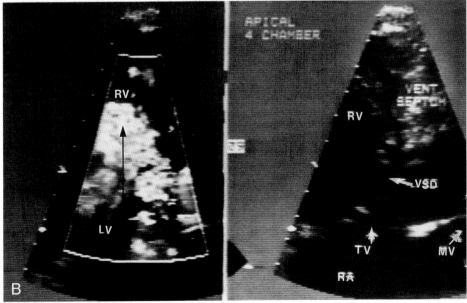

Cyanotic Patients

In a cyanotic patient, the vascularity is never normal; it must be either decreased or increased. In this discussion, no attempt is made to describe specific intracardiac lesions. The physiologic alterations produced by the lesions as manifest in the pulmonary vascularity is stressed.

Cyanosis in the presence of decreased vascularity generally indicates the severe form of pulmonic stenosis. Once you have observed cyanosis and decreased vascularity, you must decide whether or not the heart size is normal. If the overall cardiac size is normal, even in the presence of evidence of specific chamber enlargement, the most likely abnormality is severe pulmonic stenosis plus VSD (*tetralogy of Fallot;* Fig. 5.46).

A cyanotic patient with decreased vascularity and an enlarged heart is suffering from a complicated type of cardiac abnormality, usually severe pulmonic stenosis with an intact intraventricular septum. A shunt must be present to allow oxygenated blood to enter the circulation to permit survival.

If cyanosis is combined with shunt vascularity, an admixture lesion is present. In this situation, arterial and venous blood is mixed so that the aortic blood is oxygen desaturated. This occurs in *persistent truncus arteriosus* and *complete transposition of the great vessels.*

A cyanotic patient with a PVO pattern, particularly an infant, constitutes a medical emergency. The patient should be referred for immediate sonography and cardiac catheterization to determine whether a correctable lesion is present. Most of the abnormalities found in this group of patients are complex.

The cyanotic patient is summarized as follows:

- Cyanosis + Decreased vascularity + "Normal" heart size =
  Severe pulmonic stenosis + VSD (tetralogy of Fallot)
- Cyanosis + Decreased vascularity + Enlarged heart =
  Severe pulmonic stenosis + Intact ventricular septum
- Cyanosis + Shunt vascularity = Admixture lesion
- Cyanosis + Severe PVO = Severe complex abnormality; patient should be
  referred for emergency sonography and catheterization

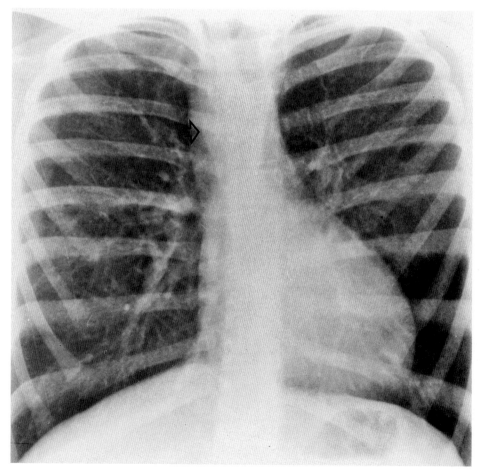

Figure 5.46. Tetralogy of Fallot. The overall heart size is normal. The pulmonary vascularity, however, is diminished. Notice the right aortic arch (*arrow*).

Chamber and Great Vessel Enlargements

The preceding sections considered the analysis of vascular patterns as the key to diagnosing congenital and acquired cardiac disease. At this point, the radiographic appearance of specific chamber enlargements is discussed briefly.

Left ventricular enlargement produces a downward and left bulge of the cardiac apex on the frontal radiograph. In the lateral view, the image of the enlarged left ventricle is seen posterior to that of the inferior vena cava. Conditions that produce pure left ventricular enlargement were discussed in the previous section (see Figs. 5.37 and 5.38).

Left atrial enlargement was also discussed previously (see Figs. 5.36, 5.43, and 5.44). *Right ventricular enlargement,* when marked, may elevate the apex of the left ventricle. This produces the so-called boot-shaped heart (see Fig. 5.46) on the frontal radiograph. On the lateral film, there is a loss of the retrosternal clear space.

Right atrial enlargement as an isolated finding is rare. It usually accompanies enlargement of the right ventricle and pulmonary arteries. Right atrial enlargement is suggested by prominence of the right cardiac border; the heart often has a boxlike appearance, as in Ebstein anomaly (Fig. 5.47).

Main pulmonary artery enlargement produces bulging of the main pulmonary artery segment along the left cardiac border (Fig. 5.48). In addition, prominent right and left main pulmonary arteries may also be observed. Peripheral enlargements were discussed in the previous section.

Various portions of the aorta may become enlarged, producing a prominence of that particular image. In addition, considerable tortuosity may occur in the descending aorta (Fig. 5.49). Tortuosity may be difficult to differentiate from aortic aneurysms on radiographs. Chest CT is much better for making that differentiation.

Congestive Heart Failure

The vascular changes in congestive heart failure have been discussed previously. To reiterate, these include dilatation of the upper lobe vessels with contraction of the lower lobe vessels. In addition, there is enlargement of the cardiac silhouette in a poorly defined pattern. Although you may presume left ventricular enlargement, it is hard to specifically identify this in view of the "flabbiness" and poor contractility of cardiac muscles.

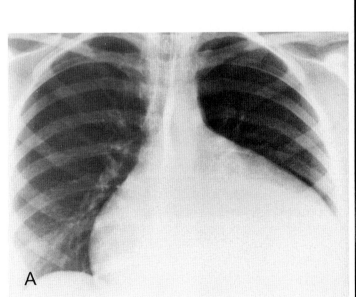
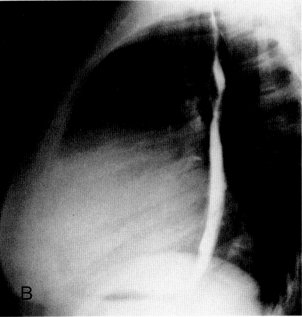

Figure 5.47.   Ebstein anomaly. Frontal **(A)** and lateral **(B)** radiographs show massive cardiomegaly that is primarily right sided.

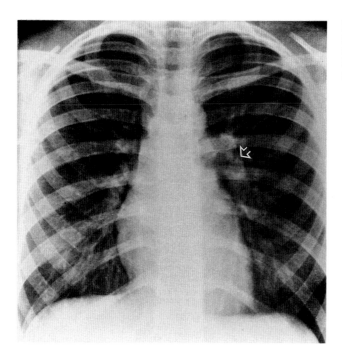

Figure 5.48. Pulmonic stenosis in an adult. There is prominence of the left pulmonary artery (*arrow*) secondary to the "jet phenomenon."

Associated findings of heart failure include interstitial and intra-alveolar edema. *Interstitial edema* occurs when the left atrial pressure increases and fluid transudes into the interstitial tissues, resulting in thickening of the interlobular septa. Kerley originally described these multiple linear densities and designated them according to their orientation:

- *Kerley A lines* are long, thin, nonbranching, linear densities obliquely directed toward the hilum.
- *Kerley B lines*, the best known and most often observed, are thin, short, transverse lines best seen near the lung bases laterally at the costophrenic angle (Fig. 5.50).
- *Kerley C lines* are actually A and B lines oriented in an AP direction. On frontal films, they appear as a fine, reticular network.

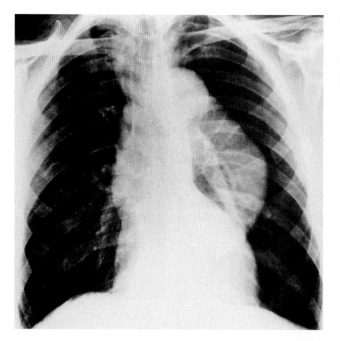

Figure 5.49. Marked tortuosity of the descending aorta. A subsequent arteriogram proved that the patient did not have an aneurysm. This appearance is distinct from that of a pseudocoarctation (see Fig. 5.38D).

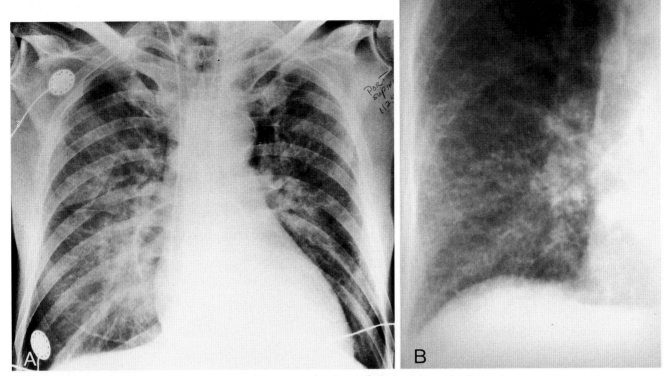

Figure 5.50.   Kerley lines in two patients with congestive heart failure. A. Frontal radiograph shows pulmonary edema is present. Notice the prominent intralobular septa (Kerley lines) throughout both lung fields. **B.** Detail view of another patient shows prominent Kerley B lines.

■ *Remember that all three types of Kerley lines represent edematous interlobular septa and not dilated lymphatic vessels.*
■ *Intra-alveolar pulmonary edema* results from further transudation of fluid into the air spaces, producing patchy, ill-defined, coalescent densities that radiate outward from the hilum. Sometimes this may have a butterfly- or bat wing–shaped distribution (Fig. 5.51). Air

Figure 5.51. Alveolar pulmonary edema. The edema in this patient is primarily central. It is not as florid as seen in Figure 5.34. Notice the engorgement of the pulmonary veins. There is left lower lobe consolidation as well.

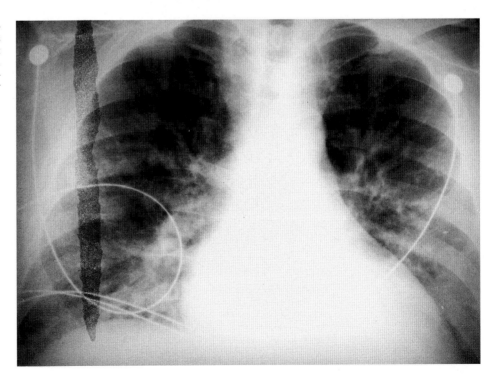

bronchograms often occur in this pattern. As with any alveolar process, the onset and clearing may be dramatic within a short time. Alveolar pulmonary edema may be asymmetric if the patient has been lying on one side before filming. The edema may also be mistaken for other causes of alveolar density such as pneumonia and hemorrhage. You should be careful to analyze the pulmonary vessels, if visible, and the cardiac size before making a diagnosis of alveolar pulmonary edema. Furthermore, edema may be present from another (noncardiac) source, such as heroin intoxication, inhalation of noxious fumes, or drowning. In these conditions, the heart is usually normal in size.

- *Pleural fluid* is another nonspecific finding that may be present in patients with congestive heart failure. If the fluid collects along a fissure, a *pseudotumor* may result (Fig. 5.52). On the lateral view, the borders are generally tapering, and the collection of fluid is oriented in a slanted configuration. These densities typically change size from day to day, depending on the amount of fluid present, and they disappear after successful therapy.

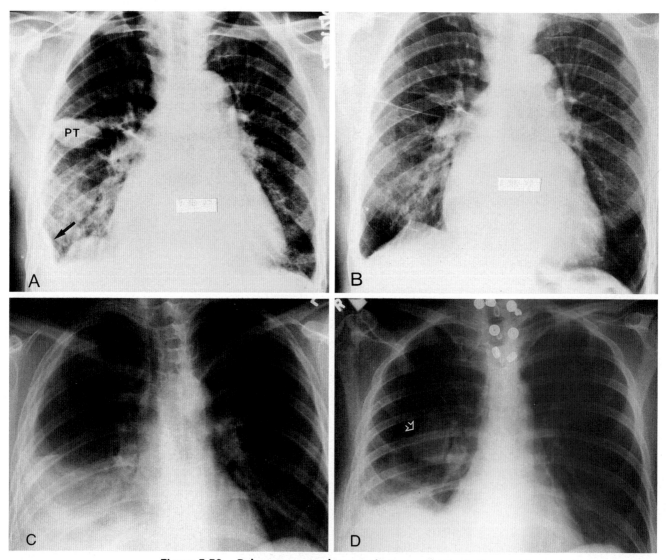

Figure 5.52.   Pulmonary pseudotumor in two patients. A. Frontal radiograph shows an oval density representing the pseudotumor (*PT*) along the minor fissure on the right side. There is loculation of pleural fluid in the right costophrenic angle (*arrow*). Notice the cardiomegaly, pulmonary venous engorgement, and Kerley lines. **B.** Four days later, the patient's cardiac status has improved. The pseudotumor is no longer present. **C.** Frontal radiograph in another patient shows a large right-sided pleural effusion. **D.** Two days later, the effusion is smaller, and a pseudotumor of loculated fluid is evident in the major fissure on the right (*arrow*).

Figure 5.53. Pericardial effusion. There is massive enlargement of the patient's cardiac silhouette. An echocardiogram (see Fig. 5.4) confirmed the presence of a large pericardial effusion.

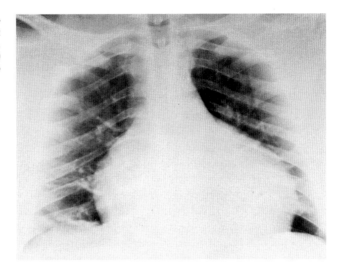

Pericardial Effusion

Pericardial effusion must always be considered when evaluating a patient with an enlarged heart. The diagnosis may be made by one or a combination of imaging studies. In general, a large heart of nonspecific configuration, particularly in the absence of pulmonary venous engorgement, should suggest a pericardial effusion (Fig. 5.53). Occasionally, the pericardium is demonstrated in normal patients as a thin, dense line separated by layers of subepicardial and mediastinal fat. In patients with pericardial effusion, this line, which never should measure more than 2 mm, is thickened.

Echocardiography is the most useful examination for detecting this condition and with the least risk to the patient. Ultrasonic shadows reflected off the pericardial and myocardial surfaces will demonstrate an abnormal collection of fluid in the pericardial sac (Fig. 5.54; see Fig. 5.4).

Figure 5.54. Pericardial effusion (*E*) demonstrated on a parasternal long-axis echocardiogram image.

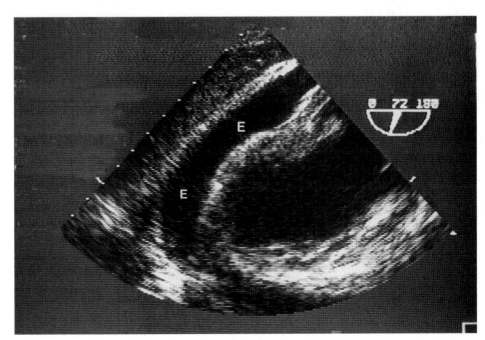

CT may be also used to diagnose pericardial effusion. A CT number near the density of water surrounding the heart ensures the diagnosis (Fig. 5.55). This diagnosis is usually made as an incidental finding in patients studied for other reasons.

Trauma

Patients who have suffered severe thoracic trauma may have an injury to the heart or great vessels. The most common mechanism for this is an accident in which the unrestrained driver of a motor vehicle strikes the steering wheel. Radiographically, the most common finding is a widened superior mediastinal shadow that is *fuzzy*. You should remember, however, that a supine radiograph in a large patient can simulate this appearance. With this in mind, you should make every effort to obtain an *erect film*. CT of the thorax is now used routinely on patients with suspected injury to the great vessels to look for evidence of mediastinal hemorrhage (see Fig. 5.56). The study is performed after intravenous injection of a bolus of contrast. CT has replaced the aortogram (Fig. 5.57) in trauma centers in the United States.

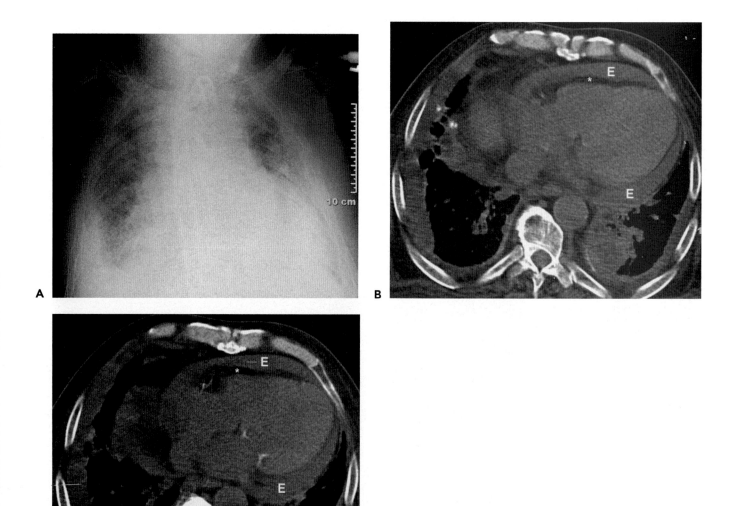

Figure 5.55. Pericardial effusion demonstrated by CT. **A.** Chest radiograph shows enlargement of the cardiac silhouette. **B and C.** CT images show a fluid collection (*E*) surrounding the heart. Notice the epicardial fat (*).

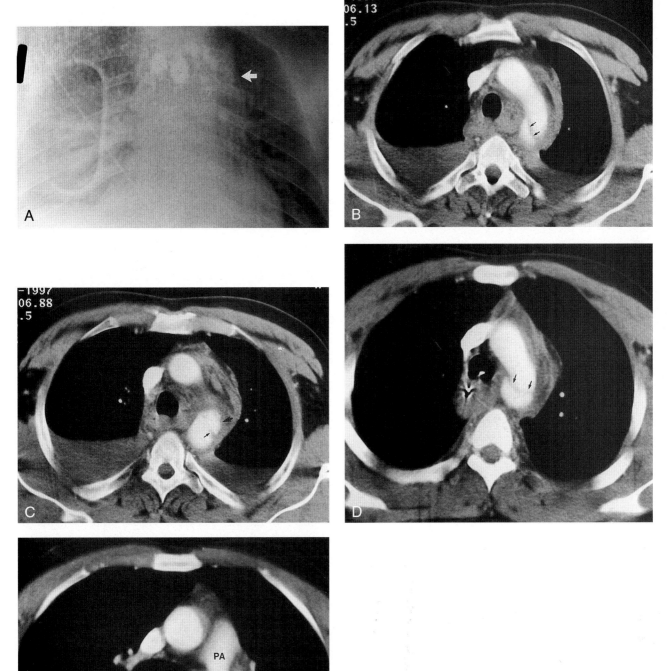

Figure 5.56. CT demonstrating aortic injuries in two patients. A. Portable chest radiograph shows widening of the superior mediastinum and irregularity of the aortic knob region (*arrow*). **B.** CT image at the level of the aortic knob demonstrates an intimal flap in the descending aorta (*arrows*). Notice the mediastinal widening from unopacified blood. **C.** CT image slightly distal shows the intimal flap (*small arrow*) as well as a pseudoaneurysm (*large arrow*). **D.** CT image in another patient shows mediastinal widening and an intimal flap in the descending aorta (*arrows*). **E.** CT image at level of carina shows a large pseudoaneurysm (*PA*) that is opacified. This indicates active bleeding. The findings in both patients were confirmed at surgery.

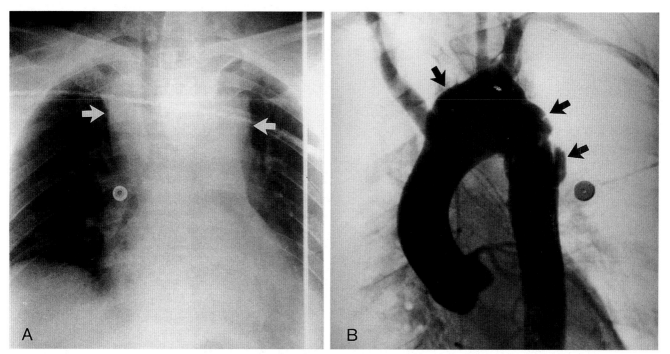

Figure 5.57. Posttraumatic aortic tear in an unrestrained driver. A. Frontal radiograph shows widening of the superior mediastinum (*arrows*). Notice the tracheal deviation to the right. **B.** Arteriogram shows the pseudoaneurysm (*arrows*). Notice the irregular contour of the aortic arch.

Changes Following Cardiac Surgery

Chapter 4 discussed some of the radiographic findings that may be encountered in the thorax following surgery. Various surgical procedures performed on the heart leave characteristic radiographic changes. Foremost of these is coronary artery bypass graft surgery. Several techniques are used in which saphenous venous grafts are used to bypass stenotic or occluded coronary arteries. These may be recognized by the presence of sternal wire sutures as well as by surgical clips in the anterior mediastinum or over the heart (Fig. 5.58). Some surgeons use metallic rings to mark the locations of the grafts. These make future coronary angiograms easier to perform because the openings of the grafts are easily visible on the fluoroscopic screen. A variation, known as minimally invasive coronary bypass surgery, is performed using a thoracoscope through small incisions in the chest wall ("keyhole procedure"). This type of surgery leaves no tell-tale sternal wires, but the surgical clips around the grafts are visible on radiographs.

One of the newest frontiers of interventional radiology and nonsurgical cardiology is the use of *intravascular stents*. These are being used in greater frequency and have the radiographic appearance of a tubular structure with a chicken-wire mesh (Fig. 5.59). Newer stents are not as dense as the older ones and may not always be seen on radiographs. All stents are demonstrated on CT.

Another procedure that leaves characteristic radiographic findings is one in which a portion of the *latissimus dorsi* muscle is wrapped around an area of the heart that has been weakened by previous myocardial infarction(s). The radiographic appearance is that of a density arising from the left or right axilla and extending to the heart (Fig. 5.60). The fact that the density does not follow the normal anatomic contours of the lungs, coupled with the presence of pacemaker leads, is the radiographic clue that this procedure has been performed.

Patients with heart disease may also have various *pacemakers* in place (Fig. 5.61). The intracardiac variety are usually of two types: unipolar, with a single lead in the right ventricle, or bipolar, with one lead in the right ventricle and the other in the coronary sinus portion of the right atrium. Another device seen in heart patients is the automatic implantable cardiac

Figure 5.58. Changes following cardiac bypass surgery. Notice the presence of sternal wire sutures, surgical clips over the cardiac surface, and metal rings (*arrows*) marking the sites of the vascular grafts.

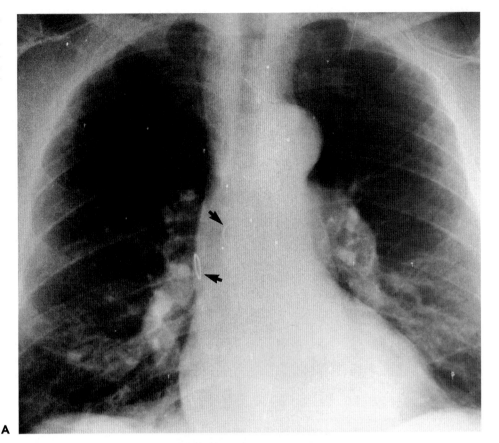

A

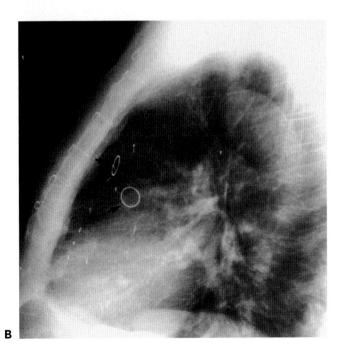

B

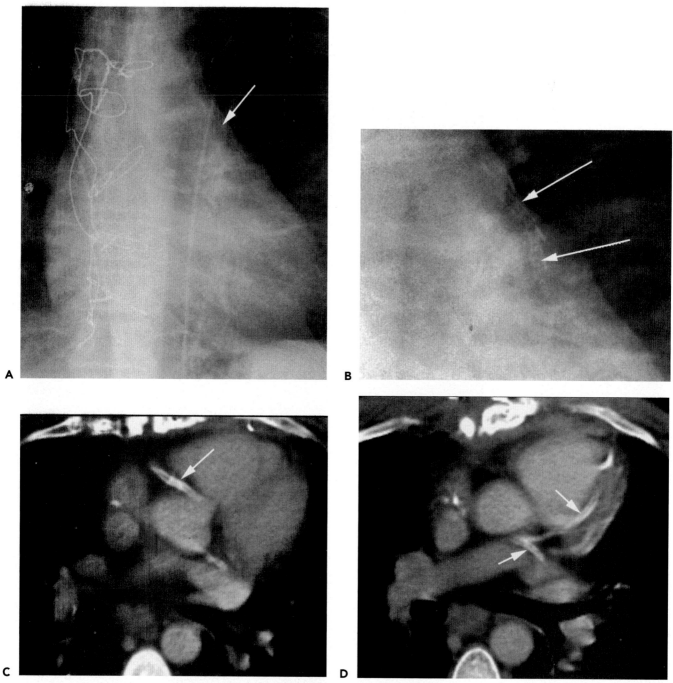

Figure 5.59. Coronary artery stents (*arrows*). A. Detail of chest radiograph shows a stent along the left cardiac border. **B.** Magnified view shows several stents in place. **C.** CT image shows a stent in the right coronary artery. **D.** CT image on the same patient shows stents in the circumflex and left anterior descending arteries. (Courtesy of Carl Fuhrman, MD, Department of Radiology, University of Pittsburgh School of Medicine.)

defibrillator (AICD; Fig. 5.62). The defibrillating leads in this device are in the superior vena cava and the right ventricle. Often an AICD is combined with a pacemaker.

Finally, cardiac *transplantation* is a proven procedure. There is nothing characteristic about the postoperative appearance of a patient following transplantation. Typically, the patient has a median sternotomy and a pacemaker. The greatest clue to the presence of a heart transplant is found by reviewing old chest radiographs, which reveal distinct differences in the cardiac silhouette.

Figure 5.60. Latissimus dorsi muscle transfer procedure. The transplanted muscle shows as a linear density in the left hemithorax (*arrow*). Notice the pacemaker wires attached to the graft.

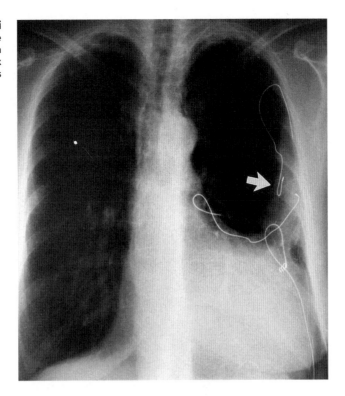

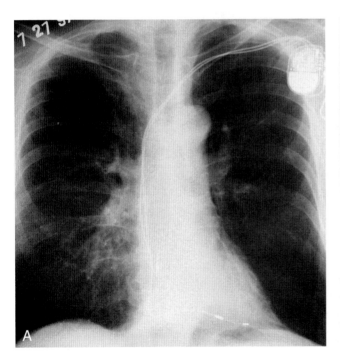

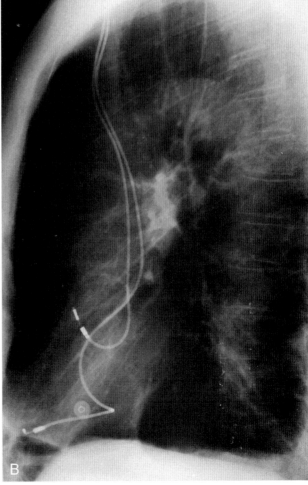

Figure 5.61. Transvenous cardiac pacemaker. A. Frontal radiograph shows the pacing box in the left subclavicular area. The pacing leads are in the right ventricle and the coronary sinus. **B.** Lateral view shows the position of the pacing leads.

Figure 5.62.   Implantable cardiac defibrillators. A and B. Epicardial variety are seen as thin boxlike wires over the right and left surfaces of the heart (*small arrows*). Notice the intracardiac (*open arrows*) and epicardial (*large arrows*) pacemaker leads. *(continues)*

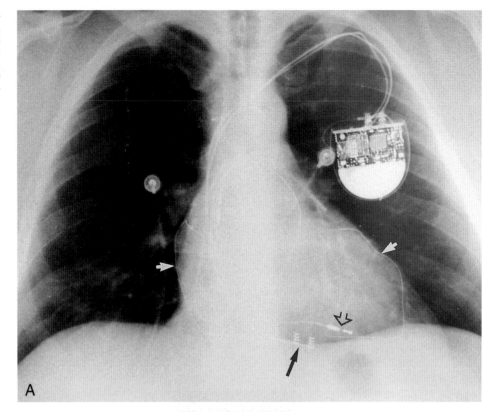

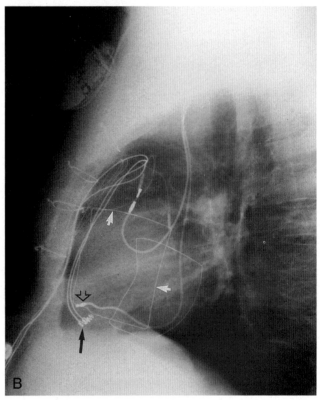

Figure 5.62. *(continued)* **C and D.** Automated implantable cardiac defibrillator. The leads are intracardiac, and the power box is over the left hemithorax.

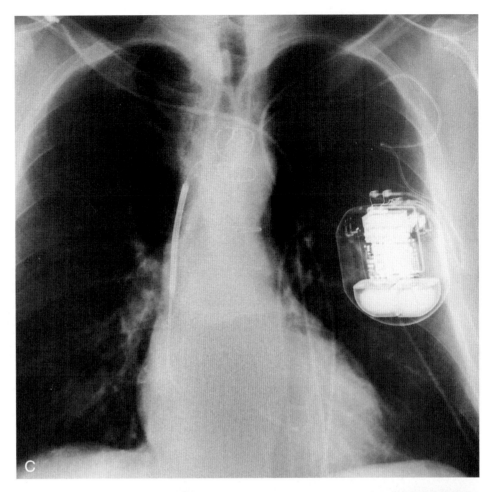

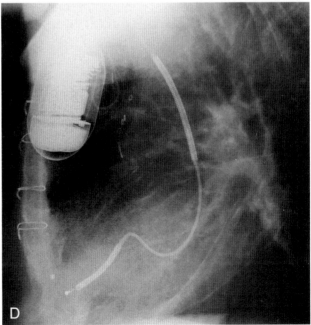

Changes in the Chest With Aging

The normal aging process is reflected in visible changes on serial chest radiographs, including a change from a more horizontal to a vertical position of the heart from youth into adulthood, tortuosity of the aorta and brachiocephalic vessels, calcification within the aortic arch, and occasionally, increasing tortuosity of the descending aorta. These findings are illustrated in Figure 5.63. Many older patients will have calcification of the coronary arteries visible on the lateral chest radiograph (Fig. 5.64). This finding may also be present in younger individuals with severe atherosclerosis, such as patients with diabetes. In addition, degenerative changes may be observed in the thoracic vertebrae. Postmenopausal women often demonstrate osteopenia and may, on occasion, show evidence of collapse of one or more thoracic vertebrae. The lungs themselves may show change with age. Hyperinflation, so-called senile emphysema, may sometimes occur. Scarring from subclinical pulmonary infections may be seen over both apices.

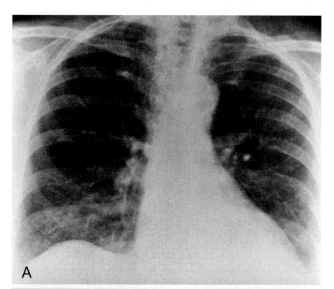
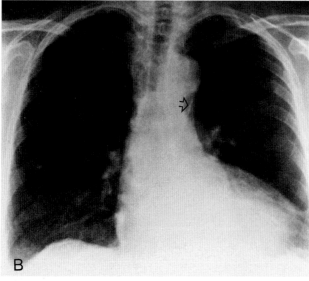

Figure 5.63. Age-related changes in cardiac silhouette in a patient with known hypertension. A. Frontal radiograph shows mild left ventricular prominence. **B.** Radiograph made 20 years later shows an increase in the size of the left ventricle. There is increased tortuosity of the descending aorta. Calcification of the descending aorta is also evident (*arrow*).

Figure 5.64. **Coronary artery calcification** (*arrows*) **in an elderly man.**

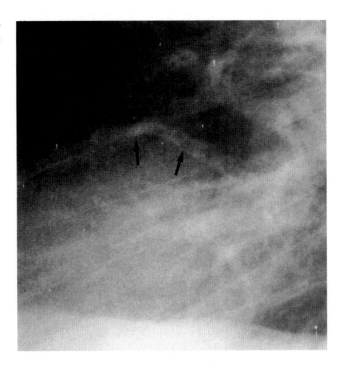

SUMMARY AND KEY POINTS

■ Cardiac imaging is primarily performed by cardiologists. However, radiography remains the initial screening imaging study for most patients.

■ This chapter focused on the analysis of chest radiographs based on the physiologic alterations they produce.

■ The configuration of the pulmonary vasculature as well as the findings of specific chamber enlargements permits the diagnosis of specific diseases.

■ Chamber enlargements, congestive heart failure, pericardial effusion, trauma, and age-related changes all produce characteristic changes on chest radiographs.

■ CT and MR imaging are playing a greater role in assessing disease of the coronary arteries.

SUGGESTED ADDITIONAL READING

Baron MG. Plain film diagnosis of common cardiac anomalies in the adult. Radiol Clin N Am 1999;37:401–420.

Baron MG, Book WM. Congenital heart disease in the adult: 2004. Radiol Clin N Am 2004;42:675–690.

Chen JTT, Capp MP, Johnsrude IS, et al. Roentgen appearance of pulmonary vascularity in the diagnosis of heart disease. AJR 1971;112:559–570.

Crean A, Dutka D, Coulden R. Cardiac imaging using nuclear medicine and positron emission tomography. Radiol Clin N Am 2004;42:619–634.

DeMaria AN, Blanchard DG. The echocardiogram. In: Alexander RW, Schlant RC, Fuster V, et al., eds. Hurst's the Heart, Arteries, and Veins. 9th Ed. New York: McGraw-Hill, 1998:415–517.

Elliott LP, ed. Cardiac Imaging in Infants, Children, and Adults. Philadelphia: JB Lippincott, 1991.

Feigenbaum H. Echocardiography. Philadelphia: Lea & Febiger, 1994.

Gutierrez FR, Brown JJ, Mirowitz SA. Cardiovascular Magnetic Resonance Imaging. St. Louis: Mosby-Year Book, 1991.

Hagen-Ansert SL. Textbook of Diagnostic Ultrasonography. St. Louis: Mosby-Year Book, 1995:1117–1389.

Higgins CB. Essentials of Cardiac Radiology and Imaging. Philadelphia: JB Lippincott, 1992.

Lipton MJ, Boxt LM. How to approach cardiac diagnosis from the chest radiograph. Radiol Clin N Am 2004;42:487–495.

Poutschi-Amin M, Gutierrez FR, Brown JJ, et al. How to plan and perform a cardiac MR imaging examination. Radiol Clin N Am 2004;42:497–514.

Schoepf UJ, Becker CR, Hofmann LK, Yucel EK. Multidetector-row CT of the heart. Radiol Clin N Am 2004;42:635–649.

Steiner RM, Levin DC. Radiology of the heart. In: Braunwald E, ed. Heart Disease: A Textbook of Cardiovascular Medicine. 5th Ed. Philadelphia: WB Saunders, 1997:204–239.

Breast Imaging

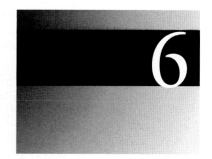

6

Breast cancer is the second most common cause of death from malignancy in American women. The American Cancer Society estimates that one of every eight women will get cancer of the breast in her lifetime. Fortunately, breast cancer can be diagnosed at an early and highly curable stage by the appropriate use of mammography. In recent years, breast cancer mortality has decreased because of a rise in the frequency of early diagnosis. Indeed, patients with screening-detected breast cancer have a survival rate at least 30% greater than symptomatic patients. The following are guidelines established by the American Cancer Society and endorsed by the American College of Radiology (ACR) regarding screening for breast cancer and the appropriate use of mammography.

Asymptomatic Women

- Women 20 years of age and older should perform breast self-examination monthly.
- Women age 20 to 40 should, in addition, have a physical examination of the breasts every 3 years.
- Women at age 40 should have a baseline mammogram.
- Women 40 years of age and older should have a mammogram and a physical examination of the breasts every year.

Symptomatic Women

- Symptomatic women with a dominant breast mass, persistent discomfort, skin dimpling, or nipple discharge should have a thorough breast examination that includes mammography and any other diagnostic study (ultrasound) to determine if cancer is present. These studies should be performed regardless of the patient's age.

Further Recommendations

- The ACR and the Food and Drug Administration further recommend that the mammographic technique used produce the greatest anatomic detail and resolution possible.
- These tests are to be provided with the lowest possible radiation dose needed to produce high-quality images. Mammography should be performed and interpreted by experienced, well-trained individuals using modern, carefully monitored equipment. All practices certified by the ACR conform with these high standards. The mammographic findings should be correlated carefully with thorough physical examination. However, there are limitations of mammography and clinicians must be aware of them. They should remember that the mammogram is a complementary procedure to a physical exam and ultrasound of the breast. Patients with palpable masses and an unremarkable mammogram should undergo ultrasound examination of the breast before biopsy is performed.

The largest breast cancer–screening project was performed by the American Cancer Society in conjunction with the National Cancer Institute in the 1970s under the Breast Cancer Detection Demonstration Project. In this study, more than 275,000 female volunteers were evaluated by physical examination and x-ray mammography at 27 centers nationwide. The results supported the value of mammography as a screening tool as well as a diagnostic method for detecting early breast cancer. Almost immediately after the study began, controversy developed regarding the safety of mammography because of the radiation dose involved. The controversy was based on several studies of women who had received extremely high doses of radiation to the breast in early childhood and who belonged to three separate populations: women exposed to the atom bombs of Hiroshima and Nagasaki, those with tuberculosis who received repeated chest radiographs and fluoroscopic examinations, and a group of women who were treated with radiation for postpartum mastitis. The controversy spurred the development of improved equipment and improved screen and film products (low dose) to further decrease the radiation dose. As a result, mammography is a safe diagnostic procedure when used by experienced personnel. For a more in-depth discussion on aspects of breast cancer, its detection, and the issue of radiation carcinogenesis, refer to the text by Kopans.

TECHNICAL CONSIDERATIONS

As previously mentioned, x-ray mammography has been proven to have the greatest efficacy for detecting occult breast cancer. Modern mammograms use either low-dose technology or digital radiography (Fig. 6.1), which lowers the dose even further. Mammography is also used to localize a mass for surgical excision (Fig. 6.2). Diagnostic ultrasound is used once a mass is detected to determine if it is cystic or solid (Fig. 6.3). Ultrasound is also used to localize breast lesions for percutaneous biopsy. Lesions that are seen only on a mammogram undergo biopsy using stereotactic techniques (Fig. 6.4).

Several other imaging procedures, such as thermography, transillumination, and magnetic resonance (MR) imaging, have also been used to evaluate breast lesions. Thermography and transillumination, although popular in the early 1970s, are no longer used because of the high incidence of false-positives and false-negatives. MR imaging is used in selected cases to locate an occult malignancy, to define the extent of an existing lesion, to assess carcinoma patients for chest wall invasion, and to monitor the response of a tumor to preoperative chemotherapy.

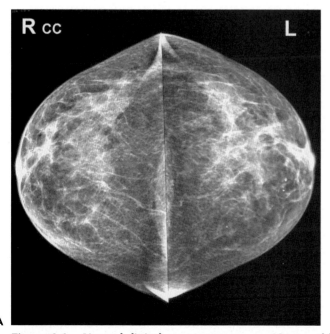

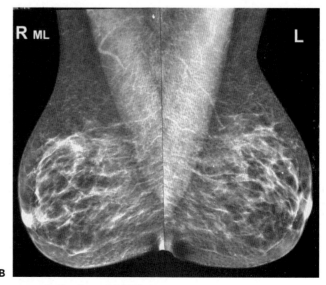

A

B

Figure 6.1.   Normal digital mammogram on a 63-year-old woman. A. Craniocaudal (CC) view.
B. Mediolateral (ML) view. Notice the exquisite detail the digital image provides.

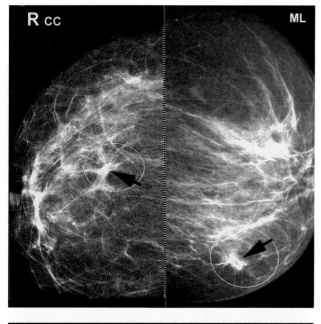

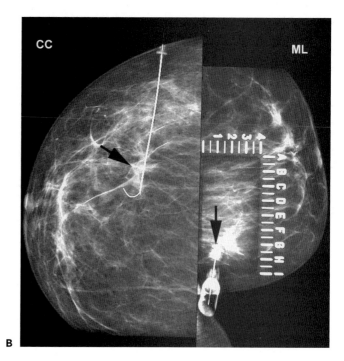

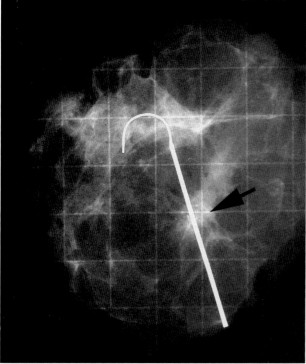

Figure 6.2. Use of mammography for needle localization. **A.** Craniocaudal (CC) and mediolateral (ML) digital mammograms show a spiculated mass with microcalcifications (*arrows*). **B.** Needle localization film shows the needle and wire in position through the mass (*arrows*). **C.** Specimen radiograph shows the mass and microcalcifications transfixed by the needle and wire. Diagnosis: ductal carcinoma in situ.

X-ray mammography is performed using a radiographic film and screen combination that provides high detail with a relatively low radiation dose. The diagnostic accuracy is identical to that of xerography, a technique used extensively in the 1970s and early 1980s. Although xerography provided exquisite soft tissue detail, it is no longer used today because of the high radiation dose required to produce the images.

Digital mammography (see Fig. 6.1) is replacing conventional film-screen mammography in many departments. The greatest advantage of digital mammography is its ability to provide improved image contrast over all regions of the breast. As a result, it is possible to find smaller lesions (Fig. 6.5). In addition, the digital images can be electronically manipulated to make certain areas more prominent. Because of this, fewer repeat images are required for technical

Figure 6.3. Breast sonography of a 2-cm simple cyst. There is a sonolucent mass representing a benign cyst (*C*). Notice the shadowing (*) beneath the cyst.

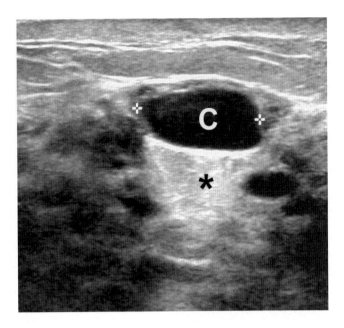

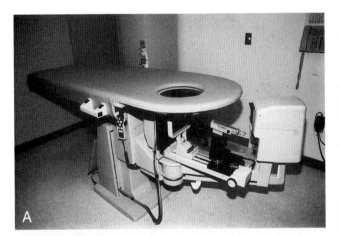

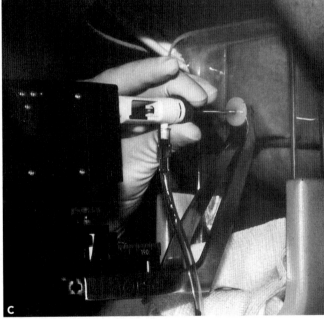

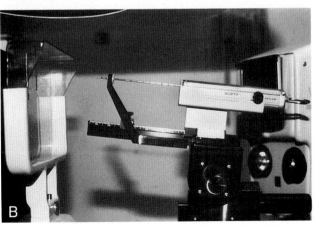

Figure 6.4. Stereotactic breast biopsy. A. Table and biopsy apparatus. The patient lies prone with the affected breast protruding through the hole in the tabletop. **B.** View of the biopsy apparatus fixed in front of a mammography tube and compression device. **C.** Mammographer guides the biopsy needle into place. (continued on page 224)

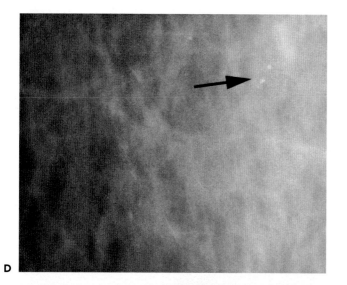

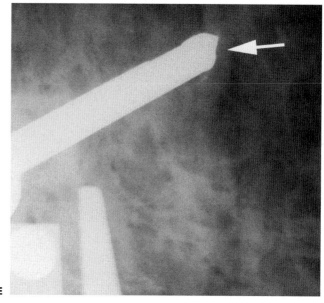

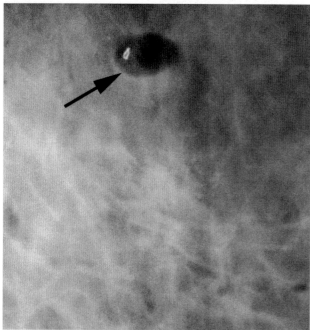

Figure 6.4. *(continued)* **D.** Detail of a mammogram showing microcalcifications in a small mass *(arrow)*. **E.** Placement of the core biopsy needle into the lesion *(arrow)*. **F.** Following biopsy, the mass and calcifications are gone and a small surgical clip is present at the excision site *(arrow)*.

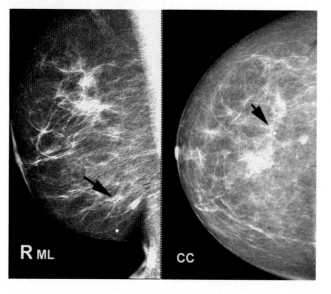

Figure 6.5. Digital mammogram in a 67-year-old woman showing a small (5-mm) carcinoma *(arrows)* **at the site of a palpable lump, delineated by radiopaque skin markers.** CC, craniocaudal view; ML, mediolateral view.

reasons. In addition, digital mammography allows images to be sent via teleradiology, facilitating mammography services in areas that do not have radiologists. Finally, digitization allows computer-aided diagnosis.

ANATOMIC AND PHYSIOLOGIC CONSIDERATIONS

The breast is actually a modified skin gland derived from the superficial layer of fascia beneath the skin. This layer divides into a superficial layer and a deep layer that forms a fibrous capsule containing the breast parenchyma. Just as the lung is divided into segments beginning at the bronchus, the breast is divided into segments. Each segment is drained by a major lactiferous duct that terminates at its orifice in the nipple (Fig. 6.6). Just as in the lung, the ducts branch into a series of terminal lobules that contain glandular lactiferous acini. The organization of segments is somewhat random and heterogeneous, making it difficult to precisely locate a lesion in a particular segment. Fortunately, this does not affect diagnostic accuracy.

The glandular tissue is supported by a crisscrossing network of fibrous tissue. Its fibrous stroma joins the superficial layer of fascia. Because of the malleable nature of the breast, imaging of the entire breast is complicated by the location of this cone-shaped structure on the cylindrical support of the chest wall. Breast tissue may be found as far medially as the sternal margin, laterally extending high into the axilla, and inferiorly into the inframammary fold. As a result, breast images are never completely free of chest wall structures—a distinct disadvantage to two-dimensional imaging. Although the standard mammogram relies on two views, craniocaudal and mediolateral oblique, additional views in selected cases are sometimes necessary to fully image the breast.

Imaging the breast is further complicated by the physiologic changes that occur in relationship to the patient's age and stage in the menstrual cycle. The breast in a young woman is extremely dense and consists mostly of glandular tissue. This glandular tissue is even more dense in a lactating woman. The tissue also increases in density and size during the later part of the menstrual cycle. As a woman ages, the glandular tissue is slowly replaced by fat. Because breast cancer is most common in older women whose breasts contain larger amounts of fat, the lesions are easier to detect than in younger women, in whom the dense glandular material often masks a tumor.

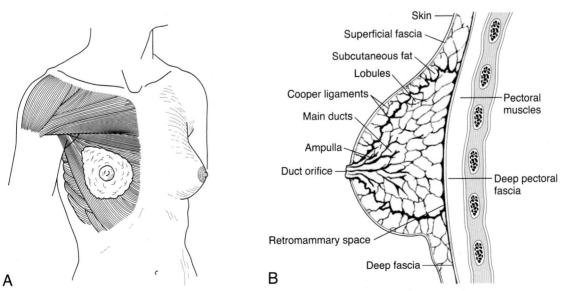

Figure 6.6.   Breast anatomy. A. Position of the breast on the pectoral muscles. **B.** Breast anatomy in longitudinal section.

PATHOLOGIC CONSIDERATIONS

Benign Lesions

A large variety of benign histologic changes occur in the breast. Many of these changes likely represent variations of normal parenchyma relating to hormonal status. The term *fibrocystic disease* is a catchall category of changes that include the presence of cysts, benign fibrous tissue, and dilated ducts in various configurations. The anatomy of the breast is such that a clinician palpating what is believed to be either a cyst or mass may, in fact, be feeling normal glandular tissue or fat surrounded by the fibrous stroma.

As a rule, benign lesions are round with smooth, well-defined margins (Figs. 6.7 and 6.8) and usually do not distort the normal breast architecture. They are often multiple and bilateral. Benign calcifications are usually coarse and are easily detectable with the unaided eye (Fig. 6.9). Macrocysts are cystic dilatations of the lactiferous duct. They are increasingly common in women in their mid-to-late 30s and are most commonly found in the premenopausal years. They generally regress after menopause. Cysts are usually distinguishable from solid tumors by ultrasound (see Fig. 6.8B). The fluid within the cysts varies in color, being clear, brown, green, or even black.

The most common solid benign tumor of the breast is the *fibroadenoma*. These tumors are hormonally sensitive and are found more commonly in young women. They are the solid lesions of the breast that undergo biopsy most frequently in women up to the mid-30s. The reason for their frequent biopsy is that they cannot be distinguished from well-circumscribed carcinomas, either by physical examination or imaging methods. Involution of fibroadenomas in postmenopausal women produces coarse calcifications.

Malignant Lesions

Ninety percent of breast cancer begins in the ductal epithelium. The histologic variety of ductal carcinomas is large. Although the carcinoma may be confined within the ductal tissue,

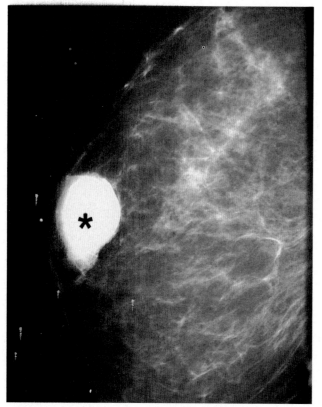

A

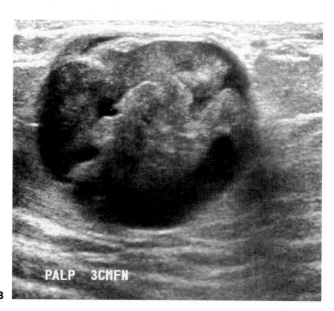

B

Figure 6.7.   Benign fibroadenoma in a 16-year-old patient.
A. Mediolateral mammogram shows a smooth, benign-appearing mass (*). **B.** Sonogram shows the mass to be solid, with smooth outer walls and no evidence of invasion.

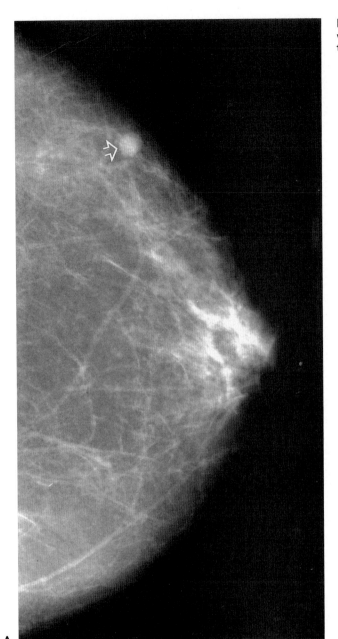

A

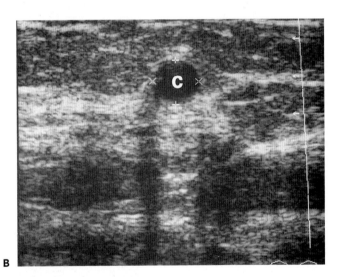

B

Figure 6.8.   Benign breast cyst. A. Craniocaudal view shows a well-defined mass with smooth margins (*arrow*). **B.** Ultrasound shows the sonolucent cyst (*C*) with shadowing and no internal echoes.

ultimately it will invade through the duct wall and spread via the lymphatic and vascular systems with resultant lymphatic and hematogenous metastases. The most common areas of lymphatic spread are to the axillary and internal mammary lymph nodes. If, at the time of detection, the axillary lymphatics are uninvolved, the 5-year survival is given as approximately 95%. This survival decreases to approximately 75% if axillary lymph nodes are involved. It is only 20% if distant metastases are present.

The radiographic findings of malignancy are those of a mass with ill-defined or irregular margins (Fig. 6.10). Other signs include a lobulated margin (Fig. 6.11), distortion and invasion of surrounding parenchyma (Fig. 6.12), clustered microcalcifications (Fig. 6.13), asymmetric density, asymmetric dilated ducts, and nipple retraction. Skin thickening and retraction are frequently found late in the disease and result from the desmoplastic effect of the tumor on the ligamentous support of the breast. Finally, enlargement of axillary lymph nodes may also be detected in a patient whose carcinoma has spread beyond the breast.

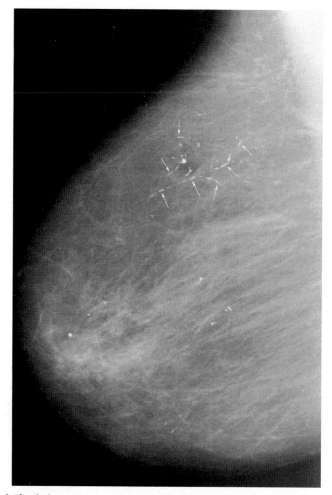

Figure 6.9. **Calcified ducts** (*arrows*). Fine, linear calcifications are present in a branching pattern. More-coarsened calcifications are located inferiorly.

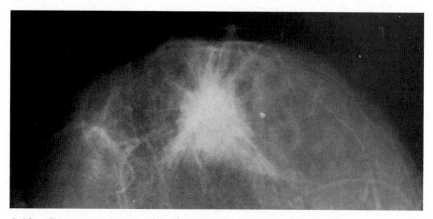

Figure 6.10. **Breast carcinoma showing classic spiculated, irregular margins.** Craniocaudal view shows distortion of normal breast parenchyma.

Figure 6.11. Breast carcinoma. Lobular margins and spiculated borders. Again, note the distortion of breast parenchyma anteriorly. The dense dot adjacent to the lesion is a marker placed by the technologist at the point the mass was palpated.

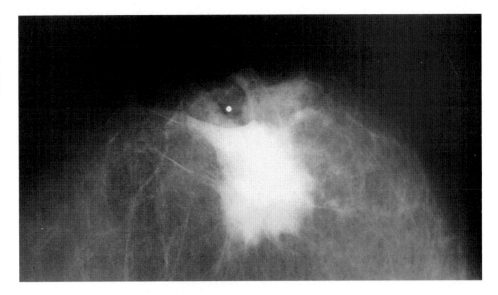

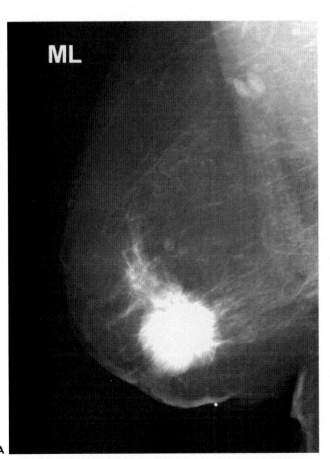

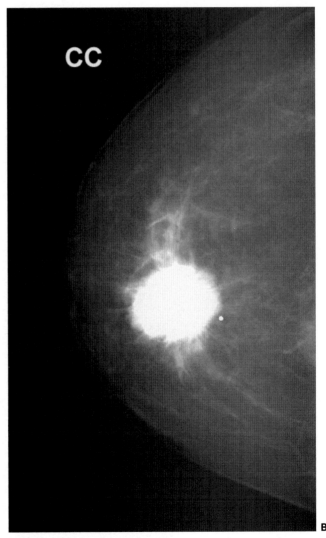

Figure 6.12.   Invasive ductal carcinoma in a 52-year-old patient. A. Mediolateral (*ML*) view. **B.** Craniocaudal (*CC*) view. These digital mammograms show the irregular dense mass with distortion and skin thickening at the site of a palpable mass, typical of carcinoma.   *(continued on page 230)*

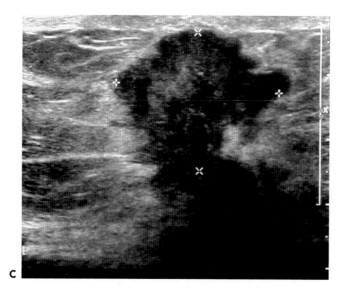

Figure 6.12. *(continued)* **C.** Ultrasound shows lobulated solid mass.

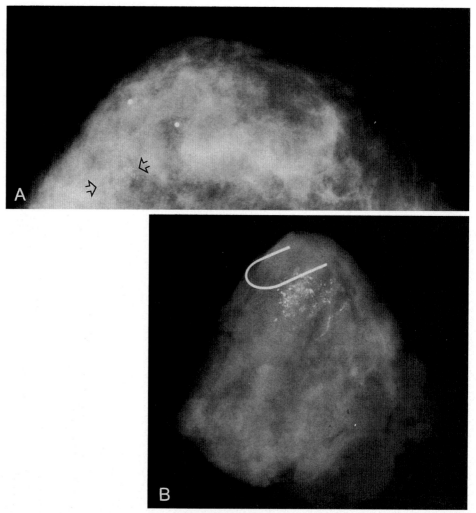

Figure 6.13.   Breast carcinoma with microcalcifications. A. Craniocaudal view shows clustered microcalcifications (*arrows*). The lesion sits deeper to the palpable masses that are identified by the two small dense pieces of shot anteriorly. Extensive fibrocystic disease is present. **B.** Radiograph of the surgical specimen. A localizing wire is present through the margin of the lesion. The entire lesion has been excised.

SUMMARY AND KEY POINTS

- Breast cancer is one of the most common malignancies in women.
- The mortality may be diminished by self-examination, clinical examination, and x-ray mammography.
- A baseline mammogram should be obtained on all asymptomatic women at age 40. Women ages 40 and older should have a yearly mammogram according to the most recent guidelines by the American Cancer Society and the American College of Radiology.
- Mammography should be performed only by skilled technologists under the supervision of an equally qualified radiologist to produce an examination of high diagnostic quality and with a low radiation dose.

SUGGESTED ADDITIONAL READING

American College of Radiology. ACR Practice Guideline for Performance of Diagnostic Mammography. Reston, VA: American College of Radiology, 2002.

American College of Radiology. ACR Practice Guideline for Performance of Magnetic Resonance Imaging (MRI) of the Breast. Reston, VA: American College of Radiology, 2004.

American College of Radiology. ACR Practice Guideline for Performance of Screening Mammography. Reston, VA: American College of Radiology, 2004.

American College of Radiology. ACR Practice Guideline for Performance of Stereotactically Guided Breast Interventional Procedures. Reston, VA: American College of Radiology, 2005.

American College of Radiology. ACR Practice Guideline for Performance of Whole Breast Digital Mammography. Reston, VA: American College of Radiology, 2001.

American College of Radiology. ACR Standard Practice Guideline for the Performance of Ultrasound-Guided Percutaneous Breast Interventional Procedures. Reston, VA: American College of Radiology, 2005.

Bassett L, Jackson V, Fu K, Fu Y. Diagnosis of Diseases of the Breast. 2nd Ed. Philadelphia: WB Saunders, 2005

Kopans DB. Breast Imaging. 2nd Ed. Philadelphia: Lippincott-Raven, 1998.

National Institutes of Health. Breast cancer screening for women ages 40–49. NIH Consensus Statement 1997;15(1):1–35.

Abdominal Radiographs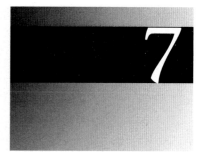

Computed tomography (CT) of the abdomen is being used extensively for diagnosing acute abdominal disorders. However, the abdominal radiograph is still an important examination for evaluating patients with suspected intra-abdominal disease. The lack of significant contrast among the abdominal viscera is considered by some a disadvantage in diagnosing disease (compared with the natural contrast occurring in the chest). This relatively unsophisticated imaging technique is highly sensitive and still provides a wealth of information from single or multiple abdominal radiographs, provided you know the anatomy and applied pathophysiology. Furthermore, the abdominal radiograph involves much less radiation exposure than does CT and costs considerably less than other studies.

There are certain principles that may help you to make a correct diagnosis in a patient with suspected abdominal disease and may guide you to perform additional diagnostic studies. As with any imaging study, you should always consider the diagnostic possibilities before ordering an abdominal radiograph. For example, abdominal radiographs are ordered in patients with known or suspected bleeding from esophageal varices, peptic ulcers, or the colon. Radiographic abnormalities are rare in these instances, and endoscopic or contrast examination is required to make the diagnosis. However, abdominal radiographs will, for example, provide diagnostic information concerning obstructions, gallstones, renal calculi, appendicoliths, and abscesses.

TECHNICAL CONSIDERATIONS

The type of radiographic examination of the abdomen should be tailored to the individual patient. For example, when searching for a missing sponge after surgery, a single supine film of the abdomen will suffice. The single film examination is also satisfactory to ascertain the presence of foreign bodies and to detect most intra-abdominal calcifications.

The *standard* abdominal radiograph, or KUB (a film showing the *kidneys, ureters,* and *bladder*), consists of a supine view, the so-called flat plate. The origin of the latter term is traced to a time when glass plates were used instead of film. At that time, stereoscopic examination was popular. Obtaining a single view of the abdomen, not in stereo, required ordering a "flat plate," an obsolete term replaced by *abdominal radiograph.*

For most patients suspected of having acute abdominal disease, an *upright film* will also be made. The purpose of this view is twofold: to identify the presence of free intraperitoneal air and to detect the presence of intestinal air-fluid levels. This study is made by having the patient stand or sit. The principle involved is the use of a *horizontal beam.* If the patient cannot stand or sit, a horizontal beam study may be performed by placing the patient in the *left lateral decubitus position* (left side down, right side up). This study is especially useful in severely ill patients who are suspected of having free intraperitoneal air. It is important that the patient be placed on the left

Figure 7.1. Pneumoperitoneum demonstrated on a left lateral decubitus radiograph. A large collection of free air is along the right flank. Notice air on both sides of the bowel wall (*open arrows*). The air-fluid levels (*small arrows*) indicate that this is a horizontal beam radiograph.

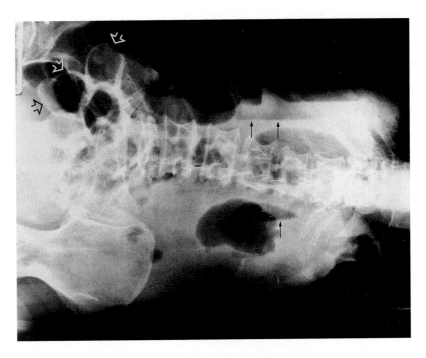

side for several minutes to allow any free air to rise over the dome of the liver. This technique can detect as little as 1 mL of free air. Once again, because of the horizontal beam, intestinal air-fluid levels may be detected. Figure 7.1 shows a patient with a pneumoperitoneum demonstrated in the left lateral decubitus position.

Because most patients with acute abdominal conditions will be admitted to the hospital, it is also desirable to obtain a *chest radiograph*. The order of filming in these patients should be as follows: abdominal left lateral decubitus, upright posterior-anterior (PA) of the chest (to allow any free air to rise under the diaphragm and be seen), and a supine abdomen.

As with any other radiologic study, you should first examine the film for *proper identification and technical quality*. A film that is too light or too dark is of little diagnostic value. Motion obscures soft tissue images and blurs the outline of a gas-filled bowel, calcifications, and other structures. As a rule, portable radiographs are helpful in detecting only gross intra-abdominal abnormalities.

Abdominal CT is one of the best technical advances for making a diagnosis of intra-abdominal disease. Multidetector CT technology has enhanced the value of the technology, speeding the examination to allow an abdominal scan to be performed in under 30 seconds. As mentioned previously, the lack of sufficient tissue contrast between the various abdominal organs is a handicap to routine radiographic diagnosis. However, the abdominal CT scan can differentiate organ densities better than radiographs, can outline these organs, and can detect subtle abnormalities that may escape diagnosis on abdominal radiographs (Figs. 7.2 and 7.3).

Finally, *ultrasonography* is an important adjunct in the evaluation of abdominal disease. It is most useful for evaluating masses and aortic aneurysms (Fig. 7.4) and detecting biliary and renal disease. Ultrasound is used in trauma patients to detect liver and splenic injuries, as well as intraperitoneal blood.

ANATOMIC CONSIDERATIONS

Figure 7.5 shows a *normal supine abdominal radiograph* of a young woman. The abdominal gas pattern is normal. Under normal circumstances, small quantities of gas are present within the stomach and portions of the small bowel and colon. The caliber of these loops is normal.

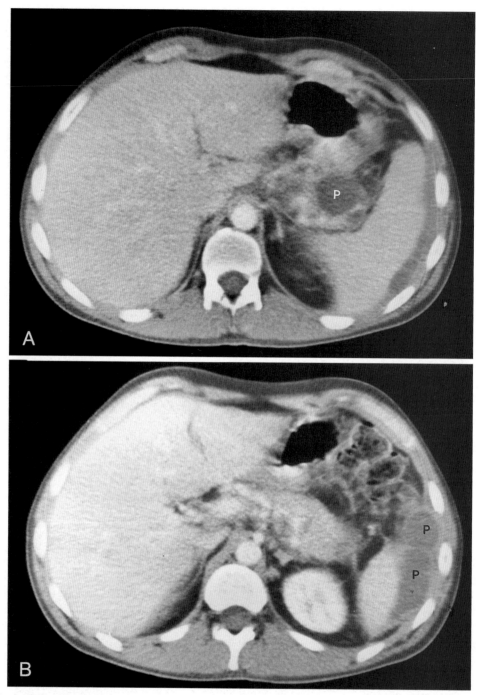

Figure 7.2.   Pancreatic pseudocyst. A. Computed tomography (CT) image shows the pseudocyst (*P*) in the tail of the pancreas. **B.** Image slightly more distal shows multilocular pseudocysts surrounding the lateral aspect of the spleen.

There is no evidence of mucosal thickening. The normal small bowel valvulae conniventes and colonic haustra should not exceed 3 mm in thickness when outlined by air. The exact anatomy of these loops is defined by the mucosal pattern (Fig. 7.6).

Images of the kidneys, spleen, liver, and psoas muscles should be sought on all abdominal radiographs (see Fig. 7.5). These are identifiable because of the small amounts of fat that surround them. In evaluating hepatic or splenic size, remember that one is really only seeing the posterior margin of each organ because of the location of the adjacent extraperitoneal perivisceral fat.

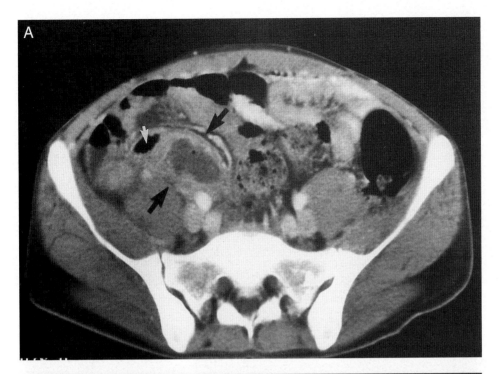

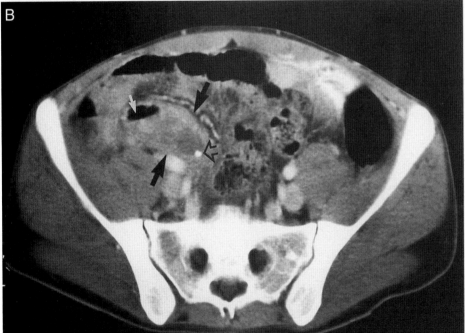

Figure 7.3. Appendiceal abscess. A. CT image demonstrates a mass in the right lower quadrant with a lucent center (*black arrows*). Notice the gas collection anteriorly (*white arrow*). **B.** Image slightly more distal shows similar findings with an associated fecalith (*open arrow*).

The *properitoneal flank or fat stripe* outlines the *margins of the abdomen* lateral to the ascending and descending colon. This stripe appears as a lucent line separating the soft tissues of the skin from the abdominal cavity. The line is often obliterated in inflammatory conditions of the abdomen (appendicitis, peritonitis, etc.).

Under normal circumstances, *gas patterns* should change over a period of several minutes when serial films are made. This indicates normal peristaltic activity. Absence of this activity, particularly when there is absolutely no change in the appearance of the bowel, is strongly suggestive of bowel infarction.

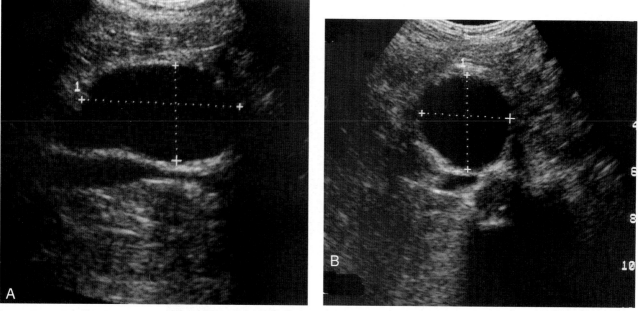

Figure 7.4. Abdominal aortic aneurysm. Longitudinal **(A)** and axial **(B)** ultrasound sections demonstrate a large saccular aneurysm that measures 27.00 cm in the longitudinal plane and 13.65 cm in the axial plane.

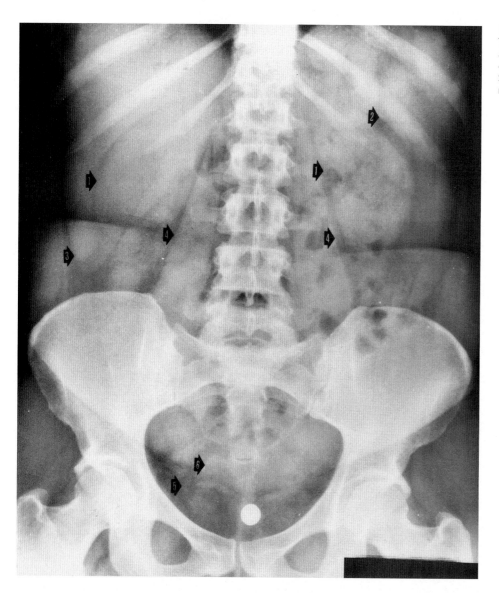

Figure 7.5. Normal abdomen. The bowel gas pattern is unremarkable. The following soft tissue shadows are visible: (*1*) Kidneys. (*2*) Spleen. (*3*) Liver margin. (*4*) Psoas muscles. (*5*) Bladder. (*6*) Uterus.

Figure 7.6. Normal mucosal patterns. From top to bottom: stomach, small intestine, colon. The horizontal mucosal folds running the length of the stomach are the *gastric rugae.* The vertical mucosal folds of the small intestine are the *valvulae conniventes.* The vertical mucosal folds of the colon are the *haustra.*

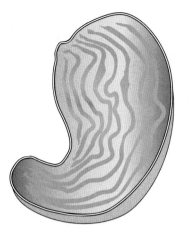

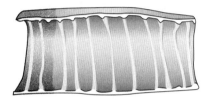

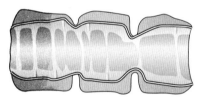

The *bony structures* encountered on an abdominal **radiograph** include the lower thoracic and lumbar vertebrae, sacrum, lower ribs, pelvis, and hips. Frequently, degenerative changes will be present in the spines of older individuals.

Finally, one should be aware that there is a significant amount of the *lower lobe of each lung* visible on abdominal radiographs. It is not uncommon for pneumonia in these extreme basal portions of the lungs (Fig. 7.7) to manifest as acute abdominal pain, particularly in a child. Furthermore, tumors may occasionally be demonstrated on an abdominal radiograph (Fig. 7.8).

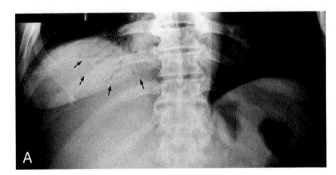

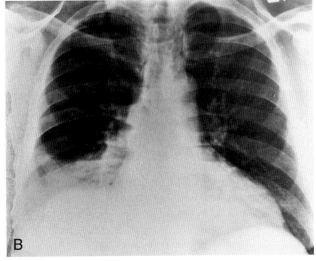

Figure 7.7. Right lower lobe pneumonia seen on an abdominal radiograph. A. Abdominal radiograph shows multiple air-bronchograms (*arrows*) behind the liver image. **B.** Chest radiograph shows the consolidation in the right lower lobe.

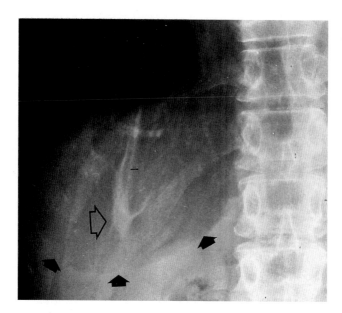

Figure 7.8. Carcinoma (*open arrow*) of the extreme base of the right lower lobe (*solid arrows*).

PATHOLOGIC CONSIDERATIONS

Pathologic alterations seen on the plain film include the following:

- Abnormal gas and mucosal patterns
- Abnormalities of soft tissue images
- Abnormal calcifications
- Abnormal fluid—ascites
- Bone and joint abnormalities
- Postoperative changes

Abnormal Gas and Mucosal Patterns

Intraluminal Gas

The gas demonstrated on abdominal radiographs is either *intraluminal* or *extraluminal*. The abnormalities produced by *intraluminal gas* include distension or dilation of one or more bowel loops, the presence of air-fluid levels (Fig. 7.9), and the presence of mucosal thickening (Fig. 7.10). Intraluminal gas, when mixed with bowel content, frequently gives a bubbly appearance, particularly in the colon. In infants and children, however, this "adult stool pattern" is never normal, and the patient should be studied further to determine the source of the abnormality.

How can you, the clinician, determine whether a loop or multiple loops of bowel are *dilated*? No firm answers or numerical limits are listed in references. However, two rules of thumb may help you decide: (1) a single air-filled loop of small bowel or colon that is distinctly much larger than the others on serial films may represent local dilation, and (2) multiple air-filled loops of small bowel or colon that give the abdomen a distinctive "gas bag" appearance usually represent ileus or obstruction. In many instances, you will have to use your judgment and experience in looking at these examinations to make a determination of bowel distension. As always, whenever in doubt, consult your radiologist.

Distended or dilated bowel may occur under a variety of circumstances. Most often this is of the so-called *adynamic ileus* type, in which peristalsis is markedly diminished. The typical appearance shows gaseous distension of the colon and small bowel in a "mild stasis" pattern. Interestingly enough, air-fluid levels may be present in these patients. These occur in both the large and small bowels in what has been termed a "balanced" (even-distribution) pattern. This

Figure 7.9. Air-fluid levels in a patient with a small bowel obstruction. Notice the dilation of the air-filled loops.

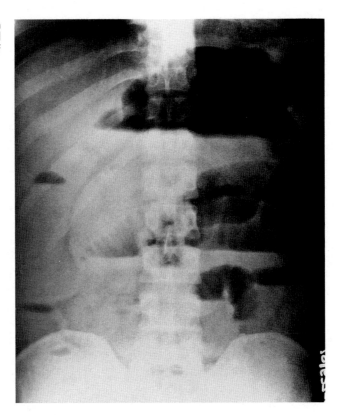

pattern occurs most commonly in patients following trauma (including surgery), with peritonitis, as a manifestation of taking drugs, in bowel ischemia, and in chronically ill, bedridden patients.

A localized ileus that persists on serial studies is suggestive of an adjacent area of inflammation. This occurs in pancreatitis (Figs. 7.11 and 7.12) and acute appendicitis and is called a *sentinel loop*.

Distended loops of bowel with air-fluid levels in a diffuse pattern are highly suggestive of a *mechanical obstruction* (see Fig. 7.9). The typical pattern shows a distended cascade of loops proximal to the obstruction and an essentially gasless distal abdomen. The bowel loops frequently have a stepwise appearance or are of the hairpin (180° turn) type. *The presence of gas within the rectum does not rule out a low obstructing colonic lesion.* Gas may be introduced into the rectum by digital examination, colonoscopy, rectal temperature determination, and enemas. In an early obstruction, the characteristic pattern may not be well developed. However, serial examinations will show the development of the characteristic loops.

The causes of a mechanical obstruction vary, depending on whether the patient is an adult or a child. In the adult, common causes include adhesions (Fig. 7.13), hernia, tumor, and volvulus (Fig. 7.14). In infants and children, intussusception (Fig. 7.15) is a common cause of obstruction. In the newborn and very young infant, duodenal atresia (Fig. 7.16) should be suspected. Each of these conditions has characteristic findings that, when present, should allow you to make a correct diagnosis. *Intussusception* occurs when a segment of intestine (the *intussusceptum*) invaginates or "telescopes" into the contiguous distal segment (the *intussuscipiens*). This produces mechanical obstruction and, if left untreated, ischemia. Approximately 90% of intussusceptions are ileocolic; the remainder are (in decreasing order of frequency) ileoileocolic, ileoileal, and colocolic. Unlike adults, in whom intussusceptions are typically caused by mesenteric neoplasms, those in the pediatric age group are idiopathic. Radiographic findings, when present, include a mass effect, targetlike lucencies in the mass (representing mesenteric fat trapped in the intussusception), and a crescent or streaks of air outlining the trapped bowel (see Fig. 7.15).

Duodenal atresia is the most common site of intestinal atresia. Two variants occur: membranous and stenosis. The abdominal radiograph typically demonstrates gaseous dilatation

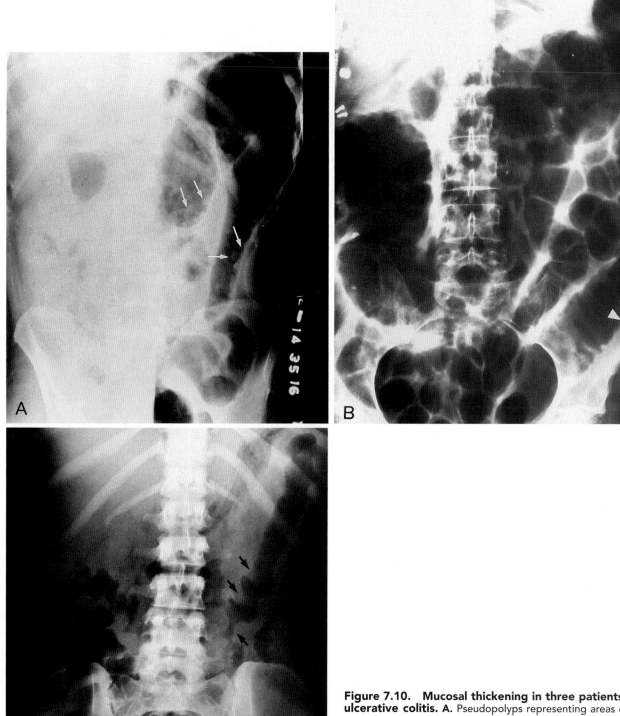

Figure 7.10.   Mucosal thickening in three patients with ulcerative colitis. A. Pseudopolyps representing areas of preserved mucosa are present throughout the bowel (*arrows*). **B.** Notice the thickened bowel wall on the left side (*arrowheads*). **C.** The thick mucosa has the appearance of "thumbprinting" (*arrows*). Notice the loss of haustral markings more proximally.

Figure 7.11. Sentinel loop of the transverse colon in a patient with pancreatitis. Notice the pancreatic calcifications (*arrows*). A bullet from a previous gunshot wound is present over the pelvis on the left side.

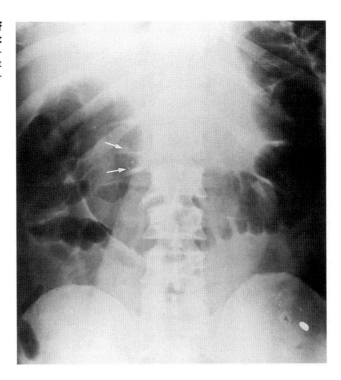

Figure 7.12. Small bowel sentinel loop in a patient with pancreatitis of the tail of the pancreas. A single dilated loop of jejunum (*arrow*) is present. Notice the increased distance between the jejunum and the contrast-filled stomach as the result of pancreatic phlegmon.

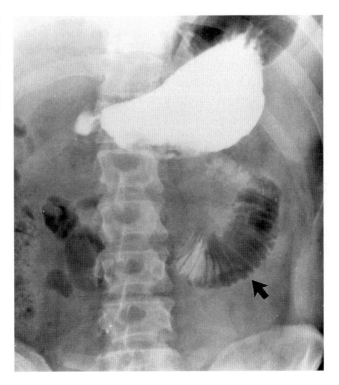

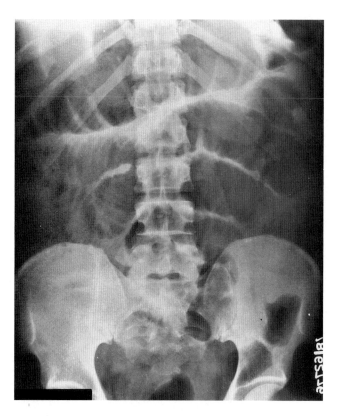

Figure 7.13. Small bowel obstruction, supine view. (This is the same patient as Fig. 7.9.) Dilated air-filled loops of small intestine are evident in a cascading pattern. The pattern is suggestive of bowel obstruction.

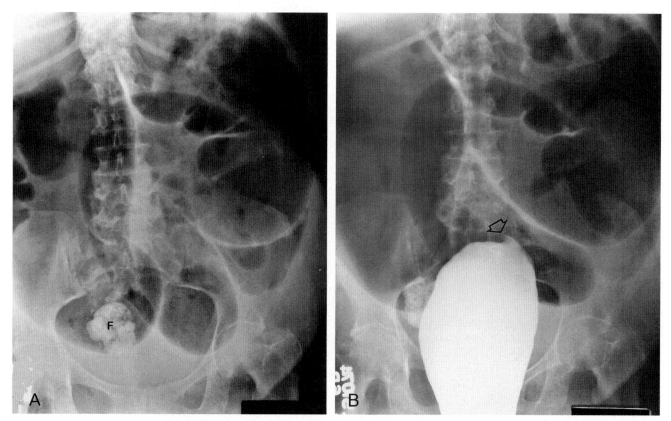

Figure 7.14. Sigmoid volvulus. A. Supine abdominal film shows massive dilatation of the colon. Incidental note is made of a calcified uterine fibroid (*F*). **B.** Barium enema shows the site of the volvulus (*arrow*).

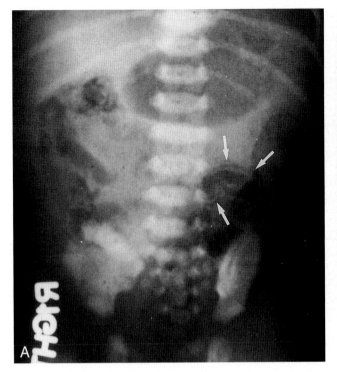

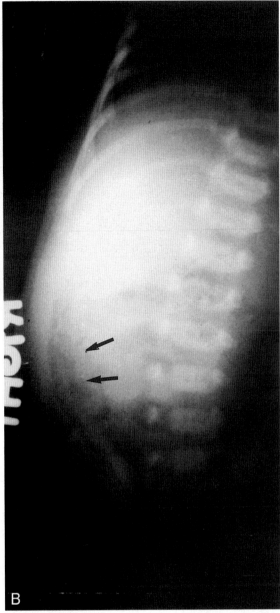

Figure 7.15. **Intussusception.** Supine **(A)** and left lateral decubitus **(B)** radiographs demonstrate crescentic streaks of air within the trapped loops of bowel (*arrows*).

of the stomach and duodenal bulb without distal gas. The appearance has been termed the "double-bubble" sign (see Fig. 7.16).

As mentioned previously, peristaltic activity, even in a patient with bowel obstruction, should be evident by changes that occur in the outline of gas-filled loops. You should always be cognizant, therefore, of the bowel loops that fail to change their configuration on serial radiographs. This finding is considered pathognomonic for dead bowel, usually the result of ischemic disease.

Inguinal hernias are fairly common entities in adults, and occasionally in children. They can be recognized by the presence of an enlarged scrotum that contains multiple loops of air-filled bowel (Fig. 7.17). Incarceration of a hernia may be the cause of obstruction.

Most abdominal radiographs are obtained to determine the presence or absence of *intestinal obstruction.* A term that is frequently used for those studies in which the findings are not positive is *nonspecific abdominal gas pattern.* This term should be abandoned because it gives little

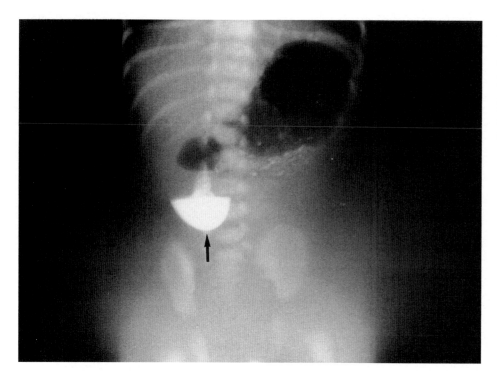

Figure 7.16. Duodenal atresia. Supine radiograph demonstrates the "double bubble" of air trapped in the stomach and the duodenal bulb. Notice the absence of other gas in the abdomen. The white density beneath the duodenal air is barium in the descending duodenum. Notice the abrupt termination of this loop at the level of the atresia (*arrow*).

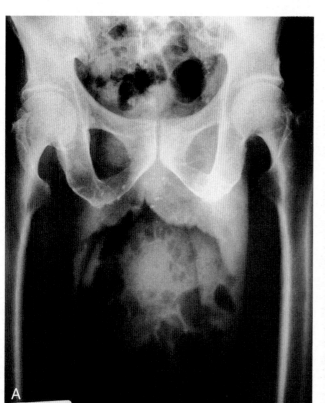

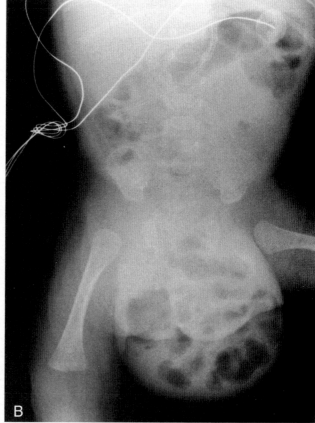

Figure 7.17. Inguinal hernia. In both an adult **(A)** and a newborn **(B)**, loops of bowel fill the scrotum.

information regarding what is actually present on the radiograph. Maglinte has suggested that the term be replaced by something more descriptive of the various intestinal gas patterns encountered. He has four categories: (1) *normal,* defined as either absence of small bowel gas or presence of gas within not more than four variably shaped loops of small intestine that are also less than 2.5 cm in diameter; (2) *mild bowel stasis,* defined as multiple slightly dilated (2.5- to 3-cm) loops with three or more air-fluid levels, without disproportionate distension of the small bowel relative to the colon; (3) *probable obstructive pattern,* defined as unequivocal dilation of multiple gas or fluid-filled loops of bowel, with multiple air-fluid levels but an element of uncertainty of the diagnosis of obstruction; and (4) *definite obstructive pattern,* in which the diagnosis is unequivocal. For small bowel obstruction, gaseous distension of small bowel is disproportionate to the colon.

Mucosal Patterns

The *natural contrast* between the soft tissues, the mucosa, and the air within the bowel allows evaluation of that bowel. A thickened bowel wall is always abnormal. Mucosal thickening is generally present when the valvulae conniventes of the small intestine or the colonic haustra are thicker than 3 mm. If the bowel is distended with air, the actual (edematous) wall may be identified by air on one side and increased soft tissue density on the other (see Fig. 7.10). Thickened mucosa are most often encountered in inflammatory bowel disease (see Fig. 7.10), bowel edema in hypoproteinemic and malabsorption states, submucosal hemorrhage of any cause, and ischemia (Fig. 7.18). These last two conditions often produce two interesting patterns of mucosal thickening: thumblike indentations in the gas-filled bowel ("thumbprinting") and a picket fence appearance of the valvulae in the small bowel (the "stacked coin" appearance). The exact cause of the thickening cannot be determined without applying important history and physical examination findings. For example, a patient with a history of sudden

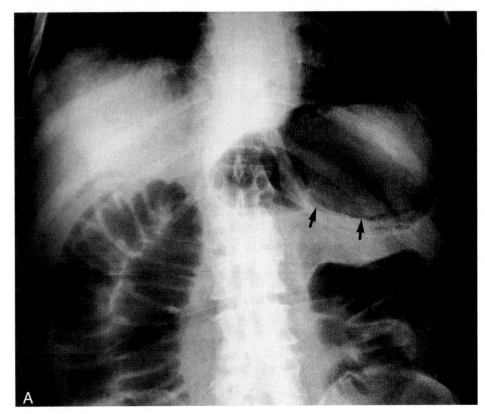

Figure 7.18. Bowel ischemia from a massive celiac and mesenteric infarction. A. Detail view of upper abdomen shows pneumatosis in the stomach wall (*arrows*). (continued on page 246)

Figure 7.18. *(continued)* **B.** View of lower abdomen shows pneumatosis of the small bowel (*arrow*). **C.** CT section shows pneumatosis (*arrows*) in a loop of small bowel. Notice how thick the wall is. *(continued on page 247)*

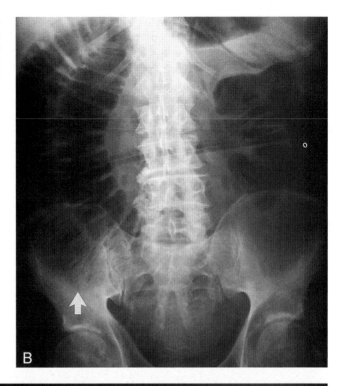

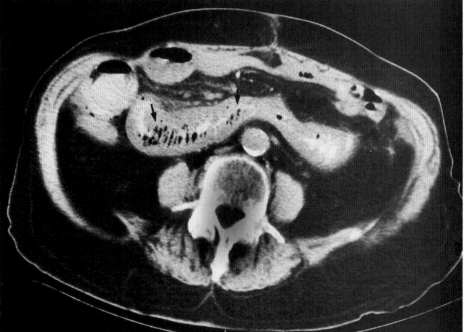

onset of abdominal pain accompanied by blood-streaked diarrhea and dilated bowel on plain film is likely to have colitis (see Fig. 7.10).

Extraluminal Gas

Extraluminal gas may be either free (*pneumoperitoneum*) or contained within an abscess cavity, the retroperitoneum, the bowel wall, or the biliary or portal venous systems of the liver.

Free intraperitoneal air in the absence of immediate previous surgery suggests a ruptured viscus. The most common cause is a perforated peptic ulcer or a colonic diverticulum. Trauma is another cause. If the perforation is intraperitoneal, gas will be seen under

Figure 7.18. *(continued)*   **D and E.** CT sections through the liver show portal venous gas (*arrows*).

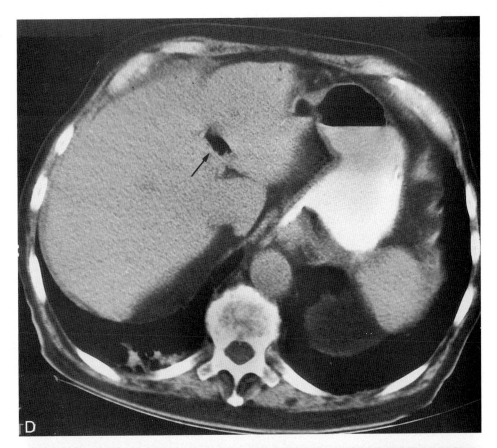

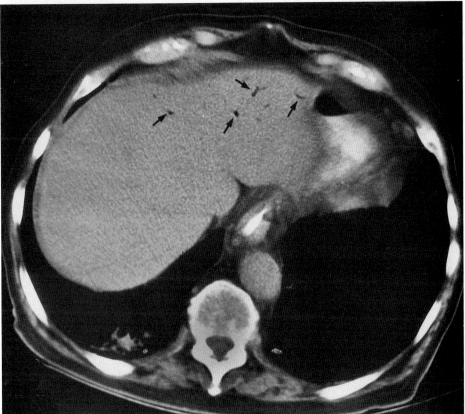

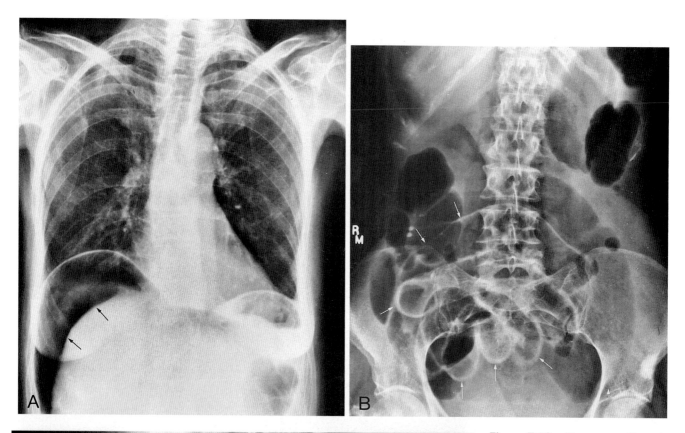

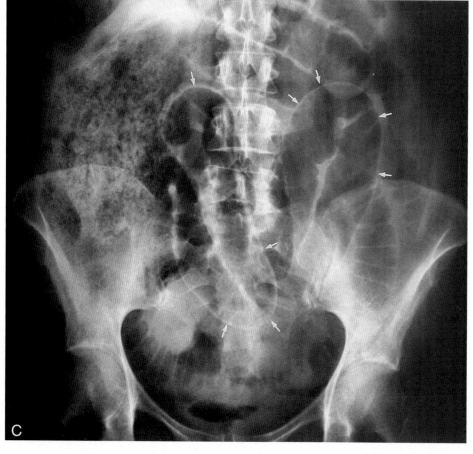

Figure 7.19.   Pneumoperitoneum.
A. Chest radiograph shows air beneath the diaphragm. The liver margin is outlined by air (*arrows*). **B.** Supine abdominal radiograph of this massive pneumoperitoneum shows air on both sides of the bowel wall (*arrows*). **C.** Supine radiograph in another patient also shows air on both sides of the bowel wall. The serosal surfaces are clearly defined (*arrows*).

both leaves of the diaphragm on an upright radiograph (Fig. 7.19A). Furthermore, decubitus positioning may also demonstrate free intraperitoneal air (see Fig. 7.1). However, it is possible to make the diagnosis of pneumoperitoneum on a supine film from the *double-wall sign*, which results when air on both sides of the bowel outlines that structure rather distinctly (see Fig. 7.19B). Under normal circumstances, the *serosal* surface of bowel is not visible because of its water density. Air within the peritoneal cavity, however, changes the radiographic density that outlines the bowel wall. In infants, who are usually examined in the supine position, free intraperitoneal air may outline the falciform ligament. Massive pneumoperitoneum may also produce the *football sign*, in which there is an overall lucency to the abdomen, much like a football with the vertebrae representing the laces (Fig. 7.20).

Retroperitoneal air, particularly from a perforated duodenal ulcer or ruptured duodenum secondary to trauma, is often manifest as a sharpening or enhancement of the psoas shadow. Occasionally, the renal image will be highlighted as well. This diagnosis may be difficult to make based on radiographs. However, on a CT scan, the presence of retroperitoneal air is easily detected.

Gas loculated within the abdomen generally indicates the presence of an *abscess*. The air may be confined to a known anatomic space (such as Morison's pouch beneath the liver), to an emphysematous gallbladder (Fig. 7.21), to the renal capsule (Fig. 7.22), to the lesser sac, or within an organ (Fig. 7.23), or it may be free within the abdominal cavity. The gas may be a small localized collection or, more commonly, may have a mottled bubbly appearance. Frequently, it is necessary to do a CT examination with oral or rectal contrast to determine the location of normal loops of bowel and to rule out the presence of an aberrant loop of bowel being responsible for the abnormal shadow. The CT scan is also the most reliable study for the diagnosis of abscesses (Figs. 7.24 and 7.25).

Figure 7.20. Pneumoperitoneum in an infant. The free air in the abdomen outlines the peritoneal cavity, giving it a football shape, with the vertebrae representing the laces.

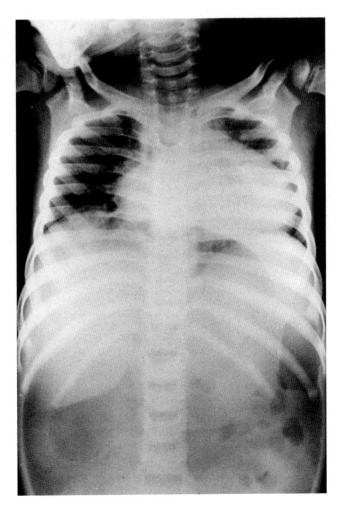

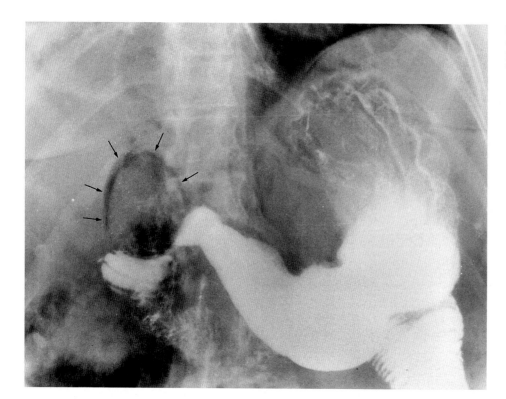

Figure 7.21. Emphysematous cholecystitis in a diabetic patient. Gas outlines the gallbladder (*arrows*).

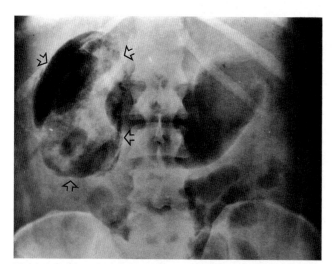

Figure 7.22. Emphysematous pyelonephritis in a diabetic patient. A large collection of gas outlines the right kidney (*arrows*). The psoas margin on the right is lost.

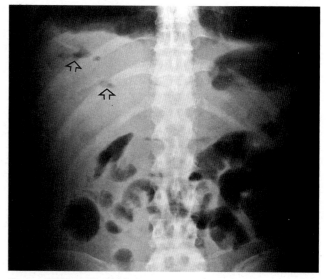

Figure 7.23. Liver abscess. Collections of gas are within the liver (*arrows*). A CT scan would confirm the extent of the lesion.

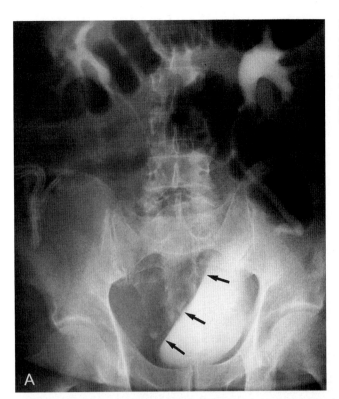

Figure 7.24. Left flank abscess.
A. Intravenous urogram shows displacement of the right ureter to the left by a large flank mass on the right. Notice the flattening and compression of the right side of the bladder wall (*arrows*). **B.** CT image shows the large abscess (*A*) compressing the right lateral wall of the bladder (*B; arrows*).

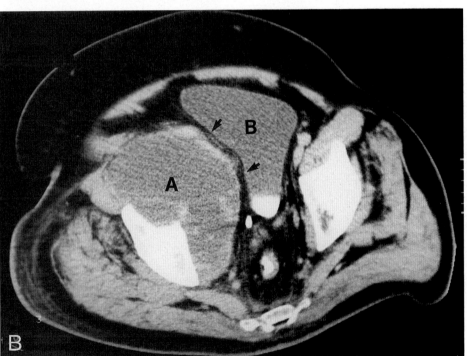

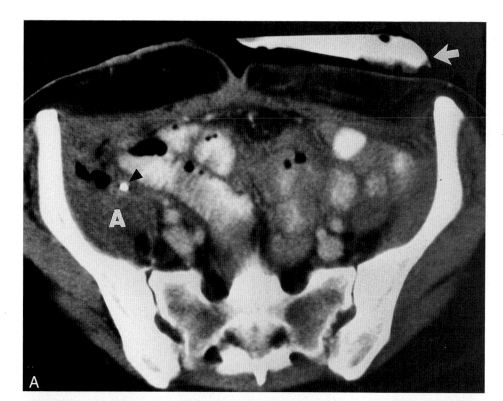

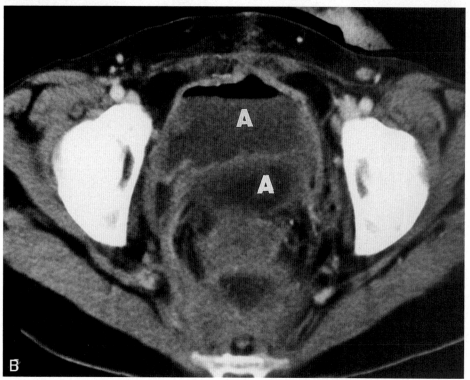

Figure 7.25. Multilocular abscesses (A) of the pelvis in a patient with regional enteritis (Crohn disease). A. Notice the colostomy bag on the abdominal surface (*arrow*). An appendicolith is adjacent to the abscess on the right (*arrowhead*). **B.** The abscess collects at the most dependent portion of the peritoneum.

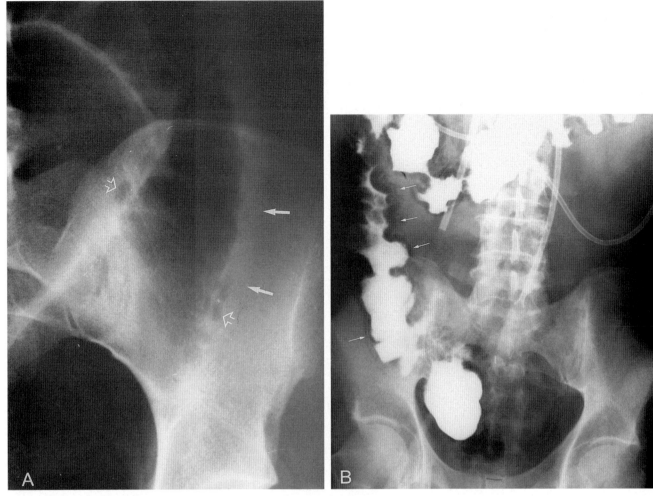

Figure 7.26.   Pneumatosis intestinalis. A. Detail view of the left lower quadrant of a patient with ulcerative colitis. Notice the thickening of the bowel wall (*solid arrows*) and the gas within the bowel wall (*open arrows*). **B.** Massive pneumatosis (*arrows*) in another patient with ischemic colitis.

Intramural gas (*pneumatosis intestinalis*) may be found in a variety of benign and pathologic conditions. A common cause of pneumatosis in older adults is microperforation of a diverticulum. Gas appears as streaky densities surrounding the bowel (Fig. 7.26). Occasionally, a giant air cyst will occur. CT also demonstrates intramural gas (Fig. 7.27). Intramural gas may also be found in bowel infarction in older patients and particularly in premature newborn children with necrotizing enterocolitis (Fig. 7.28). In both types of patients, gas may be found within the portal system of the liver.

Gas in the *biliary tree* may occur following endoscopic papillotomy (Fig. 7.29), following surgery in which the common bile duct is anastomosed to the small bowel, or in infection. Portal gas is usually located in the periphery, whereas biliary gas in seen more centrally. Correlation with the clinical findings is necessary to properly interpret this observation.

Abnormalities of Soft Tissue Images

Soft tissue abnormalities include displacement or misplacement, enlargement, presence of a mass, and loss of margins. Although CT, ultrasound, and, to some extent, magnetic resonance (MR) examinations provide more detailed information regarding these abnormalities, the radiograph can detect most of them. In my experience, abdominal abscesses produce radiographic abnormalities in up to 70% of cases.

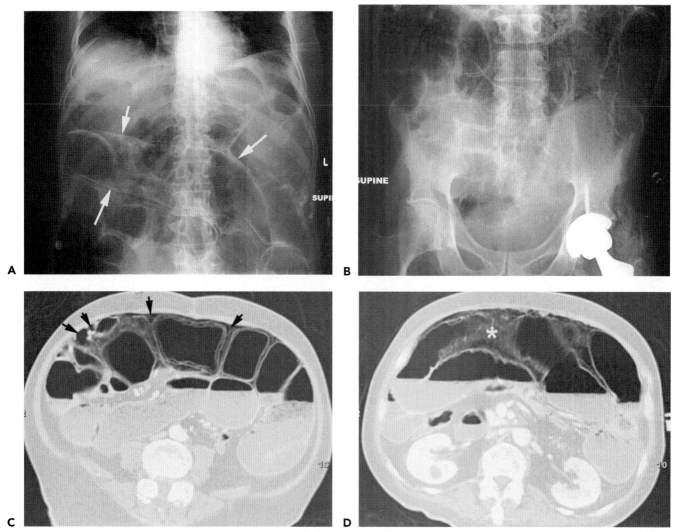

Figure 7.27.   Intramural gas and pneumoperitoneum caused by a bowel infarction. A and B. Supine radiographs show dilated loops of the small and large bowels. Both sides of the bowel wall can be seen in A (*arrows*). **C.** CT image shows dilated loops of bowel anteriorly with gas in the walls. Notice the pneumoperitoneum between the dilated loops (*arrows*). **D.** CT image shows pneumatosis (*) in the wall of the dilated loop of small bowel.

Enlargement of the abdominal organs may cause displacement of other organs. For example, splenomegaly will displace the gastric air shadow medially (Fig. 7.30). Enlargement of the pancreas will cause anterior displacement of the stomach (demonstrated on an upper gastrointestinal series). The renal image may be displaced inferiorly by an enlarged adrenal gland or tumor and laterally by enlarged paraspinal lymph nodes.

Certain *congenital anomalies*, particularly of the urinary tract, may result in abnormal position of the kidneys. In a patient with a horseshoe kidney, the lower poles are oriented toward the midline. Malposition of a kidney may result in the absence of the normal renal outline on the plain film, especially if the kidney is within the pelvis.

Abdominal masses are frequently revealed by the displacements or distortion of normal viscera (Fig. 7.31). The most common mass encountered in the pelvis is a distended bladder. If you doubt the diagnosis, a repeat radiograph should be made after the patient has successfully voided. CT is recommended for confirmation of all masses.

The *loss of the margin* of a soft tissue structure is a valuable sign in evaluating patients with abdominal disease. The loss of a renal outline or psoas margin (see Fig. 7.22) generally indicates an inflammatory condition in the retroperitoneum. The loss of the psoas margin accompanied by scoliosis is a nonspecific finding that may be seen in acute appendicitis,

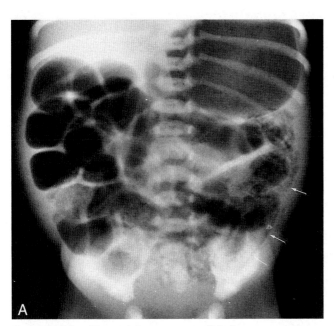 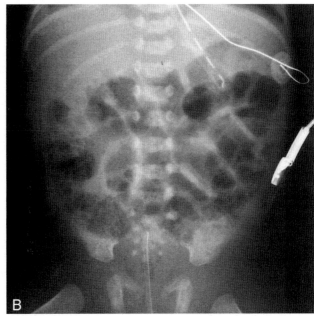

Figure 7.28.   Necrotizing enterocolitis in a premature newborn. A. Pneumatosis intestinalis is on the left side (*arrows*). **B.** A similar pattern appears bilaterally in another patient. The adult stool pattern is always abnormal in an infant.

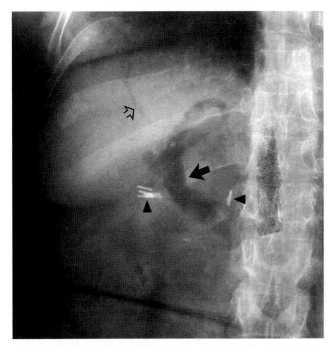 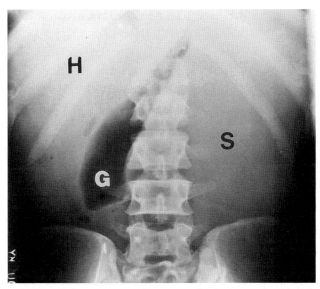

Figure 7.30.   Hepatosplenomegaly in a patient with Hodgkin disease. Notice the enlargement of the liver (*H*) and spleen (*S*). The gastric air bubble (*G*) is displaced to the right of midline.

Figure 7.29.   Pneumobilia in a patient following endoscopic papillotomy. Notice the air in the dilated common bile duct (*solid arrow*), common hepatic ducts, and intrahepatic ducts (*open arrow*). Surgical clips (*arrowheads*) from a previous cholecystectomy are evident.

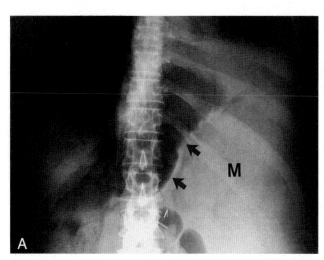
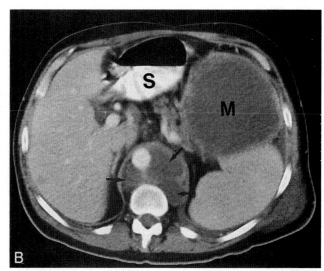

Figure 7.31.   Mass effect caused by splenic metastases. A. Detail of an abdominal radiograph shows a large mass (*M*) displacing and compressing the greater curvature of the stomach (*arrows*). **B.** CT section shows the mass (*M*) to be in the anterior pole of the spleen. Notice the relationship of the mass to the stomach (*S*) as well as the necrotic para-aortic lymph nodes (*arrows*).

urinary calculus, or perforated viscus. As mentioned previously, the loss of the properitoneal fat line may also be seen in several inflammatory conditions, particularly appendicitis.

Abnormal Calcifications

The list of calcifications that may be found on abdominal radiographs is long and beyond the scope of this text. However, certain physiologic conditions frequently produce calcifications seen on abdominal studies. These include the costal cartilages, vascular calcifications (such as phleboliths in the pelvic venous plexus), atherosclerotic plaques of the aortoiliac vessels, prostatic calcifications, and old granulomas of spleen and lymph nodes. Several of these are illustrated in Figure 7.32. Abnormal calcifications include biliary (Fig. 7.33) and urinary calculi (Fig. 7.34), calcified aneurysms (Fig. 7.35), pancreatic calcifications (Fig. 7.36), calcified uterine fibroid tumors, and calcified appendiceal fecaliths (Fig. 7.37). In addition, foreign bodies may often be seen. These may include ingested foreign materials (e.g., tablets; Fig. 7.38) or traumatic foreign bodies (e.g., bullets, buckshot, or shrapnel). You may, on occasion, see a patient with a self-introduced rectal foreign body (Fig. 7.39). On occasion, fragments of antacid tablets may collect in a gastric ulcer (Fig. 7.40).

Abnormal Fluid—Ascites

The classic appearance of ascites has been described as diffuse, "ground glass" density of the abdomen. Generally, by the time this has occurred, ascites is clinically apparent and need not be diagnosed by radiographic means. However, small amounts of peritoneal fluid (ascites or blood) may appear in a subtle manner.

The accumulation of several hundred milliliters of ascitic fluid may be apparent on the supine radiograph as a collection of water-density material overlying the sacrum above the bladder. This occurs because the fluid collects posteriorly in the pelvis. With increasing volume, however, the ascites extends superolaterally out of the pelvis, producing bilateral collections on either side of the main fluid bulk, giving the appearance of "dog ears." Further increase in the amount of fluid (to more than 500 mL) will extend up along the lateral gutters, displacing the colon medially from the radiolucent flank stripes (Fig. 7.41). As the amount of fluid increases, the liver and spleen are displaced from the body wall. Finally, floating loops of bowel may be seen in the "sea of ascites." CT and ultrasound are more useful in diagnosing ascites.

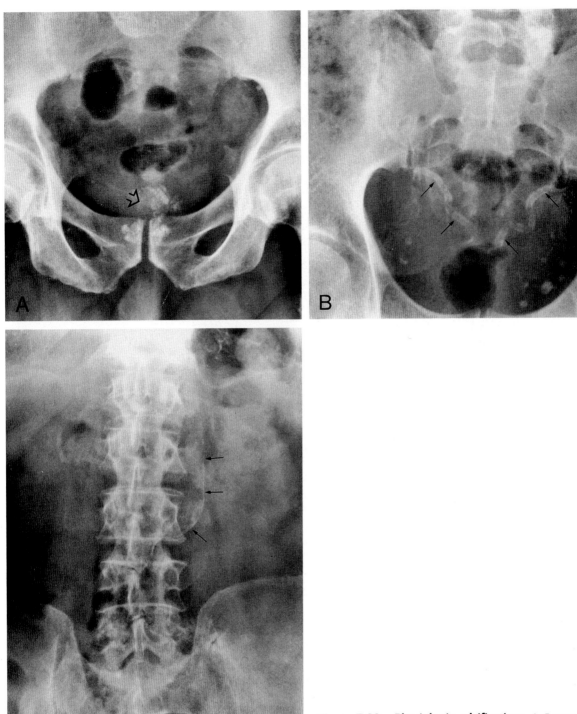

Figure 7.32.   Physiologic calcifications. A. Prostate (*arrow*). **B.** Vasa differentiae (*arrows*) in a diabetic man. **C.** Abdominal aortic aneurysm (*arrows*).

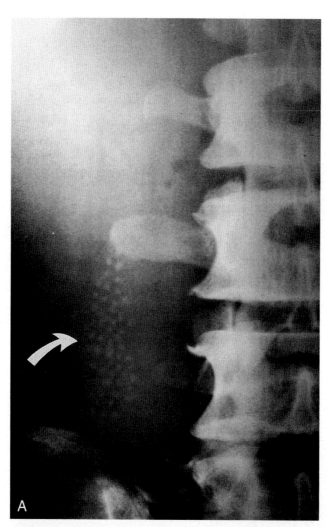

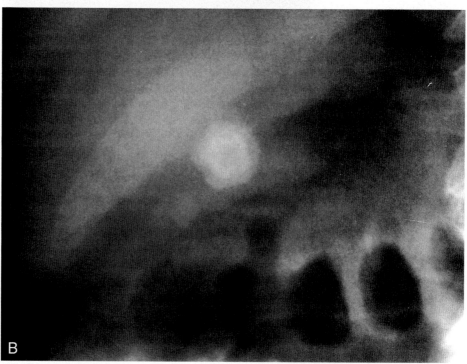

Figure 7.33. Calcified gallstones. A. Multiple small stones (*arrow*). **B.** A single stellate laminated stone.

Figure 7.34. Calcified urinary stones. A. Scout film shows multiple intrarenal calculi (*arrowheads*). A large calculus adjacent to the transverse process of L3 on the right (*open arrow*) is in the ureter. **B.** An intravenous urogram shows this calculus (*arrow*) to be partly obstructing the kidney and proximal ureter. Notice the dilation of the renal calyces, pelvis, and ureter on the right.

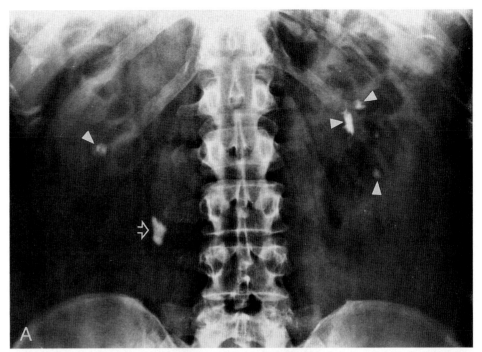
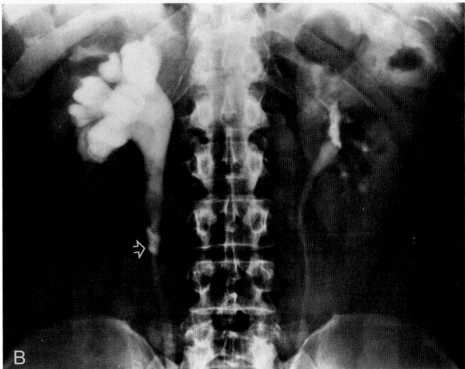

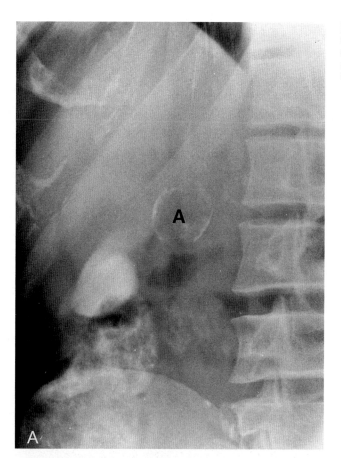

A

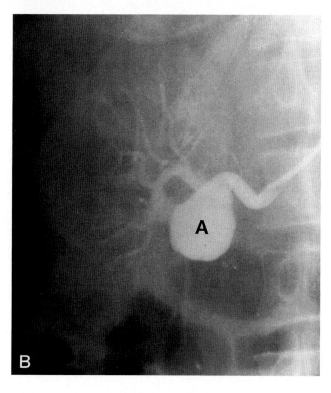

B

Figure 7.35. Renal artery aneurysm. A. Scout film from a cholecystogram shows the calcified aneurysm (A). **B.** Renal arteriogram shows the aneurysm to advantage.

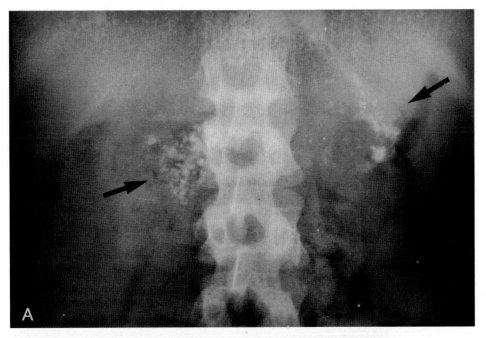

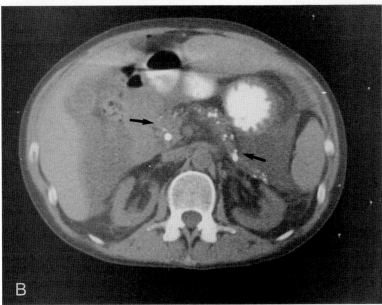

Figure 7.36.   **Pancreatic calcifications (*arrows*). A.** Detail of a plain film. **B.** CT image.

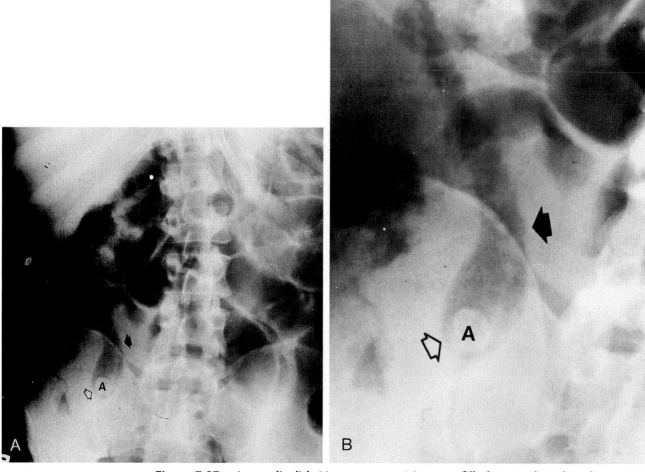

Figure 7.37. Appendicolith (*A; open arrow*) in a gas-filled appendix (*closed arrow*). **A.** Abdominal film. **B.** Detail view.

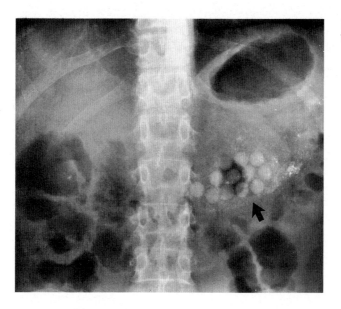

Figure 7.38. Ferrous sulfate tablets in the stomach (*arrow*).

Figure 7.39. Rectal foreign body.

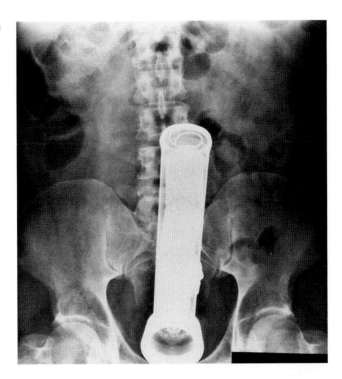

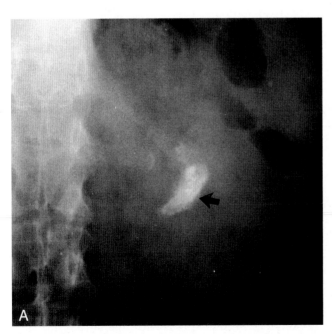

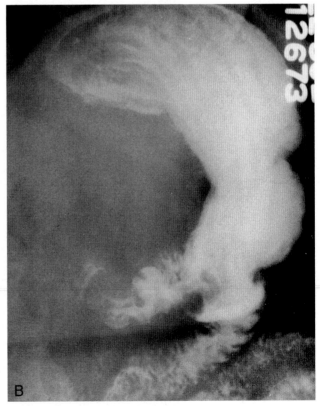

Figure 7.40.   Antacid fragments in a gastric ulcer. A. Detail view of the left upper quadrant shows dense material to the left of midline (*arrow*). **B.** Detail view of an upper gastrointestinal examination shows barium in the large ulcer on the greater curvature (*arrow*). Notice how the ulcer shape conforms to the shape demonstrated in A.

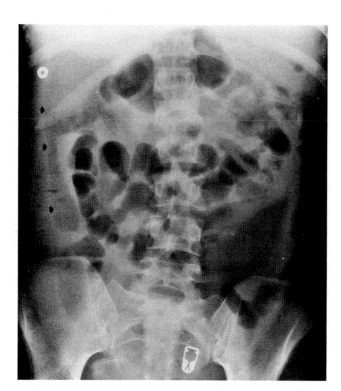

Figure 7.41. Ascites. Notice the displacement of gas-filled bowel (*arrows*) from the flank stripe and clustering centrally.

Bone and Joint Abnormalities

When looking at an abdominal radiograph, it is possible for several changes in the bones and joints to provide clues regarding intra-abdominal pathology. Although some of these changes are discussed in more detail in Chapter 11, several deserve mention at this point.

Many intra-abdominal disorders have well-recognized skeletal manifestations. Inflammatory bowel disease (regional enteritis, ulcerative colitis) frequently have an associated *spondyloarthropathy* that affects the lumbar vertebrae and the sacroiliac joints. In these patients, asymmetric *syndesmophyte* formations may occur along the vertebral end plates. Syndesmophytes are distinguished from the more common *osteophytes* by the direction in which the spurring points. Syndesmophytes represent ossification of Sharpey fibers of the disc annulus and are oriented in a vertical plane. Osteophytes are simple bone spurs that extend horizontally initially before pointing vertically. As a rule, syndesmophytes are more delicate and thinner than osteophytes. Another manifestation of the spondyloarthropathy of inflammatory bowel disease is *sacroiliitis* that may be symmetric or asymmetric. In many instances, bowel mucosal changes may be appreciated in addition to the bony changes (Fig. 7.42).

Other musculoskeletal manifestations include osteolytic or osteoblastic metastatic lesions from a variety of abdominal and/or pelvic malignancies. Large lytic lesions suggest renal carcinoma; blastic lesions suggest prostate carcinoma in a man or carcinoid tumor in either gender. Dense bones with smudged, thickened trabeculae are characteristic of renal osteodystrophy. In such an instance, look for evidence of dialysis catheters or of a renal transplant.

Postoperative Changes in the Abdomen

It is important to recognize the signs of previous surgery in the abdomen. Wire sutures or surgical clips in the abdomen are typical indicators. In this era of laparoscopic surgery, metallic clips may be the only evidence that a surgical procedure has been performed. The position of the sutures or staples frequently can give an idea of what type of surgery was performed. For example, wire sutures extending obliquely from the midline toward the right flank may indicate that the patient has had biliary surgery. Metallic clips in the region of the esophagogastric junction indicate previous vagotomy; those in the right upper quadrant indicate cholecystectomy (Fig. 7.43; see Fig. 7.29). Multiple surgical clips in the pelvis indicate gynecological

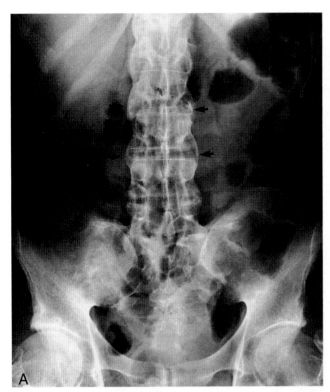
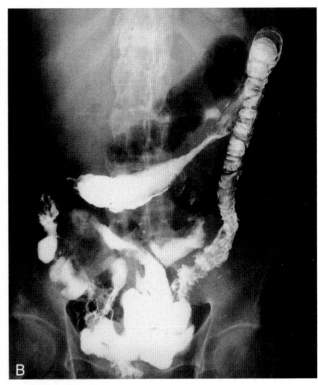

Figure 7.42.   Spondyloarthropathy of inflammatory bowel (Crohn) disease. A. Abdominal radiograph shows ankylosis of the sacroiliac joints. Compare with Figure 7.41. There are also syndesmophytes bridging the vertebral discs (*arrows*). **B.** Barium enema shows loss of haustra and irregularity of the transverse colon and terminal ileum, typical of Crohn disease (see Chapter 8).

Figure 7.43. Postoperative appearance following cholecystectomy. Notice the surgical clip (*arrow*) in the right upper quadrant. The patient also has a gastric bezoar, accounting for the mottled appearance to the stomach.

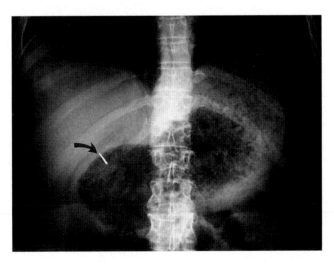

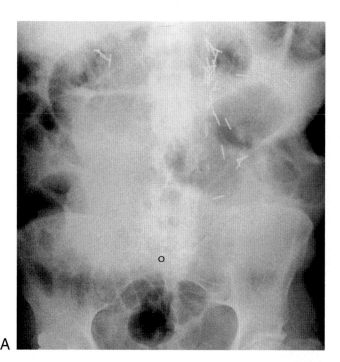

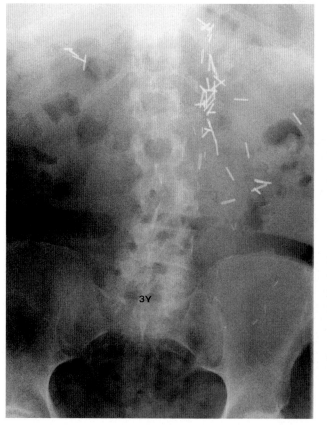

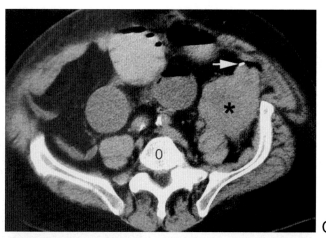

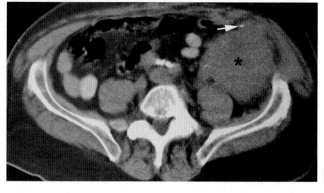

Figure 7.44. Recurrent tumor. A. Radiograph shows surgical clips in the left flank. **B.** Follow-up radiograph 3 years later shows the clips have become splayed apart. **C.** CT of the area made at same time as radiograph in A shows the mass (*). A surgical clip (*arrow*) is present along the anterior margin of the mass. **D.** CT made at the same time as radiograph in B shows the mass (*) to have enlarged. Notice the shift of the clip (*arrow*) anteriorly.

surgery in a woman or prostate surgery in a man. Multiple fine staples in a circular array indicate that a bowel resection has been performed. If an organ has been removed, its image will no longer be present. Ostomy devices (see Fig. 7.25A) are easily demonstrated, as are dialysis catheters.

Surgical clips in the abdomen or pelvis form valuable landmarks for evaluation of some diseases. In patients with known lymphomas or other tumors, the displacement of clips is an important indication of lymph node enlargement or tumor recurrence (Fig. 7.44). Furthermore, displacement of clips or of a foreign body such as a bullet may provide clues to the diagnosis of an intra-abdominal abscess. Scarring and fibrosis will result in the clips moving together.

SUMMARY AND KEY POINTS

- Abdominal radiographs are highly sensitive for detecting acute and chronic abnormalities.
- The key to diagnosing intra-abdominal abnormalities rests in recognizing abdominal gas patterns and mucosal images.
- Once there is radiographic evidence of pathology in the abdomen, a follow-up examination with ultrasound and/or CT is recommended.
- The follow-up of suspected lesions in the gastrointestinal and urinary tracts are discussed in Chapters 8 and 9, respectively.

SUGGESTED ADDITIONAL READING

Brant WE, Helms CA. Fundamentals of Diagnostic Radiology. 2nd Ed. Philadelphia: Lippincott Williams & Wilkins, 1999: 651–667.

Buonomo C, Taylor GA, Share, JC, et al. Gastrointestinal tract. In: Kirks DR, Griscom NT, eds. Practical Pediatric Imaging: Diagnostic Radiology of Infants and Children. 3rd Ed. Philadelphia: Lippincott-Raven, 1998:821–1007.

Federle M, Jeffrey R, Anne V. Diagnostic Imaging: Abdomen. Philadelphia: WB Saunders, 2005.

Frimann-Dahl J. Roentgen Examinations in Acute Abdominal Diseases. 3rd Ed. Springfield, IL: Charles C. Thomas, 1974.

Maglinte DDT. Nonspecific abdominal gas pattern: an interpretation whose time is gone. Appl Radiol 1997;26:5–8.

Margulis AR, Burhenne HJ, eds. Alimentary Tract Radiology. 5th Ed. St. Louis: Mosby-Year Book, 1997.

Meyers MA. Dynamic Radiology of the Abdomen: Normal and Pathologic Anatomy. 5th Ed. New York: Springer, 2000.

Gastrointestinal Imaging

8

Gastroenterology, like radiology, has undergone significant technical and therapeutic changes in the past 25 years. As often happens, technical advances in one specialty radically change another. Four such developments have changed the way physicians evaluate the gastrointestinal (GI) system.

The first of these developments was the perfection of and improvements in *flexible fiberoptic endoscopy*. Endoscopic evaluation of the stomach, duodenum, and colon has resulted in a significant decrease in the number of contrast studies of the GI tract. However, improvements in double-contrast techniques have also increased radiologic diagnostic accuracy. Although barium studies and endoscopy have similar sensitivities in finding diseases of the GI tract, endoscopy has become the standard diagnostic modality for several reasons. First, clinicians are now referring their patients directly to gastroenterologists for colon cancer screening and for diagnosis of other GI abnormalities. Second, improvements in endoscopy training and equipment have made the procedure safer. Third, if an abnormality, such as a colon polyp, is found on a barium study, the patient will be referred for endoscopic biopsy and/or excision.

Endoscopy is not without risks. Most of these studies are performed using conscious sedation. In addition, there is always the risk of perforation of the bowel during the procedure.

The issue of cost-efficiency must also be addressed. Cost-effectiveness is determined by the total cost of obtaining a diagnosis in the shortest period of time. A normal double-contrast barium enema is relatively less expensive than a colonoscopy. However, an abnormal barium study results in a colonoscopic examination, which increases the cost of finding the polyp or carcinoma. Finally, it should be noted, that in many parts of the world where endoscopy is not or cannot be performed, barium examinations remain the main investigative modality for suspected diseases of the GI tract.

The second advance was the emergence of *computed tomography (CT)*. This allowed noninvasive detection of hepatic and pancreatic abnormalities (Fig. 8.1) as well as detection of traumatic solid visceral rupture (Fig. 8.2). The speed of modern multidetector CT scanners now allows a complete examination of the abdomen to be performed in less than a minute. This is important when breath holding is needed during the scan. "Virtual colonoscopy" is a type of CT examination in which a sophisticated computer program produces three-dimensional images of the interior of the colon. Initial reports suggest an accuracy approaching that of colonoscopy for detecting polyps and colon carcinoma. However, the technique has not attained widespread use and, at the time of this writing, is considered by many to remain experimental. Finally, CT has made guided-needle biopsy possible.

The third advance was the improvement in *diagnostic ultrasound technology*. The use of ultrasound has resulted in the complete abandonment of oral and intravenous cholecystography. Ultrasound is now the investigative method of choice for evaluating the biliary system. Furthermore, ultrasound is now a vital component for monitoring biliary lithotripsy, the fragmentation of gallstones using sound waves.

Figure 8.1. Pancreatic pseudo-cyst. Computed tomography (CT) image shows the pseudocyst in the tail of the pancreas (*arrows*), adjacent to the spleen.

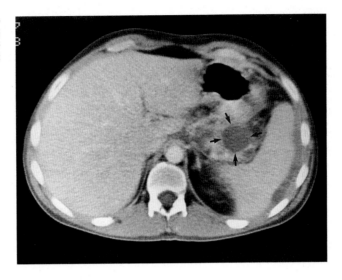

The final technical advance that affects GI diagnosis is *magnetic resonance (MR) imaging.* MR imaging is now used to investigate many GI disorders, including those of the hepato-biliary system and metastases. Magnetic resonance cholangiopancreatography (MRCP) is now being performed for suspected biliary obstruction. Its accuracy approaches that of endoscopic retrograde cholangiopancreatography (ERCP), a procedure performed by gastroenterologists. However, MRCP is entirely noninvasive and, therefore, is without the complication rate of ERCP.

The real impact of newer imaging forms can best be appreciated in light of how many intra-abdominal lesions were evaluated as little as 25 years ago. Although intrinsic lesions of the GI tract have always been evaluated by contrast examinations and subsequently by endoscopy, suspected intra-abdominal masses were evaluated by studies that showed the *effect* of the mass on surrounding organs by detecting their displacement when filled with barium or some other contrast. Furthermore, once a mass was detected, angiography was often employed to determine if there were any parameters that suggested malignancy. Diagnostic ultrasound, CT, and MR imaging now afford us the opportunity to directly identify the masses themselves rather than their secondary effects.

Chapter 7 showed that abdominal radiographs are valuable preliminary diagnostic studies. However, it is necessary to opacify the GI tract with contrast material to determine the presence of intrinsic abnormalities. Three examinations are used for primary evaluation of the GI tract: upper GI examination, small bowel "follow through," and barium enema. Ancillary studies such as CT scanning, ultrasound, MR imaging, and ERCP are particularly useful for examining the liver and pancreas.

Figure 8.2. Hepatic (*open arrow*) and splenic (*arrowhead*) fractures in a trauma patient. In addition, there is a large hematoma in the tail of the pancreas (*P*). Notice the fluid (blood) surrounding the spleen.

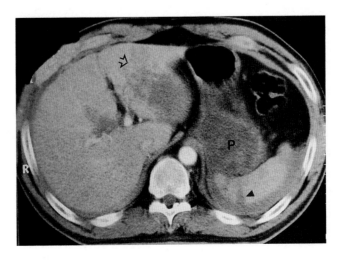

TECHNICAL CONSIDERATIONS

Bowel Preparation

The optimal way to study any hollow viscus filled with contrast material is to have that viscus *completely empty* of any other content. Similarly, it is also necessary for the stomach and bowel to be empty for an endoscopic evaluation. For examination of the upper GI tract, an overnight fast is usually sufficient to produce this effect. Food within the stomach after a documented overnight fast is abnormal and usually indicates gastric outlet obstruction, most often secondary to peptic ulcer disease (Fig. 8.3). In this situation, the stomach may be studied after inserting a nasogastric tube and suctioning out the remaining content. With infants and children, it is necessary to withhold food or drink only for the usual interval between feedings, because a child who is not hungry will not drink barium and one who has fasted too long will usually be too irritable to cooperate.

Obtaining a clean colon is a different matter. Many preparations have been used to cleanse the colon of most of its content. These include laxatives, enemas, and flushing by ingestion of massive quantities of fluids. In most patients, the use of hypertonic laxatives the night before the study and a cleansing enema the morning of the study produces the desired results. These measures may have to be more vigorous during hot summer months, when fluid loss through the skin hampers the osmotic effects of many types of bowel preparations. Furthermore, any barium left from a previous examination should be removed. The degree of bowel cleanliness should be determined by a scout radiograph of the abdomen. *Patients who are suspected of having toxic megacolon, acute ulcerative colitis, or obstruction should not have cleansing enemas and should be studied directly by colonoscopy.* It is not necessary to vigorously cleanse the colon in children because usually the clinician is not looking for small mucosal lesions, such as those found in adults.

Order of Studies

There is a *logical order* in which studies of the GI tract should be performed. Barium enema and upper GI examination may be performed on the same day, in that order. The idea is to do the study that requires the greatest amount of clarity in the abdomen before introducing additional contrast material. An upper GI series may be performed immediately after the barium enema if the patient has adequately evacuated the colon. If the patient is to have a motility study or exam of the small bowel, that is done before a colon examination.

Information Exchange

It is important for the clinician to give as much *clinical information* as possible to the referring radiologist. The request should always contain pertinent information and a tentative diagnosis.

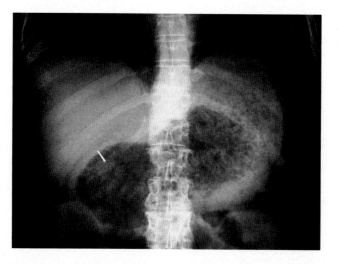

Figure 8.3. Gastric bezoar. The stomach appears mottled and bubbly.

The radiologist should question the patient and ask about symptoms necessitating the examination. It is not unusual, however, for a patient to go for an examination without understanding the reason for the study or with few or no complaints referable to the area of the body under examination.

Pediatricians should inform the parents that they will probably be allowed to be in the room while their child is examined. In some instances, they may even assist in holding the child and giving reassurance.

The patient should also be informed that the clinician, after receiving the results of the examination from the radiologist, will notify the patient of the findings. This removes the onus from the radiologists of having to report serious findings such as colon cancer to patients they may not know well. Radiologists should make it a practice to inform a patient when a study is normal, however, because most patients are apprehensive about the condition for which they are studied. Quite often, the patient will not see the referring physician for several hours or perhaps days or weeks following the examination. To make a patient worry about a diagnosis of cancer or some other serious illness when the study is normal is simply not in anybody's best interests.

Procedures

Under normal circumstances, two modes of radiographic recording are used: fluoroscopy and radiography. Fluoroscopic examination is important to determine the swallowing mechanism and the motility of the GI tract (peristalsis), as well as to position the patient so that all parts of the organs being studied are examined. Detail radiographs or *spot films* are obtained of several strategic areas under direct fluoroscopic control: the esophagogastric junction, the duodenal bulb area, the ileocecal area, and the flexures and the rectosigmoid junction of the colon. The exact number and variety of spot films will vary from examiner to examiner. Furthermore, if an abnormality is found at fluoroscopy, additional spot films are taken. Occasionally, the fluoroscopic portion of the examination is recorded on videotape for later playback and evaluation. After the fluoroscopic portion of the study, overhead radiographs are taken with the patient in various positions for further delineation of whole organs, such as the stomach or colon. Delayed radiographs are usually added to examinations of the small bowel and of the colon (following evacuation of barium).

The preferred method for routine study is to use a thick preparation of barium and to distend the stomach or colon with gas (*air contrast study*). In the first situation, a gas-releasing preparation is ingested with the oral barium. In the second, air is introduced through the rectal tube. The resulting study portrays the mucosa in detail and is usually sufficient to reveal subtle abnormalities. Often these studies are performed after pharmacologic enhancement, using glucagon to hinder peristalsis and to relax spastic bowel.

Water-soluble contrast is used to study patients with suspected perforations of the GI tract. This includes postoperative patients in whom an anastomotic leak is suspected. Barium outside the confines of the bowel produces an extremely desmoplastic reaction within surrounding tissues. The only contraindication to the use of water-soluble contrast agents is in a patient with suspected esophago-airway communication. In that situation, the water-soluble contrast produces a severe chemical pneumonitis in the lungs—a reaction that can be fatal. Oil-soluble contrast or barium should be used for that group of patients.

Ultrasound is used frequently to evaluate patients with suspected biliary and pancreatic disease. The examination is a reliable noninvasive method with a high degree of accuracy. Furthermore, the study may be performed after cholecystokinin enhancement. Ultrasonography has replaced oral cholecystography.

Abdominal *CT examinations* are commonly used in studying patients with jaundice, pancreatic disease, and suspected hepatic metastases from other intra-abdominal malignancies. CT is also used for staging malignancies of the GI tract because it can demonstrate local invasion as well as abnormal lymph node metastases. Many studies have shown the complementary nature of CT with ultrasound in evaluating patients suspected of having pancreatic or biliary disease. Ultrasound is the less expensive procedure; however, because modern CT is much more rapid than in the past, increased throughput (patients per hour) may result in decreased

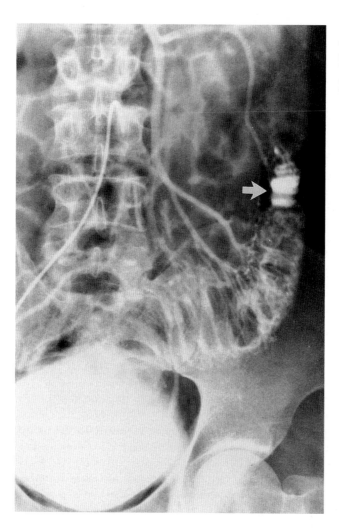

Figure 8.4. Mesenteric arteriogram in a patient with lower gastrointestinal bleeding. Delayed film shows a "stain" of contrast (*arrow*) at the site of a bleeding diverticulum in the descending colon.

costs for that procedure. A CT scan provides more definitive information, particularly in pancreatic disease. Intravenous contrast enhancement is a common adjunct to CT.

Angiography is used to evaluate the GI tract primarily for diagnosis and therapy in patients with acute GI hemorrhage. The bleeding site may be localized by selective catheterization of celiac or mesenteric branches and a vasopressor infused to control or stop the bleeding (Fig. 8.4). Angiography is also used to evaluate patients with portal hypertension before a contemplated transjugular intrahepatic portosystemic shunt (TIPS) procedure (see Chapter 3) or shunt surgery and in mapping hepatic metastases if partial hepatectomy or infusion chemotherapy is being considered.

Percutaneous cholangiography with the thin-walled (Chiba) needle is used by radiologists to study patients with obstructive jaundice. Contrast material injected through the needle, which has been placed in a dilated biliary duct, is used to localize the site of the obstruction (Fig. 8.5). Following this, a catheter may be inserted for percutaneous decompression and drainage, or a stent may be introduced, as mentioned in Chapter 3.

ERCP is a procedure in which the ampulla of Vater is cannulated under direct endoscopic control. The examination takes a skilled endoscopist, most often a gastroenterologist. After cannulation, contrast material is injected into the ductal system, and fluoroscopic spot and overhead radiographs are made. A stent or drainage catheter may be left in place as part of this procedure. The endoscopist also can perform a papillotomy. ERCP is being supplanted in some institutions by MRCP because the latter procedure is noninvasive.

Two commonly used nuclear imaging studies to investigate abnormalities of the GI tract are hepatobiliary imaging and gastrointestinal bleeding localization. The biliary scan uses technetium−99m–labeled mebrofenin and iminodiacetic acid derivatives to investigate uptake and excretion physiology of the liver as well as kinesis of radio-labeled bile in the extrahepatic

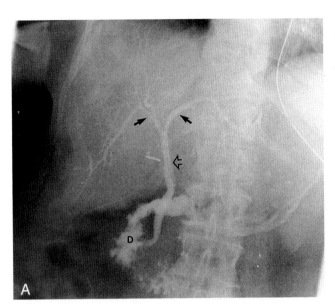
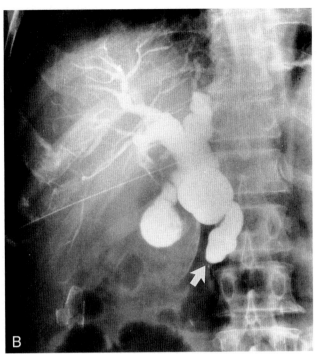

Figure 8.5.   Cholangiograms. A. Normal intra-operative examination demonstrates normal-sized hepatic (*small arrows*) and common bile (*open arrow*) ducts. Contrast flows freely into the duodenum (*D*) and refluxes into the stomach. **B.** Percutaneous transhepatic cholangiogram shows massive dilation of the common bile duct and hepatic ducts in this patient with obstruction near the distal common bile duct (*arrow*). This was subsequently percutaneously decompressed with a catheter.

biliary tree. The radiotracer is administered intravenously and then removed from the blood by the liver and concentrated in the bile. Under normal circumstances, the agent can be detected in the gallbladder within 10 to 15 minutes of administration (Fig. 8.6). It is excreted through the common bile duct into the duodenum within 30 to 45 minutes. An obstruction of the cystic duct will prevent the passive filling of the gallbladder (Fig. 8.7), thus yielding a

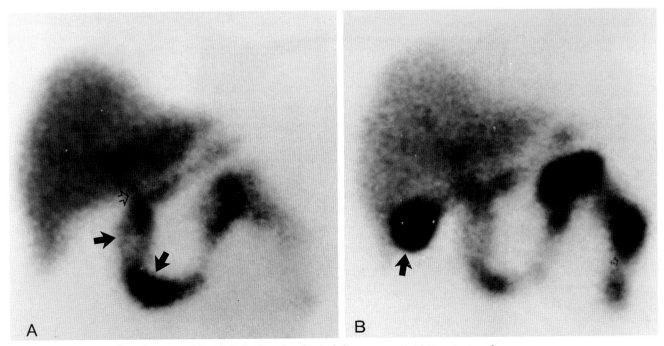

Figure 8.6.   Normal technetium-99m–labeled mebrofenin biliary scan. A. Thirty minutes after injection, the isotope is being excreted by the liver through the common bile duct (*open arrow*) into the duodenum (*closed arrows*). **B.** At 60 minutes, the isotope fills the gallbladder (*arrow*).

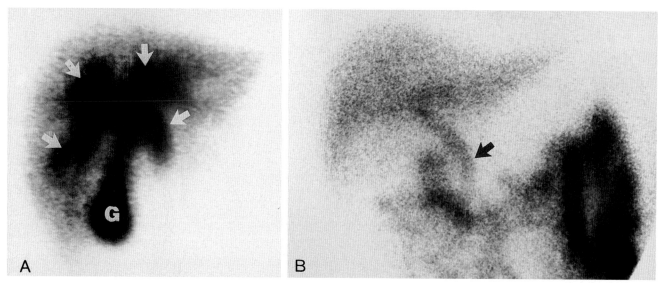

Figure 8.7.   Abnormal technetium-99m–labeled mebrofenin biliary scans. A. Patient with a common duct stone. Ninety minutes after injection, the isotope is in the liver and gallbladder (G). There is no excretion into the duodenum, and the biliary tree is dilated (*arrows*). **B.** Patient with acute cholecystitis from cystic duct stone. No gallbladder filling occurs at 60 minutes. The isotope passes freely into the duodenum through the common bile duct (*arrow*).

diagnosis of acute cholecystitis. In the setting of acute cholecystitis, a hepatobiliary imaging study has a 95% positive and negative predictive value. The predictive value of this study is improved by concordant ultrasound imaging of the right upper quadrant for anatomic correlation. Hepatobiliary imaging is also useful in the setting of biliary surgery or trauma to diagnose intraperitoneal biliary leaks. Finally, hepatobiliary imaging with additional chemical challenges using cholecystokinin can help in the diagnosis of biliary dyskinesia or acalculous cholecystitis.

Technetium-99m–tagged autologous red blood cells are used to investigate active gastrointestinal bleeding. In patients who have lower gastrointestinal bleeding in an acute setting

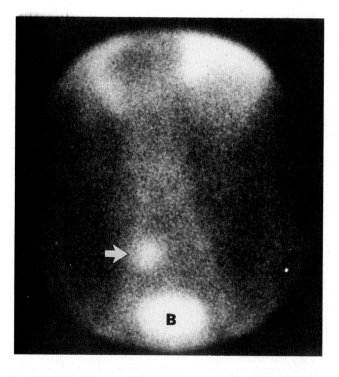

Figure 8.8.   Bleeding Meckel diverticulum. Increased isotope concentration in the ileocecal region (*arrow*) is caused by bleeding. B, bladder.

Figure 8.9. Magnetic resonance cholangiopancreatogram (MRCP). Notice the normal hepatic ducts (*thin white arrows*), common bile duct (*large white arrow*), and ampulla of Vater (*black arrow*) in the descending duodenum (*D*).

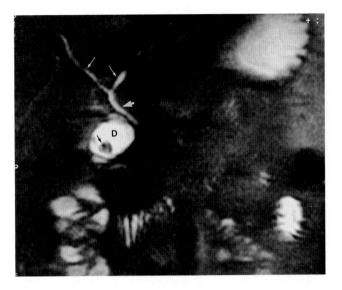

along with some hemodynamic instability, a nuclear medicine bleeding scan is very helpful in localization of the site of bleed. This study is more sensitive than invasive angiography and can, in fact, help plan the therapeutic angiography if necessary. A gastrointestinal bleeding scan will detect as little as 0.1 mL/min of active extravasation into the gastrointestinal lumen compared with the 1 mL/min flow usually cited for angiographic evaluation.

A technetium-99m pertechnetate scan, also known as a Meckel's scan, is used primarily in the pediatric setting for diagnosis of Meckel diverticulum, a common congenital malformation of the ileocecal region. Although most of these diverticula are asymptomatic, some contain gastric mucosa, which may occasionally result in lower gastrointestinal bleeding. In pediatric patients who present with intermittent lower intestinal bleeding manifesting as "currant jelly" stools, a bleeding scan is very helpful. The "free" technetium-99m pertechnetate is excreted in the gastric mucosa. Using this physiology, localization of an abnormal gastric mucosal site in the right lower quadrant is easily achieved.

MR imaging has increasing applications for evaluation of the GI tract. It is used primarily to evaluate the liver, biliary tree (Fig. 8.9), and to a lesser extent, the pancreas. Advances in MR technology now allow studies without significant motion artifacts from respiration, aortic pulsations, and peristalsis, all of which adversely affect the image. MR studies may be augmented by intravenous use of gadolinium-diethylenetriamine pentaacetic acid (Gd-DTPA), a paramagnetic contrast agent.

Before deciding which of these special studies to perform, you should thoroughly discuss the case with a radiologist to determine the optimal study and, if multiple studies are needed, the order in which they should be performed. In this way, you save time between making the diagnosis and beginning treatment and eliminates more costly and less productive studies.

ANATOMIC CONSIDERATIONS

It is important for you to recognize the normal anatomy of the GI tract and the variations that may occur. For example, six indentations may be seen on the *esophagus* as it courses from the pharynx into the abdomen. The uppermost is the indentation of the cricopharyngeus muscle posteriorly at the level of C6. Other indentations occur at the thoracic inlet, at the aortic arch at the level of T4 to T5, at the left mainstem bronchus, proximal to the diaphragmatic hiatus by the descending aorta, and at the esophagogastric junction (Fig. 8.10).

The *stomach* may assume various positions, lying either vertically or horizontally within the abdomen. This depends mainly on the patient's body habitus. The radiologic anatomy of the

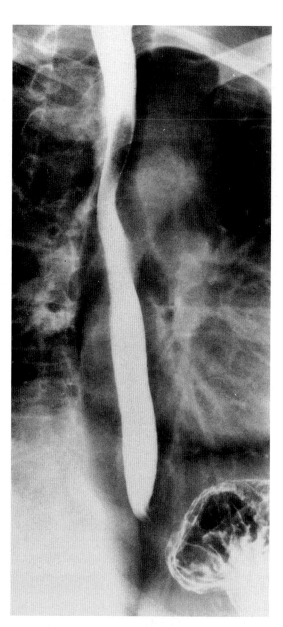

Figure 8.10. **Normal esophagus.** A small amount of air is present in the upper esophagus. Notice the indentation at the level of the aortic arch.

normal stomach includes the fundus, body, antrum, prepyloric region, and pylorus (Fig. 8.11). The gastric mucosa (*rugae*) appears as linear parallel folds extending along the length of the stomach (Fig. 8.12). There is wide variation in the size of the rugae.

The *duodenum* begins at the pylorus. The first portion is the bulb, which appears as a triangular-shaped structure with the base toward the pylorus. The duodenum then sweeps downward (the second or descending portion), curves medially (third portion), and twists back upward (fourth portion), terminating at the ligament of Treitz. Occasionally, on a normal duodenal examination, a small indentation representing the ampulla of Vater may be observed along the medial border of the descending portion.

The *jejunum* begins at the ligament of Treitz, gradually merging with the *ileum*, which enters the *cecum* via the ileocecal valve. It is usually possible to differentiate the jejunum from the ileum by the mucosal pattern. In normal persons, the cecum is in the right lower quadrant of the abdomen. The wormlike (vermiform) *appendix* typically projects downward from the cecum. In some people, however, it may be oriented cranially (retrocecal appendix). Usually, the ileocecal valve is on the medial aspect of the cecum.

The *colon* ascends, forming two looplike structures in the right and left upper quadrants known as the hepatic and splenic flexures, respectively. The descending colon terminates in the

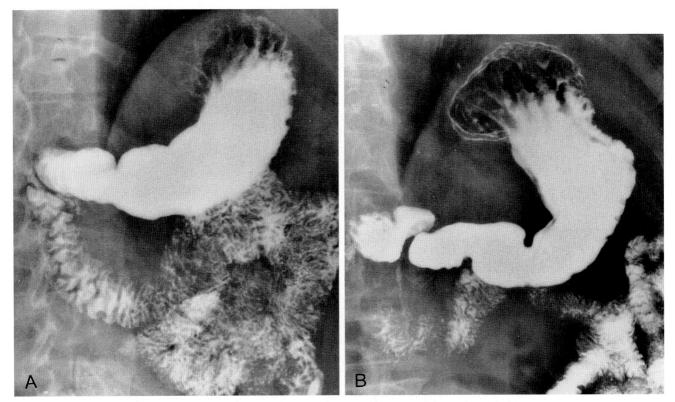

Figure 8.11. Normal stomach, duodenum, and proximal small bowel. Variations in normal appearance in two patients.

Figure 8.12. Normal mucosal patterns. A. Stomach. **B.** Small intestine. **C.** Colon.

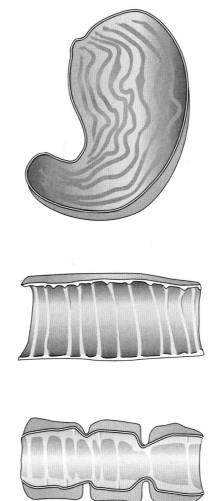

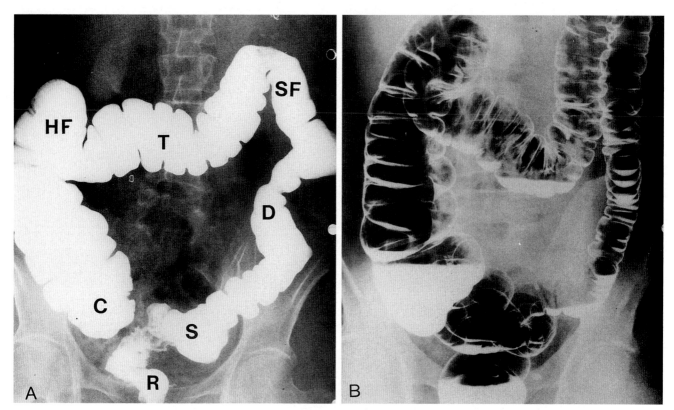

Figure 8.13.   Normal barium enema. A, single contrast. *C,* cecum; *HF,* hepatic flexure; *T,* transverse colon; *SF,* splenic flexure; *D,* descending colon; *S,* sigmoid colon; *R,* rectum; **B,** double contrast.

sigmoid colon, which is often quite redundant, particularly in older patients. The sigmoid colon continues on to the rectum (Fig. 8.13). Under normal circumstances, the rectum can be distended with barium greater than half the distance between the walls of the pelvis.

In addition to assessing the anatomy of the GI tract, the clinician must also be concerned with its physiology—that is, its *motility.* The causes of motility disorders are varied and complex.

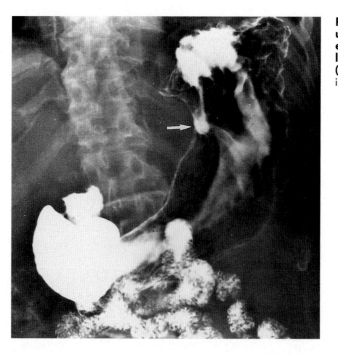

Figure 8.14.   Double-contrast upper gastrointestinal (GI) examination of a patient with a lesser-curvature gastric ulcer (*arrow*). Notice the folds radiating into the ulcer crater.

Figure 8.15. Double contrast barium enema in a patient with ulcerative colitis. Notice the lack of haustra and narrowing of the rectum and sigmoid.

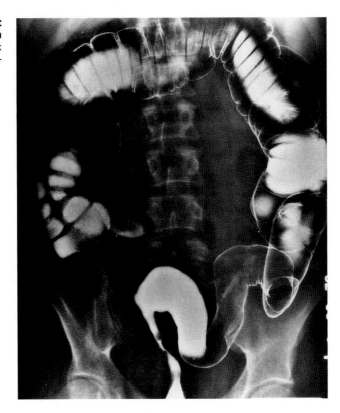

Suffice it to say that in the normal esophagus, a stripping wave should be seen propagating a bolus of barium in a smooth, progressive motion. Peristalsis continues in the stomach from the fundus extending down to the pylorus. In the duodenum, peristalsis is slightly different: the stripping motion found in the esophagus and stomach is not present. Instead, there is distension of the duodenal bulb, which opens at its apex and contracts forcibly as a unit moving the bolus through. Propulsive contractions are observed throughout the small intestine and colon.

In the colon, several areas of normal or physiologic narrowing may be exaggerated with spasm. These are found in the transverse colon near the flexures and in the descending colon. When significant spasm of the GI tract is evident, particularly in the colon, a pharmacologically enhanced study is required. Glucagon injected intravenously in 0.5- to 2-mg doses will produce relaxation of the GI tract through its antivagal action. Glucagon may also be used to relax the GI tract for double-contrast examinations (Figs. 8.14 and 8.15) to aid in finding subtle abnormalities.

PATHOLOGIC CONSIDERATIONS

Because the GI tract is a tube, *pathologic alterations found in one segment appear identical when encountered in any other segment.* For example, a mucosal tumor of the esophagus has an appearance identical to a similar-sized tumor of the stomach, small intestine, or colon. The incidence of these lesions varies from location to location, and you must learn the common locations of these lesions in each segment. However, remember that for practical purposes, *these lesions all have a similar appearance, no matter where they occur.* (Using the same concept, a broad generalization may be made that similar-appearing lesions are also found in other tubular structures such as the urinary tract, bronchi, and blood vessels.)

There are six basic pathologic alterations that can be recognized:

1. Polypoid lesions
2. Mucosal masses
3. Ulceration
4. Diverticula
5. Extrinsic compression
6. Benign strictures

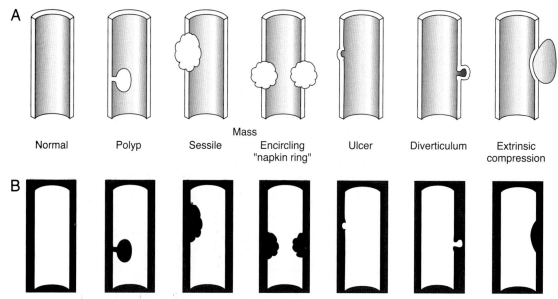

Figure 8.16. Schematic drawing illustrating pathologic alterations affecting the GI tract.
A. Gross appearance. **B.** Radiographic appearance.

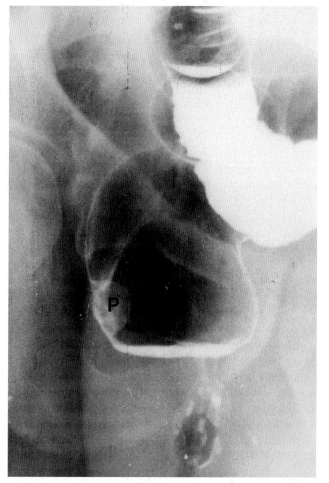

Figure 8.17. Sessile polyp (*P*) of the rectum.

Figure 8.18. Pedunculated polyp (*P*) of the descending colon. Notice the stalk of the polyp (*arrows*).

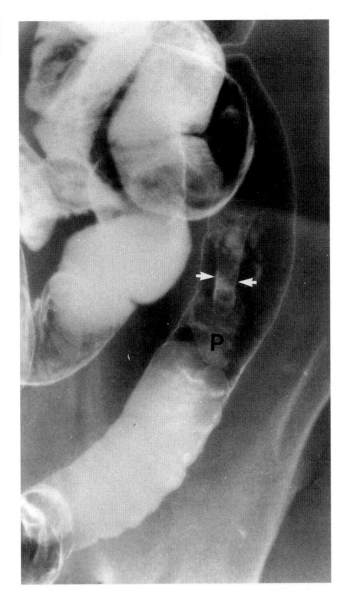

The first five of these are illustrated in Figure 8.16. In addition, motility disorders and dilatation may be encountered in any portion of the GI tract.

Polypoid lesions appear as small, rounded, filling defects in the lumen. They may be broad based (*sessile;* Fig. 8.17) or on a stalk (*pedunculated;* Fig. 8.18). They are true mucosal lesions, and when observed end-on, their outer margins are indistinct, being obscured by surrounding barium. In contrast, diverticula profiled end-on have discernible outer margins but indistinct inner margins (Fig. 8.19).

Figure 8.19. The difference between the radiographic appearances of a polyp (*P*) and a diverticulum (*D*). A. Profile view. **B.** End-on view. The mnemonics for distinguishing these two lesions when seen end-on are FOP (fuzzy outside = polyp) and FIT (fuzzy inside = tic).

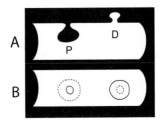

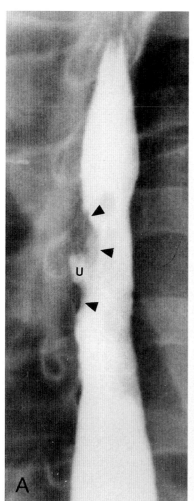

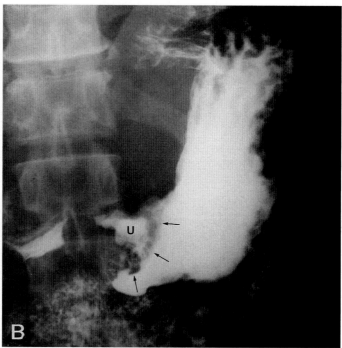

Figure 8.20.   Mucosal masses. A. Ulcerating esophageal carcinoma. An ulcer crater (*U*) is present within the mucosal mass (*arrowheads*). **B.** Ulcerating malignancy of the gastric antrum. The ulcer (*U*) is within the mucosal mass (*arrows*). **C.** Polypoid colonic carcinoma presents as an irregular filling defect. **D.** Sessile colon carcinoma (*arrowheads*). Notice the abrupt margin between normal mucosa and tumor.

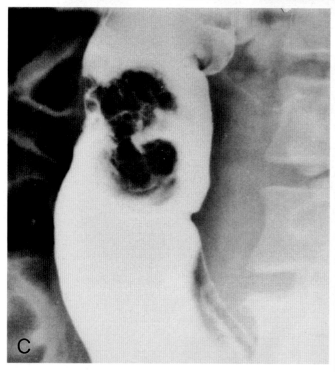

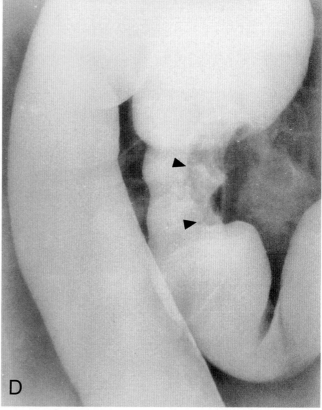

Mucosal masses frequently begin as small polyps. As a polyp enlarges, its surface may become irregular. Puckering may occur near the base of the lesion. There is an abrupt change of the mucosa from normal to tumor (Fig. 8.20). This frequently produces a "shoulder" of tumor at the mucosal transition point. Further growth results in encasement as the tumor grows completely around the lumen, producing the classic "napkin ring" or "apple core" appearance (Fig. 8.21). Such lesions do not transmit the normal peristaltic wave, and their appearance remains constant when observed on serial radiographs. Many malignant masses may ulcerate.

There are two other varieties of filling defects that may be observed in the GI tract: mucosal hypertrophy (Fig. 8.22) and varices (Fig. 8.23). With both these entities, it is important not to misinterpret them as tumors.

Ulceration of the GI tract results in a collection of barium being found outside the normal lumen. Frequently, the ulcer is surrounded by an edematous ulcer collar or mound. In benign ulcers, particularly of the stomach, mucosal folds may be observed radiating into the ulcer crater. The inflammatory mass leading up to the ulcer is smooth with gradually sloping margins. Occasionally, a smooth collar of inflamed mucosa is present between the lumen and the crater (*Hampton's line*). This is also considered a sign of a benign ulcer because a tumor does not show this feature. Penetration of the ulcer beyond the normal lumen is another sign of a benign lesion. As mentioned previously, ulcerations may also occur within masses. You should remember that *there are no malignant ulcers; there are ulcerating malignancies.* Patients with multiple or recurrent ulcers should be studied for Zollinger-Ellison syndrome to search for gastrin-producing tumors. Several ulcers are illustrated in Figures 8.24 through 8.26. Table 8.1 lists the radiologic differential features between benign gastric ulcers and ulcerating gastric malignancies.

Diverticula are benign outpouchings of the wall of the GI tract that are covered by all layers of the bowel wall. They may be relatively small, as in the colon (Fig. 8.27), or quite large, as a Zenker diverticulum of the esophagus (Fig. 8.28). Occasionally, they contain foreign material. Figures 8.29 through 8.31 show various diverticula.

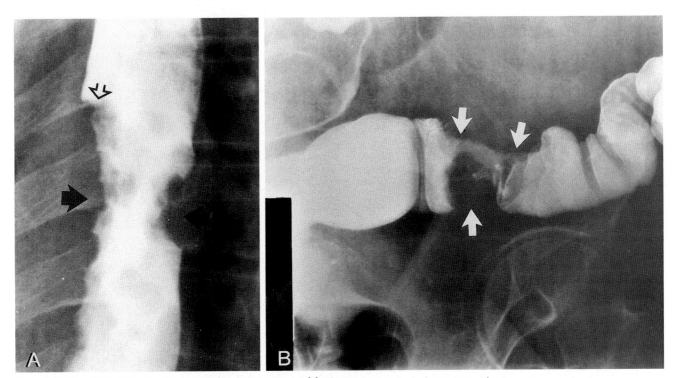

Figure 8.21. "Napkin ring" or "apple core" mucosal lesions. A. Esophageal carcinoma shows the constricting lesion (*solid arrows*) with abrupt mucosal margins, termed a "tumor shoulder" (*open arrow*). **B.** Colon carcinoma (*arrows*). Notice the similarity of these lesions.

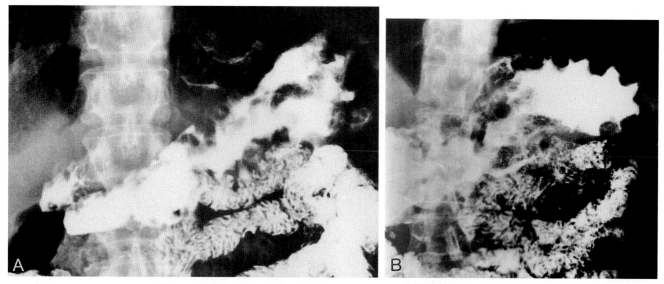

Figure 8.22. Hypertrophic gastric mucosal folds. Two views (**A and B**) show multiple filling defects in the stomach representing hypertrophic mucosa. Endoscopy was required for confirmation.

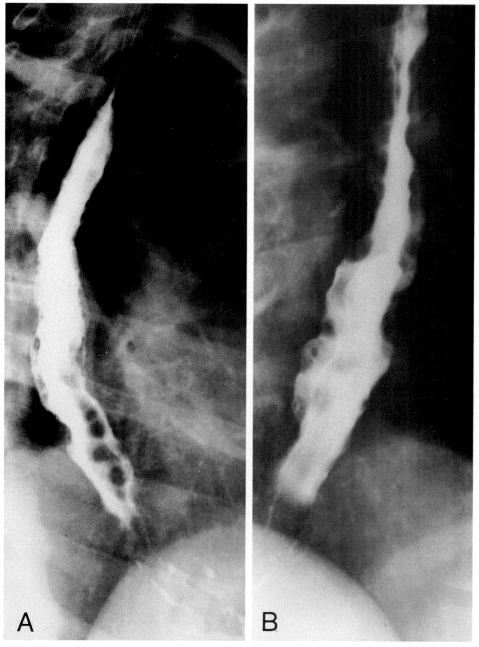

Figure 8.23. Esophageal varices. Multiple wormlike filling defects in two patients with histories of chronic alcohol abuse.

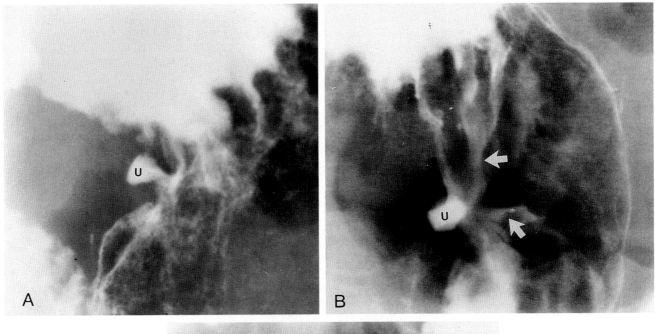

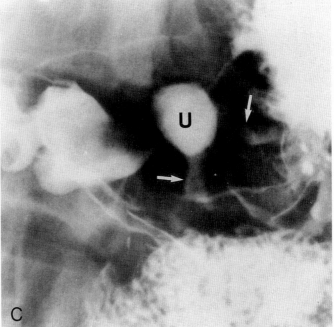

Figure 8.24. Benign gastric ulcers (*U*). Ulcers in three patients. Folds radiate into the ulcer crater in B and C (*arrows*).

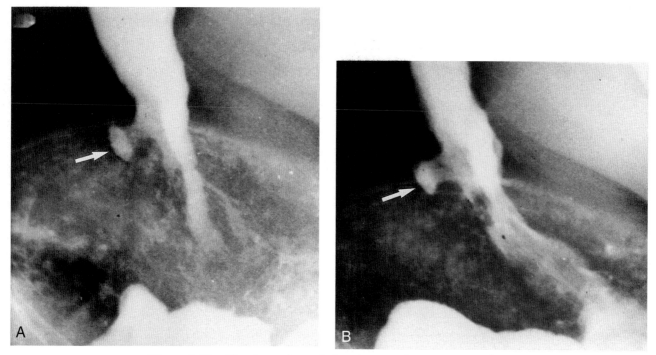

Figure 8.25.   Distal esophageal ulcer (*arrows*) in a patient with gastroesophageal reflux. A small collar of edematous mucosa leads up to the ulcer crater.

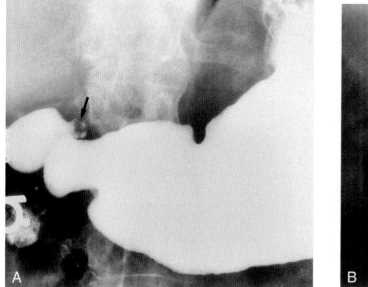 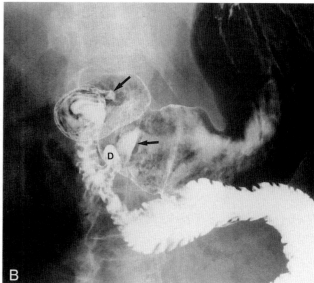

Figure 8.26.   Duodenal ulcers (*arrows*). A. Single-contrast study shows a small filling defect within the ulcer crater that represents a blood clot. **B.** Double-contrast study demonstrates two ulcers as well as a duodenal diverticulum (*D*).

TABLE 8.1

COMPARATIVE FEATURES OF BENIGN GASTRIC ULCERS AND ULCERATING MALIGNANCIES

Benign Gastric Ulcers	Ulcerating Malignancies
Penetration beyond lumen	Intraluminal crater located between abrupt points of transition (in contrast to intraluminal crater in mound of even edematous surrounding tissue)
Mucosal folds radiate to crater edge	Crater shallow, width exceeds depth
Hampton's line	Absent Hampton's line
Ulcer collar	Ulcer irregularly shaped
Ulcer mound, gradual tapering to normal mucosa	Eccentric location of ulcer in mass
Normal distensibility and pliability	Fixation of affected area
Peristalsis transmitted through area	Peristalsis not transmitted through area
Single, centrally located blood clot in crater base	Irregular base of crater

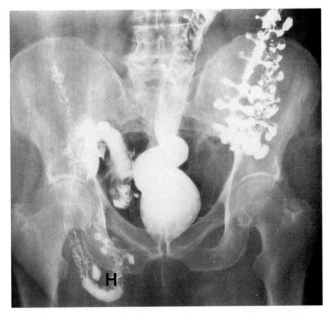

Figure 8.27.   Colonic diverticulosis. A postevacuation radiograph shows the diverticulosis to be worse on the left. Notice the inguinal hernia (*H*) on the right.

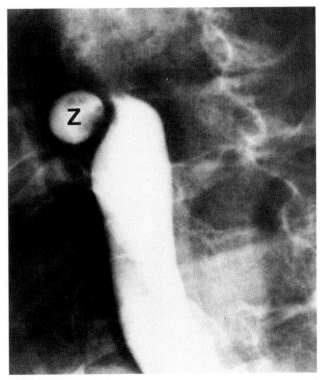

Figure 8.28.   Zenker diverticulum (*Z*) of the proximal esophagus.

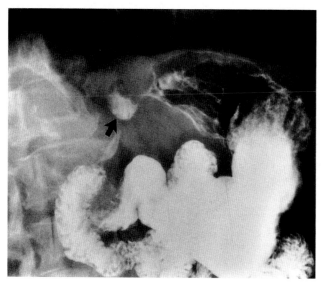

Figure 8.29. Gastric diverticulum (*arrow*).

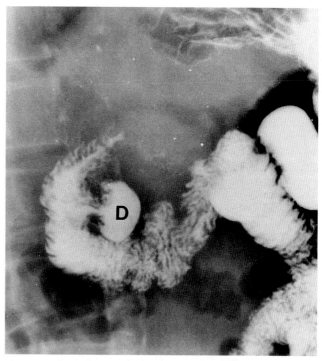

Figure 8.30. Duodenal diverticulum (*D*) in its typical location in the descending duodenum, at the level of the ampulla of Vater.

Extrinsic compression (Fig. 8.32) appears as a smooth indentation of the bowel wall with gradually tapering margins. On palpation during fluoroscopy, the mucosa can be seen to be intact. It may be difficult to differentiate this from an intramural lesion causing compression.

A *benign stricture* appears as a concentric or eccentric narrowing of the lumen (Fig. 8.33). The margins should be smooth and tapering, and the mucosa generally should be intact. A stricture is often difficult to differentiate from carcinoma, which usually has a nodular appearance and often a "shoulder" of tumor (Fig. 8.34).

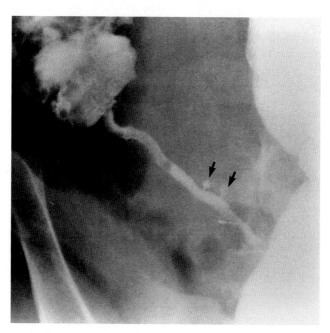

Figure 8.31. Appendiceal diverticula (*arrows*). The small lucency within the appendix is an air bubble.

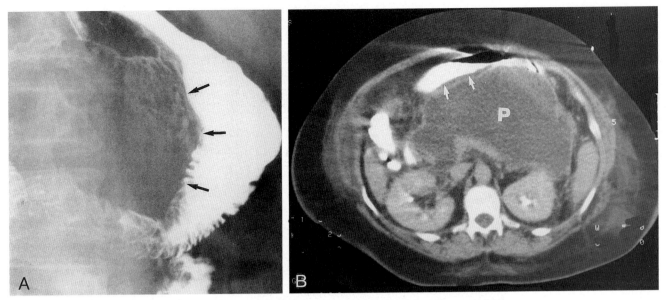

Figure 8.32. Pancreatic pseudocyst. A. A spot film from an upper GI examination shows extrinsic compression of the stomach by a large pancreatic pseudocyst (*arrows*). **B.** CT image shows the pseudocyst (*P*). Notice the compression of the contrast-filled stomach (*arrows*).

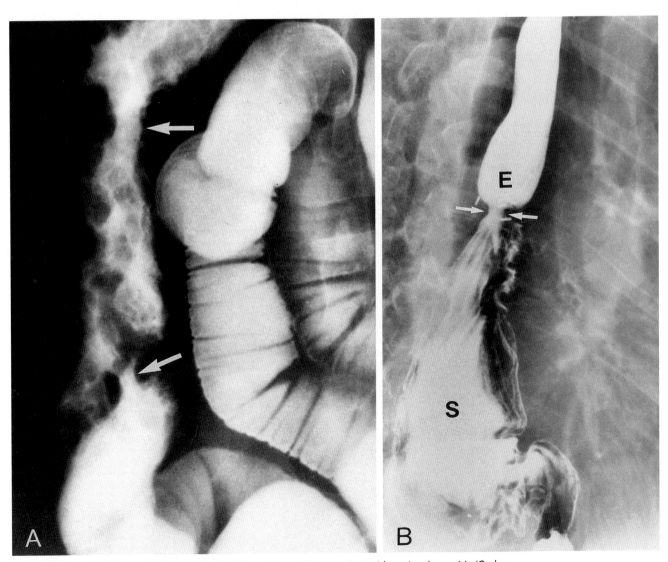

Figure 8.33. Strictures. A. Small bowel strictures (*arrows*) in a patient with regional enteritis (Crohn disease). Notice the abnormal mucosa in the involved segment. **B.** Stricture (*arrows*) at the site of anastomosis of esophagus (*E*) and stomach (*S*) in a patient who has undergone gastroesophagostomy. *(continued on page 290)*

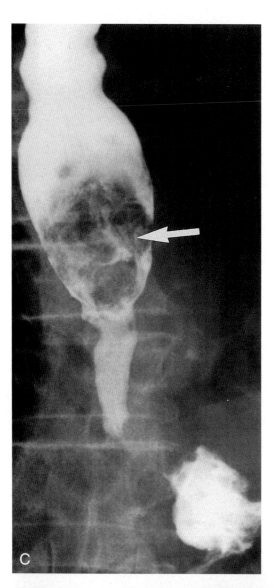

Figure 8.33. *(continued)* **C.** Distal esophageal stricture in a patient with chronic gastroesophageal reflux. A large bolus of food (*arrow*) is in the dilated portion of the esophagus just above the stricture.

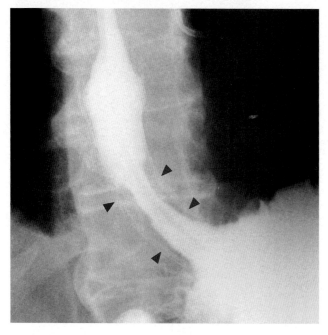

Figure 8.34. Malignant stricture of the distal esophagus in a patient with a stent placed for carcinoma. The tumor has grown through the stent (*arrowheads*) to narrow the lumen.

Inflammatory Bowel Disease

Inflammatory bowel disease is a term that is applied to both *ulcerative colitis* and *Crohn disease* (regional enteritis) of the bowel. Both diseases produce a spectrum of pathologic changes, including ulceration; obstruction; and formation of pseudopolyps, strictures, and fistulas. In addition, chronic ulcerative colitis is prone to undergo malignant change.

Both chronic inflammatory bowel conditions are of unknown origin. However, they share many clinical, epidemiologic, pathologic, radiographic, and even immunologic features. Some authorities feel that each entity represents a different pathologic response to a common cause; others believe both diseases represent different parts of the spectrum of a single disease process.

The definitive diagnosis of both diseases is best made by endoscopy with or without biopsy. Nevertheless, classic radiographic findings have been described for each of these diseases and will be briefly contrasted here.

The typical case of *ulcerative colitis* has radiographic manifestations that directly reflect the pathologic manifestations, including exudative inflammation involving primarily the bowel mucosa and submucosa. Classically, the muscularis is spared. Edema of the bowel wall gives the impression of thickened bowel. Ulcerations are shallow and coalescent (Fig. 8.35), often isolating islands of normal mucosa that are termed *pseudopolyps* (Fig. 8.36).

In the acute stages, spasm and irritability are evident fluoroscopically. Edema results in smudging and haziness of the mucosal folds. The disease characteristically involves the entire colon. Occasionally, the terminal ileum is involved (*backwash ileitis*); however, this more commonly occurs in Crohn disease.

Long-standing disease results in the chronic or "burned-out" stage, which produces foreshortening of the colon and narrowing of the lumen. The barium enema reveals a very tubular ("pipestem") appearance of the colon with a loss of normal haustral markings (Fig. 8.37). Colon carcinoma may develop in as many as 5% of patients with long-standing ulcerative colitis (Fig. 8.38).

Figure 8.35. "Collar button" ulcers (*arrows*) in a patient with ulcerative colitis.

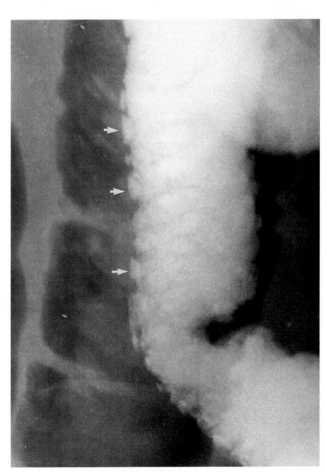

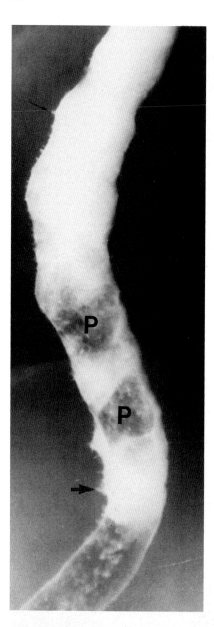

Figure 8.36.   Pseudopolyps (*P*) in a patient with ulcerative colitis. Irregular ulcers appear along the colon margin (*arrows*).

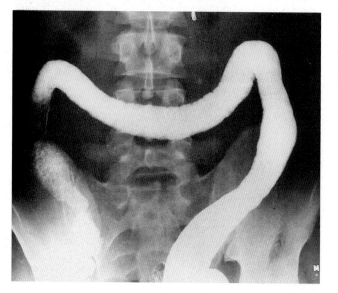

Figure 8.37.   Appearance of the colon in long-standing ulcerative colitis. The colon is fairly rigid, devoid of haustral markings, and foreshortened. Compare with Figure 8.13.

Figure 8.38. Colon carcinoma in a patient with long-standing ulcerative colitis. (This is the same patient as in Fig. 8.37, 7 years later.) A "napkin ring" lesion is present in the midtransverse colon (*arrows*).

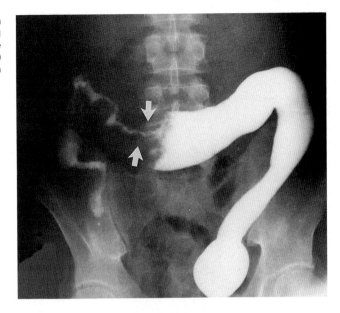

Crohn disease of the colon (*granulomatous colitis*) is identical to *regional enteritis* that occurs elsewhere in the GI tract. Crohn disease classically involves *all* layers of the bowel wall. This results in strictures and obstruction as well as enteroenteric, enterocutaneous, and enterovertebral fistulas (Fig. 8.39).

The radiographic manifestations in most instances are distinct from those of ulcerative colitis. The barium enema generally demonstrates patches of involved bowel with normal intervening mucosa—the so-called skip lesions (Fig. 8.40). Longitudinal ulcers with trans-

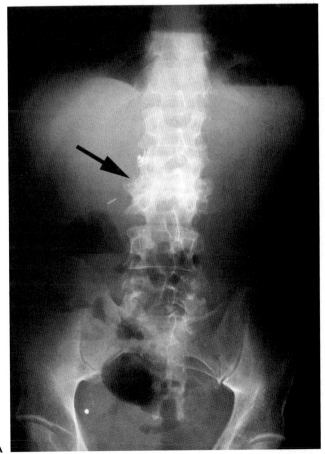

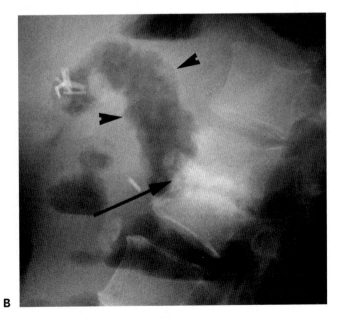

Figure 8.39. Crohn disease with enterovertebral fistula. Patient presented with clinical findings of a disc space infection. **A.** Abdominal radiograph shows sclerosis and loss of disc height at L2–L3 (*arrow*). **B.** Lateral spot film following small bowel barium study shows an abnormal loop of small bowel (*arrowheads*) lying adjacent to the L2–L3 disc space. Notice the "cobblestone" mucosal pattern in the dilated loop. The disc space (*arrow*) is narrowed, has irregular borders, and is sclerotic. The disc space infection resulted from an enterovertebral fistula.

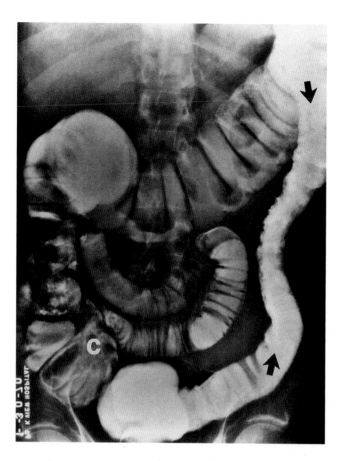

Figure 8.40. Crohn disease of the colon demonstrating skip lesions. The involved segment of bowel is the descending colon (*arrows*). C, cecum.

verse fissures give a typical "cobblestone" appearance (Fig. 8.41). Typically, the rectum is spared but the right colon is more severely involved. The terminal ileum is involved in almost every instance (Fig. 8.42). Fistulous tracts are often demonstrable (see Figs. 8.39 and 8.42). Unlike ulcerative colitis, development of colon carcinoma is unusual.

Table 8.2 contrasts the two diseases.

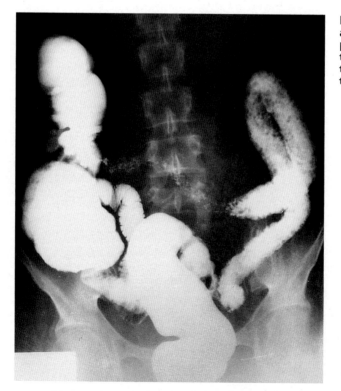

Figure 8.41. "Cobblestone" appearance of the colon in a patient with Crohn disease. This typical pattern is best appreciated in the splenic flexure. Compare with the hepatic flexure (see Fig. 8.13).

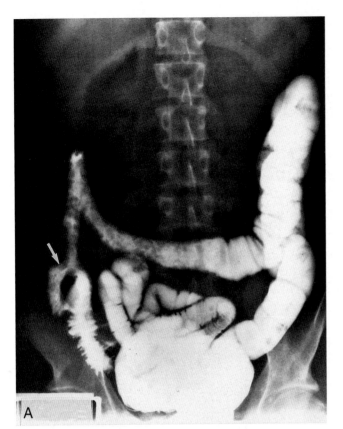
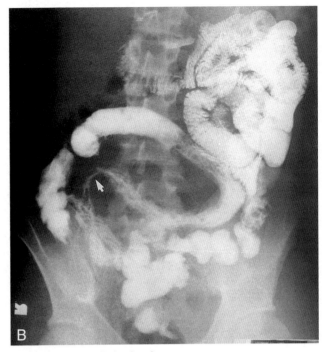

Figure 8.42. **Ileal involvement and fistula formation (*arrows*) in two patients with Crohn disease.** Notice the "mass effect" of the inflammatory process on the loop of bowel above the stricture in B.

TABLE 8.2		
COMPARISON OF ULCERATIVE COLITIS AND CROHN DISEASE		
Feature	**Ulcerative Colitis**	**Crohn Disease**
Clinical		
Fever, malaise	+	++
Rectal bleeding	++	±
Tenderness	±	++
Diarrhea	+++	+++
Abdominal mass	−	+++
Abdominal pain	−	+++
Fistulas	−	+++
Endoscopic		
Rectal disease	+++	+
Linear ulcers	−	+
Continuous disease	+++	−
Skip lesions	−	+++
Radiographic		
Continuous disease	+++	−
Skip lesions	−	+++
Ileal involvement	+	+++
Strictures	−	+
Fistulas	−	++
Carcinoma	+++	−
Pseudopolyps	+++	−
"Collar button" ulcers	+++	+
"Cobblestone" pattern	−	+++

Postoperative Appearance of the Gastrointestinal Tract

Surgical procedures alter the appearance of the barium-filled GI tract in several ways. These are briefly described and illustrated in this section.

Esophageal bypass surgery for carcinoma or stricture is done primarily using *gastroesophagostomy*. In this procedure, sometimes called an esophagogastrectomy, the stomach is mobilized, preserving its blood supply, and is brought into the chest where it is anastomosed with the resected end of the esophagus. On a chest radiograph or esophagogram, this appears as a soft tissue density that may contain air or mottled fluid just to the right of the cardiac silhouette (Fig. 8.43A, B). Frequently, the gastric rugae identify this structure. On the lateral film, the transposed stomach is in an anterior position. In some instances, a segment of transverse colon may be used (see Fig. 8.43C, D, and E). Another palliative procedure for this disease is the use of *stents* in an attempt to keep the esophageal lumen open (Fig. 8.44).

A number of procedures, many of which are performed through a laparoscope, have been designed to treat esophageal reflux with or without a hiatal hernia. Most of these (Belsey, Thal, Nissen) involve *fundoplication*, in which the gastric fundus is sutured around the esophagus to create a tighter sphincter. This results in the radiographic appearance of a mass with smooth, intact mucosa near the esophagogastric junction (Fig. 8.45). This finding should alert the flu-

Figure 8.43. Appearance after esophageal bypass surgery. A and B. Gastroesophagostomy. **A.** Frontal radiograph shows an air-containing mass in the right paratracheal region (*arrows*). Surgical clips are evident. **B.** Esophagogram shows that the "mass" is the result of the transposed stomach. **C, D, and E.** *(continued on page 297)*

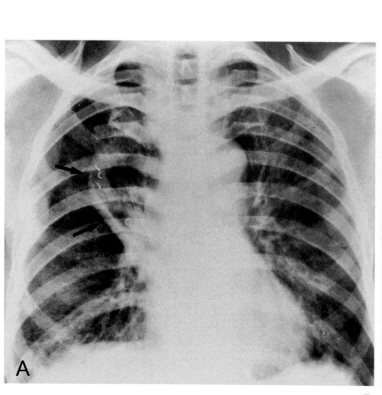

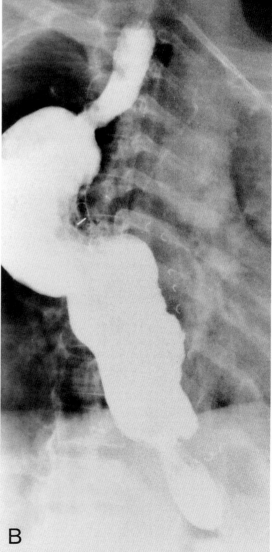

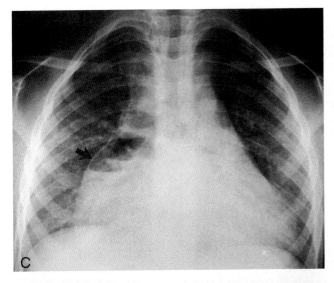

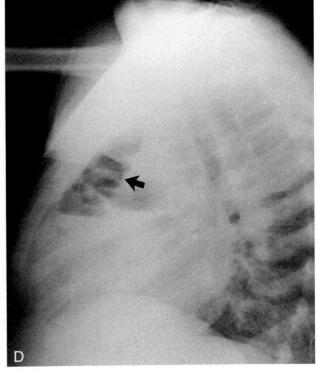

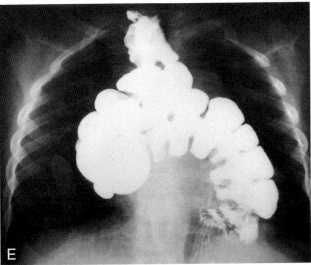

Figure 8.43. *(continued)* Colonic interposition. Frontal and lateral chest radiographs (C and D) show an air-containing mass (*arrows*) to the right of the cardiac border and substernally, respectively. A barium study (E) shows the interposed segment of transverse colon. In this patient, the proximal anastomosis is at the thoracic inlet.

oroscopist to the type of procedure performed. There are usually surgical clips in the vicinity of the esophagogastric junction.

Surgical procedures developed for treating morbid obesity (bariatric surgery) involve *gastric bypasses*, in which the gastric antrum is anastomosed directly to a portion of distal ileum to prevent absorption of large quantities of nutrients. Other procedures include *gastric stapling* or *gastric banding*, in which the overall volume of the stomach is made smaller by closing off a portion of the fundus and body (Fig. 8.46). These procedures may be recognized by the location of surgical staple lines located at the anastomotic or operative sites. A careful history from the patient is usually sufficient to determine if the patient has had one of these procedures. Complications of these procedures include anastomotic leaks (Fig. 8.47) and obstruction, both of which may be demonstrated with the appropriate contrast examinations.

Surgery for peptic ulcer disease may take several forms. One popular procedure is *vagotomy and pyloroplasty*. Previous vagotomy may be recognized by the presence of midline surgical clips at the level of the diaphragm. A pyloroplasty performed at the same time results in a deformity in the antral and pyloric regions. This may often be confused with severe scarring from previous ulcer disease. An alternate form of drainage procedure is *gastrojejunostomy*, in which a loop of jejunum is anastomosed with the greater curvature of the stomach.

Patients who have had repeated episodes of severe peptic ulcer disease with or without perforation may require a *subtotal gastrectomy*, especially if they show signs of obstruction.

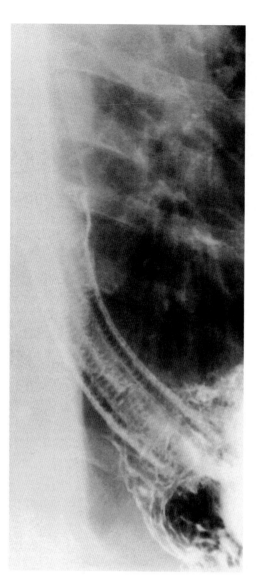

Figure 8.44. Esophageal stent placed for carcinoma. (This is the same patient as in Fig. 8.34.) Notice the corrugated appearance of the stent.

Figure 8.45. Appearance after Nissen fundoplication procedure for esophageal reflux. A. Close-up view of epigastric region of a chest radiograph shows a mass (*arrow*) in the gastric fundus. **B.** Upper GI examination shows narrowing of the esophagogastric junction and the mass (*arrow*) representing the plicated portion of the gastric fundus.

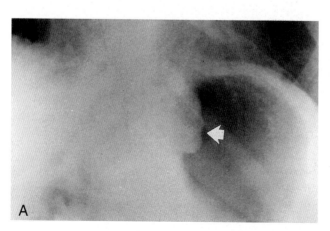

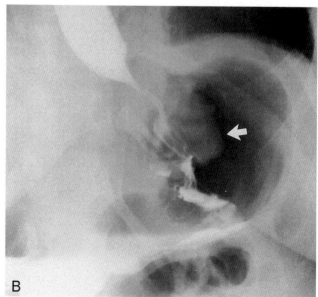

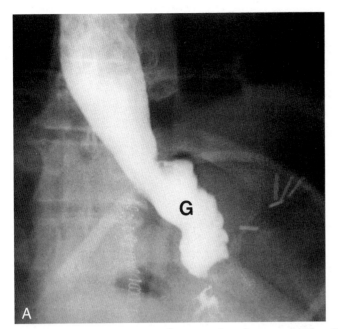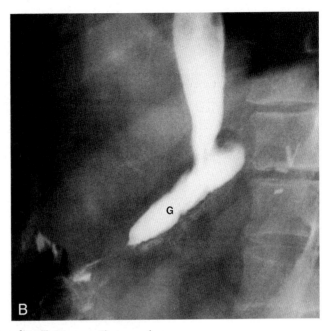

Figure 8.46.   Appearance after gastric volume reduction ("banding") surgery. The procedure leaves a small gastric pouch (G). Notice the suture lines to the left (**A**) and just below the pouch (**B**).

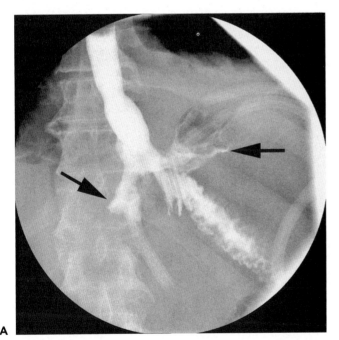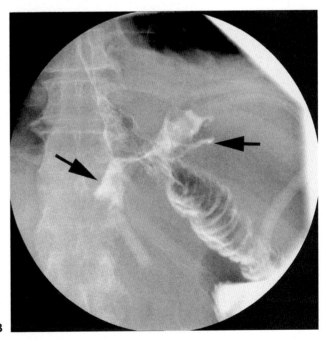

Figure 8.47.   Anastomotic leak following bariatric surgery. A, B, and C. Fluoroscopic spot films show the leakage of contrast (*arrows*). *(continued on page 300)*

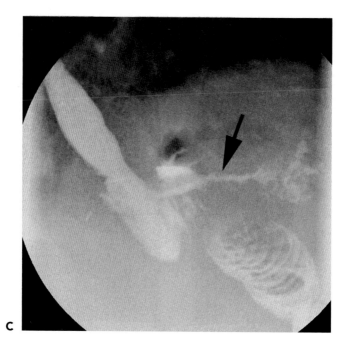

Figure 8.47.   *(continued)*

C

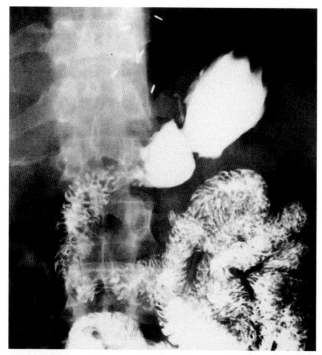

Figure 8.48.   Appearance after Billroth I subtotal gastrectomy and gastroenterostomy. Notice the absent duodenal bulb.

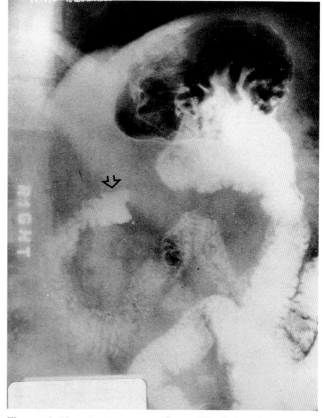

Figure 8.49.   Appearance after Billroth II subtotal gastrectomy and gastroenterostomy. Notice the blind ending of the afferent loop (*arrow*).

Although several procedures have been designed, they are referred to as either a Billroth I or Billroth II subtotal gastrectomy. A Billroth I procedure (Fig. 8.48) is recognizable as a direct continuation of an amputated distal stomach with the duodenum. The base of the duodenal bulb is removed at the time of surgery. In a Billroth II procedure (Fig. 8.49), a subtotal gastrectomy is performed, with anastomosis of the gastric stump to a loop of jejunum. An afferent loop drains the pancreatobiliary system through the duodenum. The base of the duodenal bulb usually is removed in this procedure.

Anastomoses between the distal ileum and colon (ileocolostomy) are performed for inflammatory bowel disease or carcinoma. These are easily recognized by the filling of small bowel from a portion of colon other than the cecum. A ring of staples marks each anastomosis (Fig. 8.50). Whenever an anastomotic leak is suspected, examination with water-soluble contrast is indicated (Fig. 8.51).

CT is used extensively to evaluate patients after surgery. The prime indications for this procedure are for detecting infections and abscesses, for recurrence or local spread of a known malignancy (Fig. 8.52), and for metastases (Fig. 8.53).

Accessory Digestive Organs

The accessory digestive organs are the gallbladder, liver, and pancreas. These organs are best evaluated by diagnostic ultrasound, CT, and occasionally by MR imaging.

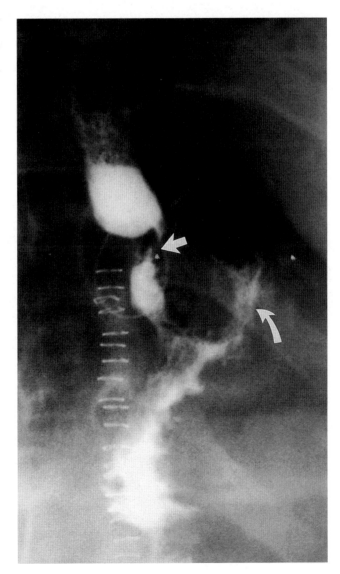

Figure 8.50. Appearance of anastomoses after ileoesophageal interposition for morbid obesity. Notice the anastomosis with the esophagus (*short arrow*) and the gastric pouch (*curved arrow*).

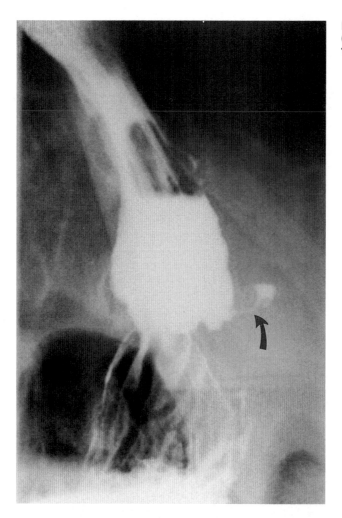

Figure 8.51. Anastomotic leak (*arrow*) in a patient after gastric "banding."

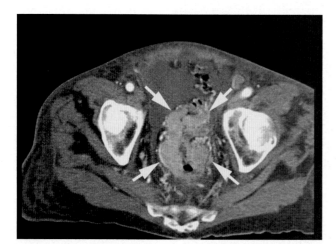

Figure 8.52. Recurrent colon carcinoma. CT image of the pelvis shows recurrent perirectal masses (*arrows*). The tissue planes in the area are indistinct owing to local invasion.

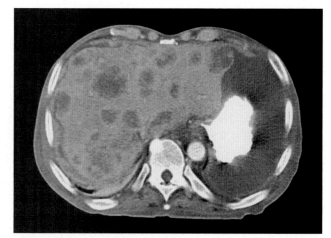

Figure 8.53. Metastases from colon carcinoma. (This is the same patient as in Fig. 8.52.) CT image through the liver demonstrates multiple round and irregular areas of low density, representing metastases.

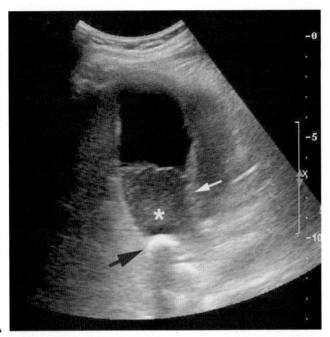
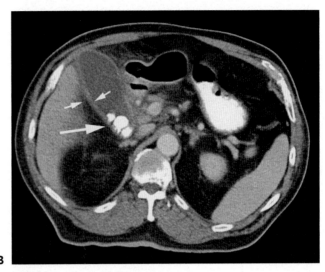

A   **B**

Figure 8.54.   Cholecystitis. A. Ultrasound shows thickening of the gallbladder wall (*small white arrow*) with many internal echoes representing "sludge" (*). A large stone is present (*large black arrow*). Notice the shadowing beneath the stone. The obstructing calculus is not demonstrated in this study. **B.** CT image shows the thickened gallbladder wall (*small arrows*) and multiple stones (*large arrow*).

As previously mentioned, the *biliary tract* may be visualized either by ultrasound, biliary scintigraphy, or CT. The most common abnormalities encountered in the biliary tract are cholecystitis (Fig. 8.54; see Fig. 8.7) and cholelithiasis with or without obstruction (Figs. 8.55 and 8.56).

The most common abnormalities encountered in the *liver* are obstructive jaundice and metastases (Fig. 8.57). Both of these may be evaluated by ultrasound and CT. The CT scan, however, is particularly advantageous in evaluating metastases and may be used to guide percutaneous biopsy of metastatic or other masses of the liver (Fig. 5.58). Although MR imaging also may be used to evaluate hepatic metastases, CT is much more efficient. However, MR imaging is particularly useful in evaluating patients with hemangiomas (Fig. 8.59). In these patients, the vascular lesion has an extremely high signal. MR may also be used to diagnose

Figure 8.55.   Multiple calcified gallstones. One of the stones (*arrow*) is near the neck of the gallbladder.

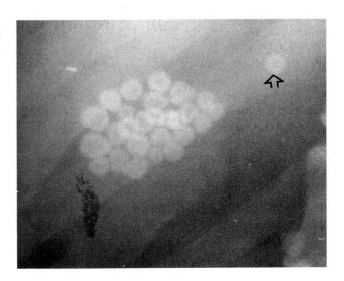

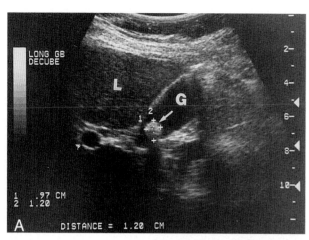
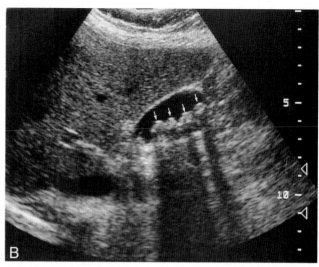

Figure 8.56. Cholelithiasis. A. Ultrasound shows a single stone (*arrow*) measuring 1.2 × 0.97 cm in the dependent portion of the gallbladder. L, liver; G, gallbladder. **B.** Ultrasound showing multiple stones (*arrows*). Notice the shadowing (sonolucent areas) in each patient.

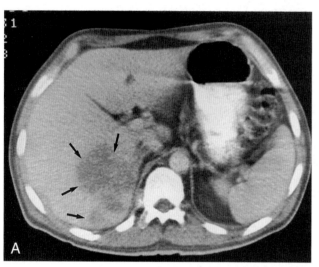
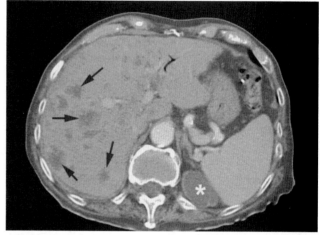

Figure 8.57. Liver metastases in two patients. A. Patient with renal carcinoma. **B.** Patient with rectal carcinoma. Both CT images show multiple lucent areas within the liver (*arrows*). Notice the hydronephrosis of the left kidney (*) as a result of ureteral obstruction from recurrent tumor in the pelvis.

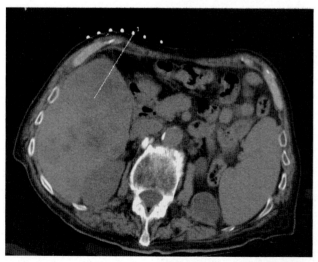
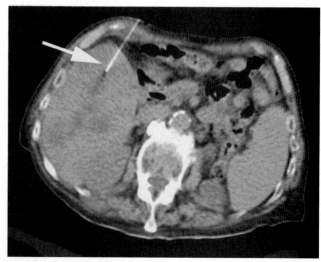

Figure 8.58. CT-guided biopsy of a liver metastasis. (This is the same patient as in Fig. 8.57B.) **A.** Preliminary CT image used to calculate direction and depth of puncture. Notice the multiple metastatic lesions in the liver. **B.** Biopsy needle (*arrow*) is advanced into a lesion.

Figure 8.59. Hepatic hemangioma. This T2-weighted MR image shows the hemangioma (*H*) as a rounded area of very high (bright) signal against the darker background of the normal liver tissue. Notice the coexistent metastatic lesion (*M*) from a left renal tumor (*T*) and pleural effusion (*PE*) that have a lower signal than the hemangioma.

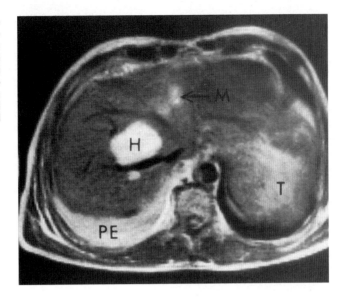

hemochromatosis of the liver by demonstrating the iron-laden liver as having a low signal on both T1- and T2-weighted images (Fig. 8.60).

The *pancreas* was one of the most elusive organs to image in the past. Although pancreatitis and pancreatic pseudocysts make themselves clinically apparent at a relatively early stage of the disease, pancreatic carcinoma often does not. Once the patient with pancreatic carcinoma becomes symptomatic, he or she is usually beyond cure from either surgery or radiation therapy. Direct pancreatic imaging, therefore, has become one of the major advances in medical diagnosis in the last three decades. The pancreas lends itself readily to evaluation by either ultrasound or CT (Figs. 8.61 to 8.63).

The evaluation of *appendicitis* (Figs. 8.64 and 8.65) and intra-abdominal abscess from any cause has been greatly facilitated by the development of CT and ultrasound. Although most *abdominal abscesses* demonstrate abnormalities on abdominal radiographs, a definitive diagnosis may be made by CT examination (Fig. 8.66). Furthermore, CT-guided drainage is now possible (see Fig. 3.19).

Finally, CT has made it easier to diagnose traumatic injuries to the liver, spleen, and pancreas (Fig. 8.67). Modern CT machines are now able to scan the abdomen in 10 to 20 seconds, making it possible for most patients to cooperate by breath holding to obtain an ideal study.

Figure 8.60. Hemochromatosis. Inversion recovery image shows the liver to have a low signal (black). T1- and T2-weighted images (not shown) demonstrated identical findings.

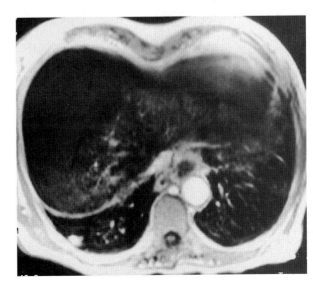

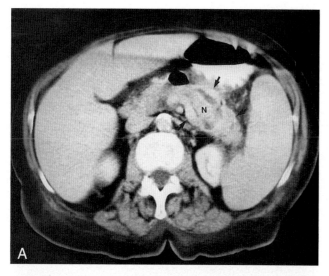

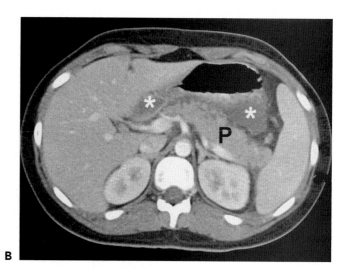

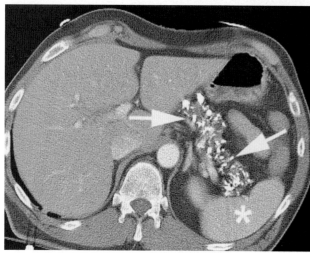

Figure 8.61. Pancreatitis in three patients. A. CT image shows enlargement of the pancreas (*arrow*) and a necrotic focus (*N*) in the central portion of the pancreas. **B.** CT image shows enlargement of the pancreas (*P*). There are fluid collections (*) anterior to the pancreas. **C.** CT image of a patient with chronic pancreatitis shows multiple calcifications in the pancreas (*arrows*). Notice how the tail of the pancreas ends in the hilus of the spleen (*).

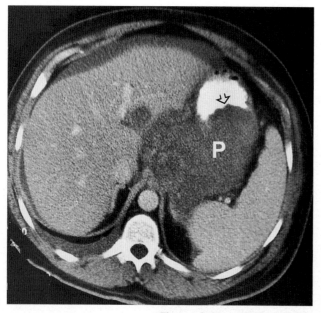

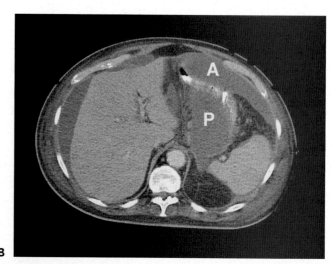

Figure 8.62. Pancreatic pseudocysts. A. CT image shows a large pseudocyst (*P*) compressing the posterior gastric wall (*arrow*). **B and C.** Pseudocyst (*P*) in another patient with ascites (*A*). *(continued on page 307)*

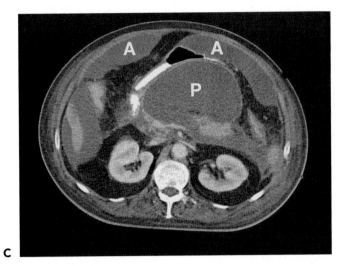

C

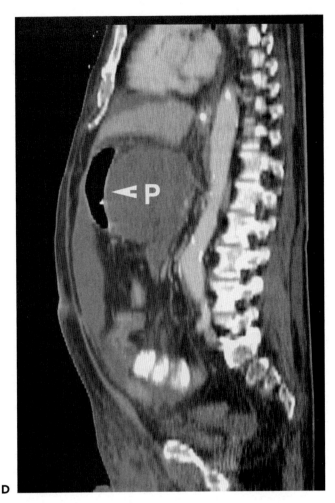

D

Figure 8.62. *(continued)* **C.** Pseudocyst (*P*) in another patient with ascites (*A*). **D.** Sagittal reconstructed CT image shows the pseudocyst (*P*) pressing on the stomach (*arrowhead*).

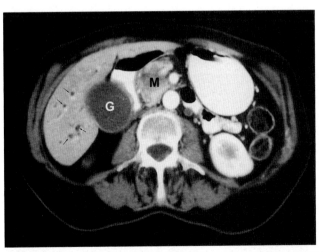

A

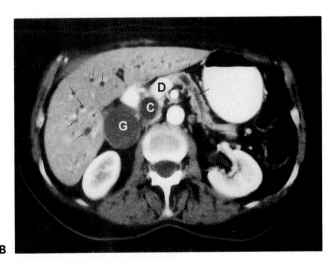

B

Figure 8.63. **Pancreatic carcinoma in two patients. A.** CT image shows a mass (*M*) in the head of the pancreas. The gallbladder (*G*) is massively dilated, as are the intrahepatic biliary ducts (*arrows*). **B.** CT image slightly higher demonstrates dilation of the common bile duct (*C*), pancreatic duct (*long arrows*), gall bladder (*G*), and intrahepatic biliary ducts (*short arrows*). Notice the relationship of the duodenum (*D*) to the pancreas and common bile duct. The contrast-enhanced inferior vena cava lies between the common bile duct and the liver. *(continued on page 308)*

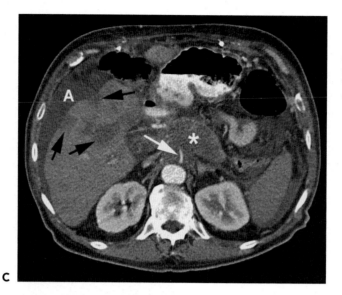

Figure 8.63. *(continued)* **C.** CT image in another patient shows a mass (*) in the head of the pancreas surrounding and compressing the celiac artery (white *arrow*). Notice the multiple liver metastases (*black arrows*) and ascites collection (*A*).

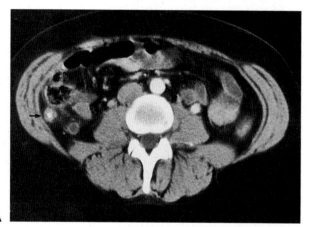

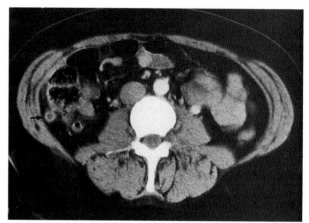

Figure 8.64. **Appendicitis. A.** CT image shows a fecalith in a thickened appendix (*arrow*). **B.** Image slightly higher shows the thickened appendiceal wall (*arrow*).

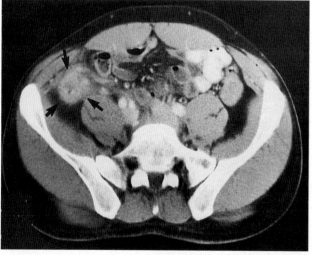

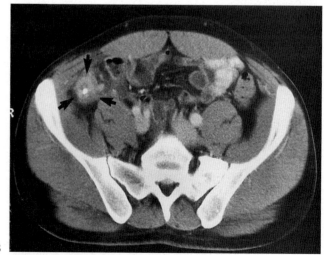

Figure 8.65. **Appendicitis with abscess. A.** CT image shows a soft tissue inflammatory mass in the right lower quadrant (*arrows*). **B.** Image slightly lower shows a calcified fecalith within the thickened appendix (*arrows*).

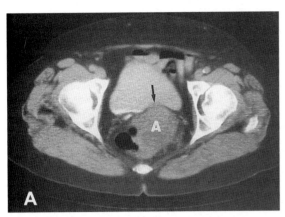
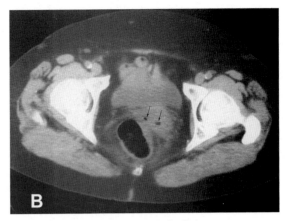

Figure 8.66. Perirectal abscess. A. Pelvic CT image shows a large abscess (*A*) compressing the floor of the bladder (*arrow*). The air-containing rectum is displaced to the right. **B.** Slightly lower, the abscess contains gas (*arrows*).

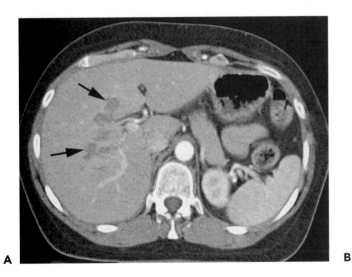
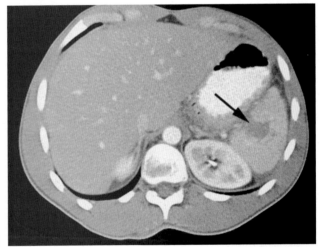

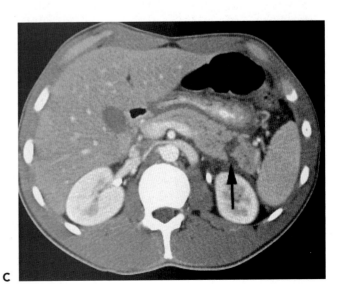

Figure 8.67. Abdominal visceral injuries depicted by CT.
A. Liver laceration in the central portion of the right lobe (*arrows*).
B. Splenic laceration (*arrow*). **C.** Pancreatic laceration (*arrow*).

Special Pediatric Considerations

A large variety of disorders affect the GI tract and accessory organs of digestion in the pediatric age group. A complete description would be beyond the aim and scope of this text. However, several disorders occur in sufficient frequency as to merit special mention. These are esophageal foreign body, pyloric stenosis, Hirschsprung disease, and intussusception. Each has characteristic imaging features that should be easily recognizable.

Infants and small children frequently put *foreign objects* in their mouths and all too often end up swallowing them. In most instances, the object (coins are most common) readily passes through the GI tract without incident. Occasionally, the object lodges within the esophagus, usually at the level of the thoracic inlet (Fig. 8.68). Irregular and sharp foreign bodies are more likely to cause complications, such as perforation. The radiographic evaluation of every patient suspected of swallowing a foreign object should include radiographs of the chest and abdomen. Small children can usually be studied with a single film. If the object is a coin, it can safely be removed in the radiology department using a Foley catheter, as long as there is no evidence of airway obstruction or mediastinal inflammation.

Hypertrophic pyloric stenosis is the result of hypertrophy and hyperplasia of the circular muscle layer of the pylorus. It is a common cause of persistent vomiting in infants. Although the diagnosis is made primarily on clinical grounds, ultrasound and barium studies are used to confirm the diagnosis (Fig. 8.69). An abdominal radiograph on a patient with pyloric stenosis may, on occasion, show distension of the stomach with a paucity of distal gas.

Intussusception occurs when a segment of intestine (the *intussusceptum*) invaginates or "telescopes" into the contiguous distal segment (the *intussuscipiens*). This produces mechanical obstruction and, if left untreated, ischemia. The majority (approximately 90%) of intussusceptions are ileocolic. The remainder are (in decreasing order of frequency) ileoileocolic, ileoileal, and colocolic. Unlike intussusceptions in adults, which are caused by mesenteric neoplasms, those in the pediatric age group are idiopathic. Radiographic findings, when present, include a mass effect, targetlike lucencies in the mass (representing mesenteric fat trapped in the intussusception), and a crescent or streaks of air outlining the trapped bowel (Fig. 8.70). If there is no evidence for either pneumoperitoneum or peritonitis, an air or barium enema may be performed for both diagnostic purposes as well to reduce the

Figure 8.68.   Esophageal foreign bodies. A. Jack. **B.** Coin.

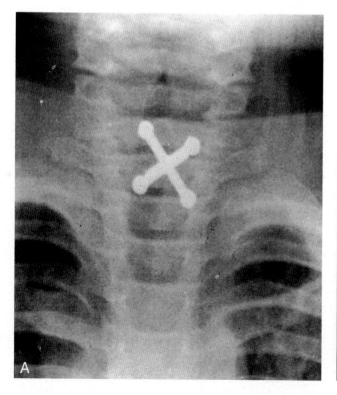

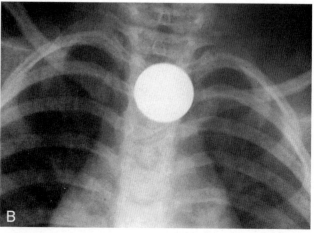

Figure 8.69.   Pyloric stenosis. Ultrasound examination of the pyloric region shows a narrowed lumen (*L*) and thickening of the wall of the pylorus (*sonolucent area between the white ×'s and +'s*).

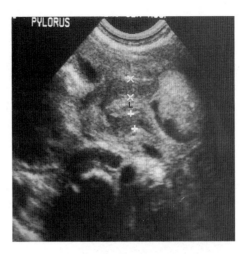

Figure 8.70.   Intussusception. Supine **(A)** and left lateral **(B)** decubitus radiographs demonstrate crescentic streaks of air within the trapped loops of bowel (*arrows*).

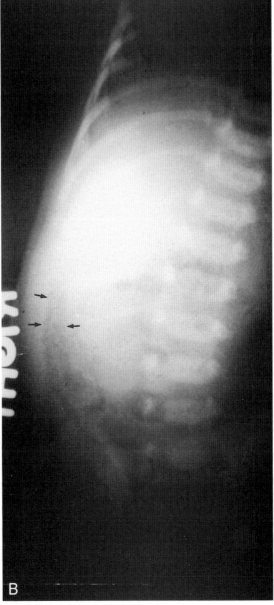

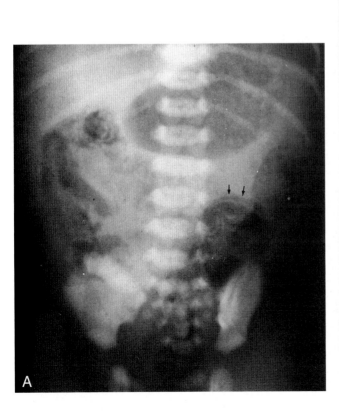

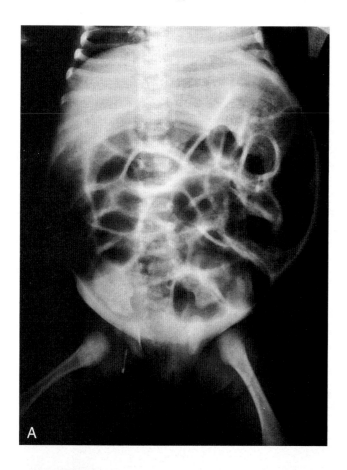

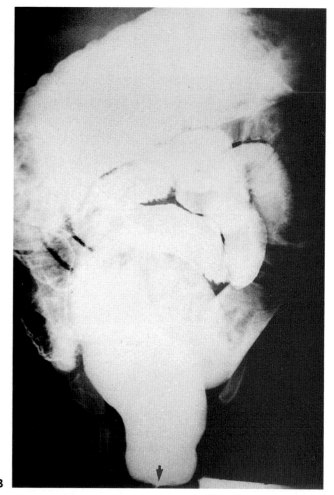

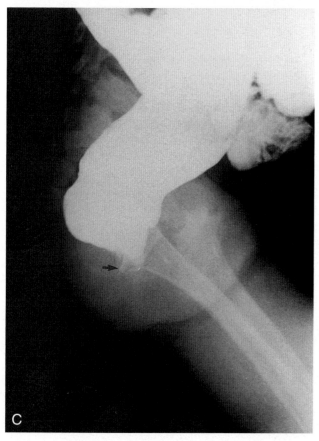

Figure 8.71. Hirschsprung disease. A. Abdominal radiograph demonstrates massive dilatation of large and small bowel. Frontal **(B)** and lateral **(C)** barium enema images demonstrate dilated colon ending in a small, tapered, atonic segment at the rectum (*arrows*).

intussusception. Current practices prefer the air enema to reduce the likelihood of barium-induced peritonitis in the setting of possible colonic rupture as an adverse outcome of an attempted intussusception reduction. Using fluoroscopic guidance and a pressure valve–equipped catheter, air is instilled into the colon progressively until the obstructing component of the intestine or small bowel is pushed back and reduced into the anatomically normal location.

Hirschsprung disease is the result of congenital absence of the intramural ganglion cells in the distal bowel. It is more common in boys than in girls. The absence of the distal ganglion cells results in the inability of the peristaltic wave to pass through the abnormal bowel segment and thus produces an obstructive clinical picture, manifested primarily as chronic constipation. Radiography is beneficial in making the diagnosis. Abdominal radiographs reveal an obstructive pattern in infants and evidence of fecal impaction in older children (Fig. 8.71A). A barium enema may demonstrate the atonic bowel segment as an area of abrupt tapering of the lumen (see Fig. 8.71B, C).

SUMMARY AND KEY POINTS

- The gastrointestinal tract is a tubular structure that allows recognition of patterns of disease that may occur in any portion.
- Typical abnormalities include polypoid lesions, mucosal tumors, ulcerations, diverticula, extrinsic compression, and benign strictures.
- Although the appearance of these lesions will be quite similar from segment to segment, the incidence varies depending on the disease.
- Special imaging procedures and their applications to the gastrointestinal tract were also discussed.
- Endoscopy has replaced conventional barium imaging in the United States.

SUGGESTED ADDITIONAL READING

Blickman JG. Pediatric Radiology: The Requisites. St. Louis: Mosby, 1994: 57–110.

Brant WE, Helms CA. Fundamentals of Diagnostic Radiology. 2nd Ed. Philadelphia: Lippincott Williams & Wilkins, 1999: 651–767.

Buonomo C, Taylor GA, Share JC, et al. Gastrointestinal tract. In: Kirks DR, Griscom NT, eds. Practical Pediatric Imaging: Diagnostic Radiology of Infants and Children. 3rd Ed. Philadelphia: Lippincott-Raven, 1998:821–1007.

Donnelly LF. Fundamentals of Pediatric Radiology. Philadelphia: WB Saunders, 2001: 97–140.

Donnelley LF, Jones BV, O'Hara S, et al. Diagnostic Imaging: Pediatrics. Philadelphia: WB Saunders, 2006.

Federle MP, Jeffrey RB, Anne V. Diagnostic Imaging: Abdomen. Philadelphia: WB Saunders, 2005.

Gore RM, Levine MS, Laufer I. Textbook of gastrointestinal radiology. Philadelphia: WB Saunders, 1994.

Laufer I, Levine MS. Double Contrast Gastrointestinal Radiology. 2nd Ed. Philadelphia: WB Saunders, 1992.

Margulis AR, Burhenne HJ, eds. Alimentary Tract Radiology. 5th Ed. St. Louis: Mosby-Year Book, 1997.

Rao PM, Rhea JT, Novelline RA, et al. Effect of computed tomography of the appendix on treatment of patients and use of hospital resources. N Engl J Med 1998;338:141–146.

Ziessman HA. O'Malley JP, Thrall JH. Nuclear Medicine: The Requisites. 3rd Ed. St. Louis: Mosby, 2006.

Urinary Tract Imaging

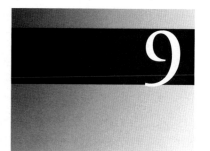

Urinary tract imaging has undergone a tremendous change in the past two decades. Whereas urography was considered the primary investigative tool in the past, it is now used infrequently in the United States and has a subservient role relative to ultrasound and computed tomography (CT). Nevertheless, urography is still an important diagnostic tool.

Imaging of the urinary tract is designed principally to evaluate two basic types of abnormalities: "physiologic" and morphologic. The so-called *physiologic abnormalities* include various diseases referred to collectively as the *medical nephropathies*. These include diseases of the glomeruli, tubules, and interstitial tissues. Also included are forms of tubular and cortical necrosis. In patients with these diseases, intravenous urography shows poor function or none at all, and the diagnosis is best determined by biopsy. Furthermore, intravenous urography may be detrimental.

The *morphologic abnormalities* constitute the other large group in which imaging is definitely of value. These will be discussed in the "Pathologic Considerations" section.

TECHNICAL CONSIDERATIONS

Basically, nine types of studies are commonly used to evaluate the urinary tract: the intravenous urogram (IVU); the retrograde urogram; the cystogram, which is often combined with a study of the urethra as a voiding cystourethrogram; the nephrostogram; ultrasound; CT scanning; magnetic resonance (MR) imaging; renal angiography; and isotope studies. CT, with contrast enhancement, is replacing the urogram for most applications.

Intravenous urography, often inaccurately called intravenous pyelography, is an infrequently performed examination in the United States, having been replaced, for the most part by CT. However, in many parts of the world, the IVU is still commonly used. Before starting an IVU, an abdominal radiograph should be obtained to look for calculi that may be obscured by the excretion of contrast material and to determine the degree of bowel cleanliness. As with the colon examination, preparation of the bowel is necessary to eliminate overlying gas and fecal material that may obscure the renal outlines.

Before ordering any study that uses contrast, it is imperative that you question the patient regarding a history of allergy in general and allergy to iodinated radiopaque drugs in particular. It is very important to ask these patients if they have ever had their kidneys x-rayed before. A history of feeling warm after a contrast injection should not be considered evidence of allergy but rather a normal physiologic reaction. This symptom may be prevented by using low-osmolar contrast agents. If a history of a previous true reaction to contrast material is elicited, the radiologist, in consultation with the referring physician, must decide whether the study requested is absolutely necessary or whether an alternative study, such as ultrasound or noncontrasted CT, can be performed. If it is deemed that the study is needed, the patient may be "prepared" by the referring physician: 2 days of dosing with prednisone and a dose of antihistamine (diphenhydramine) immediately before the study. The use of low-osmolar contrast agents reduces but does not totally eliminate adverse reactions. The IVU should not be performed on a patient with evidence of renal failure because the contrast agent may worsen that condition.

The indications for intravenous urography in adults and children are primarily to gain morphologic information, to assess renal function, to localize obstructions, and to evaluate postoperative changes of the urinary tract. In children, an IVU is used to evaluate girls with wetting problems that may be caused by an ectopic ureter. On occasion, the urogram may be used after an ultrasound examination to provide additional information on abnormalities found on that study.

During the typical urogram, tomography of the kidneys should be used routinely to show renal outlines that may otherwise be obscured by overlying gas or bowel content (Fig. 9.1). The filming sequence uses tomography during the earliest or "nephrogram" phase, when contrast material is in the small vessels and nephrons. This method offers the best opportunity to evaluate the renal parenchyma as well as the renal size and shape. Two or more static radiographs (without tomography) are obtained, usually at 5-minute intervals, to examine the collecting systems, the ureters, and the bladder. Additional views of the kidneys or of the bladder are taken as needed to delineate any areas still in question. Occasionally, oblique views will be obtained. In this way, the examination is "tailored" to each patient.

Retrograde examinations are performed on the urethra, bladder, ureters, and renal collecting system. The *urethrogram* is used mainly to study strictures or trauma to the male urethra. The cystogram is performed to determine the integrity of the urinary bladder as well as to search for evidence of vesicoureteral reflux. A retrograde study of the ureters and the renal collecting system—*retrograde ureteropyelogram*—is performed when there is clinical suspicion of obstruc-

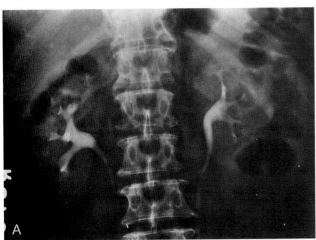

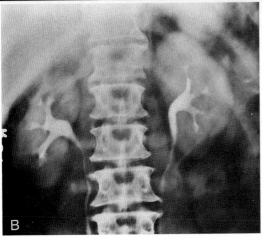

Figure 9.1. Use of nephrotomography during intravenous urography. A. Detail view of kidneys shows bowel gas obscuring renal borders. **B.** Nephrotomography blurs the overlying gas and bowel content, revealing smooth, normal-appearing renal borders.

Figure 9.2.   Normal renal ultrasound. A. Longitudinal image. The kidney has a reniform shape (*arrows*). The corticomedullary areas are relatively sonolucent. The collecting system and renal pelvis produce echoes. L, liver **B.** Coronal image showing the sonolucent renal sinus pyramids.

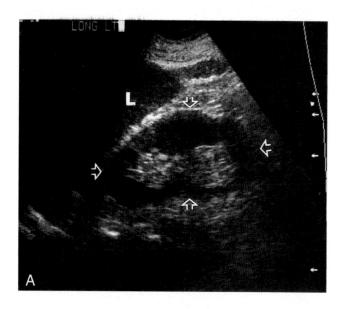

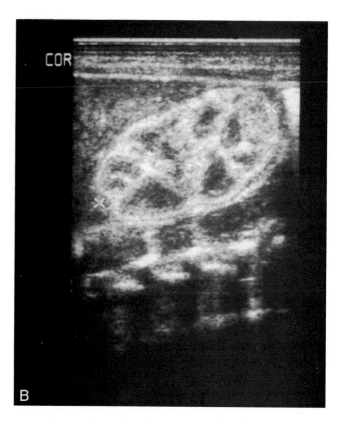

tion from stones, strictures, or tumor. This examination is performed by a urologist in the operating room.

Once the bladder is filled, the patient may be asked to void, and during this process, a *voiding cystourethrogram* (*VCUG*) is done to determine proper physiologic function as well as the presence or absence of vesicoureteral reflux. This study is most often performed on children and is indicated to study patients with recurrent urinary tract infections, hydronephrosis or hydroureter, hematuria, or day and night wetting in a previously continent boy; it is also used to evaluate patients with complex anomalies. A variation of the standard VCUG called *cyclic VCUG* is a technique in which several cycles of filling and voiding with a catheter in place are performed. This variation is useful for demonstrating reflux, particularly in patients with massive urinary tract obstruction.

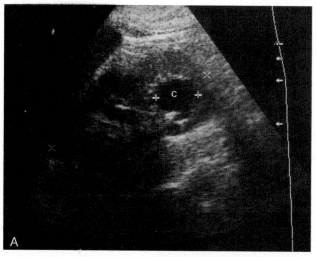

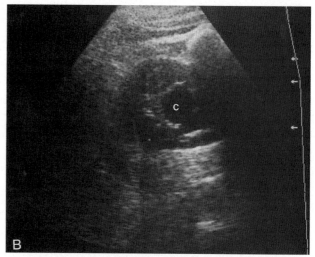

Figure 9.3.   Renal cyst. A. Longitudinal image shows the sonolucent cyst (*C*). Notice the increased echoes beneath the cyst ("through transmission"). **B.** Axial image again shows the cyst (*C*) and the "through transmission."

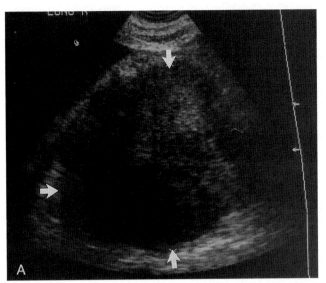

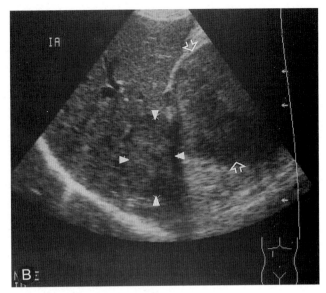

Figure 9.4. Renal carcinoma in upper pole of right kidney. (This is the same patient as in Fig. 8.57A.) **A.** Longitudinal ultrasound image shows gross distortion of the renal outline by a large mass (*arrows*). Notice the internal echoes in the upper portion of the tumor. Contrast this with the cyst in Figure 9.3. **B.** Longitudinal scan slightly higher again shows the renal mass (*arrows*). Notice the invasion of the right lobe of the liver (*arrowheads*).

Nephrostograms are performed to diagnose obstruction or extravasation after a surgical or percutaneous nephrostomy. Contrast is injected into the nephrostomy catheter, and the flow of the contrast is monitored fluoroscopically. If an obstruction or extravasation is encountered, the site of the abnormality is documented with spot radiographs and the procedure is terminated. Delayed images may be obtained to determine any progress of the flow of contrast through the area of obstruction.

The urinary tract is easily studied by real-time and Doppler *ultrasonography*. In many instances, this technique has replaced the IVU as the initial study for evaluating renal size and renal shape. Figure 9.2 shows a scan of the right kidney. Renal ultrasound is also used in assessing the nature of renal masses by searching for internal echoes within the masses. Renal cysts with only fluid in them have no internal echoes and are referred to as *sonolucent* (Fig. 9.3). Tumors, on the other hand, frequently show internal echoes, indicating their solid nature (Fig. 9.4). Doppler ultrasound is used to screen for renal artery stenosis in patients with hypertension (Fig. 9.5).

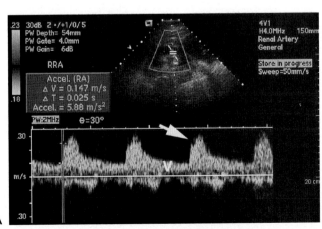

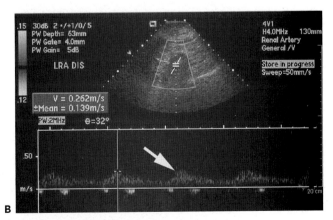

Figure 9.5. Renal artery Doppler examinations. A. Normal Doppler waveform of an arcuate branch of the right renal artery. The slope (*arrow*) of the systolic upstroke is normal (>300 cm/sec^2). Velocities (*V*) in the normal right renal artery are less than 180 cm/sec, consistent with no significant renal artery stenosis. **B.** Doppler waveform of an arcuate branch of the left renal artery in the same patient shows slow systolic upstroke and delay to peak (*parvus tardus* morphology; *arrow*) distal to a significant stenosis. (Courtesy of H. Scott Beasley, MD, Department of Radiology, Western Pennsylvania Hospital.)

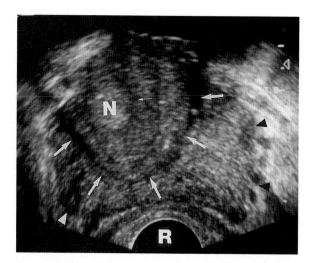

Figure 9.6. "Normal" prostate ultrasound in an elderly man. Two distinct areas are delineated. The peripheral zone is the area immediately adjacent to the rectum (*R*). This is surrounded by the true capsule (*arrowheads*). The central zone is outlined by the surgical capsule (*large arrows*). Within this zone are the urethra (*small arrow*) and some smaller septations. A small adenomatous nodule (*N*) is present.

Ultrasound is also used to evaluate the prostate gland. The development of the transrectal ultrasound transducer makes it possible to study the internal anatomy of the prostate (Fig. 9.6). Ultrasound may differentiate benign prostatic hypertrophy from carcinoma (Fig. 9.7). However, the diagnosis should always be confirmed by biopsy of suspicious areas of the prostate using a special transrectal ultrasound biopsy device. These techniques hold promise to reduce the morbidity and mortality rate of prostatic carcinoma.

Abdominal CT scanning is used for evaluating renal masses as well as for determining the origin of masses that distort or displace the normal urinary tract, such as enlarged abdominal lymph nodes. CT is also the best method of evaluating renal trauma (Fig. 9.8). The CT characteristics of renal cysts show that they are of low density and of CT numbers that correspond to the numbers of urine. On intravenous injection of contrast material, there is no enhancement of the mass, which appears as a prominent "lucency" against the contrast-containing parenchyma (Fig. 9.9). Renal cell carcinoma is, on the other hand, generally isodense (i.e., its density is the same as renal tissue) on the unenhanced scan and with enhancement may show hypervascularity, manifested by increased density of the lesion (Fig. 9.10). Contrast enhancement often aids in demonstrating necrotic areas within the mass. It is often possible to determine the extent of extrarenal

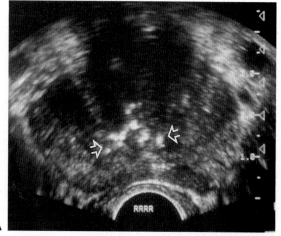

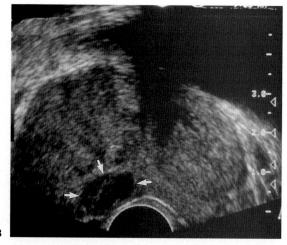

Figure 9.7. Prostate abnormalities. A. Benign prostatic hypertrophy. The gland is diffusely enlarged. There are many small calcifications (*arrows*) that cast echo shadows. **B.** Prostate carcinoma. A sonolucent area immediately adjacent to the rectum (*arrows*) represents a carcinoma. All such lucent nodules should undergo biopsy, even though only 25% turn out to be cancerous. This nodule was palpable.

Figure 9.8. Renal trauma showing a shattered kidney on the left. Notice the general absence of function and the large mass representing the intrarenal and perinephric hematoma.

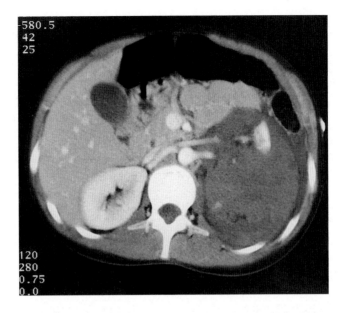

Figure 9.9. Renal cysts. (This is the same patient as in Fig. 9.3.) Computed tomography (CT) image shows a large cyst (*C*) in the posterior portion of the right kidney. Notice the two smaller cysts (*arrows*) on the left.

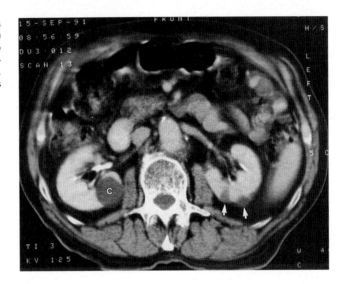

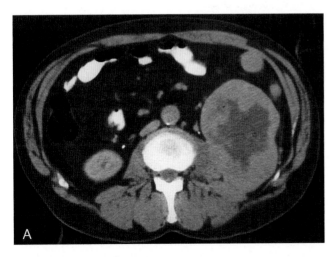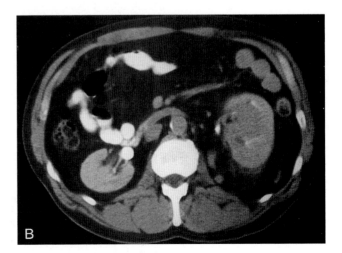

Figure 9.10. Renal carcinoma. A. CT image shows enlargement of the left renal outline. The left kidney is devoid of normal internal markings. The low-density area within the left kidney represents necrosis. **B.** Image slightly lower clearly shows the difference between the two kidneys.

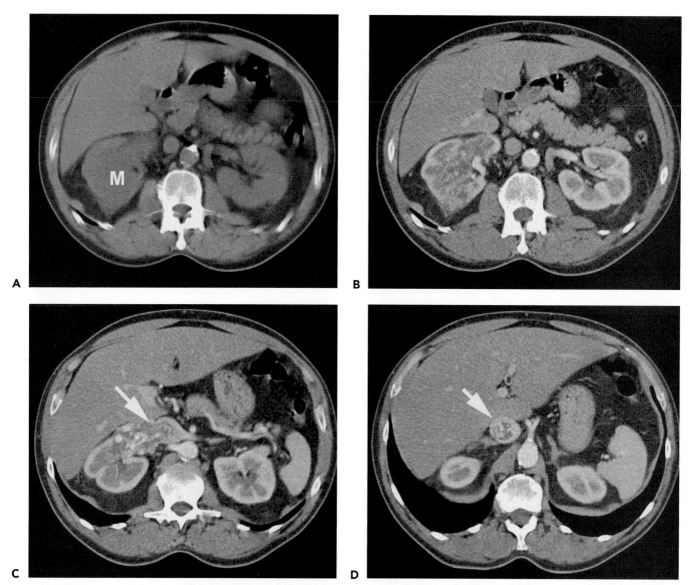

Figure 9.11. Renal carcinoma with renal vein and inferior vena cava invasion. A. CT image before contrast shows a mass (*M*) in the right kidney. **B.** Contrast-enhanced image shows the mass to advantage. **C and D.** Additional images show the tumor invading the renal vein and the inferior vena cava (*arrows*).

involvement by tumor (Fig. 9.11), including invasion of the renal veins and the inferior vena cava (Fig. 9.12). In most large medical centers, CT is the procedure of choice for evaluating patients suspected of having urinary calculi that cause obstruction (Fig. 9.13).

MR imaging of the urinary tract is used to evaluate renal masses, the effects of pelvic neoplasms on the bladder (Fig. 9.14), and renal transplants (Fig. 9.15). The ability of MR to image in coronal and sagittal planes is also useful for evaluating the kidneys and surrounding structures. This is especially true in demonstrating invasion of the renal vein or the inferior vena cava by renal carcinoma. Most recently, MR imaging of the prostate has been performed (Fig. 9.16). Initial studies suggested the technique might be useful in differentiating benign prostatic hypertrophy from prostatic carcinoma. However, further experience showed that, like ultrasound, MR imaging did not offer that level of differentiation. Therefore, all suspicious prostate nodules found on MR images should undergo biopsy.

Renal scintigraphy is also used for assessing urinary tract abnormalities in both adults and children. Compounds of technetium-99m are used to evaluate vesicoureteral reflux, to study renal cortical morphology, to determine whether a dilated ureter or renal collecting system is obstructed, and to screen for renal artery stenosis in patients with hypertension.

Figure 9.12. Renal carcinoma with extrarenal invasion. CT image shows a mass in the left kidney (*arrows*). The mass extends beyond the confines of the kidney into the renal vein (*RV*) and into the inferior vena cava (*VC*). Compare the size of the vena cava with that of the adjacent aorta (*A*). The vena cava should be the same size. Notice the relationship of the pancreas (*P*) to the left kidney.

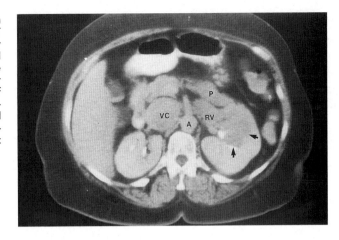

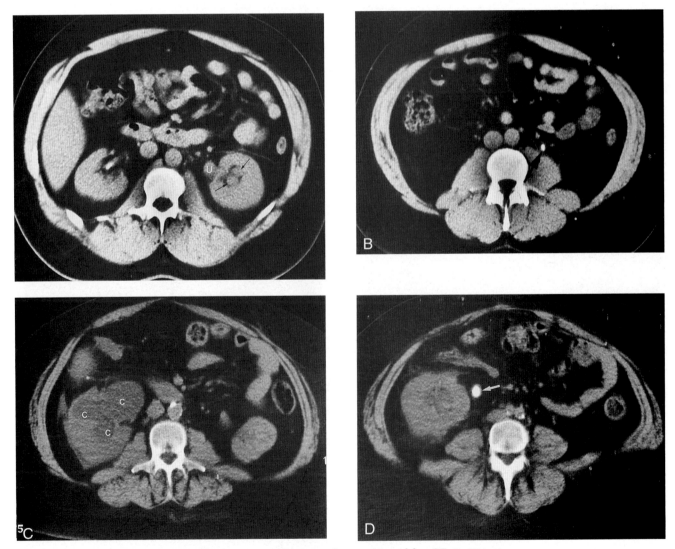

Figure 9.13. Obstructive uropathy in two patients as demonstrated by CT. A. CT image shows dilation of the ureter (*U*) as well as the calyces (*arrows*). **B.** Image more distally shows the calcified stone in the ureter (*arrow*). **C.** CT image in another patient shows massive calyceal dilation (*C*). **D.** Image more distal shows the large obstructing stone in the ureter (*arrow*). The lower pole of the kidney is enlarged.

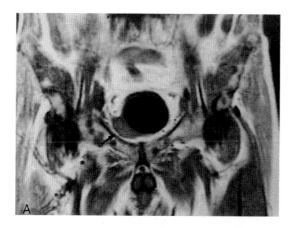

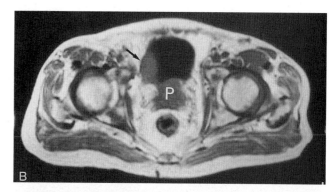

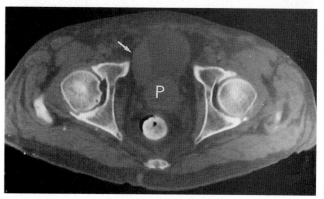

Figure 9.14. Prostatic carcinoma. A. Coronal T1-weighted magnetic resonance (MR) image shows a mass (*arrow*) invading the floor of the bladder on the right side. **B.** Axial image shows the mass (*arrow*) invading the bladder floor. Notice the enlarged prostate (*P*). **C.** CT image shows identical findings (*arrow*).

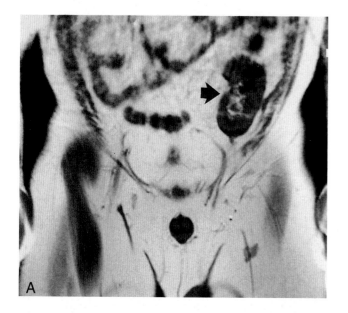

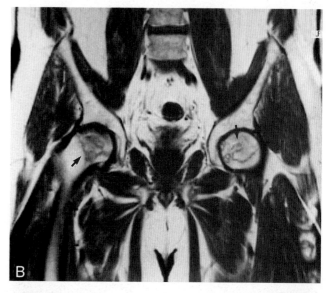

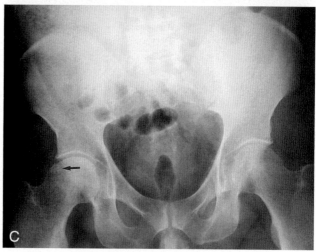

Figure 9.15. Renal transplantation with avascular necrosis of the femoral heads. A. Coronal T1-weighted MR image shows the transplanted kidney in the left iliac fossa (*arrow*). **B.** Image more posteriorly shows serpentine areas of low signal in both femoral heads (*arrows*), representing areas of avascular necrosis. **C.** Pelvic radiograph shows partial collapse of the right femoral head (*arrow*). The left is normal.

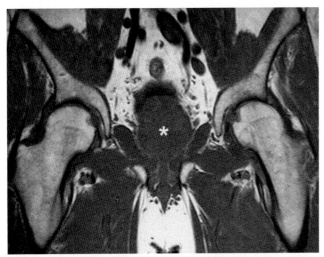
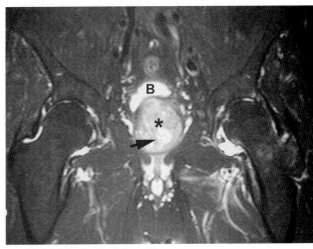

A   B

Figure 9.16.   Benign prostatic hypertrophy with nodule (*arrow*) demonstrated by MR imaging. T1-weighted **(A)** and T2-weighted **(B)** MR images show the enlarged prostate (*) pushing up on the floor of the bladder (*B*). Notice the nodule in B (*arrow*). Biopsy was necessary to determine that the nodule was benign.

ANATOMIC CONSIDERATIONS

The *kidneys* in a normal adult measure 11 to 14 cm from pole to pole. They are invested in their own fascia, with their upper poles oriented slightly medially. There may be a normal difference in size between the right and left kidneys; the left kidney is often 0.5 to 1.5 cm longer than the right.

The *collecting system* consists of three to five infundibula, each draining one or more calyces. The calyx forms a sharply defined "cup" around the papilla, which it drains (Fig. 9.17). The

Figure 9.17.   Detail view of a normal right kidney during intravenous urography. Notice the delicate cupping of the calyces (*arrows*).

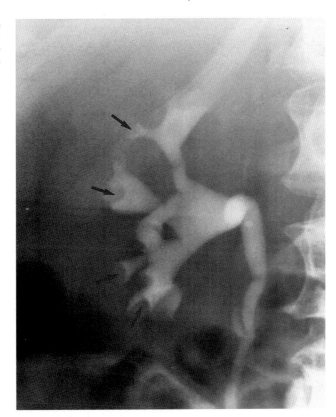

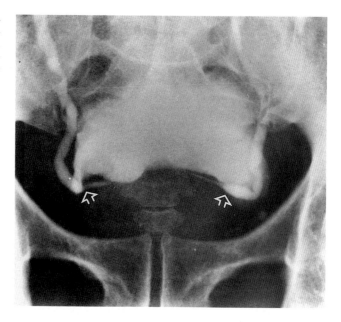

Figure 9.18. Prostatic enlargement. The floor of the bladder is elevated by the enlarged prostate. Notice the "fish hooking" of the distal ureters (*arrows*) as they enter the bladder.

calyces are easily discernible on the normal urogram. The infundibula unite to form the renal pelvis, which terminates in the ureter.

The *ureters* course down the retroperitoneal surface on either side of the vertebral column, generally in a vertical pattern, until they reach the bony pelvis, where they may make a slight lateral deviation before turning medially to enter the posterior aspect of the bladder at the trigone. The ureters are not bound down by fascia and are relatively free to move, a fact that is useful in the evaluation of retroperitoneal disease.

The *urinary bladder* should be smooth and ovoid without trabeculation or other mucosal markings. Normal variations in the shape of the bladder occasionally result in a lobular configuration.

The *prostate* lies immediately inferior to the bladder in males and, when enlarged, may indent and elevate the floor of the bladder (Fig. 9.18). The urethra courses through the prostate. The membranous portion of the male urethra between the prostatic and bulbous urethra is fixed in the urogenital diaphragm. This area is subject to laceration from trauma to the pelvis.

The *vascular supply* to the kidney generally consists of a single pair of renal arteries. However, occasionally two or more arteries to each kidney are present. A single renal vein drains each kidney. On the right, the vein drains directly into the inferior vena cava without anastomosis with other veins. On the left, the renal vein communicates with the left adrenal and gonadal veins. These two communications form a collateral pathway for blood to drain the kidney in the event of renal vein thrombosis. Collateral channels in the arterial system may enlarge when there are stenotic lesions of the renal artery. The foremost of these is the ureteric artery.

PATHOLOGIC CONSIDERATIONS

As previously mentioned, the so-called physiologic abnormalities uniformly result in a decrease or absence of renal function. The only morphologic change that may be discerned is a decrease in the size of the kidneys. This discussion concentrates on diseases that produce recognizable morphologic abnormalities, including the following:

- Congenital abnormalities
- Obstructive lesions
- Infections
- Masses—cysts and tumors

- Vascular lesions
- Traumatic lesions
- Extrinsic compression
- Renal transplantation

This list is not comprehensive. You should understand that many entities fall into a "crossover" category. For example, obstruction of the ureteropelvic junction is considered the most common congenital obstruction of the urinary tract. This entity could be categorized as both congenital and obstructive. Multicystic dysplastic kidney could be discussed with renal cystic diseases. However, the origin of this disorder is severe obstruction, occurring during embryonic life. In keeping with the philosophy of this text, the discussion that follows covers the *concepts* of each pathologic category. For details of the specific imaging findings for a particular entity, consult one of the texts listed at the end of this chapter.

Congenital Abnormalities

Congenital anomalies of the urinary tract occur frequently. The complex development of the genitourinary tract in embryonic life provides many opportunities for anomalous development to occur. Anomalies may be relatively benign, such as duplication of the collecting system (Fig. 9.19) and an uncomplicated horseshoe kidney (Fig. 9.20); or they can be severe, such as posterior urethral valves with secondary megacystis, hydroureter, and hydronephrosis in a newborn male infant. Other anomalies include ectopic kidneys and ectopic ureteroceles.

Dilation of the distal end of the ureter results in formation of a *ureterocele.* Two types occur: simple and ectopic. The *simple* ureterocele results from dilation of only the distalmost end of the ureter and produces a cobra-head–like filling defect in the contrast-filled bladder (Fig. 9.21). An *ectopic* ureterocele is the masslike, dilated submucosal distal portion of an ectopic ureter, usually resulting from a duplicated collecting system (see Fig. 9.19). Ectopic ureteroceles appear as sausage-shaped filling defects in the contrast-filled bladder (Fig. 9.22). On ultrasound, they have a similar appearance.

Posterior urethral valves are considered the most common cause of urethral obstruction in male children. This abnormality obstructs the flow of urine out of the bladder and frequently results in impaired renal function in as many as one third of patients with the disorder. The disorder may be initially diagnosed with prenatal ultrasound, particularly when the obstruction is severe and results in oligohydramnios. On a VCUG or retrograde urethrogram, the classic appearance is that of dilation of the posterior urethra producing the so-called spinnaker sail sign (Fig. 9.23).

Figure 9.19. Duplication of the upper collecting system. Notice the double renal pelvis from the upper pole of each kidney and the duplicated ureter. This duplication extended to the ureterovesical junction (not shown on this film).

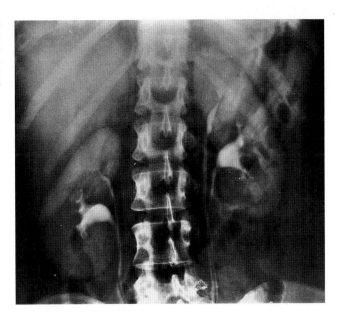

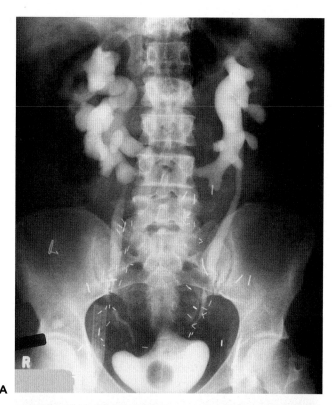

A

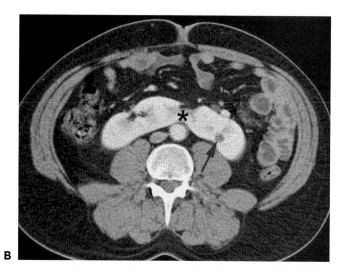

B

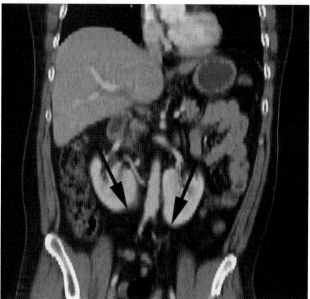

C

Figure 9.20. Horseshoe kidney. A. Intravenous urogram (IVU) shows dilation of the urinary collecting system bilaterally. Notice the alteration of orientation of both renal poles. A pair of kidneys orientated in this manner should suggest the diagnosis. **B.** CT axial image shows the contrast-enhanced isthmus (*). Notice the small renal cyst on the left (*arrow*). **C.** Coronal reconstructed image shows the kidneys oriented with their bottoms pointing medially (*arrows*).

There are numerous congenital abnormalities of position, rotation, and fusion. *Renal ectopia* is a term used to denote the abnormal position of one kidney with regard to the other. When the affected kidney is located on the other side of the abdomen (usually beneath the normal kidney), it is termed *crossed renal ectopia*. Renal malrotation is a common and not significant renal abnormality in which the renal hilus becomes directed more medially and slightly more anteriorly than normal. Ureteropelvic obstruction is the most common complication of this condition. *Horseshoe kidney* is the most common type of congenital renal fusion abnormality. The fusion occurs in the lower poles of the two kidneys across the midline, forming an isthmus that lies anterior to the aorta and inferior to the vena cava. On urograms, ultrasound, and CT

Figure 9.21. Simple ureterocele presenting as a "cobra head" filling defect in the bladder (*arrows*). The kidneys above are normal. Compare with Figure 9.22A.

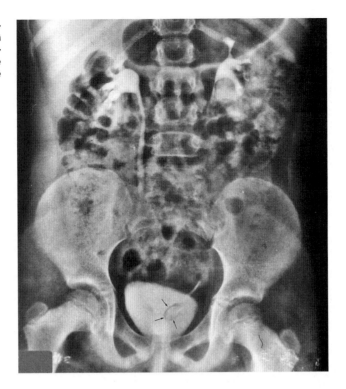

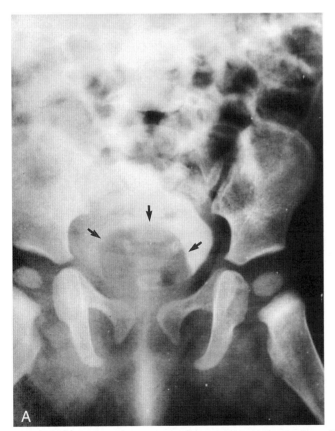

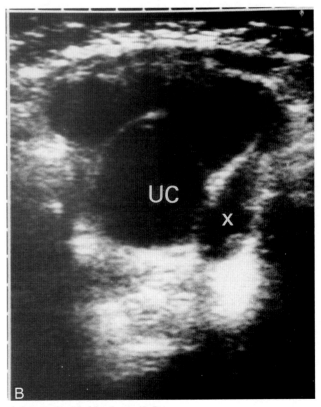

Figure 9.22. Ectopic ureterocele. A. Urogram shows a large filling defect in the bladder (*arrows*). **B.** Ultrasound image on another patient shows a large ureterocele (*UC*) as well as a dilated ureter (×) on the left.

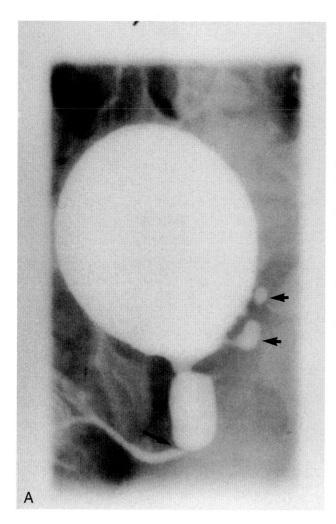

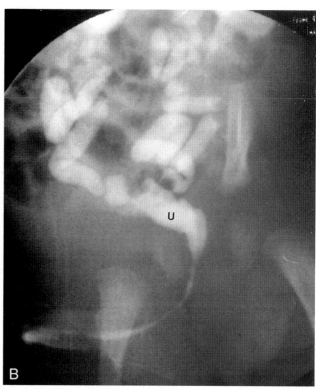

Figure 9.23.   Urinary obstruction from posterior ure-thral valves in two patients. A. Cystourethrogram shows the valve (*long arrow*), dilated proximal urethral segment, and bladder diverticula (*short arrows*). **B.** Cystourethrogram in another patient shows the dilated urethra (*U*) as well as serpentine dilation of both ureters above.

examinations, the fusion is easily recognized by the abnormal orientation of the renal collecting systems as well as by the isthmus itself (see Fig. 9.20).

For an in-depth discussion of these and other congenital disorders, consult Kirks and Griscom's *Practical Pediatric Imaging.*

Obstructive Lesions

Obstruction of the urinary tract may be either congenital or acquired. The congenital causes of obstruction were discussed previously. The acquired variety is more common and is usually the result of urinary calculi (Fig. 9.24). Other causes are tumor (Fig. 9.25) and operative manipulation. Whatever the cause, obstruction produces a series of pathophysiologic changes that result in characteristic radiographic appearances, depending on the degree of renal parenchymal destruction.

Acute obstruction results in one of two types of urographic changes: (1) initial nonopacification of the renal collecting system with subsequent delayed appearance of contrast on the abnormal side, or (2) prompt visualization, with evidence of dilation (*caliectasis*) of the collecting system (see Fig. 9.24B). CT will show a dilated ureter (see Fig. 9.24D) and frequently will show the stone (see Fig. 9.24E). Frank *hydronephrosis* usually indicates a long-standing obstruction. Frequently, when a stone is the cause of the obstruction, that stone will be demonstrated. It is occasionally necessary to obtain oblique views to be certain that any calcifications present on the abdominal radiograph are indeed within the urinary tract. Acute obstruction may also result in alternative drainage of contrast through the renal veins or lymphatics (*pyelovenous* or *pyelolymphatic transflow,* respectively; see Fig. 9.24F).

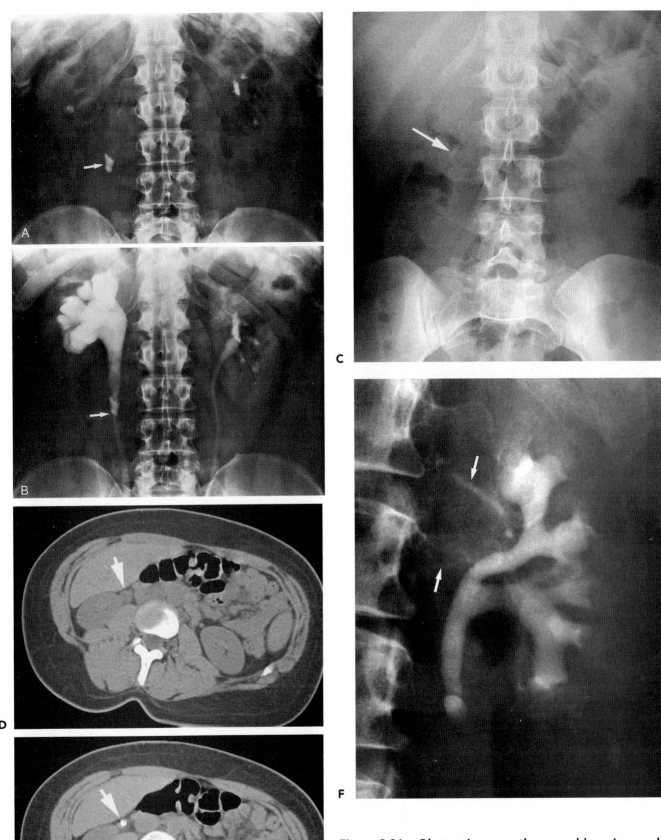

Figure 9.24. Obstructive uropathy caused by urinary calculi. A. Abdominal radiograph shows multiple calculi overlying the renal shadows. Notice the large calculus adjacent to the L3 interspace on the right (*arrow*). **B.** IVU demonstrates partial obstruction on the right secondary to the ureteral stone (*arrow*). The left kidney is not obstructed. **C.** Radiograph in another patient shows a faint calcified stone (*arrow*). **D.** CT image shows a dilated ureter on the right (*arrow*). **E.** CT image slightly inferiorly shows the stone in the ureter (*arrow*).**F.** Detail view of the left kidney in another patient shows pyelolymphatic transflow (*arrows*) as well as obstructive calyceal changes.

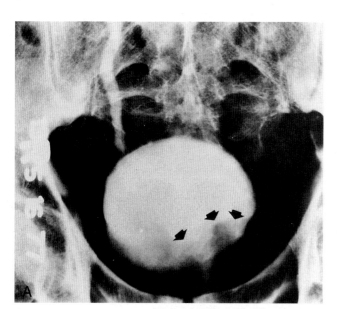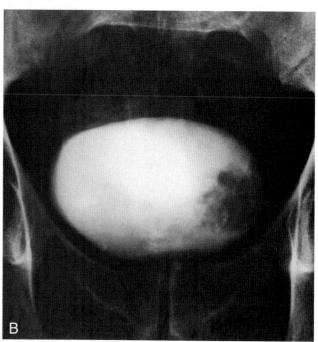

Figure 9.25.   Bladder carcinomas in two patients. A. Obstruction of the left ureter (*arrows*) is complete. The right ureter is not affected. **B.** A villous lesion is on the left.

Ultrasonography and CT are also useful techniques for diagnosing hydronephrosis (Figs. 9.26 and 9.27). Ultrasound is the procedure of choice for evaluating newborns and infants with palpable abdominal masses, because as already mentioned, many such masses are caused by urinary abnormalities.

Urinary *calculi*, the most common causes of obstruction, may be opaque or nonopaque. Populations of certain areas, such as the Southeast and Southwest United States, have a high incidence of urinary stones. Interestingly, the composition of stones varies with the locale. In the so-called stone belt of North Carolina, 85% of the urinary stones are formed of oxalate, whereas only 40% of stones among patients in New York State are of that composition.

Most stones contain a mineral deposit embedded in an inorganic matrix. This matrix has been found to be elevated in the urine of patients with hyperparathyroidism, renal infection, patients taking thiazide diuretics, and patients undergoing steroid therapy in an amount that ranges from 3 to 15 times that of normal patients.

Urinary stones may be found in the kidneys (Fig. 9.28) as well as in the ureter and the bladder (Fig. 9.29). Bladder stones are often the result of long-standing infection and/or presence of a foreign body. Large renal stones that coalesce in hydronephrotic collecting systems are called *staghorn calculi*, after their branched, antler-like appearance (Fig. 9.30).

Urinary stones must be differentiated from *nephrocalcinosis*, a pathophysiologic condition in which calcium is deposited within renal tissue. It results from an underlying disease that elevates the serum calcium level. In most instances, the calcification is limited to the distal convoluted tubules. These calcifications appear as fine, stippled deposits that should be easily differentiated from stones by their appearance and location (Fig. 9.31). There are many causes of this condition, but the most common ones include medullary sponge kidney, hyperparathyroidism, renal tubular acidosis, and milk-alkali syndrome.

Infections

Infection is a common disease of the urinary tract. It is often found as a complication of obstruction. Acute *pyelonephritis* may be difficult to recognize radiographically because of the subtle changes it produces on the collecting system. Occasionally, this condition may be detected on a radiograph if it produces a large swollen kidney. More commonly, however, the

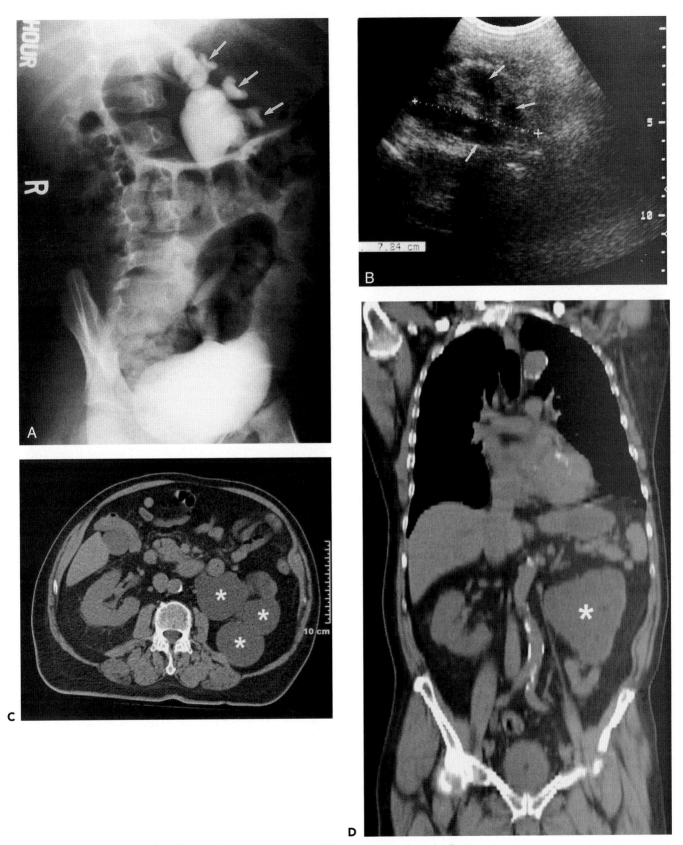

Figure 9.26. Hydronephrosis. A. Oblique image from an IVU shows a dilated renal collecting system with blunt calyces (*arrows*). **B.** Ultrasound image of the same patient shows the dilated calyces as sonolucent areas (*arrows*). **C.** Axial CT image in another patient shows three massively dilated calyces (*) in the left kidney. **D.** Coronal CT reconstructed image shows the hydronephrotic mass (*) on the left.

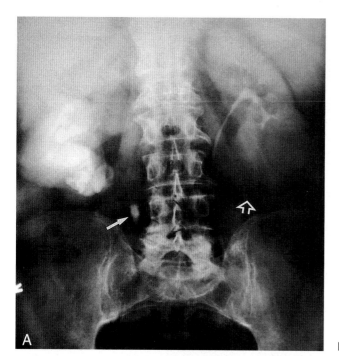

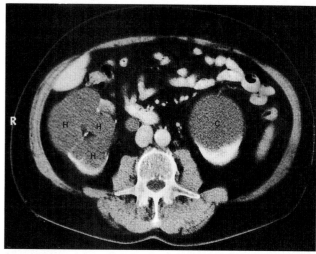

Figure 9.27. Hydronephrosis of the right kidney. A. Urogram shows a large ureteral stone on the right (*solid arrow*). Notice the hydronephrotic changes in the right kidney. The left kidney shows a normal collecting system. A large soft tissue mass (*open arrow*) projects from the lower pole. **B.** CT image shows the hydronephrotic collecting system (*H*) on the right. The mass on the left is a renal cyst (*C*).

effects of chronic pyelonephritis are encountered. These include marked cortical irregularity, focal cortical scarring, clubbed irregular calyces, and loss of renal volume (Fig. 9.32). Other complications of infections in the collecting system include the development of a renal carbuncle or abscess (Fig. 9.33), pyonephrosis, emphysematous changes in diabetics (Fig. 9.34), and papillary necrosis. The latter condition results from anoxia of the renal papilla, causing

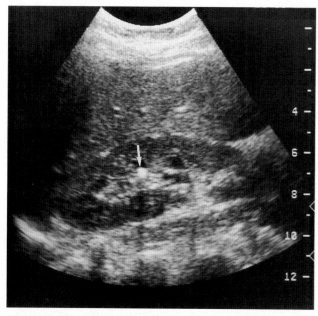

Figure 9.28. Ultrasound image demonstrating a renal calculus (*arrow*). Notice the shadowing below the stone.

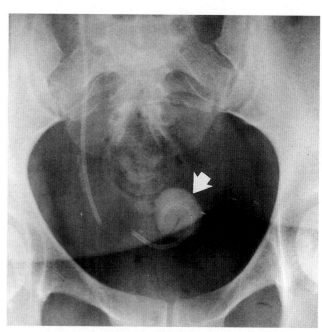

Figure 9.29. Bladder calculus (*arrow*) surrounding the broken end of a urinary stent.

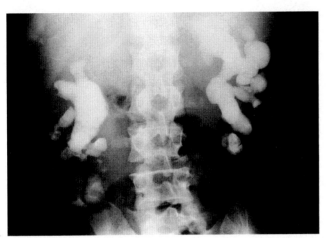

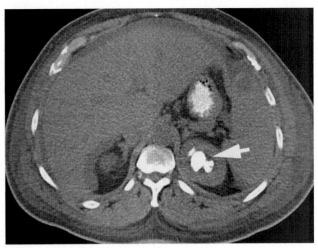

Figure 9.30.   Staghorn calculi. A. Radiograph shows bilateral staghorn calculi. **B.** CT image of another patient shows the dense central calcification in the left kidney (*arrow*). No intravenous contrast was injected in either patient.

sloughing of that papilla. Characteristic findings include a filling defect in a calyx, a ring of contrast surrounding a filling defect, and an abnormal blunted calyx (Fig. 9.35). Often excretion of the contrast medium by the abnormal kidney is poor.

Renal tuberculosis is occurring more commonly today, making its deadly comeback in patients with acquired immune deficiency syndrome (AIDS). Tuberculosis of the kidney in its early stages may produce nonspecific changes such as papillary necrosis. With progression of the disease, the more characteristic findings of stricture of an infundibulum, calyceal amputation, and cavitation may occur. Tuberculosis also causes ureteral strictures. A combination of renal and ureteral abnormalities such as strictures should suggest the diagnosis. The end stage of renal tuberculosis is a small, shrunken, nonfunctioning kidney that often contains calcific debris (*"putty kidney"*; Fig. 9.36).

Changes of chronic inflammation of the bladder (*cystitis*) include thickening and irregularity of the wall secondary to muscular and mucosal hypertrophy. Obstructive disease and ureterovesical reflux in association with chronic cystitis may be evaluated by diuretic renal scintigraphy and radionuclide voiding cystourethrography.

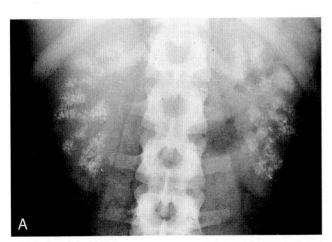

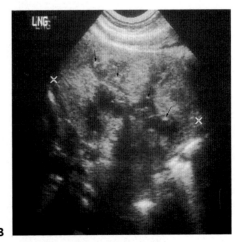

Figure 9.31.   Nephrocalcinosis. A. Radiograph shows fine deposition of calcium within the renal pyramids of both kidneys. **B.** Ultrasound image shows multiple small calcifications (*arrows*). This is a reversible condition.

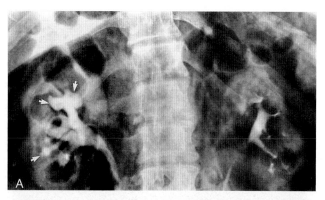 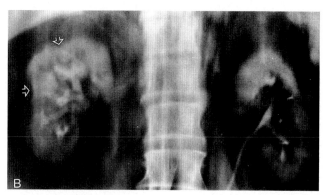

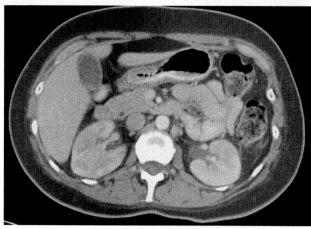

C

Figure 9.32.   Pyelonephritis. A. Chronic pyelonephritis. IVU shows blunting and clubbing of the calyces in the right kidney (*arrows*). The left kidney is normal. **B.** Nephrotomogram in the same patient shows marked cortical irregularity (*arrows*). **C.** CT image of another patient with acute pyelonephritis shows enlargement of the right kidney and loss of the normal architectural landmarks.

Figure 9.33.   Renal gas infection. Detail view of the right kidney in a diabetic patient reveals gas outlining the collecting system of the upper pole of the kidney.

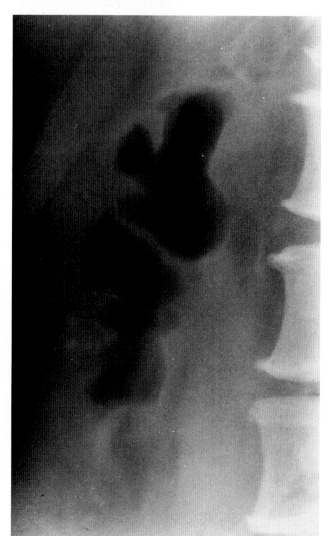

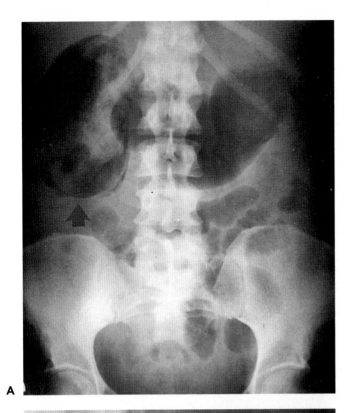

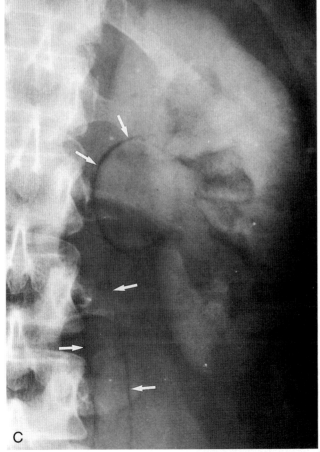

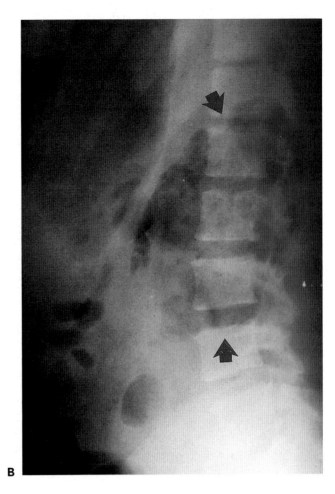

Figure 9.34. Emphysematous pyelonephritis in two diabetic patients. A. Frontal radiograph shows a large reniform gas collection on the right (*arrow*). **B.** Lateral view shows the gas collection (*arrows*) to be located posteriorly. **C.** Detail view of the left kidney of another patient shows gas outlining the renal pelvis and the ureter (*arrows*).

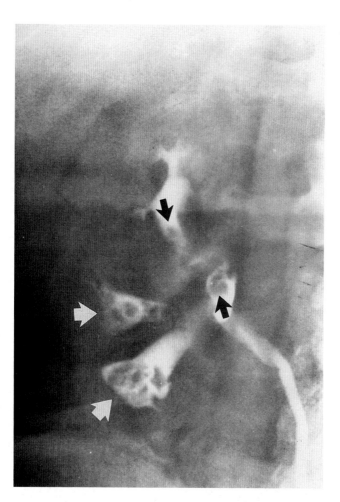

Figure 9.35. Renal papillary necrosis. Multiple filling defects (*arrows*) represent sloughed papillae within the collecting system.

Masses—Cysts and Tumors

Masses in or around the kidneys represent either cysts, tumors, or inflammatory lesions. Filling defects elsewhere in the urinary tract generally are tumors. The manner in which you encounter renal masses depends on the initial type of imaging examination performed. Some masses may be found on an abdominal radiograph; others on an IVU or abdominal CT scan. In many instances, the mass may be an incidental finding on a CT performed for another purpose (abdominal trauma, suspected appendicitis, etc.). The imaging principles for differentiating cystic from solid masses, however, remain the same no matter what the initial imaging study.

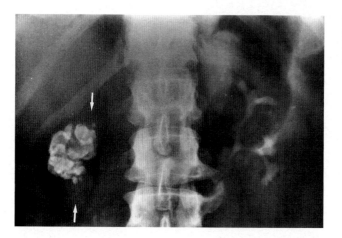

Figure 9.36. Renal tuberculosis. A small nonfunctioning right kidney containing calcific debris ("putty kidney") is present (*arrows*).

Once a *renal mass* is detected, the next logical step is an ultrasound examination to determine whether the mass is cystic or solid (Fig. 9.37). However, if the patient has hematuria, a CT examination should be performed. In some instances in which the mass was discovered on a CT, the differentiation may be obvious.

Renal cysts are extremely common in older patients and are found in a high percentage of autopsies. They are frequently incidental findings on abdominal CT scans. The CT appearance of a benign renal cyst includes a homogenous, smooth, rounded appearance of uniform radiographic density with a low CT value. Cysts do not enhance after intravenous injection of contrast material (Fig. 9.38). Renal cysts appear as bulges along the cortical margin (Fig. 9.39) or as rounded absent portions of the renal parenchyma. Frequently, a thin, beaklike collection of contrast material representing compressed parenchyma may be seen along the margin (see Fig. 9.39). A cyst may also displace the intrarenal collecting system.

A solid *renal tumor* (in either an adult or child), on the other hand, has a considerably different imaging appearance. On an ultrasound examination, the mass appears as a solid lesion with many internal echoes (Fig. 9.40A). This is contrary to the echo-free picture found in a simple renal cyst (see Fig. 9.37A, B).

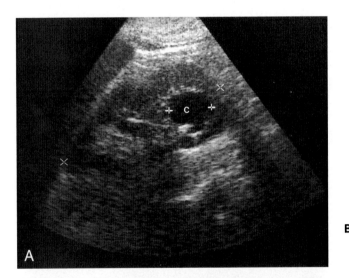

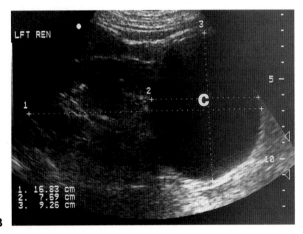

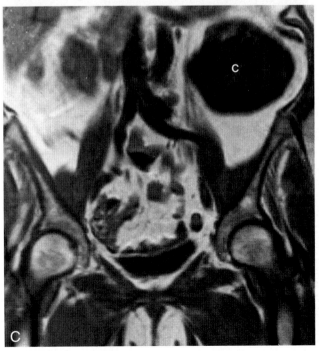

Figure 9.37.   Renal cysts. A. Longitudinal ultrasound scan shows the sonolucent cyst (*C*) with increased through transmission beneath. There are no internal echoes in the cyst. Compare with Figure 9.39A. **B.** (This is the same patient as in Fig. 9.27.) Large cyst (*C*) of the lower pole of the left kidney. Notice the measurements. **C.** T1-weighted MR image of the same cyst (*C*) shows it to have uniform low signal.

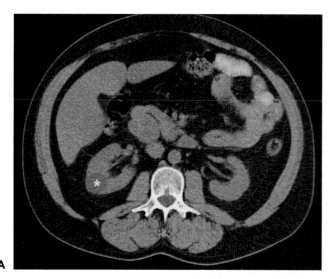
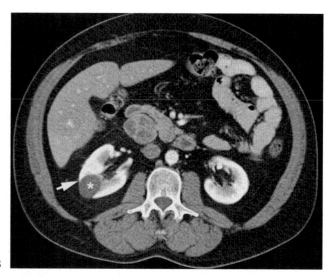

Figure 9.38. Renal cyst, CT appearance. A. Unenhanced scan shows a cyst (*) in the posterior aspect of the right kidney. **B.** After intravenous contrast injection, the cyst (*) is well defined without evidence of enhancement. Notice the beaklike appearance on the right (*arrow*).

CT has contributed greatly to the differentiation between renal cyst and tumor. On an unenhanced study, distortion of the renal architecture may be apparent (see Fig. 9.40B). When intravenous contrast material is injected, the lesion becomes denser, indicating that it is hypervascular, a finding common to solid renal tumors, especially *hypernephroma*. This is contrary to the appearance of a cyst (see Fig. 9.38). Furthermore, on a CT image, there may be evidence of extrarenal invasion by a large tumor (see Figs. 9.11 and 9.12).

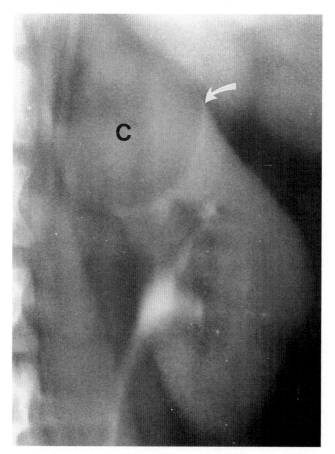

Figure 9.39. Renal cyst. The cyst (*C*) produces a bulge along the upper pole of the kidney. Notice the beaklike appearance along the parenchymal margin of the cyst (*arrow*).

Figure 9.40.   Renal carcinoma.
A. Longitudinal ultrasound shows gross distortion of the renal outline with many internal echoes anteriorly. A relatively sonolucent posterior portion represents necrotic tissue. **B.** CT scan shows enlargement of the right kidney with a large mass posteriorly (*open arrows*). Notice the area of necrosis (*N*) in the mass. The normal portion of the kidney is seen anteriorly (*solid arrow*).

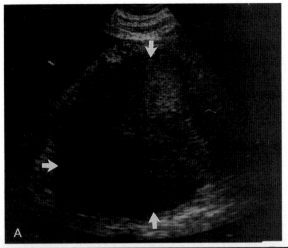

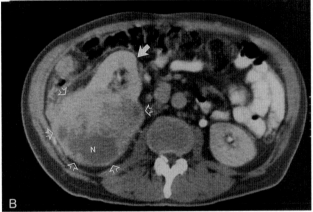

Cyst puncture is a procedure used for evaluating renal masses. It is performed under ultrasonic or CT guidance. Whatever the method, the purpose of cyst puncture is to aspirate cyst content, which is then sent for cytologic and chemical analysis. If the fluid is clear or straw colored, has a specific gravity of urine, and is free of cellular debris containing malignant cells, you may be assured you are dealing with a benign cyst. A cystic malignancy, on the other hand, generally has a hemorrhagic aspirate that contains malignant cells and often other debris and has a high fat content.

Renal cysts and solid tumors appear similar on MR imaging as on CT. Most renal cysts have the typical appearance of fluid—that is, a uniform low signal on a T1-weighted image that is intensely bright on a T2-weighted image. A solid tumor, on the other hand, has a mixed low signal at T1 that typically increases at T2. The inhomogeneous makeup of renal tumors—namely, calcification or necrosis within them—is responsible for the mottling. An MR image may also show invasion of the renal veins or inferior vena cava (Fig. 9.41). Table 9.1 lists the differential imaging features in the diagnosis of renal cysts versus renal tumors.

Simple renal cysts in children are unusual but not unheard of. Their imaging appearances are identical to those found in adults. There are two forms of *polycystic disease* in children. The first is the autosomal recessive type (Potter type 1) and occurs with no previous familial history of renal disease. The second form is the autosomal dominant type (Potter type 2) and is also known as adult polycystic disease of the kidneys and liver, in which there may be a familial history. Both forms are characterized by multiple renal and hepatic cysts of varying sizes (Figs. 9.42 and 9.43). In the late stages of the disease, little or no renal function remains.

Two types of solid tumors affect children: Wilms tumor and neuroblastoma. *Wilms tumor,* or *nephroblastoma,* is a highly malignant neoplasm of embryonic origin that contains epithelial, blastemal, and stromal elements. This tumor accounts for approximately 10% of childhood malignancies, similar to neuroblastma. It is the most common *solid* abdominal mass of childhood and occurs predominantly between the ages of 1 and 5 years. The most common

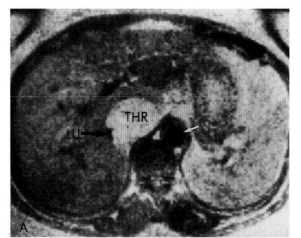

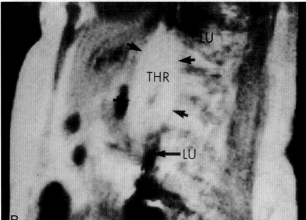

Figure 9.41. Renal carcinoma with extrarenal invasion. (This is the same patient as in Fig. 9.12.) **A.** T2-weighted axial MR image demonstrates a large tumor thrombus (*THR*) within the inferior vena cava. The lumen of the cava (*LU*) is markedly narrowed. Compare the size of the cava with the adjacent aorta (*white arrow*). **B.** T2-weighted parasagittal image shows the tumor thrombus (*THR*) within the enlarged inferior vena cava (*arrows*). Notice the patent lumen (*LU*) above and below the thrombus.

TABLE 9.1

IMAGING CRITERIA IN DIFFERENTIATING RENAL CYST AND RENAL CELL CARCINOMA

Examination	Renal Cyst	Renal Cell Carcinoma
Ultrasound	Interior sonolucent (no internal echoes)	Many internal echoes
	Well-defined border	Less well-defined border
Computed tomography	Smooth, well-defined border	Less well-defined border
	Density low	May be isodense (same as kidney)
	Avascular on contrast enhancement	Usually enhances, may show areas of necrosis
	No invasion of perirenal tissues	Invasion of perirenal tissue
Cyst puncture	Clear, straw-colored fluid	Cloudy or hemorrhagic fluid
	No cellular debris, negative cytologic evidence	Cellular debris, positive cytologic evidence
Magnetic resonance	Uniform low signal at T1, bright at T2	Mottled low signal at T1
		Mottled increase in signal at T2
Angiography	Avascular mass	Usually vascular
	No neovascularity	Neovascularity
	Vessels stretched and displaced	Irregular, nonuniform, serpentine; pooling of contrast medium; early venous filling; aneurysm-like dilations
	Vasoconstriction with epinephrine injection	No responce to epinephrine injection

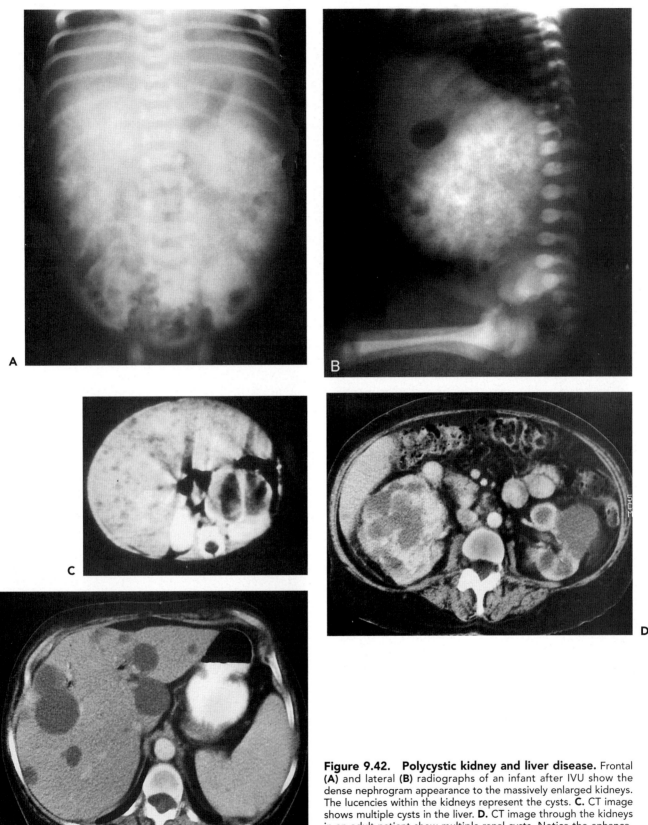

Figure 9.42.   Polycystic kidney and liver disease. Frontal
(**A**) and lateral (**B**) radiographs of an infant after IVU show the
dense nephrogram appearance to the massively enlarged kidneys.
The lucencies within the kidneys represent the cysts. **C.** CT image
shows multiple cysts in the liver. **D.** CT image through the kidneys
in an adult patient show multiple renal cysts. Notice the enhancement of the surrounding renal parenchyma after intravenous contrast administration. **E.** Image through the liver in the same patient
shows multiple cysts.

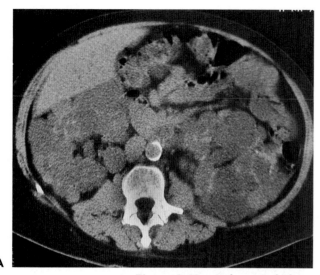

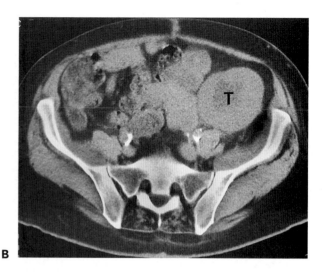

Figure 9.43. Polycystic kidney disease with renal failure. A. CT image shows multiple renal cysts. **B.** CT image through the pelvis shows a transplanted kidney (*T*).

clinical presentation is as an asymptomatic abdominal mass. It may be bilateral in as many as 5% of cases and unilateral but multicentric in approximately 7%.

From an imaging standpoint, Wilms tumor resembles other large renal tumors. The abdominal radiograph frequently shows a large soft tissue mass that displaces bowel. Calcification may be in the mass, but to a lesser degree than with neuroblastoma. An IVU would reveal distortion and stretching of the renal collecting system (Fig. 9.44) and, on

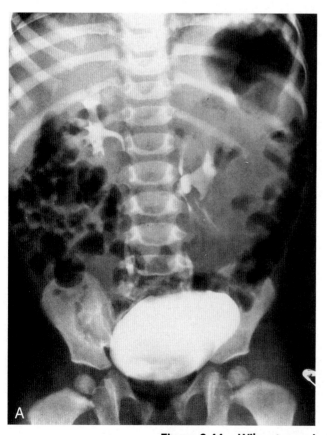

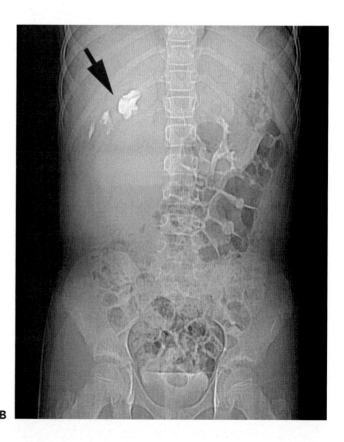

Figure 9.44. Wilms tumor in two patients. A. IVU shows a mass in the left kidney distorting the renal architecture. **B.** Digital abdominal scout view for a CT scan on another patient shows upward displacement of the contrast in the right kidney (*arrow*). The abdomen appears to be filled with a mass.

occasion, obstruction at the ureteropelvic junction. Ultrasound would show a large tumor of increased echogenicity with many cystic areas that may represent hemorrhage. CT is the procedure of choice to determine the extent of the mass and determine the degree of local or adjacent spread (Fig. 9.45). Typically, intravenous contrast results in inhomogeneous enhancement caused by the necrosis that frequently occurs within the tumor. The typical Wilms tumor shows a distinctive "beak" at the tumor–kidney interface, indicating its intrarenal origin. This serves to differentiate Wilms tumor from neuroblastoma, which originates outside the kidney. In many children's hospitals, MR is replacing CT as the imaging modality of choice because it can show evidence of vascular invasion.

Neuroblastoma is a malignant tumor of primitive neural crest cells (neuroblasts). It also accounts for approximately 10% of childhood neoplasms and is considered second only to Wilms tumor in incidence in the abdomen. It may arise anywhere along the sympathetic chain or in the adrenal medulla. It thus can involve not only the abdomen but also the thorax and neck. Metastases to lungs, bones, and the liver occur early in the disease. Neuroblastoma usually presents either as an abdominal mass or, after metastases, produce symptoms elsewhere.

Radionuclide imaging with I-123 metaiodobenzylguanidine (MIBG) is used routinely for initial staging of neuroblastoma as well as restaging after chemotherapy. Once the disease has been diagnosed, MIBG imaging is extremely helpful in assessment, because the radioisotope is specific for malignancies of neuroendocrine origin. In current practice, PET studies are also being investigated for use in imaging of neuroblastoma.

Other imaging findings are influenced by the tendency of this tumor to undergo necrosis and calcification. Abdominal radiographs or urograms frequently will show a large, calcified mass displacing the viscera (Fig. 9.46) in at least 50% of patients. Once calcifications appear on an abdominal radiograph, CT (Fig. 9.47) or MR (Fig. 9.48) is the preferred imaging procedure to be performed next. Either examination will show a large inhomogeneous mass, usually arising from the retroperitoneal paraspinal region frequently showing calcifications. The "beak" sign seen in Wilms tumors is not present because the mass began in the extrarenal tissues. There may be evidence of metastatic disease to the liver, regional lymph nodes, vertebrae, or other kidney.

Tumors of the adrenal glands may be primary adenomas, adenocarcinomas, or metastases. Metastatic lesions are more common and most frequently arise from lung carcinomas. CT is the imaging procedure of choice to demonstrate these lesions and typically shows an irregular mass of varying size involving the adrenal (Fig. 9.49).

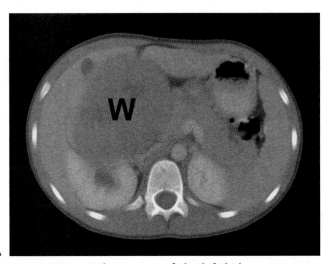
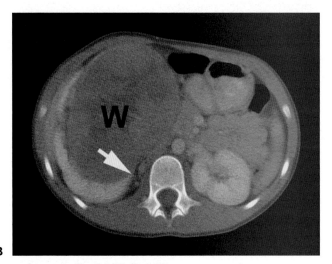

A   B

Figure 9.45.   Wilms tumor of the left kidney. (This is the same patient as in Fig. 9.44B). Two CT images show the large right renal mass (*W*). Notice the "beak" sign at the junction of the tumor with normal kidney in B (*arrow*).

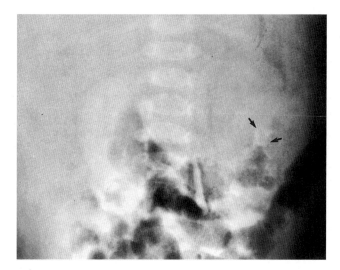

Figure 9.46. Neuroblastoma. IVU shows a suprarenal mass displacing the left kidney downward. There are scattered calcifications in the mass (*arrows*).

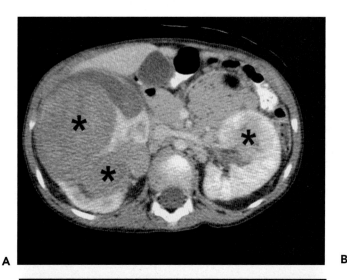

A

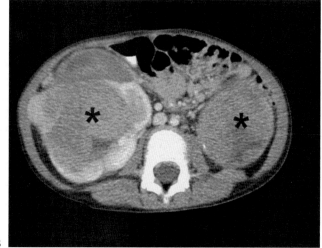

B

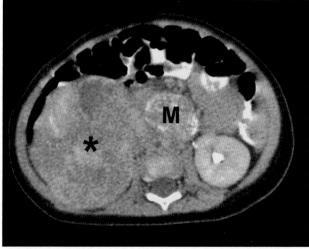

C

Figure 9.47. Neuroblastoma involving both kidneys. A and B. CT images show multilobular masses in both kidneys (*). Notice the absence of a "beak" sign. **C.** Slightly lower are nodal metastases (*M*) in addition to the left renal mass (*).

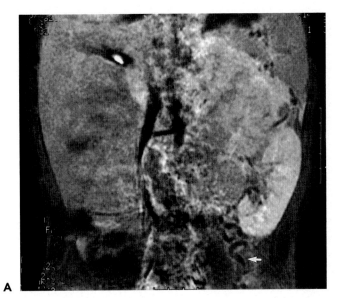

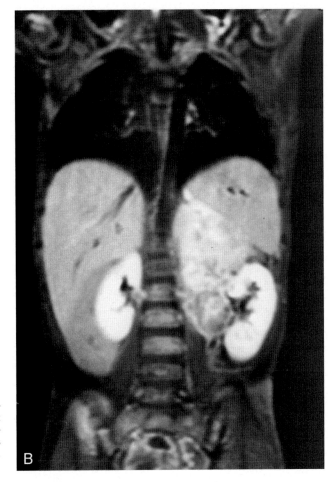

Figure 9.48. Neuroblastoma demonstrated on MR examination. A. Coronal T1-weighted image shows a large mass on the left displacing the kidney laterally. Notice the serpentine dilatation of the ureteral vein (*arrow*). **B.** Coronal T1-weighted image after intravenous enhancement with gadolinium shows the vascular nature of the tumor. Notice how brightly the kidneys enhance.

Vascular Lesions

The most common renal vascular lesion you will encounter is occlusive disease of the renal arteries. In most instances, this will be discovered in patients you are evaluating for hypertension. The most common cause of renal artery stenosis is the atherosclerotic plaque that most commonly occurs near the origin of the vessel. However, intrinsic diseases of the renal arteries, such as fibromuscular dysplasia, and a whole spectrum of other stenosing abnormalities, may result in renovascular hypertension.

An estimated 1% to 4% of hypertensive patients have renovascular hypertension. The evaluation of the hypertensive patient has undergone tremendous evolution over the past few years. Newer technical developments in Doppler ultrasound and MR angiography now make it easier to identify the patient with a curable renovascular lesion among those patients with essential hypertension. The primary diagnostic tool for imaging patients with suspected renovascular hypertension is renal artery Doppler ultrasound (Fig. 9.50). This noninvasive technique can rapidly determine if there is an obstruction to renal blood flow and identify patients needing further imaging by angiography. Nuclear imaging may also be used as the initial screening study. Both studies have a high degree of sensitivity and specificity in identifying patients who need renal angiography. Patients with severe (malignant) hypertension are usually studied by angiography, combined with renal vein renin sampling as an initial study. Furthermore, once a renal stenotic lesion is identified, it may be possible to dilate the abnormal vessel through transluminal angioplasty.

The radionuclide renogram uses the chelate technetium-99m diethylenetriamine pentaacetic acid. Studies are obtained before and after administration of an angiotensin-converting enzyme (ACE) inhibitor such as captopril (orally) or enalaprilat (intravenously). These

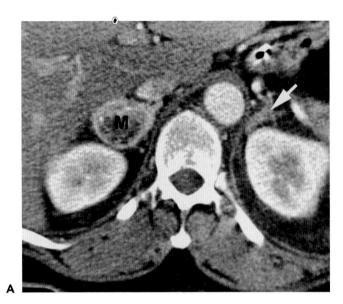

A

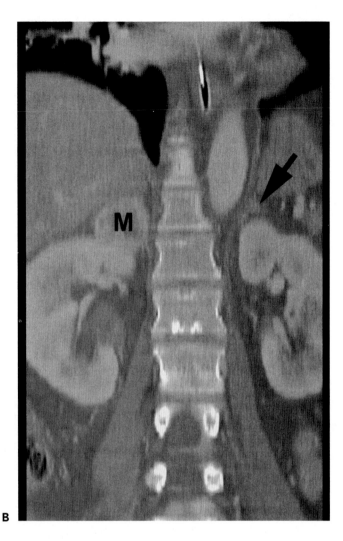

B

Figure 9.49. Metastatic lesion to the right adrenal.
Axial **(A)** and coronal **(B)** reconstructed CT images show the mass
on the right (*M*) and the normal adrenal on the left (*arrows*).

drugs enhance the discrepancy in renal uptake and excretion between the normal and abnormal kidney in patients with unilateral renal artery stenosis.

In the typical radionuclide renogram, the isotopes are rapidly injected intravenously after a scintillation camera with computer-defined regions of interest has been placed over each kidney to allow for comparison. Computer-acquired data generate the renogram curves and enhance the findings. The normal curve has three phases (Fig. 9.51): a *vascular phase* with a rapid slope; a *secretory or functional phase,* usually 2.5 to 4.5 minutes; and an *excretory phase,* during which the labeled material is excreted. Generally, a plateau is reached in 20 minutes. If the initial study is normal or near normal, the ACE inhibitor is administered to the patient and the

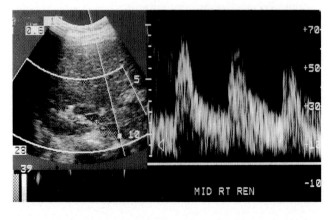

Figure 9.50. Normal Doppler examination of the right renal artery demonstrating low-resistance waveform and peak systolic velocity of 70 cm/sec.

Figure 9.51. Normal radioiso-tope renogram. (*1*) Vascular phase. (*2*) Secretory or functional phase. (*3*) Excretory phase. The graph for each kidney superimposes.

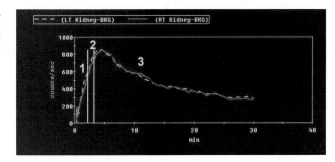

isotope study is repeated after reinjection of the radionuclides. A positive study shows prolongation of the second phase (Fig. 9.52). Other criteria include delayed peaking of counts over a kidney, delayed drainage from a kidney, and differences in renal size.

Traumatic Lesions

Trauma to the urinary tract is a common complication of major trauma to the abdomen and pelvis. The proximity of the kidneys to the twelfth ribs and to the lumbar vertebral column in an area of maximal motion often results in renal damage. Although the psoas muscles and perirenal fat provide some cushioning effect, this is insufficient to prevent serious injury as a result of major abdominal trauma. Similarly, the urinary bladder and male urethra are frequently injured as a result of fractures of the pelvis. The proximity of those structures to the pubic bones makes them particularly vulnerable to shearing injuries or puncture by a shard of displaced bone. One of the purposes of the abdominal CT examination in trauma patients is to determine whether the patient has two functioning kidneys, in addition to reveal visceral injuries.

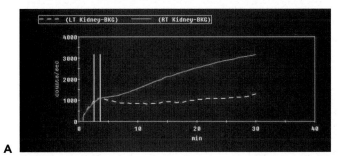

A

Figure 9.52. Renovascular hypertension caused by stenosis of the renal arteries. A. Abnormal radioisotope renogram shows poor function in the right kidney (*solid line*) and no function on the left (*broken line*). **B.** MR angiogram shows stenosis in both renal arteries (*arrowheads*). The left is more severely involved than the right, reflecting the changes in the renogram. No intravenous contrast was used for this examination.

B

Injury to the urinary tract may result from various causes. These include blunt trauma from a direct blow; penetrating injuries by a bone fragment, a foreign object (e.g., a bullet or knife), instrumentation, or a biopsy; or pathologic rupture or fracture of a diseased kidney.

Trauma to the urinary tract may be very slight, such as a renal contusion, or catastrophic, such as a shattered kidney (Fig. 9.53) or ruptured bladder (Fig. 9.54). As previously mentioned, these conditions occur as a result of major trauma to the abdomen and pelvis. Urethrocystography and CT are the preferred methods of evaluating bladder and urethral injury and renal trauma, respectively.

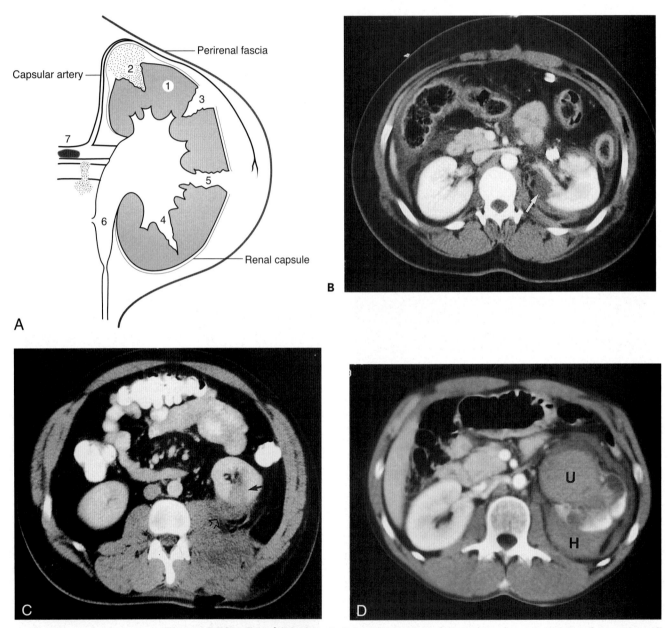

Figure 9.53.   Renal injuries. A. Drawing of various forms of renal trauma: (*1*) Renal contusion. (*2*) Laceration with intracapsular hematoma (notice the stretching of the capsular artery). (*3*) Laceration extending across the renal capsule. (*4*) Internal laceration communicating with the collecting system. (*5*) Renal fracture ("shattered kidney"). (*6*) Pelvic rupture, usually in patients with ureteropelvic obstructing lesions. (*7*) Vascular pedicle injury. Injuries 3 and 5 generally result in enlargement of the renal outline with extensive hemorrhage into the perirenal spaces. **B.** CT image shows a contusion of the left kidney manifest as an area of low density (*arrow*). **C.** Renal laceration on the left (*solid arrow*) from a stab wound to the left flank. The site of the stab wound is visible posteriorly. Notice the small perirenal hematoma (*open arrow*). **D.** Massive left renal injury with perinephric hematoma (*H*) and large peripelvic urinoma (*U*). There is extravasated contrast between the hematoma and the urinoma. (*continued on page 349*)

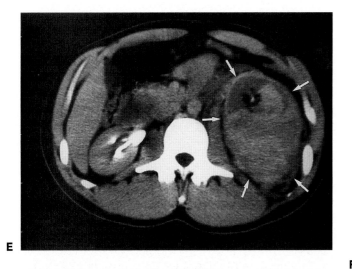

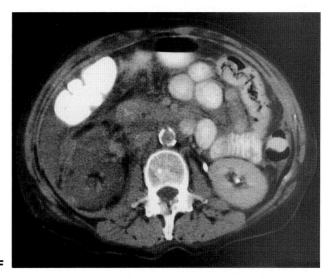

E

F

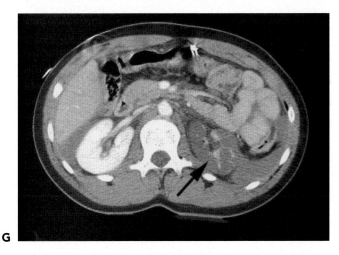

G

Figure 9.53. *(continued)* **E.** Shattered kidney. There is enlargement of the left renal outline (*arrows*). Even though this is an enhanced scan, no renal function is evident. However, areas of enhancement within the renal capsule represent fragments of renal tissue. **F.** Nonfunctioning right kidney caused by renal vein thrombosis secondary to trauma. The left kidney functions normally on this contrast-enhanced study. **G.** Nonfunctioning left kidney (*arrow*) caused by renal artery thrombosis. The dense streaks in the left kidney are the result of contrast that refluxed through the renal vein.

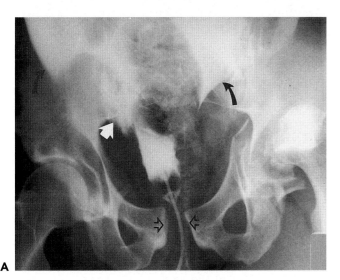

A

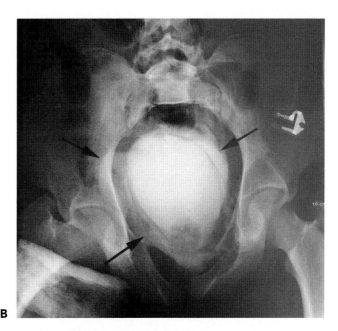

B

Figure 9.54. Pelvic fractures with bladder rupture. A. The patient has suffered a severe pelvic injury with dysraphism of the pubic symphysis (*open arrows*) and a comminuted fracture of the left acetabulum with hip dislocation. This cystogram demonstrates extraperitoneal (*white arrow*) as well as intraperitoneal (*curved arrows*) extravasation of contrast from the ruptured bladder. **B.** Another patient with disruption of the pubic symphysis and fractures of the left pubic arches. Contrast is seen outside the bladder (*arrows*).

Extrinsic Compression

Diseases in organs adjacent to the urinary tract often produce morphologic alterations on it. These include displacement of a kidney by a suprarenal mass, displacement of a ureter by enlarged lymph nodes, compression of a ureter with obstructive uropathy secondary to abdominal or pelvic masses, compression of the bladder by pelvic masses, and elevation of the bladder floor by an enlarged prostate (see Fig. 9.18). Abdominal CT scanning and ultrasound are the preferred methods of diagnostic imaging (Fig. 9.55).

Renal Transplantation

Renal transplantation is now a common surgical procedure in most large medical centers. You will undoubtedly treat many of these patients throughout your medical career. Imaging studies are used to evaluate the transplanted kidneys, determine their function (Fig. 9.56), search for signs of rejection, assess the blood supply (Fig. 9.57), and look for secondary complications such as avascular necrosis of bone (see Fig. 9.15).

Three critical conditions may affect the function of a transplanted kidney. The first is the rejection process, which will ultimately lead to a decrease in or absence of function in the transplanted kidney. Obstruction at the site of ureteric reanastomosis is a second cause of decreased function. Third, a vascular abnormality, usually renal artery stenosis, at the graft site (see Fig. 9.57) may adversely affect the function of the transplanted organ. Major imaging improvements in diagnosing stenosis of the vessels use Doppler ultrasound and MR angiography. The spectrum of diagnostic examinations performed on normal kidneys is also performed on renal transplants.

Vesicoureteral Reflux

Vesicoureteral reflux is often found in patients (usually children) being studied for recurrent urinary tract infections. It remains a controversial topic despite the changes that have occurred in its diagnosis and management over the past decades. The reflux generally occurs during voiding and thus may be demonstrated at that time by either the VCUG or radionuclide cystogram. The latter study has a lower radiation dose and is preferred for screening children whose siblings have a history of reflux as well as for follow-up of patients with known disease. Unrecognized and untreated vesicoureteral reflux may result in renal medullary scarring.

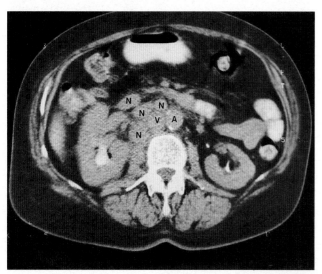
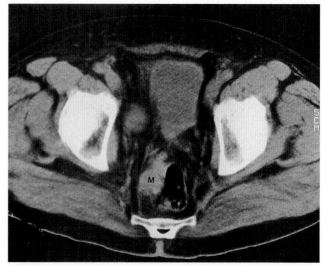

A   **B**

Figure 9.55.   Retroperitoneal tumors. A. Enlarged lymph nodes in a patient with lymphoma. CT image shows multiple enlarged lymph nodes (*N*) in the vicinity of the right renal pelvis. Notice the vena cava (*V*) and abdominal aorta (*A*). **B.** Perirectal tumor (*M*) recurrence from prostate carcinoma.

Figure 9.56. Normal renal transplant in the left iliac fossa.

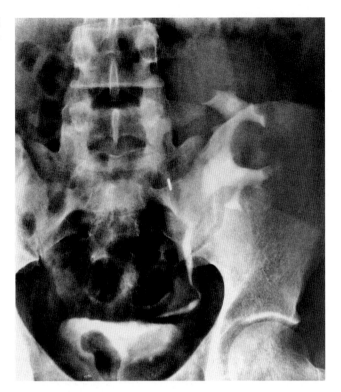

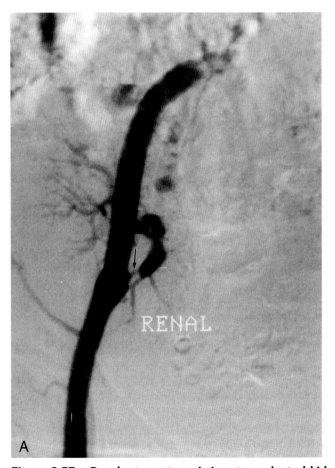

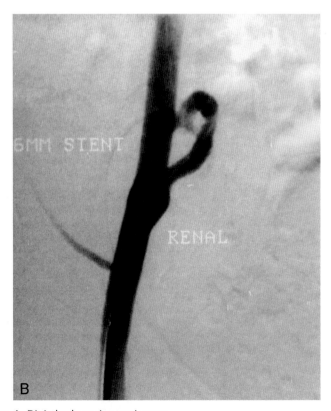

Figure 9.57.   Renal artery stenosis in a transplanted kidney. A. Digital subtraction angiogram shows stenosis of the transplanted renal artery (*arrow*). **B.** After placement of a stent, the lumen of the transplanted artery is restored.

SUMMARY AND KEY POINTS

- The urinary tract is an area of the body where many different imaging procedures are used.
- Intravenous urography, once the mainstay of uroradiology, has been replaced by CT and ultrasound in the United States. MR imaging is a useful adjunct.
- The diagnostic accuracy of these studies when used in combinations is exceedingly high.
- The various types of pathologic abnormalities you will encounter in a daily practice have been discussed, along with their differential diagnoses.
- Many urinary abnormalities, such as renal cysts, are found incidentally on CT examinations done for other purposes.

SUGGESTED ADDITIONAL READING

Amis ES, Newhouse JH. Essentials of Uroradiology. Boston: Little, Brown, 1991.

Barnewolt CE, Paltiel HJ, Leobwitz RL, et al. Genitourinary tract. In: Kirks DR, Griscom NT, eds. Practical Pediatric Imaging: Diagnostic Radiology of Infants and Children. 3rd Ed. Philadelphia: Lippincott-Raven, 1998:1009–1170.

Blickman JG. Pediatric Radiology: The Requisites. 2nd Ed. St. Louis: Mosby, 1998: 148–194.

Brant WE, Helms CA. Fundamentals of Diagnostic Radiology. 2nd Ed. Philadelphia: Lippincott Williams & Wilkins, 1999: 769–829, 859–979.

Donnelly LF, Jones, O'Hara S, et al. Diagnostic Imaging: Pediatrics. Philadelphia: WB Saunders, 2006.

Dunnick NR, Sandler CM, Newhouse JH, et al. Textbook of Uroradiology. 3rd Ed. Philadelphia: Lippincott Williams & Wilkins, 2000.

Federle MP, Jeffrey RB, Anne V. Diagnostic Imaging: Abdomen. Philadelphia: WB Saunders, 2005.

Katz DS, Lane MJ, Sommer FG. Unenhanced helical CT of ureteral stones: incidence of associated urinary tract findings. AJR 1996;166:1319–1322.

Smith RC, Verga M, McCarthy S, et al. Diagnosis of acute flank pain: value of unenhanced helical CT. AJR 1996;166:97–101.

Sommer FG, Jeffrey RB, Rubin GD, et al. Detection of ureteral calculi in patients with suspected renal colic: value of reformatted noncontrast helical CT. AJR 1995;165:509–513.

Williamson MP, Smith A. Fundamentals of Uroradiology. Philadelphia: WB Saunders, 2000.

Zagoria RJ. Genitourinary Radiology: The Requisites. 2nd Ed. St. Louis: Mosby, 2004.

Ziessman HA, O'Malley JP, Thrall JH. Nuclear Medicine: The Requisites. 3rd Ed. St. Louis: Mosby, 2006.

Zwiebel WJ, Pellerito JS. Introduction to Vascular Ultrasonography. 5th Ed. Philadelphia: WB Saunders, 2005.

Obstetric and Gynecologic Imaging

Diagnostic imaging of the female reproductive tract may be conveniently divided into obstetric and gynecologic imaging. The former discipline relies on the almost exclusive use of highly sophisticated diagnostic ultrasound. The latter, however, uses all the diagnostic methods available to both the radiologist and the gynecologist. Because of the complexity of the studies performed and their interpretation, this chapter reviews the highlights of obstetric and gynecologic imaging with the goal of informing you of indications for various studies and their applications to some common problems.

TECHNICAL CONSIDERATIONS

Diagnostic ultrasound is the primary tool for investigation of the gravid uterus as well as various conditions that may affect the female reproductive tract. Ultrasound is the procedure of choice because there is no ionizing radiation associated with its use to harm either the fetus or ovarian tissue. Furthermore, because of the normal relationships of the uterus and ovaries to the bladder, it is possible to image these organs by surface examination through a distended bladder without degradation of the image by bowel gas. Alternatively, the transvaginal technique is particularly useful for evaluating certain neoplasms. Other noninvasive imaging studies performed include computed tomography (CT) and magnetic resonance (MR) imaging. CT and MR are used primarily in evaluating suspected infections or neoplasms involving the ovaries or uterus. These studies are employed in much the same way they would be used to evaluate similar abnormalities elsewhere within the abdomen and pelvis.

Hysterosalpingography is an invasive procedure in which the uterine os is cannulated and water- or oil-soluble contrast is injected. It is primarily performed to evaluate patients with infertility in whom congenital uterine abnormalities or tubal occlusion of any origin may exist. Other indications include evaluation of patients with recurrent abortion, to assess the obstruction or patency of the fallopian tubes after ligation, and occasionally before artificial insemination to determine if there are any structural abnormalities present.

ANATOMIC CONSIDERATIONS

The anatomic aspects of the female reproductive tract are important because of the relationships of the uterus and ovaries to the bladder, rectum, and peritoneum. The *uterus* lies immediately posterior to and just above the urinary bladder and anterior to the rectum. It is completely extraperitoneal and is surrounded by peritoneal folds that extend between the uterus and the bladder and between the uterus and the colon (*rectouterine pouch of Douglas*). Although variations in uterine shape and position do occur, in most patients, the relationships are as just described and as shown in Figure 10.1. There are three parts to the uterus: the cervix, which projects into

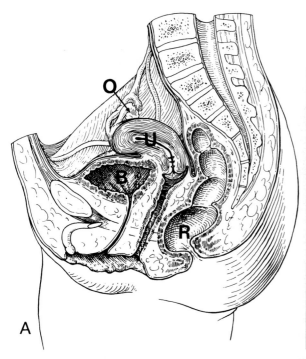

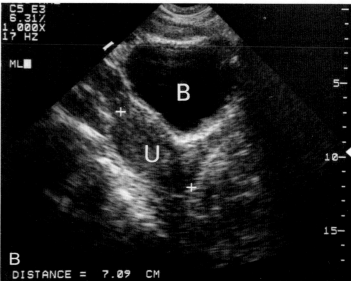

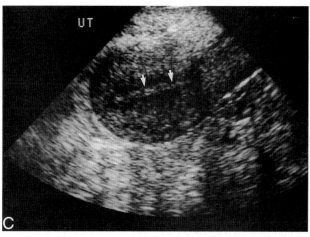

Figure 10.1.   Normal female pelvic anatomy. A. Midline sagittal drawing showing the ovary (*O*), uterus (*U*), bladder (*B*), and rectum (*R*). **B.** Normal longitudinal ultrasound showing the relationship of the uterus (*U*) and the bladder (*B*). **C.** Normal transvaginal longitudinal image of the uterus shows the endometrial surface (*arrows*).

the vagina; the body, its main portion; and the rounded end, or fundus. The *fallopian tubes* begin laterally below the level of the fundus. They are attached to the uterus by the broad ligament. The distal ends of these tubes lie close to the ovary with some of its fingerlike processes (fimbria) actually in contact with the gland. The normal *ovaries* are paired, almond-sized structures attached by the ovarian ligament to the uterus as well as to the broad ligament. They are completely shielded from the bladder anteriorly by the broad ligament.

Although the textbook depiction of the position of the ovaries is as just described, they are quite mobile and are often located lateral to the broad ligament. Figure 10.2 shows these relationships. The uterus, ovaries, and fallopian tubes are sustained by a rich vascular plexus. In addition, numerous lymphatic channels drain the area. This accounts for the intra-abdominal spread of pelvic malignancy.

The evaluation of the gravid uterus is accomplished primarily through the use of ultrasound. *Obstetric sonography is a highly complex examination that needs to be performed by a carefully trained operator and interpreted with a great degree of skill.* Early in the history of obstetric ultrasound, the primary goal was to confirm the presence of an intrauterine pregnancy, determine the location of the placenta, detect multiple gestation, determine the lie of the fetus, or estimate gestational age. Refinements and improvements in ultrasound technology have added a

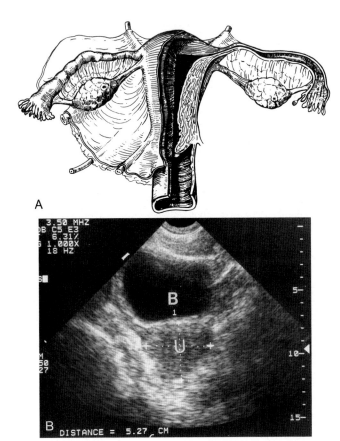

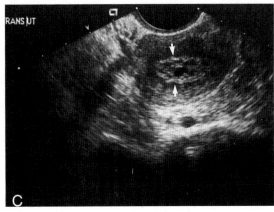

Figure 10.2.   Normal coronal anatomy. A. Cut-away section of the uterus, ovaries, and fallopian tubes. **B.** Axial ultrasound showing the relationship of the uterus (*U*) and the bladder (*B*). **C.** Transvaginal axial image shows cystic endometrium (*arrows*). The bladder is the sonolucent area above the uterus.

more important indication: detecting congenital anomalies and other abnormalities of the fetus. Indeed, many of the malpractice actions filed against obstetricians relate to failure to detect fetal abnormalities before birth.

Because ultrasound uses no ionizing radiation, it imposes no adverse biologic effects on either the mother or the fetus. However, this study, like any other, should be performed only when indicated. Table 10.1 lists the indications for obstetric sonography. Note that the indications change with time throughout the pregnancy. This discussion highlights the normal sonographic changes that may be observed at various intervals during pregnancy. In addition, several common abnormalities will be discussed. For a more in-depth treatment of the subject, see the works listed in the "Suggested Additional Reading" section at the end of the chapter.

NORMAL PREGNANCY

First Trimester

The first trimester is the time between conception and the end of the thirteenth week of gestation. Obstetricians often use the terms *gestational age* and *menstrual age* interchangeably. However, because of variations in ovulation, a 1- to 2-week discrepancy may occur between the sonographic assessment of menstrual age and the actual gestational age of the fetus. Gestational age typically is determined from the time of conception, and the menstrual age is based on the first day of the last menses. For purposes of discussion, this chapter refers only to gestational age.

A gestational sac, which may be detected as early as 3 weeks from conception, consists of a round-to-oval area devoid of echoes located within the body or fundus of the uterus (Fig. 10.3). This sonolucency represents the choriodecidual membrane that surrounds the developing embryo. The embryonic period occurs between the third and eighth weeks of gestational age. Embryonic development cannot usually be delineated in its early stages. During

TABLE 10.1
INDICATIONS FOR OBSTETRIC SONOGRAPHY

General Indications
Confirmation of intrauterine pregnancy
Estimation of gestational age
Detection of multiple gestation
Determination of placental location and texture
Detection of anatomic and functional abnormalities of the fetus
Evaluation of other pelvic masses during pregnancy

First Trimester
Uterine bleeding
Suspected threatened, incomplete, or missed abortion
Distinction between intrauterine and ectopic pregnancy
Suspected molar pregnancy
Suspected pregnancy associated with intrauterine contraceptive device

Second Trimester
Localization and evaluation of placenta
Polyhydramnios
Evaluation of fetal growth

Third Trimester
Possible placenta previa
Determination of fetal maturity to plan optimal time and mode of
  delivery

Other Indications
Maternal abdominal disorders during pregnancy
Postpartum for suspected retained products of conception

this period, all major body organs begin forming. Further growth and differentiation occur in the fetal period. The exact transition time between embryonic and fetal periods is arbitrary.

Once a fetus can be detected, the gestational age may be estimated by measuring the crown-to-rump (long-axis) length of the fetus. This method is accurate to within 1 week of gestational age (Fig. 10.4). The following normal structures can also be detected at the times indicated: arm buds, 8 weeks; leg buds, 9 to 10 weeks; fetal heart, 7 to 8 weeks; choroid plexus of the brain, 12 to 16 weeks. Other structures that can be detected during the first trimester include the umbilical stalk and the yolk sac.

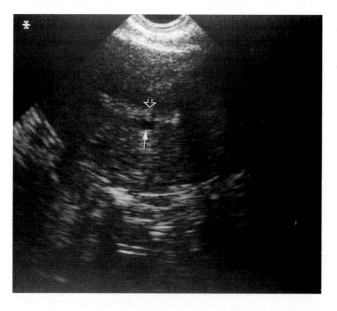

Figure 10.3. Normal 3- to 4-week gestation. Ultrasound examination shows the small gestational sac (*solid arrow*) attached to the thickened uterine wall (*open arrow*).

Figure 10.4. Normal first trimester. A. Fetal poles at 9.3 weeks of gestation. Notice the head (*open arrow*), foot (*solid arrow*), and umbilical cord (*arrowhead*). **B.** At 12.2 weeks of gestation, the crown-to-rump length (CRL) is 54.3 mm. Notice the head (*open arrow*) and upper limb (*solid arrow*).

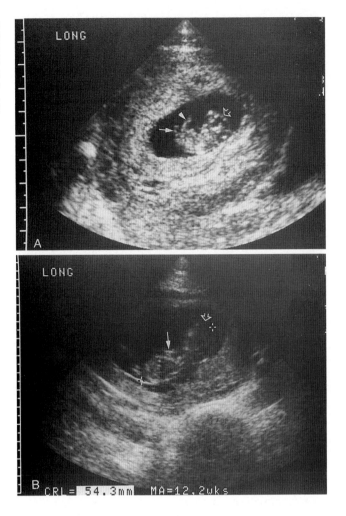

Second Trimester

The second trimester of pregnancy is the interval between the fourteenth and twenty-sixth gestational weeks. A more detailed evaluation of the fetus, uterus, and placenta is possible because of their enlargement during this time. It is in the second trimester that amniotic fluid may be detected surrounding the fetus. As a rule, the volume of amniotic fluid should equal the volume of the fetus. The location and size of the placenta can easily be determined (Fig. 10.5). The fetal organs also enlarge and are easily detectable on sonography. It is thus

Figure 10.5. Normal second trimester fetus showing the position of the placenta (*P*). Facial features are clearly visible.

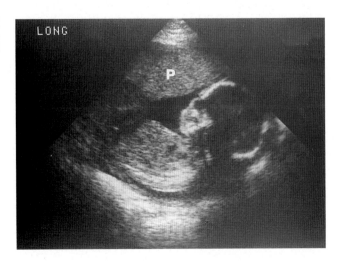

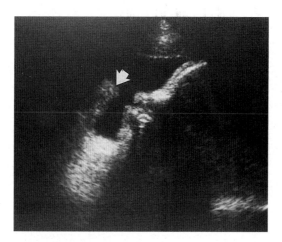

Figure 10.6. Normal third trimester fetus. Facial features are clearly visible. Is this fetus sucking its thumb (*arrow*)?

possible to determine the gross morphology and function of the heart by real-time examination. In the later portion of the second trimester, the fetal liver and kidneys can be seen, as well as the distended fetal urinary bladder. By the end of the second trimester, it is also possible to delineate the external genitalia. The extremities and their developing bones are demonstrable, and the fetal spine can be detected. It is during the second trimester that gestational age is determined from the biparietal diameter. Tables correlating biparietal diameter with menstrual age are available in every obstetric department.

Third Trimester

The third trimester of pregnancy falls between the twenty-seventh week of pregnancy up to the time of delivery (usually at 38 to 40 weeks). During this time, there is continued enlargement of both the uterus and fetus, as well as changes within the placenta. Sonography demonstrates detailed anatomy of various fetal organs (Fig. 10.6). In addition, fetal motion is visible on real-time examinations. Sonography in this period is used primarily to determine the optimal time and mode of delivery as well as to confirm or exclude the presence of a placenta previa (discussed in the next section).

PATHOLOGIC CONSIDERATIONS

Obstetric Abnormalities

A variety of abnormalities occur during pregnancy. Vaginal bleeding during the first trimester is often referred to as *threatened abortion*. There are no specific sonographic findings in this condition. However, retention of products of conception is referred to as *incomplete abortion*. In this situation, the sonographic findings may vary from a normal-appearing uterus to one that contains blood clots and/or fetal parts (Fig. 10.7).

Placenta previa is a condition in which a placenta is located either partially or completely across the cervical os (Fig. 10.8). This condition may result in maternal or fetal death from massive hemorrhage at the time of birth. The detection of placenta previa by the middle of the third trimester is necessary so that the fetus can be delivered by cesarean section before the onset of labor.

Abruptio placentae is the premature separation of the placenta from the wall of the uterus. This may be detected by sonography as a sonolucent area between the uterine wall and the placental shadows (Fig. 10.9).

Various fetal anomalies may be detected during the later stages of pregnancy. These include fetal *hydrocephalus* (Fig. 10.10), *anencephaly* (Fig. 10.11), *meningomyelocele* (Fig. 10.12), and *hydranencephaly*. Urinary abnormalities such as urinary obstruction detected by *oligohydramnios,* and multicystic or polycystic kidney disease can also be demonstrated. Abnormalities of

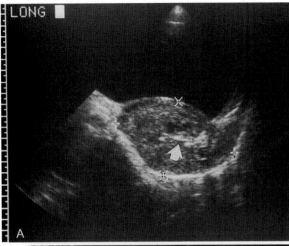

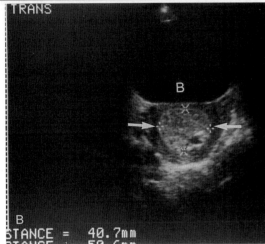

Figure 10.7.   Appearance of the uterus after incomplete abortion. A. Longitudinal scan shows retained placental products (*arrow*). **B.** Transverse scan shows the retained products of conception (*arrows*). Notice the position of the bladder (*B*) above the uterus.

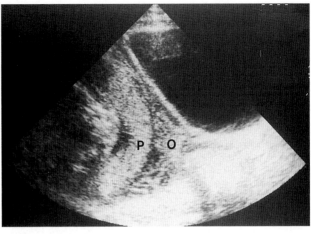

Figure 10.8.   Placenta previa. Longitudinal scan shows the placenta (*P*) lying just above the cervical os (*O*).

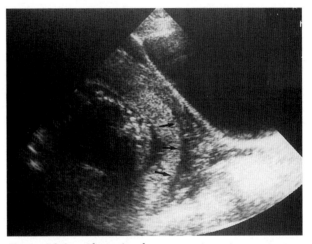

Figure 10.9.   Abruptio placentae. (This is the same patient as in Fig. 10.8.) Longitudinal scan made 1 week after Figure 10.8 shows separation of the placenta from the uterine wall (*arrows*).

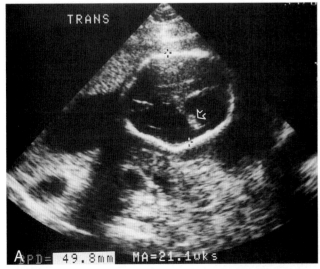

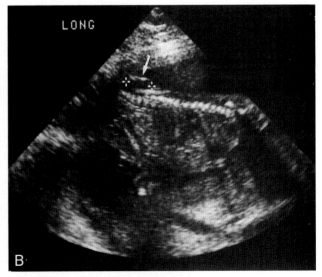

Figure 10.10.   Fetal hydrocephalus. A. Transabdominal scan shows irregularity of the skull and shift of the choroid plexus to the dependent side (*arrow*). The sonolucent area surrounding the choroid plexus is the dilated lateral ventricle. The "lemon-shaped" skull is a sign of fetal hydrocephalus. **B.** Longitudinal scan of the fetal torso shows a meningomyelocele (*arrow*) at the base of the vertebral column.

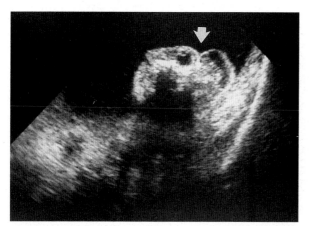

Figure 10.11. Anencephaly. Longitudinal scan shows a grossly deformed head (*arrow*).

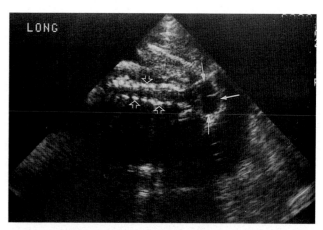

Figure 10.12. Meningomyelocele. Longitudinal scan shows the meningomyelocele (*solid arrows*) at the base of the individual vertebrae (*open arrows*).

the gastrointestinal tract that are detectable include duodenal atresia, omphalocele, and fetal ascites. Cardiac abnormalities are difficult to detect because of the cardiac motion. However, careful evaluation can result in the demonstration of certain of these anomalies. Finally, forms of dwarfism such as achondroplasia may be detected. Fractures of the fetal skeleton in utero may be the result of underlying osteogenesis imperfecta.

An *ectopic pregnancy* is one in which implantation occurs outside the uterine cavity. In most patients with this condition, the products of conception implant in a fallopian tube. Usually, there is tubal scarring as the result of previous pelvic inflammatory disease. Ectopic pregnancy is readily detectable by ultrasound (Fig. 10.13).

Gynecologic Abnormalities

Evaluation of abnormalities involving a woman's reproductive tract has benefitted greatly by the developments in body imaging. The modalities primarily used are ultrasound, CT, MR imaging, and hysterosalpingography.

As previously mentioned, ultrasound is noninvasive, uses no ionizing radiation, can be performed rapidly, and is relatively inexpensive. Thus, it is one of the initial studies to be performed in evaluation of abnormalities of the female pelvis. The ability to image in transverse,

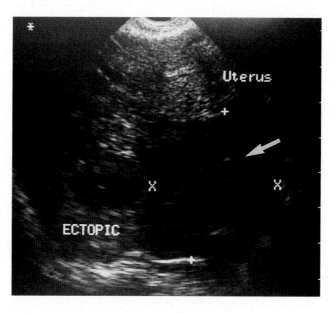

Figure 10.13. Ectopic pregnancy. Transverse scan shows an irregular collection of echoes (*arrow*) behind the uterus.

Figure 10.14. Normal hysterosalpingogram. A. After injection of contrast through the uterine os, there is spillage from both fallopian tubes (*arrows*). **B.** Delayed film shows intraperitoneal contrast outlining loops of bowel (*arrows*).

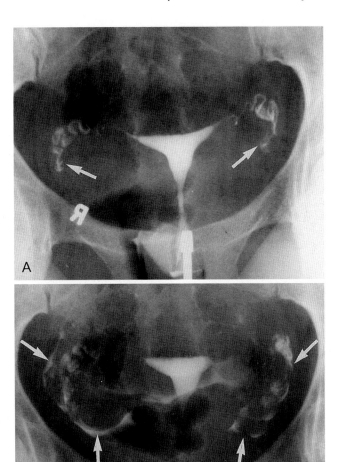

longitudinal, and transvaginal planes (see Figs. 10.1 and 10.2) is a distinct advantage over CT, which is performed in the transverse plane only. MR imaging has the advantages of both procedures and is particularly useful in evaluating pelvic neoplasms. Hysterosalpingography is the best radiologic technique for delineating the morphology of the uterine lumen as well as the patency of the fallopian tubes in evaluating patients with infertility problems (Figs. 10.14 and 10.15). Thus, the gynecologist has many imaging procedures available to diagnose abnormalities.

Figure 10.15. Abnormal hysterosalpingogram. The left fallopian tube is occluded near its origin (*large arrow*). Irregularity and scarring of the right fallopian tube (*small arrows*) is evident.

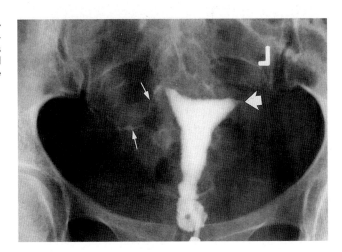

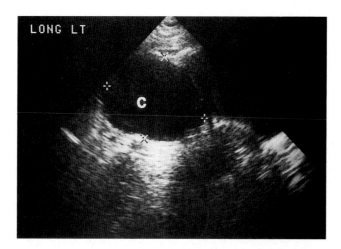

Figure 10.16. Ovarian cyst. Parasagittal longitudinal ultrasound shows the large cyst (*C*) devoid of internal echoes.

Pathologic conditions that occur within the female reproductive organs fall into four categories: congenital, physiologic, inflammatory, and neoplastic. *Congenital abnormalities* occur primarily in the uterus. Approximately 0.5% of women have congenital anomalies. These may be incidental findings of no clinical significance. However, others, such as bicornuate uterus, may result in pregnancy disorders. Congenital uterine abnormalities are often associated with renal agenesis. For this reason, it is important to image the kidneys when a uterine abnormality is encountered.

Physiologic abnormalities include cystic diseases of the ovary and endometriosis. Because of normal physiologic functions, cysts as large as 3 to 4 cm in the ovary may be simply physiologic—that is, transient and changing, depending on the phase of the menstrual cycle. However, a normal physiologic cyst that fails to regress or enlarges because of a hormonal imbalance or hemorrhage may form a functional or retention cyst. Ovarian cysts are the most common pelvic masses encountered in young women (Fig. 10.16).

Endometriosis is caused by the presence of endometrial tissue in extrauterine sites. The most common location for endometriosis is within the pelvic cavity. From an imaging standpoint, endometriosis produces cystic masses of various sizes anywhere within the pelvis (Fig. 10.17). These may implant on the colon and produce extraluminal compression defects on a barium enema.

Pelvic inflammatory disease is the result of an ascending infection from the vagina to the endometrium, the fallopian tubes, and ultimately the pelvic peritoneum. In most instances, the causal organism is gonococcal. Inflammatory collections in the pelvis may be detected

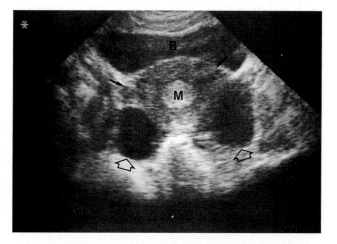

Figure 10.17. Endometriosis. Transverse ultrasound shows the bladder (*B*), the thickened uterine wall (*closed arrows*), menstrual debris (*M*), and two parauterine masses (*open arrows*) representing ectopic endometrial tissue.

Figure 10.18. Bilateral tubo-ovarian abscesses. Transverse scan shows bilateral multilocular masses of mixed echogenicity (*arrows*) on either side of the uterus (*U*).

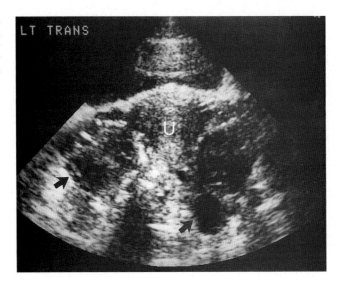

on either CT or ultrasound without difficulty. Occasionally, a tubo-ovarian abscess will be formed (Fig. 10.18).

Neoplasms of a woman's reproductive organs include both benign and malignant tumors. Common benign tumors include serous cystadenoma (Fig. 10.19), dermoid tumors (teratomas; Figs. 10.20 and 10.21), and fibroid tumors (Fig. 10.22). Dermoids often contain fat, calcifications, and occasionally dental elements, all of which are easily demonstrable by CT (see Fig. 10.21). Fibroids are extremely common and occur in up to 40% of women over the age of 35 years. They are often found as incidental calcifications on abdominal radiographs (see Fig. 10.22). In some instances they are responsible for dysfunctional uterine hemorrhage and may require hysterectomy or myotomy.

Malignant neoplasms are unfortunately common. *Endometrial carcinoma* is the most common invasive gynecologic malignancy. *Cervical carcinoma* is the second most common. It ranks sixth in cancer mortality, primarily because symptoms do not occur until late in the course of disease. *Ovarian carcinoma* is the next most common gynecologic malignant tumor. It is responsible for 50% of the deaths from gynecologic malignancy and is the fourth most frequent cause of cancer death in women (after lung, breast, and colon cancers). Malignancies of the vagina, vulva, and

Figure 10.19. Ovarian cystadenoma. Transverse scan shows a mass of mixed echogenicity (*arrows*) beneath the bladder.

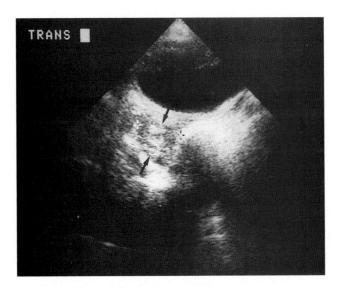

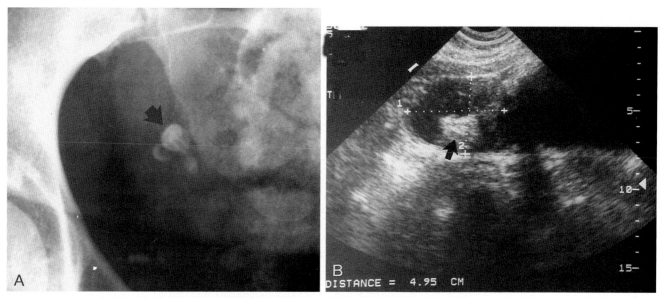

Figure 10.20. Ovarian dermoid tumor. A. Detail view of the pelvis shows toothlike calcifications in the right lower quadrant (*arrow*).
B. Ultrasound shows the dense calcified area (*arrow*) within the more cystic tumor.

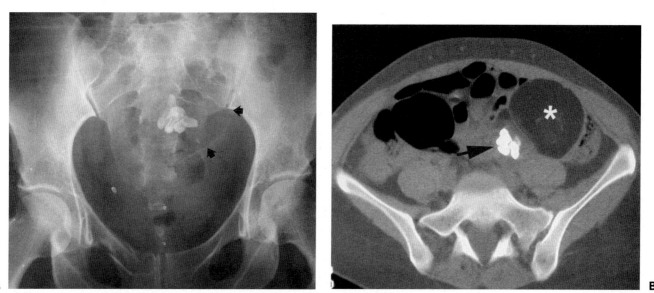

Figure 10.21. Ovarian dermoid tumor (teratoma). A. Detail view of the pelvis shows a lucent mass (arrows) on the left containing malformed teeth. **B.** CT image shows the tumor with varying fatty (*) and dental (*arrow*) components.

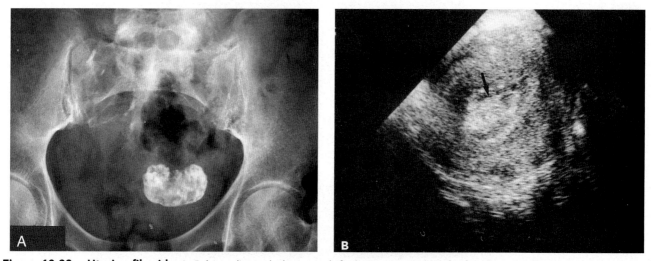

Figure 10.22. Uterine fibroids. A. Pelvic radiograph shows a calcified mass just to the left of midline. Calcifications in fibroids often look like popcorn. **B.** Ultrasound examination shows the fibroid to appear as an echogenic mass (*arrow*).

Figure 10.23. Endometrial carcinoma. Longitudinal scan shows enlargement of the uterus and echogenic material (*arrows*) immediately behind the bladder (*B*).

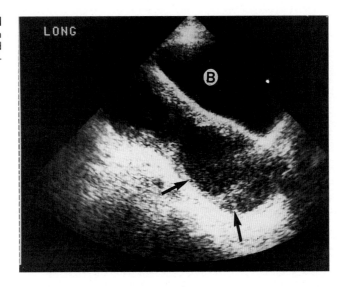

oviduct are much less common. Multimodality imaging is used in detecting, staging, and follow-up of all these neoplasms (Figs. 10.23 to 10.25). Of particular importance in the evaluation of patients with these diseases is the detection of the presence or absence of localized spread through invasion of contiguous tissues. The presence or absence of extension beyond the affected organ will determine the exact staging of the neoplasm according to the standards set by the International Federation of Gynecology and Obstetrics.

Figure 10.24. Cervical carcinoma. A. Longitudinal scan shows enlargement of the underlying cervix (*arrows*). **B.** CT image shows the mass immediately behind the bladder (*large arrow*). A small amount of gas is present within the mass (*small arrow*) secondary to necrosis. CX, cervix.

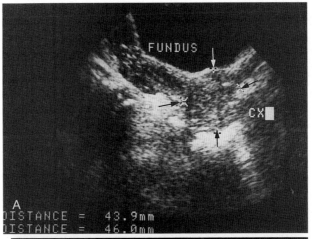

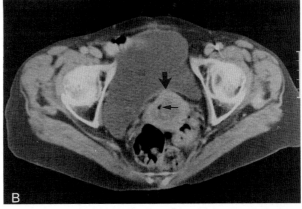

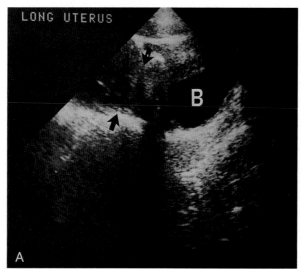

Figure 10.25. Ovarian carcinoma.
A. Longitudinal scan shows a multilocular mass (*arrows*) immediately above the bladder (*B*). **B.** Scan slightly higher shows the mass to measure 12.6 × 6.9 cm. Notice the multiple echoes within the mass.

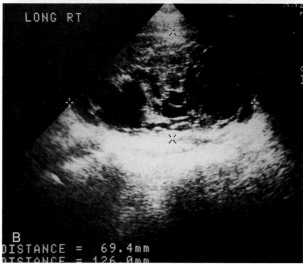

SUMMARY AND KEY POINTS

■ This chapter has dealt with the evaluation of the female reproductive tract primarily by sonography. Because of the complexity in the performance and interpretation of obstetrical sonography, the discussion has been limited to basic concepts. See the more-definitive texts listed at the end of this chapter for in-depth discussion of the sophisticated aspects of this subject.

■ Common obstetric entities include normal pregnancy, placenta previa, abruptio placentae, ectopic pregnancy, and fetal anomalies.

■ The evaluation of gynecologic abnormalities uses a multimodality imaging approach, although sonography remains a primary tool.

■ Gynecologic abnormalities include physiologic problems, such as cystic disease of the ovaries and endometriosis; pelvic inflammatory disease; and tumors. The evaluation of these abnormalities is performed in the same manner as that of other organ systems.

SUGGESTED ADDITIONAL READING

Bowerman RA. Atlas of Normal Fetal Ultrasonographic Anatomy. 2nd Ed. St. Louis: Mosby-Year Book, 1991.
Brant WE, Helms CA. Fundamentals of Diagnostic Radiology. 2nd Ed. Philadelphia: Lippincott Williams & Wilkins, 1999:881–905.

Callen PW. Ultrasonography in Obstetrics and Gynecology. 4th Ed. Philadelphia: WB Saunders, 2000.

Fleischer AC, Kepple DM. Transvaginal Sonography: A Clinical Atlas. Philadelphia: JB Lippincott, 1991.

Johnson PT, Kurtz AB. Obstetric and Gynecologic Ultrasound. St. Louis: Mosby, 2001.

Karasick S, Karasick D. Atlas of Hysterosalpingography. Springfield, IL: Charles C. Thomas, 1987.

Nyberg DA, Mahony BS, Pretorius DH. Diagnostic Ultrasound of Fetal Abnormalities. St. Louis: Mosby-Year Book, 1990.

Rumack CM, Wilson SR, Charboneau JW, et al. Diagnostic Ultrasound. 3rd Ed. St. Louis: Mosby, 2005.

Woodward PJ, Kennedy AM, Sohaey R, et al. Diagnostic Imaging: Obstetrics. Philadelphia: WB Saunders, 2005.

Musculoskeletal Imaging

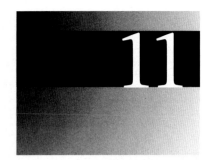

Imaging examinations of the musculoskeletal system are among the most common you will encounter. Indeed, skeletal radiographs constitute the second-largest group (after chest) of films seen in a busy radiology practice. Radiographic analysis of the skeleton provides considerable information about the overall health of the patient. In addition to obvious abnormalities of the bones and joints themselves, skeletal radiographs may provide clues to the presence of occult systemic inflammatory, metabolic, or neoplastic diseases.

This chapter outlines an approach useful in the interpretation of skeletal radiographs. In addition, the musculoskeletal applications of other imaging studies are highlighted. An important principle to remember is that, as in the gastrointestinal tract, *lesions in the skeleton appear similar to one another no matter where they are located.* The incidence may vary with the location, but the basic appearance is the same.

TECHNICAL CONSIDERATIONS

Imaging of the musculoskeletal system encompasses the entire spectrum of diagnostic radiology. Radiography remains the cornerstone for diagnosis, and thus radiographs must be obtained before ordering more-sophisticated imaging studies. Radiographs provide the road map for further investigation and diagnosis. Overall, radiographs have an intermediate sensitivity but a high specificity for diagnosing bone abnormalities. Many lesions have characteristic radiographic appearances that allow confident and accurate pathologic diagnosis, particularly when the findings are interpreted in light of clinical and/or laboratory data (Fig. 11.1). Other lesions have an indeterminate appearance that requires additional imaging or perhaps a biopsy for diagnosis (Fig. 11.2). The basic appearance and management of musculoskeletal radiography can be divided into four categories:

1. Benign, asymptomatic—"leave me alone"
2. Benign, symptomatic—elective excision
3. Malignant ("I think")—biopsy needed
4. Indeterminate—biopsy needed

Fortunately, developments in imaging technology have made the decision process easier. Using computed tomography (CT) and magnetic resonance (MR) imaging, it is possible to increase the confidence levels to put more lesions in categories 1 and 3.

CT is used extensively for evaluating musculoskeletal abnormalities. In addition to providing diagnostic information about bones and soft tissues in another plane, it is a mainstay for safe and accurate biopsy procedures (Fig. 11.3) as well as for CT-guided intervention (Fig. 11.4). CT is used to evaluate suspected tumors (Fig. 11.5); fractures, particularly of the vertebral column (Fig. 11.6); and infections (Fig. 11.7). Another use for CT is to augment arthrograms, especially of the shoulder. Multiplanar tomographic and three-dimensional reconstructions of CT examinations have been found useful by referring surgeons (Fig. 11.8).

MR imaging of the musculoskeletal system is the second most common use of this technique (after neuroimaging). MR has revolutionized musculoskeletal radiology. In addition to

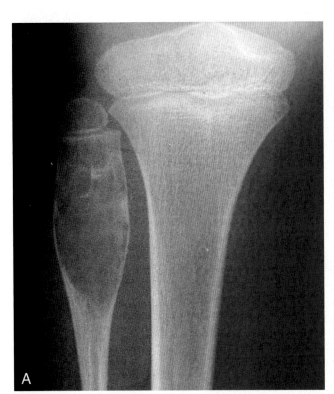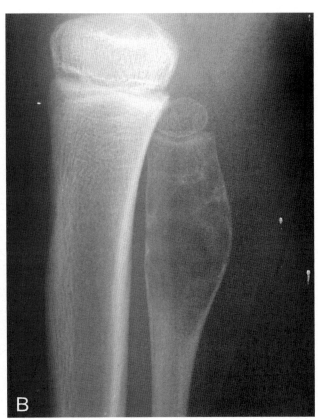

Figure 11.1.   Aneurysmal bone cyst of the proximal fibula. Frontal **(A)** and lateral **(B)** views demonstrate an expanded lesion of the diametaphyseal area of the fibula. The lesion is trabeculated and does not cross the physis. In this skeletally immature patient, the most likely diagnosis is an aneurysmal bone cyst. This lesion is radiologically characteristic enough to allow a confident diagnosis.

its ability to portray information in any plane (sagittal, coronal, axial [transverse], and unlimited oblique), it can aid in the diagnosis of primary (Fig. 11.9) and metastatic tumors (Fig. 11.10), infections (Fig. 11.11), trauma (Fig. 11.12), avascular necrosis (Fig. 11.13), tendon ruptures (Fig. 11.14), and internal joint derangements (Fig. 11.15). Indeed, MR imaging has eliminated many types of conventional arthrography. However, MR arthrography is now the procedure of choice for the definitive diagnosis of many internal joint derangements, especially of the shoulder (Fig. 11.16), because of its ability to leave little doubt as to the nature of the abnormality.

Ultrasound has been used to diagnose soft tissue lesions of the limbs such as cysts (Fig. 11.17), loose bodies (Fig. 11.18), and ligament and tendon ruptures. Throughout Europe and in many U.S. centers, it is also used for assessing tears of the rotator cuff of the shoulder (Fig. 11.19). However, the greater accuracy of MR as well as its ease of performance has resulted in poor acceptance of musculoskeletal ultrasound in the United States. Part of this relates to the orthopaedic surgeons' lack of acceptance. Ultrasound is an excellent choice for diagnosing congenital hip dysplasia in the infant whose femoral head epiphyses have not yet ossified (Fig. 11.20). Ultrasound shows the unossified cartilaginous femoral head and the acetabulum without the danger of irradiation of the pelvis and gonads. Despite the availability and the efficacy of ultrasound, pediatricians still order pelvic radiographs when they suspect congenital hip dysplasia in their patients. Ultrasound is also useful for locating nonopaque foreign bodies in soft tissues.

Nuclear imaging studies of the skeletal system include the radioisotope bone scan and indium scan. The bone scan is a valuable and useful tool for detecting areas of abnormal metabolic activity within bone. The introduction of technetium-99m–labeled phosphorus compounds (methylene diphosphonate) brought a new dimension of safety and accuracy to

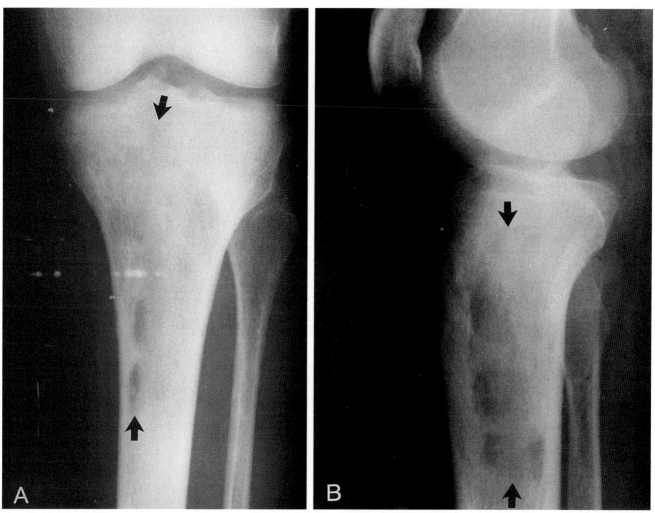

Figure 11.2.   Osteomyelitis of the proximal tibia. Frontal **(A)** and lateral **(B)** views demonstrate a destructive lesion in the diametaphyseal region of the proximal tibia (*arrows*). There is nothing characteristic about this lesion to allow confident diagnosis without a biopsy.

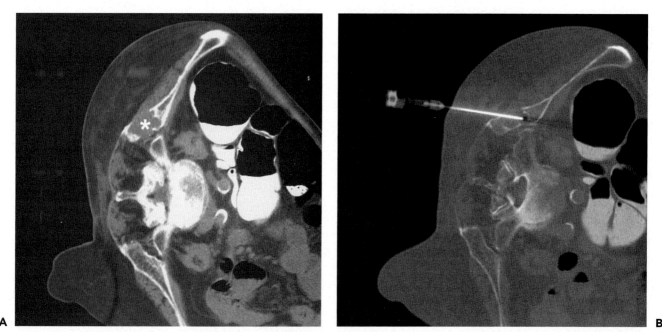

Figure 11.3.   Computed tomography (CT)–guided biopsy. A. CT image shows a destructive lesion in the right iliac bone (*). **B.** CT image shows biopsy needle in the center of the lesion. Diagnosis: metastatic lung carcinoma.

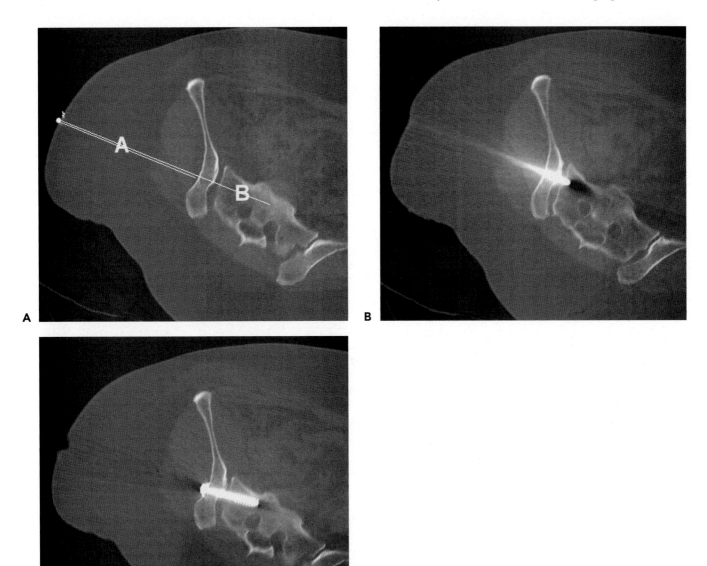

Figure 11.4. CT-guided screw placement. A. CT image shows proposed trajectory of the screw insertion. A, distance from skin to bone; B, distance from skin to desired position in the sacrum. **B.** CT image shows screw being placed. **C.** CT image shows final position of screw.

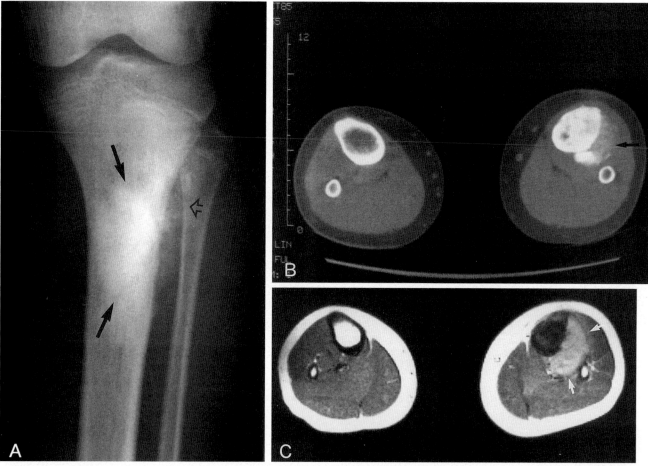

Figure 11.5. Osteosarcoma of the proximal tibia. A. Frontal radiograph shows an area of bone destruction with clouds of dense osteoid matrix (*solid arrows*). The lesion extends beyond the margin of bone into the soft tissues (*open arrow*). **B.** CT image shows the increased density caused by this osteogenic sarcoma in the left tibia. Notice the extraosseous extension into the soft tissues (*arrow*). **C.** T2-weighted MR image shows the extent of soft tissue involvement to better advantage (*arrows*). The dense osteoid tissue appears black.

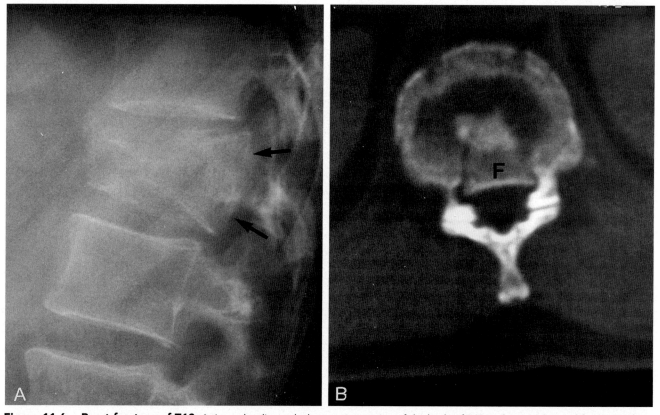

Figure 11.6. Burst fracture of T12. A. Lateral radiograph shows compression of the body of T12 and retropulsion of fragments from posterior vertebral body line into the vertebral canal (*arrows*). **B.** CT image shows the displaced fragment (*F*) narrowing the vertebral canal.

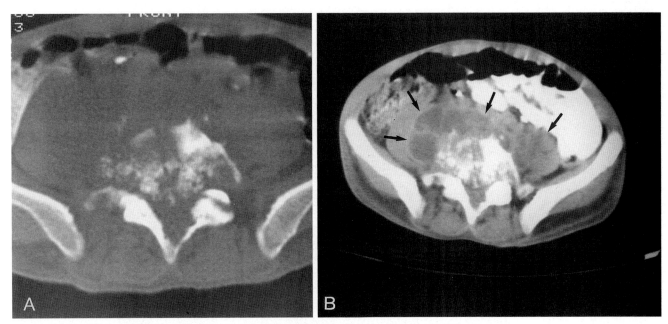

Figure 11.7. Vertebral tuberculous osteomyelitis and paraspinous abscess. A. CT image near the lumbosacral junction shows a destructive process of L5 and a paraspinal soft tissue mass in front of the vertebrae. **B.** CT image slightly lower made at soft tissue windows after intravenous contrast enhancement shows the large multilocular abscess in the soft tissues (*arrows*). The rim of the abscess is enhanced.

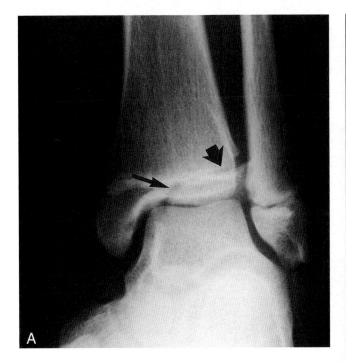

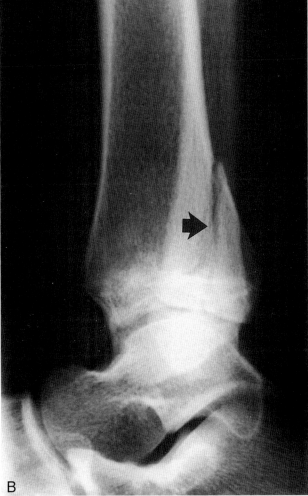

Figure 11.8. Triplane fracture of the distal tibia. A. Frontal radiograph shows fractures through the epiphysis (*thin arrow*) and the lateral physis (*fat arrow*). **B.** Lateral radiograph shows a coronal fracture of the posterior tibia (*arrow*). (continued on page 374)

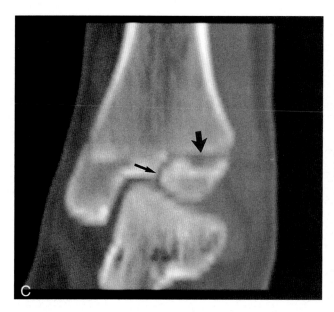

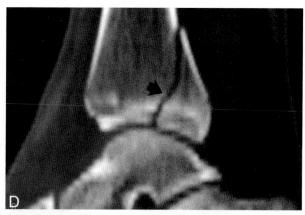

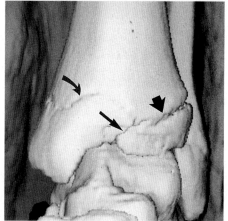

Figure 11.8. *(continued)* **C.** Coronal tomographic reconstructed CT image shows the epiphyseal (*thin arrow*) and the physeal (*fat arrow*) fractures. **D.** Sagittal tomographic reconstructed CT image shows the coronal fracture (*arrow*) actually extends to the joint surface. **E.** Three-dimensional reconstructed CT image shows the epiphyseal fracture (*thin arrow*) and physeal fracture (*fat arrow*) as well as the normal physis medially (*curved arrow*).

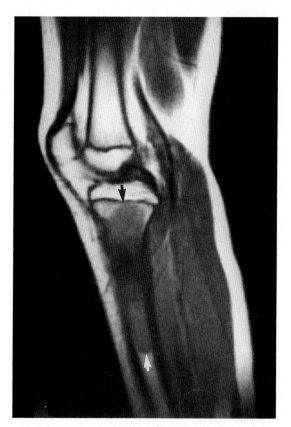

Figure 11.9. Osteosarcoma of the tibia. (This is the same patient as in Fig. 11.5.) Direct sagittal T1-weighted image shows an extensive area of marrow replacement in the proximal tibia (*arrows*). Cortical breakthrough is suggested in the darkest area near the middle.

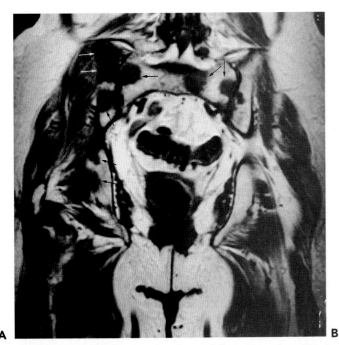
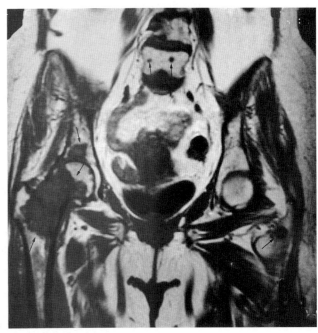

Figure 11.10.   Metastases to the pelvic region. A and B. Coronal T1-weighted images demonstrate multiple areas of low signal (*arrows*) involving the iliac bones, sacrum, both proximal femurs, and the lumbar vertebrae.

Figure 11.11. Osteomyelitis of the proximal tibia. (This is the same patient as in Fig. 11.2.) Direct coronal T1-weighted MR image demonstrates an extensive area of low signal within the marrow space of the tibia. The process extends up to the joint line but has not yet crossed it. The actual extent of marrow involvement is greater than the degree of bony destruction seen on the radiograph.

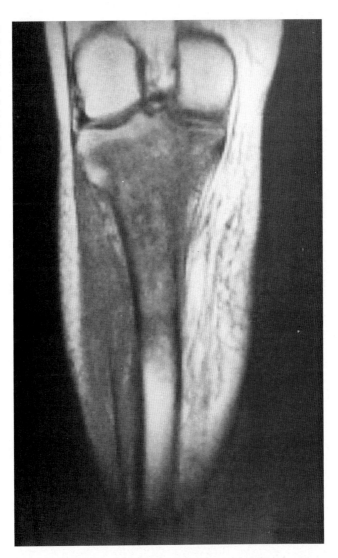

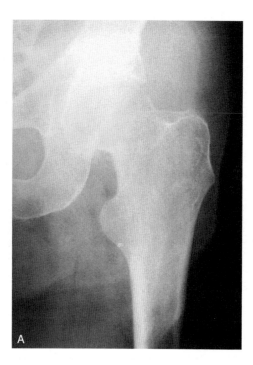

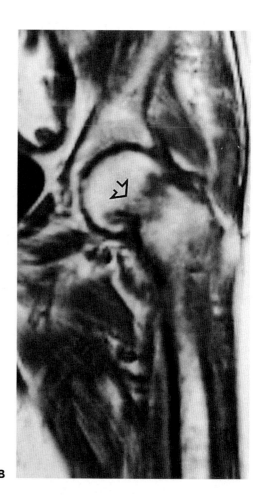

Figure 11.12. Occult hip fracture diagnosed by magnetic resonance (MR) imaging. A. Radiograph of the hip is not satisfactory for diagnosing a hip fracture in this elderly patient. **B.** T1-weighted coronal image shows a transverse line of low signal (*arrow*) representing a fracture of the femoral neck.

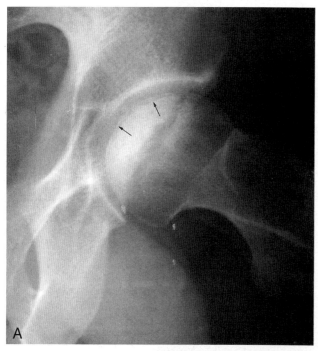

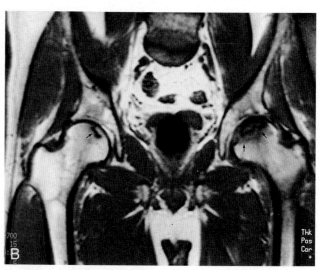

Figure 11.13. Avascular necrosis of the left femoral head. A. Frog-leg lateral radiograph of the left hip demonstrates increased density to the femoral head and subchondral lucency (*arrows*). **B.** T1-weighted image of the pelvis shows low signal within both femoral heads (*arrows*). Radiographs of the right hip were normal.

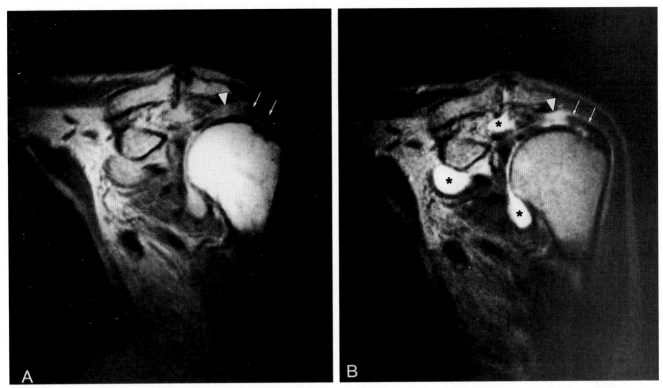

Figure 11.14.   Rotator cuff tear. A. T1-weighted oblique coronal image shows an area of interruption (*arrowhead*) of the tendon of the supraspinatus muscle (*arrows*). **B.** Gradient echo oblique coronal image shows the findings to better advantage. The globular areas of increased signal (*) represent a joint effusion. This figure shows the differences in signal between T1 and gradient echo images.

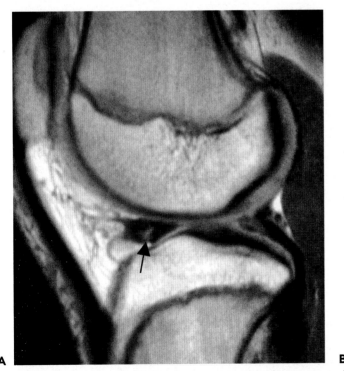

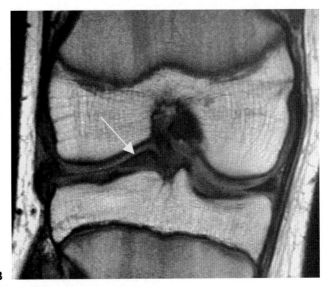

Figure 11.15.   Internal joint derangements as demonstrated by MR imaging. A. Torn anterior horn of the medial meniscus. Proton density sagittal MR image shows an area of increased signal (brightness, *arrow*) in the anterior horn of the medial meniscus. Normally, the meniscus should be a uniform black triangle. **B.** In the same patient, coronal proton density image shows the tear to be a "bucket handle" type, with a fragment of meniscus displaced into the interior of the joint (*arrow*).   *(continued on page 378)*

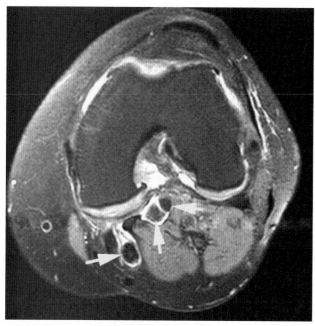

C

Figure 11.15. *(continued)*   **C.** Axial T2-weighted image shows multiple synovial loose bodies (*arrows*) in a multilocular Baker cyst.

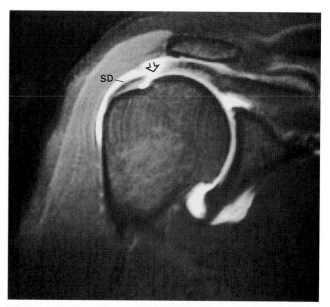

Figure 11.16.   MR arthrogram demonstrating a complete tear of the rotator cuff (*arrow*). The bright contrast flows from the glenohumeral joint space into the subdeltoid bursa (*SD*). Normally, the intact rotator cuff prevents this.

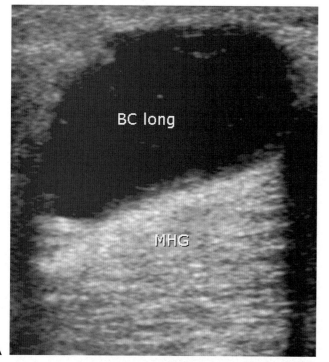

A

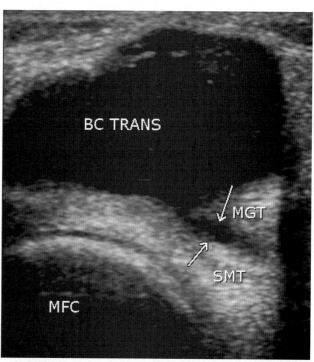

B

Figure 11.17.   Cysts diagnosed by ultrasound. Longitudinal **(A)** and axial **(B)** ultrasound studies show the Baker cyst (*BC*). Notice the extension of the cyst between the two tendons (*arrows*) in B.   *(continued on page 379)*

Figure 11.17. *(continued)* **C.** Ganglion cyst (GC) of the dorsum of the wrist on a longitudinal scan. The cyst is located just above the trapezoid and the second metacarpal (*MC II*). MFC, medial femoral condyle; MGT, medial gastrocnemius tendon; MHG, medial head gastrocnemius; SMT, semimembranosus tendon. (Courtesy of Mihra Taljanovic, MD, Department of Radiology, University of Arizona.)

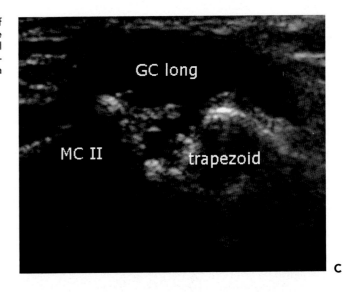

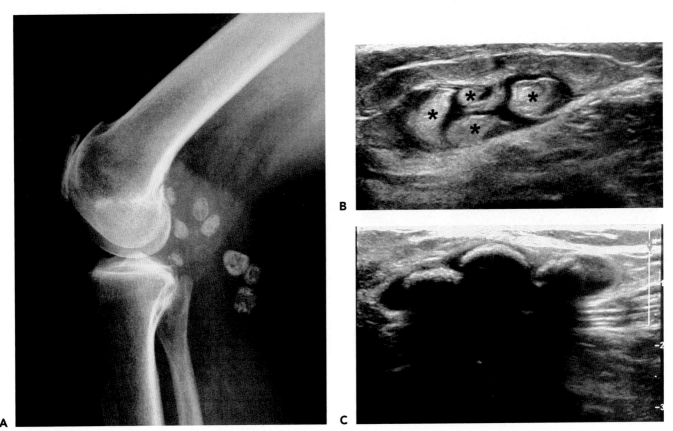

Figure 11.18.   Synovial osteochondromatosis. (This is the same patient as Fig. 11-15C.) **A.** Lateral radiograph shows multiple loose bodies in the popliteal fossa. **B.** Longitudinal ultrasound exam shows multiple bodies (*) within a cyst. **C.** Axial ultrasound exam shows shadowing from the loose bodies. This is similar to the picture seen with gallstones.   *(continued on page 380)*

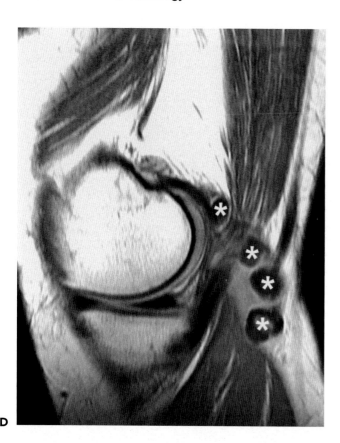

Figure 11.18. *(continued)* **D.** Sagittal proton density MR image shows the loose bodies (*) to be within a Baker cyst.

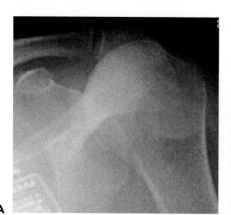

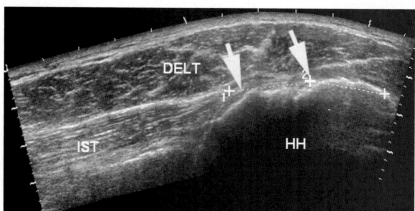

Figure 11.19.   Supraspinatus tendon rupture (rotator cuff tear). A. Radiograph shows elevation of the humeral head and impingement on the acromion. These findings are strongly suggestive of rotator cuff tear. **B.** Oblique coronal ultrasound shows a complete tear of the supraspinatus tendon and demonstrates the free ends of the torn tendon (*arrows*). DELT, deltoid; HH, humeral head; IST, infraspinatus. (Courtesy Mihra Taljanovic, MD, Department of Radiology, University of Arizona.)

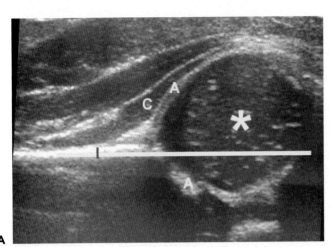

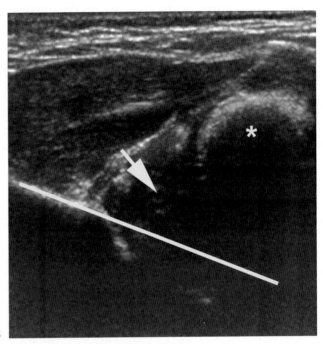

Figure 11.20.   Congenital hip dysplasia. A. Ultrasound examination shows lateral subluxation of femoral head (*) with application of pressure. Normally, an extension of a line drawn along the ischium (*I*) should pass through the center of the femoral head. **B.** Dislocation of femoral head. With pressure, the femoral head echoes disappear (*arrow*) and the echoes of the femoral neck now can be seen (*). A, acetabulum; C, cartilaginous portion of acetabular roof. (Courtesy of Leonard E. Swischuk, MD, University of Texas at Galveston.)

nuclear imaging. The phosphorus contained within the isotope is exchanged in areas of rapid bone turnover (metabolism): destructive lesions such as osteomyelitis, tumors, arthritis, and areas of growing bone. Although the scan itself is not specific for a particular disease, it indicates an area of bony abnormality to which radiography, CT, or MR may be directed. The bone scan is often positive before the conventional radiograph shows any abnormality in a particular bone. It should be used as the primary screening examination for detecting metastases (Fig. 11.21) and fractures (Fig. 11.22) and in cases of suspected child abuse (Fig. 11.23). A notable exception, when the bone scan is not useful in diffuse bone disease, is in cases of multiple myeloma. Little or no abnormal uptake of the isotope occurs in that disorder.

The typical *bone scan* is performed in three phases. First is the *vascular phase,* which consists of serial images performed at 2- to 5-second intervals to follow the flow of the isotope through the vascular system. This phase can indicate areas of increased or decreased blood flow. Second is the *blood-pool phase,* which consists of static images to determine areas of hyperemia, such as would occur in osteomyelitis. Third is the *delayed phase,* which consists of static images of the skeleton obtained 2 to 3 hours after injection to determine areas of increased tracer uptake or areas of decreased uptake (photopenia). On rare occasions, when vertebral collapse from osteoporosis or metastases is suspected, a fourth phase is obtained at 24 hours to compare the ratio of residual isotope in abnormal vertebrae versus normal vertebrae.

As mentioned previously, the *technetium scan* is often nonspecific. One area where a more specific isotope scan may be used is in suspected osteomyelitis. These studies use indium-111–labeled white cells to identify areas of inflammatory activity (Fig. 11.24). This is particularly useful in a patient who may have an infection around a metallic implant (plate, screw, rod, or prosthesis), because the metal often produces artifacts in MR imaging.

Arthrography is the study of joints, using contrast material that is injected into the joint space. Two varieties are performed. In *conventional arthrography,* iodinated contrast is injected without or with air into the shoulder to detect tears of the rotator cuff (Fig. 11.25) or into the

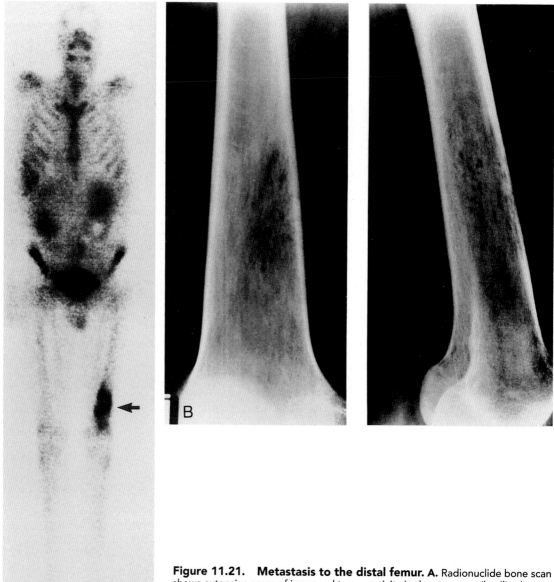

Figure 11.21.   Metastasis to the distal femur. A. Radionuclide bone scan shows extensive areas of increased tracer activity in the sternum, ribs, iliac bones, and distal left femur (*arrow*). **B.** Frontal and lateral radiographs of the distal left femur show a moth-eaten to permeative bony destructive process.

wrist for ligamentous tears (Fig. 11.26). This type of study is also used in evaluating patients with painful joint prostheses (Fig. 11.27). Although conventional arthrography has largely been replaced by MR imaging, it still is used for patients who are unable to go into the magnet. The second type of arthrography is the *MR arthrogram.* In this procedure, dilute paramagnetic agents are injected into the joint before MR examination (see Fig. 11.16). MR arthrography has the advantage over unenhanced MR imaging in that it clearly identifies tears of cartilage, tendons, and ligaments that may or may not have been demonstrated on the conventional study (Fig. 11.28).

Percutaneous bone biopsy is a procedure that diagnostic radiologists can perform using any imaging modality that will show the lesion; however, CT is the method of choice (see Fig. 11.3). In addition to obtaining tissue for pathologic diagnosis, CT-guided excision of osteoid osteomas is replacing conventional surgical excision because of its greater accuracy in localization, lower morbidity, and lower cost. Furthermore, CT-guided injections of steroids, alcohol, or methyl

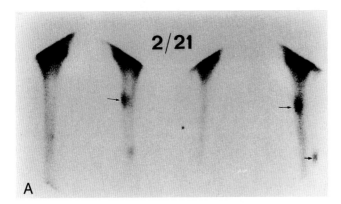

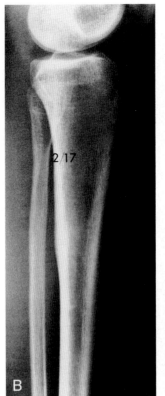

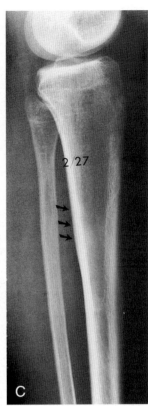

Figure 11.22.   Stress fracture of the tibia in a runner.
A. Radionuclide bone scan shows an area of tracer uptake in the proximal tibia (*long arrow*). A second area is present in the distal fibula (*short arrow*). **B.** Lateral radiograph made 4 days earlier is normal. **C.** Lateral radiograph made 10 days after the first shows periosteal new bone formation in the posterior tibia (*arrows*).

Figure 11.23.   Child abuse. Radionuclide bone scan demonstrates multiple areas of tracer activity in the ribs (*arrows*), a finding considered pathognomonic for child abuse.

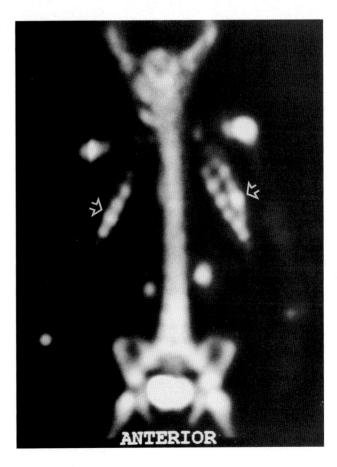

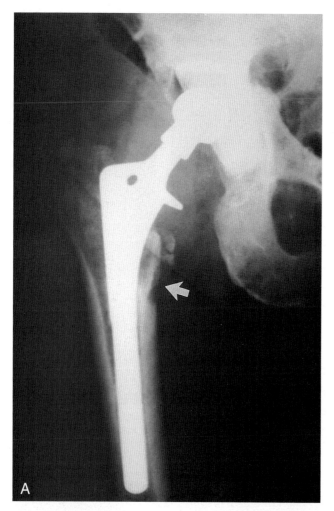

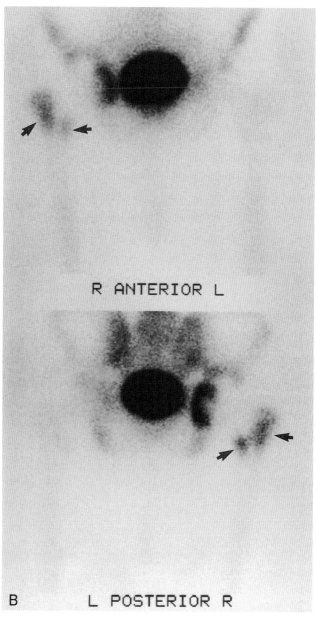

R ANTERIOR L

B   L POSTERIOR R

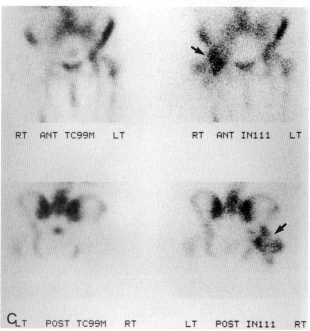

RT ANT TC99M LT   RT ANT IN111 LT

C LT POST TC99M RT   LT POST IN111 RT

Figure 11.24.   Infection at site of hip implant. A. Radiograph shows a lucency in the vicinity of the lesser trochanter (*arrow*) in a patient with a painful prosthesis. **B.** Conventional bone scan shows increased tracer activity in both trochanters (*arrows*). Is this normal postoperative change or evidence of loosening or infection? The main portion of the femoral head is photopenic because of the presence of the prosthesis. **C.** Concomitant technetium-99m bone marrow scan (left) and indium-111 white blood cell scan (right) show the marrow area of the right hip to be photopenic while there is increased white cell concentration on the indium study (*arrows*). This is considered pathognomonic for infection.

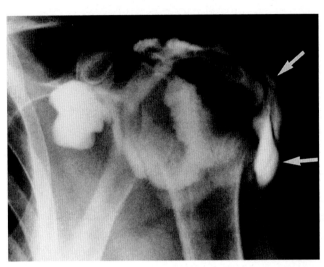

Figure 11.25. Shoulder arthrogram demonstrating a complete rotator cuff tear. Contrast injected into the glenohumeral joint has extravasated into the subacromial/subdeltoid bursa (*arrows*). An intact rotator cuff prevents this from occurring.

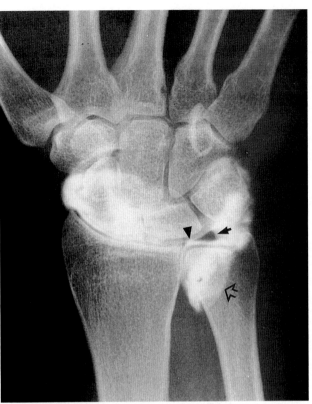

Figure 11.26. Triangular fibrocartilage tear. Wrist arthrogram demonstrates extravasation of contrast into the distal radioulnar joint space (*open arrow*). Notice the tear (*arrowhead*) in the triangular fibrocartilage (*short arrow*) at its point of origin from the distal radius.

Figure 11.27. Loose total knee implant. Subtraction film following intra-articular injection of contrast shows the contrast tracking between bone and cement at the site of implantation of the tibial component (*arrows*).

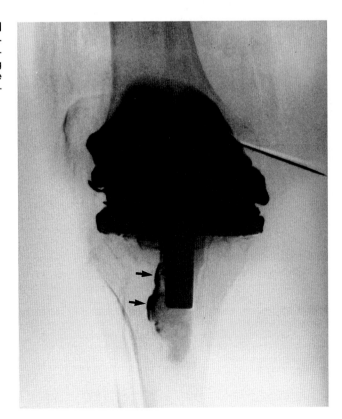

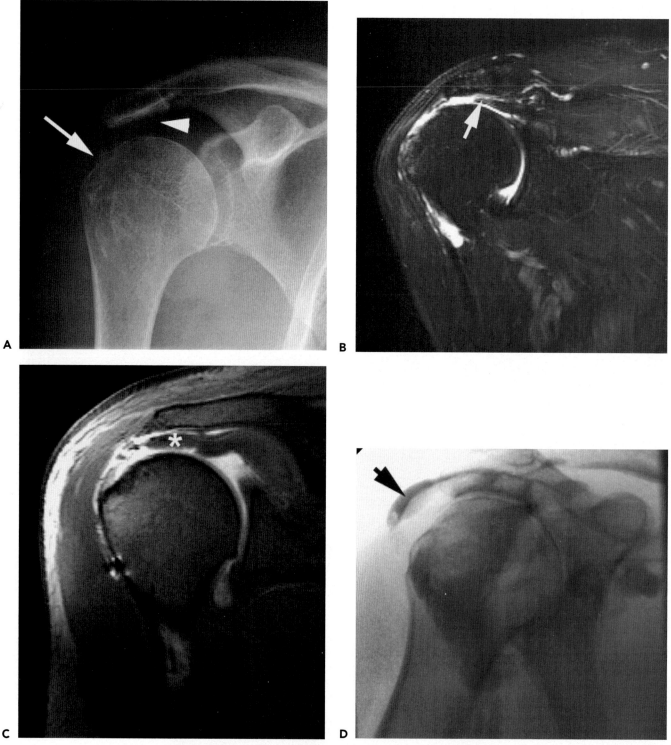

Figure 11.28.   MR arthrograms demonstrating rotator cuff tears in two different patients.
A. Radiograph shows irregularity of the greater tuberosity of the humerus (*arrow*) and the undersurface of
the acromion (*arrowhead*). These findings are typical of rotator cuff disease and impingement. **B.** Coronal
oblique MR image demonstrates extravasation of contrast into the subdeltoid bursa through a tear in the
supraspinatus tendon, which is retracted (*arrow*). **C.** Coronal oblique MR image in another patient demonstrates shredding and atrophy of the supraspinatus tendon (*) with extravasation of contrast into the
subdeltoid bursa. **D.** Radiographic spot film taken at the time of injection shows extravasated contrast
(*arrow*) in the subdeltoid bursa.

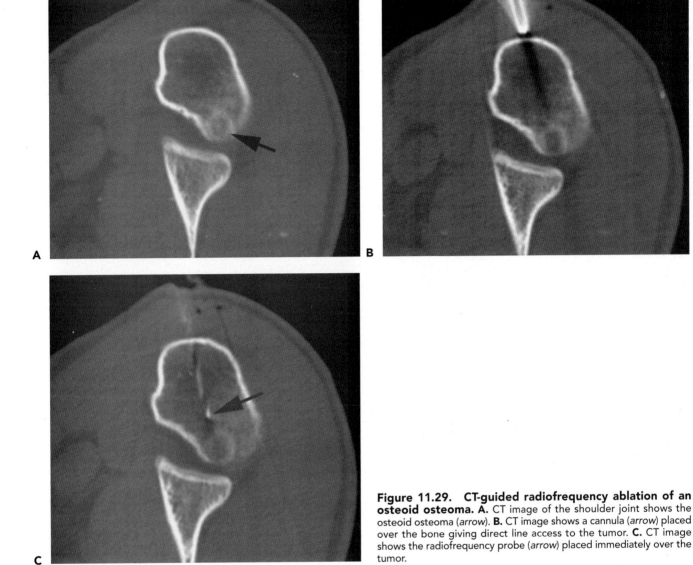

Figure 11.29. CT-guided radiofrequency ablation of an osteoid osteoma. A. CT image of the shoulder joint shows the osteoid osteoma (*arrow*). **B.** CT image shows a cannula (*arrow*) placed over the bone giving direct line access to the tumor. **C.** CT image shows the radiofrequency probe (*arrow*) placed immediately over the tumor.

methacrylate into bone tumors or tumorlike lesions is commonplace at large medical centers. A variation on this procedure is the ablation of osteoid osteomas by a radiofrequency probe placed under CT guidance (Fig. 11.29). Another variation of this procedure is CT-guided screw placement for sacroiliac instability (see Fig. 11.4) or for acetabular fractures.

Angiography is used infrequently to evaluate patients with suspected bone tumors because MR has largely superseded it for this purpose. However, in these patients, angiography may be performed to localize tumor vessels for either embolization or chemotherapy infusion. Angiography is also used to evaluate blood vessels in severe skeletal trauma where vascular injury is suspected (Fig. 11.30).

Concern for patients with osteoporosis and its subsequent morbidity and mortality has led to the development of several methods of assessing bone mineral density using imaging studies: dual x-ray absorptiometry (DXA), CT densitometry, and a sonogram device for scanning of the calcaneus. Each of these methods has advantages and drawbacks in terms of sensitivity and accuracy. However, at present, DXA scanning is the procedure of choice (Fig. 11.31). Using a database of normal bone density for comparison, this modality provides an objective assessment of a patient's bone mineral density. This is helpful in initial diagnosis and reevaluation

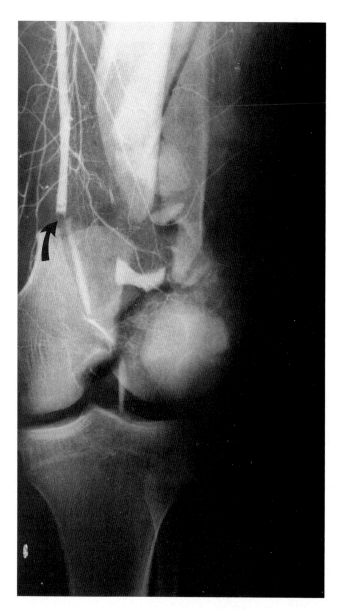

Figure 11.30. Transected femoral artery (*arrow*) in a patient with a severely comminuted intercondylar fracture of the distal femur.

after therapy is initiated. If you have a patient for whom you are considering performing a bone densitometry study, you should consult your radiologist.

ANATOMIC CONSIDERATIONS

The anatomy of each of the 206 bones in the skeleton is not reviewed here; for that purpose, you can consult an anatomy textbook. However, you should remember that because you are dealing with three-dimensional structures in the skeleton, many bony projections may overlap and produce "strange" images with which you are not familiar. The best way to avoid this confusion is to have a thorough knowledge of the anatomy of the bone being studied.

Bones are grouped into five types based on their shapes:

1. *Long bones,* which have two ends and a shaft (femur, humerus, and, interestingly, phalanges, which are miniature long bones)
2. *Short bones,* which are typically six sided (carpal and tarsal bones)
3. *Flat bones* (calvaria, ribs, os coxae, and sternum)

4. *Irregular bones,* which have many sides (vertebrae)
5. *Sesamoid bones,* which lack periosteum and develop in tendons (the largest is the patella)

Furthermore, there are two architectural types of bone: *compact* (dense) and *cancellous* (spongy). The distribution of these types of bones depends on the stress to which each bone is subjected.

There are three locations within a long bone: the *epiphysis,* or growth center; the *metaphysis,* an area that lies just beneath the *physis,* or growth plate; and the *diaphysis,* or shaft. Bone growth occurs at the physis. The blood supply to the metaphysis is the most prominent, which explains the frequent occurrence of infections and tumors at that location. Flat bones such as the os coxae have *metaphyseal equivalent* areas. As discussed later, these locations are of considerable importance in predicting the nature of some bone lesions.

PATHOLOGIC CONSIDERATIONS

The analysis of bone and joint lesions can be as simple as the ABCS:

Anatomic appearance and alignment abnormalities
Bony mineralization and texture abnormalities
Cartilage (joint space) abnormalities
Soft tissue abnormalities

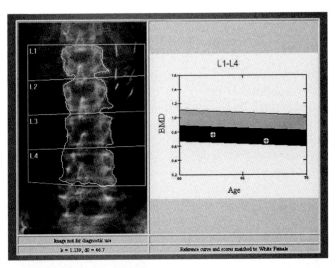

A

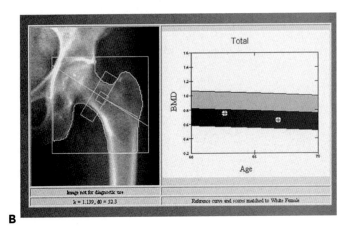

B

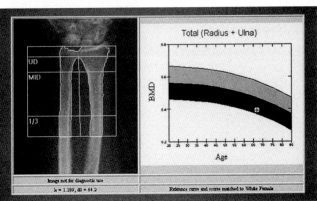

C

Figure 11.31. Dual x-ray absorptiometry bone densitometry scans. A. Lumbar scan. **B.** Right hip scan. **C.** Right wrist scan. The images show the areas studied at each level. The data from each measurement reflect the bone mineral density (BMD). A graphic printout for each level shows the patient's average density (+) at below the mean for her age. The complete scan has charts of all the measurements.

TABLE 11.1

DISTRIBUTION OF BONE DISEASE BY PATHOLOGIC CATEGORY

Category	Distribution		
	Monostotic	**Polyostotic**	**Diffuse**
Congenital	X	X	
Inflammatory	X	X	
Neoplastic	X	X	X
Metabolic	(X)	(X)	X
Traumatic	X	X	
Vascular	X	X	

Each of these will be elaborated on later in the chapter. Using this analytical approach, however, you will find how adept you will be at recognizing and diagnosing many bone and joint lesions.

There are six basic pathologic categories of skeletal disease: *congenital, inflammatory, metabolic, neoplastic, traumatic,* and *vascular.* A seventh category, *miscellaneous* or *other,* might be added to encompass diseases that do not fall strictly into one of the first six.

The logical approach to musculoskeletal radiology begins by defining the *distribution* of a lesion and by applying a number of factors that can further narrow the diagnostic choices. These factors have been termed *predictor variables.*

Distribution

The distribution of a bone or joint lesion provides important clues to the etiology of that lesion. Lesions may be *monostotic* or *monoarticular*—that is, confined to one bone or joint; *polyostotic* or *polyarticular*—that is, located in many bones or joints; or *diffuse*—that is, involving virtually every bone or joint. Applying this distribution pattern to the six pathologic categories produces the scheme shown in Table 11.1. As the table shows, only two disease categories may occur diffusely: neoplastic and metabolic. Metabolic disease by definition is a diffuse disease; however, occasionally monostotic or polyostotic forms occur. Examples of these lesions are shown in Table 11.2.

TABLE 11.2

EXAMPLES OF DISTRIBUTION: PATHOLOGIC RELATIONSHIPS

Category	Monostotic/Articular	Polyostotic/Articular	Diffuse
Congenital	Cervical rib	Cleidocranial dysplasia	
Inflammatory	Osteomyelitis, gout	Congenital lues, rheumatoid arthritis	
Neoplastic	Any primary bone tumor	Myeloma	Metastasis
Metabolic	(Paget disease)	(Paget disease, fibrous dysplasia)	Osteopetrosis, hyperparathyroidism
Traumatic	Single fracture	Multiple fractures, battered child	
Vascular	Perthes disease	Perthes disease	

TABLE 11.3

PREDICTOR VARIABLES FOR BONE AND JOINT LESIONS

Behavior of the lesion
  Osteolytic
  Osteoblastic
  Mixed

Bone or joint involved
Locus within a bone
  Epiphysis (or apophysis)
  Metaphysis (or equivalent)
  Diaphysis

Age, gender, and race of patient
Margin of lesion
  Sharply defined
  Poorly defined

Shape of lesion
  Longer than wide
  Wider than long
    Cortical breakthrough
    No breakthrough

Joint space involvement
Bony reaction (if any)
  Periosteal
    Solid
    Laminated ("onionskin")
    Spiculated, sunburst, "hair on end"
    Codman triangle
  Sclerosis
  Buttressing

Matrix production
  Osteoid
  Chondroid
  Mixed

Soft tissue changes
History of trauma or surgery

Predictor Variables

Eleven predictor variables may be applied to the radiographic appearance of any bone or joint lesion to help you make a correct diagnosis. Table 11.3 enumerates and expands these diagnostic parameters. They are also explained here.

It should become apparent from the discussion that many of these variables apply to the diagnosis of bone tumors. However, primary bone tumors, exclusive of myeloma, are rare lesions. You should recognize that, in many instances, you may not be able to make a specific diagnosis even after applying all these factors. Radiologists should be satisfied that they have done their best when they have been able to categorize a difficult lesion as either *aggressive* or *nonaggressive* and have thus decided whether the lesion needs to undergo biopsy.

Behavior of the Lesion

Bone lesions may be primarily *osteolytic* (*osteoclastic* or *bone destroying*) or *osteoblastic* (*bone forming, reactive,* or *reparative*); occasionally, you will see a mixture of the two. Lytic lesions are usually the result of increased osteoclastic activity. The pathologic entity (infection or tumor) stimulates the multinucleated osteoclasts or giant cells to literally make room for it. This explains the presence of giant cells in so many pathologic bone lesions. There are three forms of osteolytic bone destruction: geographic, moth-eaten, and permeative. *Geographic* destruction implies that large areas of bone have been destroyed and are easily visible with the unaided eye (Fig. 11.32). A *moth-eaten* appearance is one in which there are many discrete, small holes throughout the bone, similar to a piece of clothing ruined by moth larvae (Fig. 11.33). A moth-eaten appearance suggests a more aggressive lesion. A *permeative* pattern is one in which there is fine bony destruction (Fig. 11.34). Pathologically, this represents a lesion diffusely infiltrating bone through the Haversian system. In many instances, a magnifying lens is required to see the bone destruction. Permeative destruction implies a very aggressive process, such as the round cell tumors of bone (Ewing tumor, myeloma, reticulum cell sarcoma), or osteomyelitis.

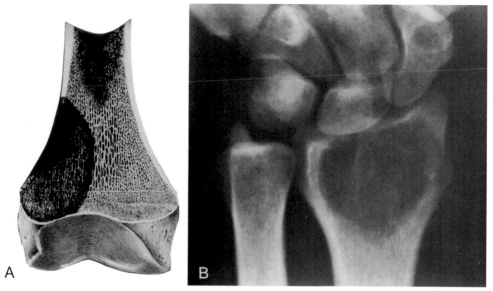

Figure 11.32.   Geographic bone destruction. A. Drawing showing a large destructive lesion that is easily seen with the unaided eye. **B.** Giant cell tumor of the distal radius, an example of a geographic lesion.

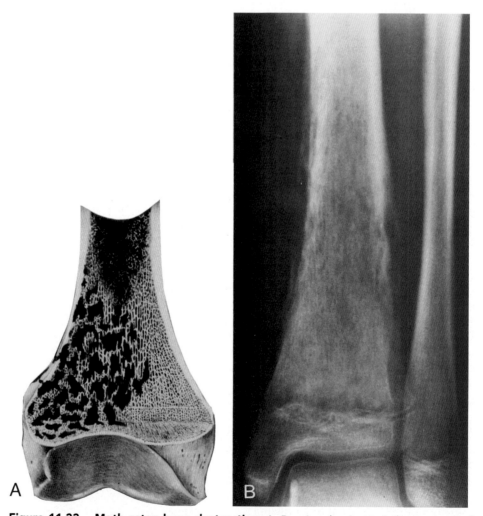

Figure 11.33.   Moth-eaten bone destruction. A. Drawing showing typical appearance of moth-eaten destruction. In most instances, this may be seen with the unaided eye. **B.** Osteomyelitis of the distal tibia, an example of moth-eaten bony destruction.

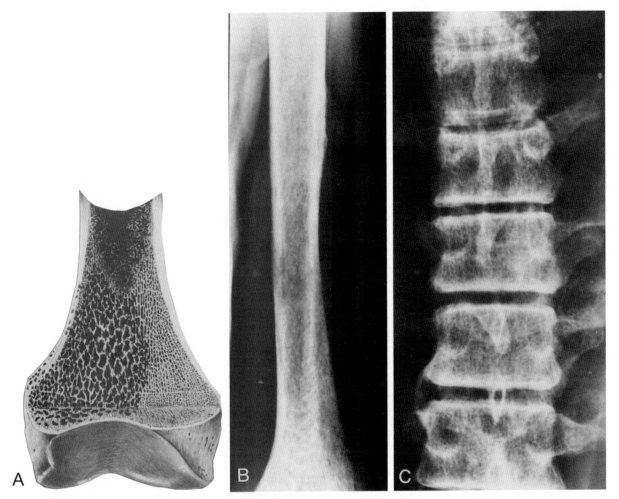

Figure 11.34.   Permeative or infiltrative bone destruction. A. Drawing showing the pathologic process is infiltrating the Haversian system. Magnification may be required to see the lesion. **B.** Permeative bony destruction in a patient with metastatic breast carcinoma involving the entire humerus. Notice the severe soft tissue wasting, an indication of cachexia in this patient. **C.** Permeative destruction of the vertebrae in a patient with multiple myeloma. At first glance, this appears like osteoporosis. On closer inspection, there is actual bone destruction.

Bone or Joint Involved

Some diseases have a predilection for certain bones or joints. Figure 11.35 illustrates the preferred locations of many common bone and joint lesions. Notice, for example, that chondrosarcomas (Fig. 11.36) favor the pelvis, whereas enchondromas (Fig. 11.37) favor the phalanges and metacarpals; Paget disease commonly affects the pelvis, skull, spine, and tibia but spares the fibula (Fig. 11.38); gout favors the bones of the hands and feet (Fig. 11.39) as does rheumatoid arthritis (Fig. 11.40); and hyperparathyroidism commonly affects the skull, distal clavicles, and the hands and feet (Fig. 11.41). It is important to remember, however, that any lesion may be found in an unusual site (for example, a chondrosarcoma of the skull base). When that occurs, the lesion usually has all the characteristics of the entity at a more typical location. When confronted by a lesion in what may seem an unusual site, mentally transfer that lesion to the knee, one of the most common locations for benign and malignant processes, and the identity may become more apparent.

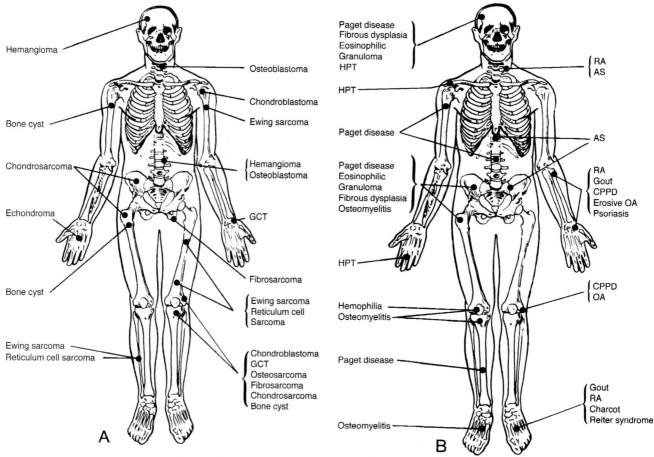

Figure 11.35.   Preferred locations for bone lesions. A. Neoplastic conditions. **B.** Non-neoplastic conditions. AS, ankylosing spondylitis; CPPD, calcium pyrophosphate deposition disease; GCT, giant cell tumor; HPT, hyperparathyroidism; OA, osteoarthritis; RA, rheumatoid arthritis.

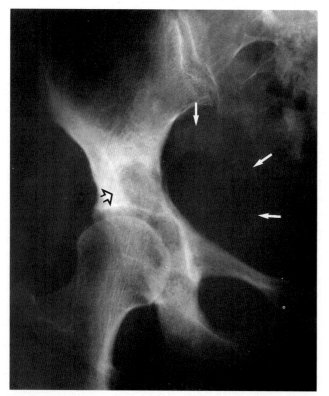

Figure 11.36.   Chondrosarcoma of the pelvis. There is a large lytic lesion just above the acetabulum (*open arrow*). An associated soft tissue mass with flocculent calcification extends into the pelvis (*closed arrows*).

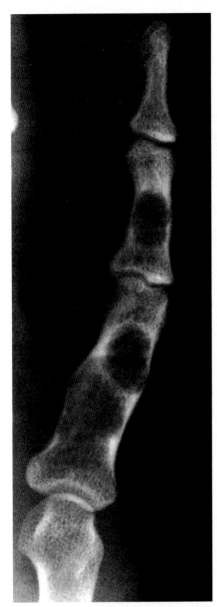

Figure 11.37. Enchondromas of the proximal and middle phalanges.

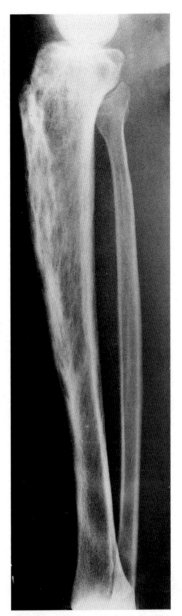

Figure 11.38.   Paget disease of the tibia. Notice that the fibula is spared.

Locus Within Bone or Joint

The location of a lesion within a bone or joint can provide an important clue to the identity. Many lesions have a predilection for the epiphysis, metaphysis, or diaphysis. The common locations of bone tumors are shown in Figure 11.42. Nonneoplastic lesions also have a predilection for favored areas of bones or joints; for example, osteoarthritis prefers the weight-bearing surfaces of the large joints (Fig. 11.43), whereas rheumatoid arthritis affects the entire surface of the same joint (Fig. 11.44). Osteomyelitis favors the diametaphyseal region where red marrow is prevalent. Similarly, Langerhans cell histiocytosis (histiocytosis X, eosinophilic granuloma) is found in areas rich in red marrow.

The various arthritides favor not only joints but also sites within and around a joint. Each synovial joint consists of three parts: a cartilage-bearing surface, an area devoid of cartilage called the "bare" or para-articular area, and a joint capsule. Both the areas with and without

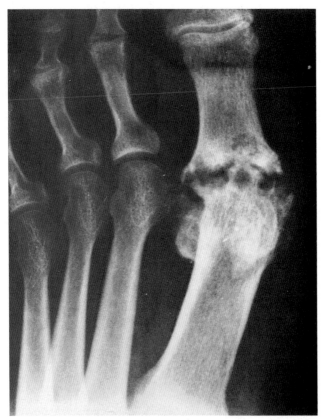

Figure 11.39.   Gout. The metatarsophalangeal joint of the great toe is severely involved in this patient with long-standing gout.

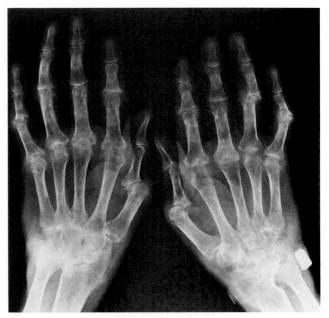

Figure 11.40.   Rheumatoid arthritis of the hands and wrists. Notice the involvement of the wrist joints, the metacarpophalangeal joints, and interphalangeal joints.

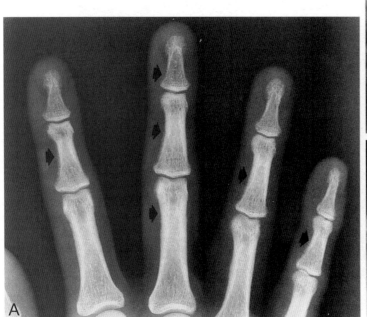

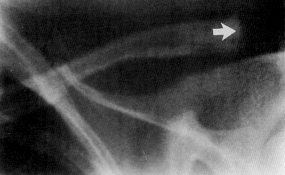

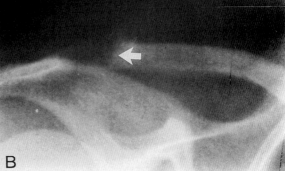

Figure 11.41.   Hyperparathyroidism. A. Detail view of the hands shows subperiosteal resorption in the phalanges (*arrows*). **B.** Detail views of both distal clavicles show subchondral resorption bilaterally (*arrows*).   *(continued on page 397)*

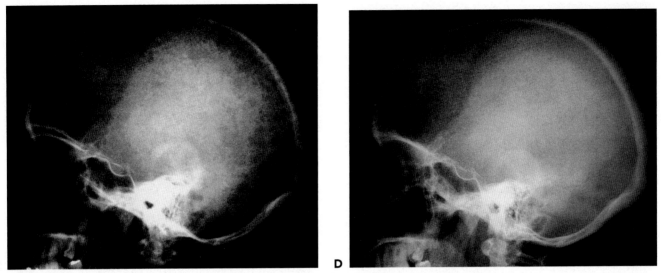

C   **D**

Figure 11.41. *(continued)* **C.** Skull radiograph shows the typical "salt and pepper" appearance caused by the osteoporosis. **D.** Skull radiograph of same patient 6 months after removal of the patient's parathyroid adenoma. The bones have returned to normal.

Figure 11.42. Common locations of bone tumors. Chondroblastoma favors the epiphysis in the skeletally immature patient. Round cell lesions favor the diaphysis. The majority of other lesions favor the metaphysis. Giant cell tumors will extend to the joint surface in a skeletally mature patient.

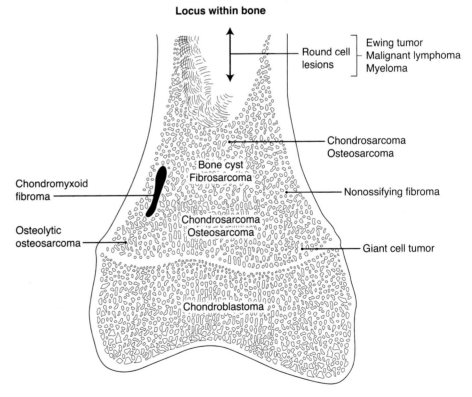

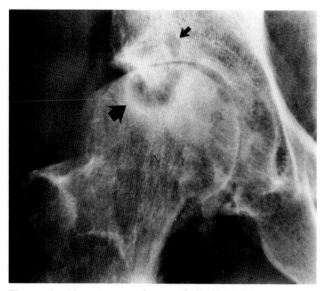

Figure 11.43.   Osteoarthritis of the hip. The hip joint has narrowed, particularly superiorly. Large degenerative synovial cysts (geodes) are present in both the femoral head (*fat arrow*) and acetabulum (*small arrow*). Notice the osteophyte formation in both the acetabulum and femoral head.

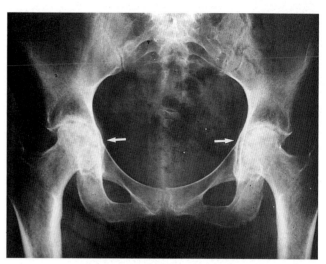

Figure 11.44.   Rheumatoid arthritis of the hips. There is medial migration of both femoral heads (protrusio acetabula, *arrows*). Notice that the entire joint is involved in rheumatoid arthritis. Compare with Figure 11.43.

cartilage are contained within the joint capsule (Fig. 11.45). Diseases such as rheumatoid arthritis and osteoarthritis primarily involve the cartilage areas (Fig. 11.46), while gout, psoriatic arthritis, and reactive arthritis affect the bare (para-articular) areas (Fig. 11.47).

Age, Gender, and Race of the Patient

The distribution of bone diseases also depends on the patient's age. A 10-year-old child with a permeative lesion of the shaft of the humerus is likely to have a Ewing tumor (Fig. 11.48). A lesion of similar appearance in a much older patient should suggest malignant lymphoma (reticulum cell sarcoma) of bone. The clinician can often predict the type of a malignant bone tumor on the basis of the patient's age. For example, the most common type of tumor in

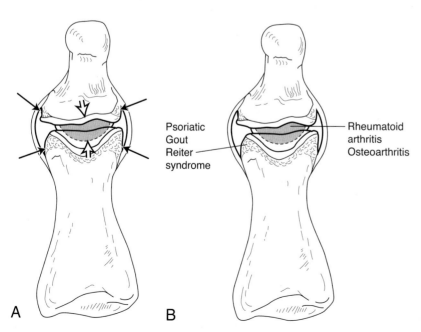

Psoriatic
Gout
Reiter
syndrome

Rheumatoid
arthritis
Osteoarthritis

A   B

Figure 11.45.   Drawings illustrating joint surfaces. A. The two areas within the joint capsule are the cartilage area (*open arrows*) and the "bare" (para-articular) areas (*solid arrows*). **B.** Rheumatoid arthritis and osteoarthritis primarily affect the cartilage areas. Psoriatic arthritis, gout, and the arthropathy of reactive arthritis affect the bare areas. In the late stages of all arthropathies, all areas of the joint are involved.

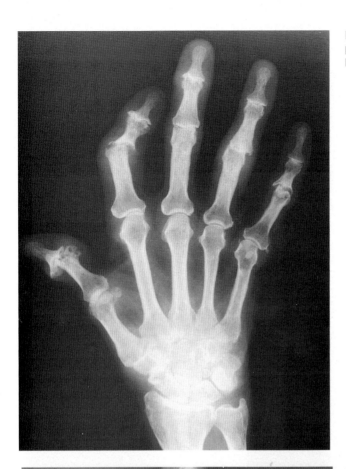

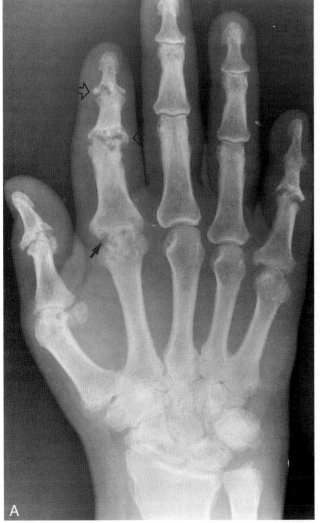

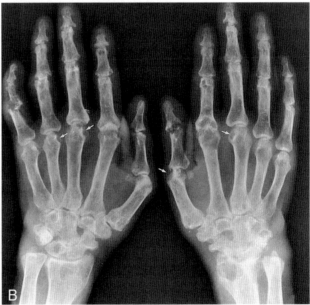

Figure 11.46. Erosive osteoarthritis. The cartilage areas are primarily affected, giving a "gull wing" appearance to the distal interphalangeal joints of the first three digits.

Figure 11.47. Involvement of the "bare" (para-articular) areas. A. Psoriatic arthropathy (advanced). The disease affects the bare areas initially, as shown in the second metacarpophalangeal joint (*solid arrow*). Notice the new bone formation at the bases of the middle and distal phalanges of the second digit (*open arrows*), giving a "mouse ear" configuration. In addition there is the "single ray phenomenon," in which all the joints of the first, second, and fifth digits are involved. **B.** Gout showing involvement of the para-articular areas of multiple distal metacarpals (*arrows*).

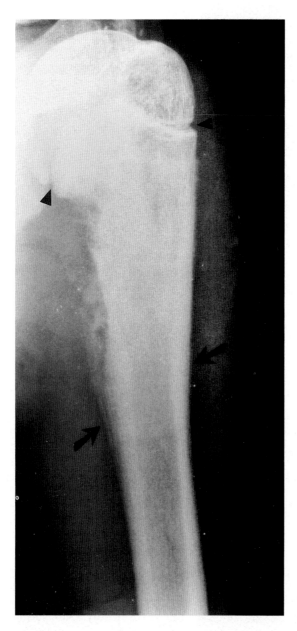

Figure 11.48. Ewing tumor of the proximal humerus. A large destructive lesion is in the diametaphyseal region. Flocculent reactive bone is present. Notice the interrupted laminated periosteal reaction (*arrows*). This lesion may easily be confused with an osteosarcoma. The open physis in the humerus (*arrowheads*) puts the patient in an age group that would favor Ewing tumor.

patients under 1 year of age is neuroblastoma; in the first decade, Ewing tumor of tubular bone; ages 10 to 30 years, osteosarcoma and Ewing tumor of flat bones; between ages 30 and 40 years, most of the malignant sarcomas; and over age 40 years, metastatic carcinoma, along with multiple myeloma and chondrosarcoma.

Certain benign lesions also occur more commonly in certain age groups. For example, Paget disease is almost never seen in patients younger than age 40 years. Infantile cortical hyperostosis (Caffey disease) does not occur in patients over age 1 year.

Many lesions also have a gender distribution. Paget disease is found more commonly in males. Rheumatoid arthritis, fibrous dysplasia, and congenital hip dysplasia favor females.

In addition to gender predominance, there is a racial predominance in some diseases, such as sickle cell disease (African descent), thalassemia (Mediterranean descent), and Gaucher disease (Ashkenazic Jewish descent).

Margin of Lesion

The border between normal and abnormal bone is called the *transition zone*. Careful attention to this area will yield a wealth of information regarding the biologic behavior of bone lesions.

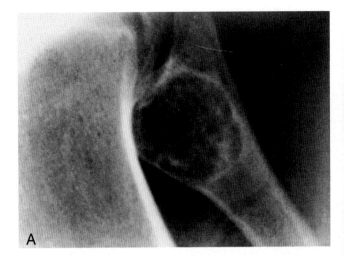

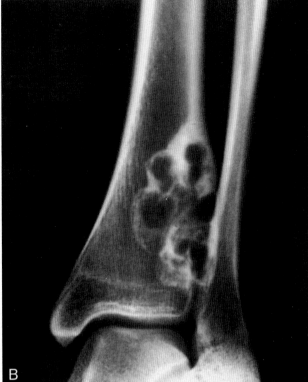

Figure 11.49.   Benign lesions demonstrating a sharp transition zone. A. Enchondroma of the head of the fibula. Notice the flocculent chondroid matrix within the lesion. **B.** Benign fibrous cortical defect (fibroxanthoma). A sclerotic border around this bubbly benign lesion clearly defines the transition between normal and abnormal bone. If asymptomatic, both of these lesions should be left alone.

In general, an abrupt transition zone that appears as a dense area of sclerosis between a lesion and normal bone or as a thin, well-defined line between normal and abnormal bone (Fig. 11.49) indicates a nonaggressive or benign process. On the other hand, a broad or wide, poorly defined zone between normal and abnormal bone indicates a more aggressive lesion (Fig. 11.50). The differences in the growth rate of these lesions account for the differences in their appearance. Slow-growing, benign lesions such as a fibroxanthoma of bone (see Fig. 11.49B) or a focus of tuberculosis progress at a rate slow enough to allow the bone to react in an attempt to contain them. An aggressive lesion, such as a malignant tumor or osteomyelitis, progresses at a rapid rate, and the bone is unable to respond adequately. Furthermore, a sclerotic margin that is thick with fuzzy borders should suggest an inflammatory lesion such as sclerosing osteomyelitis or tuberculosis.

Shape of Lesion

The shape of a lesion indicates its growth rate in the same way that the margin does. A lesion that is longer than it is wide—that is, oriented with the shaft of the bone—is likely to be a nonaggressive benign process. In this situation, the lesion is growing with bone and not faster than bone. On the other hand, a lesion that is wider than the bone, has broken out of the bone, and has extended into the soft tissues is a more aggressive type of lesion (Fig. 11.51). MR imaging is particularly useful for assessing the extraosseous extent of bone lesions.

Joint Space Involved or Crossed

If a lesion involves or crosses a joint space, it most likely has an inflammatory origin. This is generally the case, no matter how aggressive or malignant a process may appear (Fig. 11.52). Infections will extend across a joint space, but tumors will not. Tumors that have a predilection for the ends of bones, such as chondroblastoma and giant cell tumor (Fig. 11.53), will extend to the joint but will not cross it. Furthermore, even the most malignant bone tumors respect

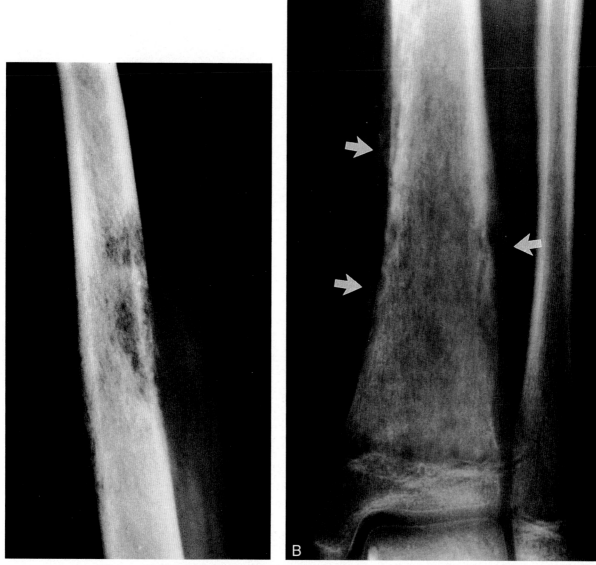

A

B

Figure 11.50.   Aggressive lesions demonstrating poor transition zone. A. Metastatic lung carcinoma. **B.** Osteomyelitis. It is impossible to tell where normal bone is. Notice the periosteal reaction (*arrows*). Each of these lesions requires a biopsy to make a diagnosis.

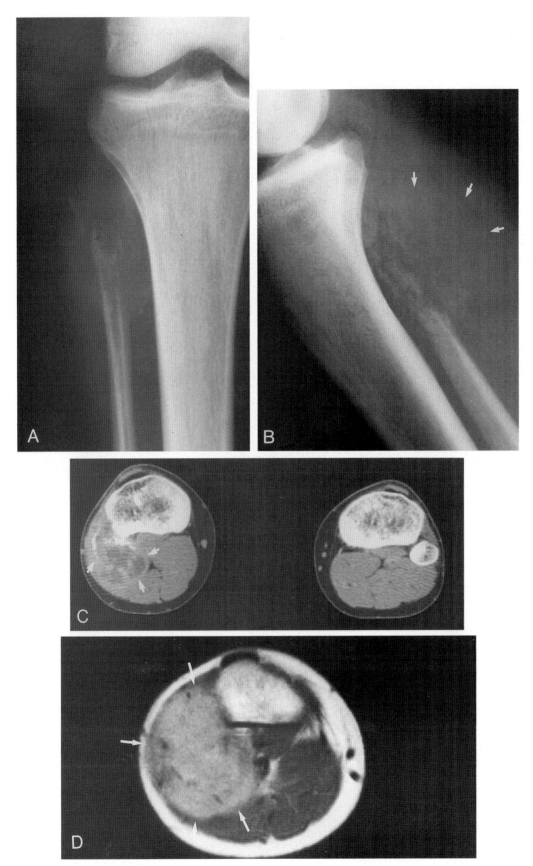

Figure 11.51. Osteosarcoma of the proximal fibula. A. Frontal radiograph shows a poorly defined destructive lesion involving the head and proximal shaft of the fibula. The lesion has broken out of bone. **B.** Lateral radiograph shows the lesion to extend into the soft tissues (*arrows*). **C.** CT image shows the lesion extending into the soft tissues on the right side (*arrows*). **D.** T2-weighted MR image shows the soft tissue involvement to better advantage (*arrows*).

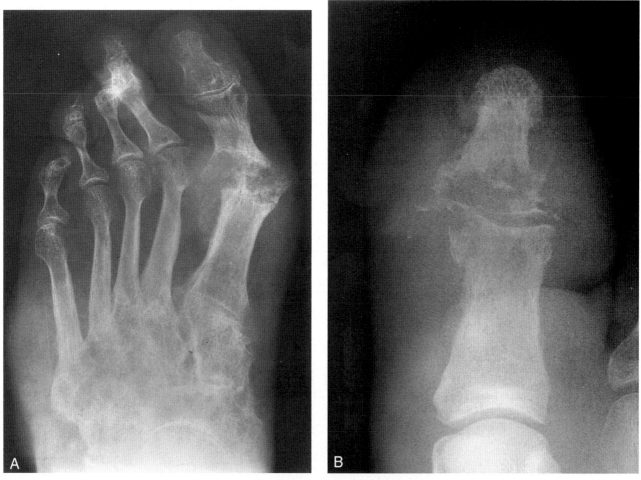

Figure 11.52. Joint space involvement. A. Tophaceous gout. **B.** Osteomyelitis and joint space infection in a diabetic patient. These extensive destructive lesions involve both sides of the joint. This signifies that the process is either an arthropathy or an infection.

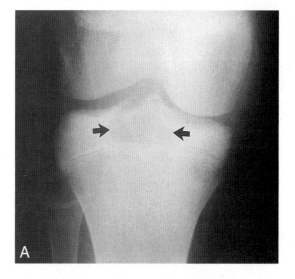

Figure 11.53. Epiphyseal tumors. A. Chondroblastoma (*arrows*) of the proximal tibia. The lesion has not crossed the physis. (*continued on page 405*)

Figure 11.53. *(continued)* **B.** Giant cell tumor of the distal tibia. This large bubbly lesion extends down to the joint line *(arrows)* but has not crossed it. As a rule, tumors respect joint surfaces and physes.

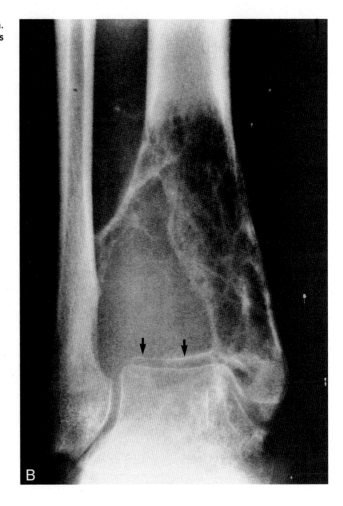

the cartilage of the physes (Fig. 11.54). On the other hand, abnormalities found on both sides of a joint that has *intact cortical margins* should suggest a polyostotic disorder rather than an arthropathy.

Bony Reaction

Bony responses to insult include periosteal reaction, sclerosis, and buttressing. *Periosteal reaction* is of four varieties: solid, laminated or onionskin, spiculated ("sunburst" or "hair on end"), or Codman triangle. *Solid* (uninterrupted, organized, or wavy) periosteal reaction (greater than 2 mm) indicates a benign process. It most often occurs in osteomyelitis (Fig. 11.55) and fracture healing. A *laminated* (layered) or *onionskin* type of periosteal reaction indicates *repetitive injury* to bone. This was previously thought to be pathognomonic of Ewing tumor or reticulum cell sarcoma of bone. However, this type of reaction also occurs in any type of repetitive injury to bone, such as in child abuse. Once again, the nature of the laminated periosteal reaction may be determined by its thickness. In a Ewing tumor, the periosteal reaction is thin, irregular, and disorganized (Fig. 11.56), whereas in a benign process such as osteomyelitis or repetitive trauma, such as child abuse (Fig. 11.57), the reaction is considerably thicker and often wavy. A *spiculated, "sunburst,"* or *"hair-on-end"* appearance is almost always associated with a malignant bone lesion (Fig. 11.58), most often an osteosarcoma. Occasionally, this type of periosteal pattern occurs in Ewing tumors and in metastatic squamous cell tumors. This form of periosteal reaction is the result of the neoplastic process breaking through a layer of periosteal new bone, followed by new periosteal response and subsequent breakthrough. The *Codman triangle* represents triangular ossification of a piece of periosteum that has been elevated (see Figs. 11.56A and 11.58B). In the

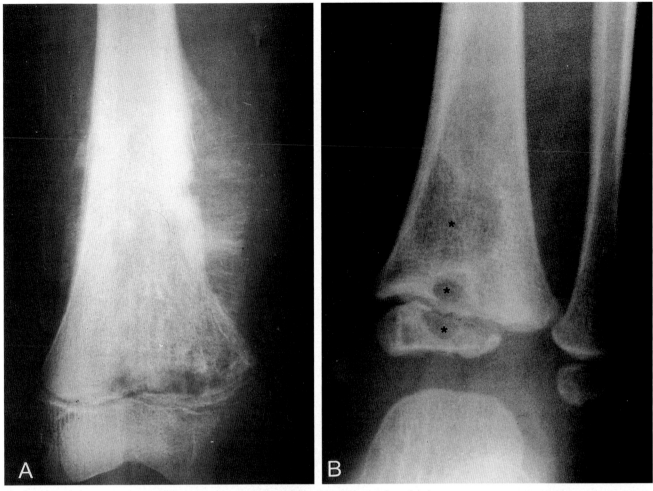

Figure 11.54. Relationship of lesions to the physis. A, osteosarcoma extends down to the physis but does not cross it. **B,** tuberculous osteomyelitis has produced cystic lesions (*) on both sides of the physis. The ankle joint is still not crossed.

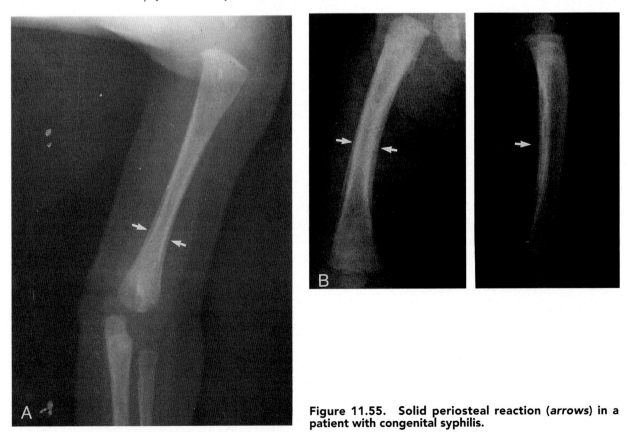

Figure 11.55. Solid periosteal reaction (*arrows*) in a patient with congenital syphilis.

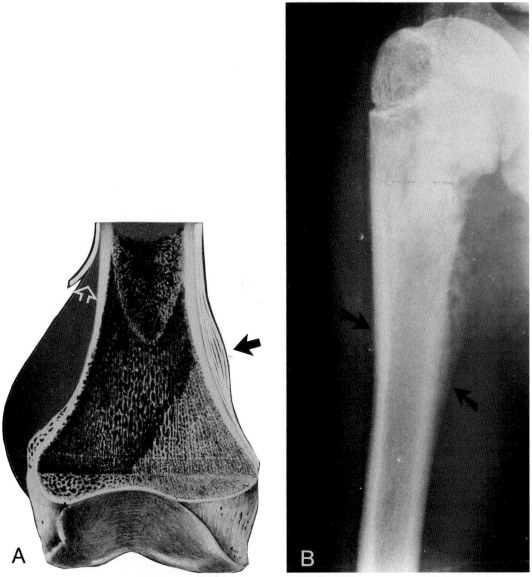

Figure 11.56.   Laminated periosteal reaction. A. Drawing showing laminations (*solid arrow*). A Codman triangle is demonstrated on the opposite side (*open arrow*). **B.** Irregular interrupted periosteal reaction (*arrows*) in a patient with a Ewing tumor.

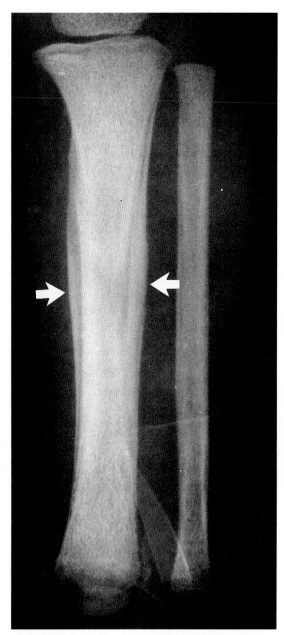

Figure 11.57.   Laminated but solid periosteal reaction (*arrows*) in an abused child.

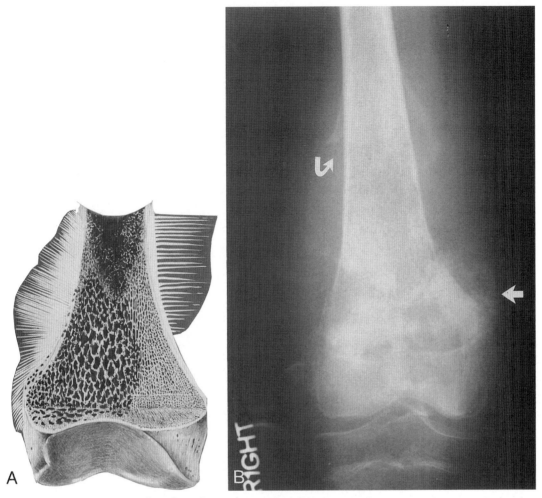

Figure 11.58.   Spiculated periosteal reaction. A. Drawing showing variations on spiculated periosteal reaction. **B.** Osteosarcoma demonstrating spiculated periosteal reaction (*straight arrow*). Notice the Codman triangle (*curved arrow*).

past, this finding was thought to be pathognomonic of tumor. However, it occurs in many benign conditions, including subperiosteal hemorrhage of any cause, such as postoperatively, in scurvy, and in child abuse.

Sclerosis is an attempt by the bone to wall off a diseased area. It generally indicates a benign process (Fig. 11.59). *Buttressing* is an attempt by the bone to reestablish architectural integrity; the term is derived from the flying buttresses of Gothic architecture (Fig. 11.60). The most common example of this is the *osteophyte* of degenerative arthritis (see Fig. 11.60B, C) or the *syndesmophyte* of inflammatory arthritis (Fig. 11.61). An osteophyte represents ossification along the corners of a joint. As a rule, it first grows horizontally before turning vertically. A syndesmophyte, on the other hand, represents ossification of Sharpey fibers in the disc. It is always oriented vertically. In ankylosing spondylitis, syndesmophytes are thin, delicate, and symmetric. In diffuse idiopathic skeletal hyperostosis, they are thicker, coarser, and usually symmetric. In other inflammatory arthropathies, such as psoriatic arthritis, reactive arthritis, or the spondyloarthropathy of inflammatory bowel disease, they are thick and asymmetric.

The *enthesophyte* is a variant of osteophytes and syndesmophytes. *Entheses* are the tendinous or ligamentous attachment points on bones. Some diseases, such as psoriatic arthropathy, produce ossification of entheses (Fig. 11.62).

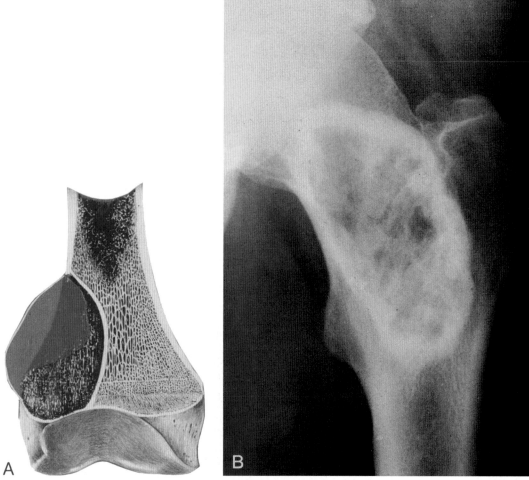

Figure 11.59.   Reactive sclerosis. A. Drawing showing sclerotic rim around a geographic lesion. **B.** Sclerosis around a focus of fibrous dysplasia of the proximal femur.

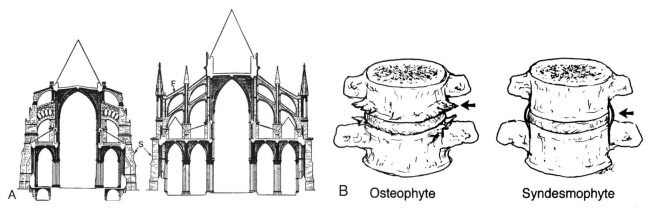

Figure 11.60.   Buttressing. A. Drawing illustrates flying (*F*) and standing (*S*) buttresses as used in Gothic architecture. **B.** Drawing illustrating the difference between osteophyte and syndesmophyte. *(continued on page 411)*

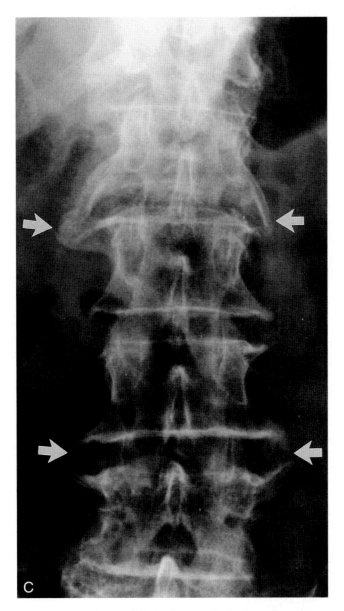

Figure 11.60. *(continued)* **C.** Detail view of the lumbar vertebral column shows large osteophytes (*arrows*) at multiple levels.

Matrix Production

Matrix is a substance produced by certain bone tumors. It may be. *chondroid* (cartilaginous), *osteoid* (bony), or mixed. Chondroid matrix appears as fine, stippled calcification; as rings, or Cs and Os; or as multiple popcornlike calcifications. Matrix frequently occurs in bulky masses of tumor within the soft tissues (Fig. 11.63). Osteoid matrix, on the other hand, is dense, usually of the same radiographic density as bone. It occurs most often in osteosarcoma (Fig. 11.64) but also may be seen in the benign ossifying condition called myositis ossificans (Fig. 11.65), in which soft tissue ossification results from injury and hemorrhage. Tumor matrix may be differentiated from the calcification of myositis ossificans by observing its distribution (Fig. 11.66). As a rule, calcified tumor matrix is concentrated in the *center* of the lesion (see Fig. 11.66A), whereas calcification of other sources (myositis ossificans or bone infarct) occurs initially in the *periphery* and then spreads centrally (see Fig. 11.66B).

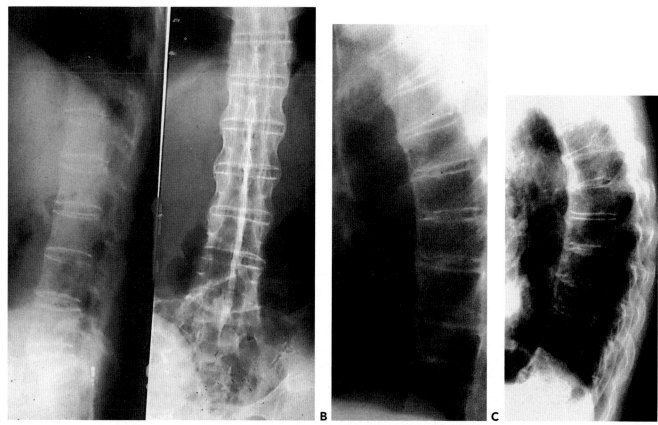

A B C

Figure 11.61. Syndesmophytes in ankylosing spondylitis and diffuse idiopathic skeletal hyperostosis. A and B. Thin, delicate syndesmophytes extend across the intervertebral discs in these two patients with ankylosing spondylitis. **C.** In a patient with diffuse idiopathic skeletal hyperostosis, the flowing syndesmophytes are coarser and primarily anterior.

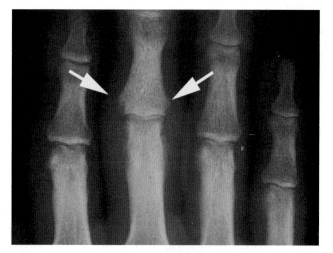

Figure 11.62. Enthesophytes in psoriatic arthropathy. Irregular new bone formation (*arrows*) is seen along the proximal portions of the middle phalanx. Similar changes are in the proximal phalanx.

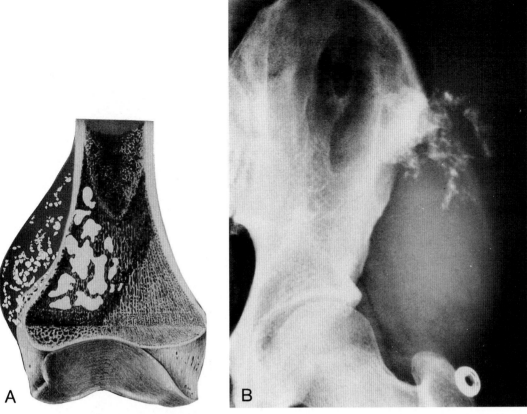

Figure 11.63. Matrix formation. A. Drawing showing lumpy and flocculent types of matrix. **B.** Chondroid matrix in a patient with chondrosarcoma. Notice the flocculent calcifications within the soft tissues adjacent to the iliac bone.

Figure 11.64. Osteosarcoma of the pelvis demonstrating osteoid matrix. Notice how dense the lesion is because of the osteoid matrix formation.

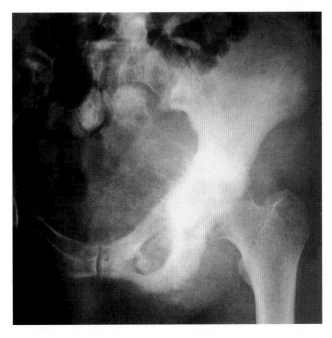

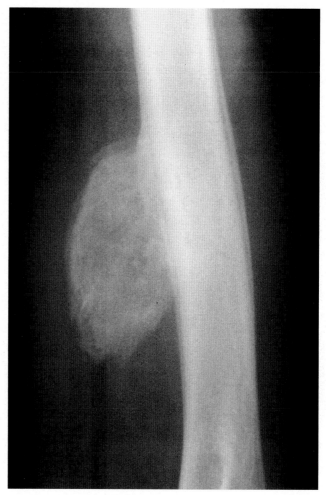

Figure 11.65.   Myositis ossificans of the humerus. The lesion is well defined, with uniform ossification that is slightly denser in the periphery. Notice the laminated but solid periosteal reaction.

Soft Tissue Changes

By analyzing the soft tissues, you may obtain important clues regarding an underlying injury, disease process, or a specific bone lesion. For example, diffuse muscle wasting suggests a patient with paralysis, primary muscle disease, or severe inanition caused by disseminated carcinomatosis or AIDS. The presence of soft tissue swelling may be indicative of a mass (Fig. 11.67), hemorrhage, inflammation, or edema. The loss or displacement of fat lines normally found in the soft tissues is another indication of adjacent abnormality. For example, displacement or obliteration of the pronator quadratus fat line in the wrist (Fig. 11.68) usually indicates a fracture of the wrist. Elevation or displacement of the fat pads of the elbow indicates fluid within the joint capsule, usually the result of trauma (Fig. 11.69), but sometimes is found in inflammatory conditions such as rheumatoid arthritis. The presence of a *lipohemarthrosis* or fat-fluid level in the suprapatellar space on a horizontal beam lateral radiograph of the knee is indicative of a fracture communicating with the joint (Fig. 11.70). Lipohemarthroses are also commonly found on CT examinations of fractures (Fig. 11.71).

Calcifications within the soft tissues may be the result of old trauma or connective tissue disorders. Occasionally, old parasitic disease will be manifest by soft tissue calcifications.

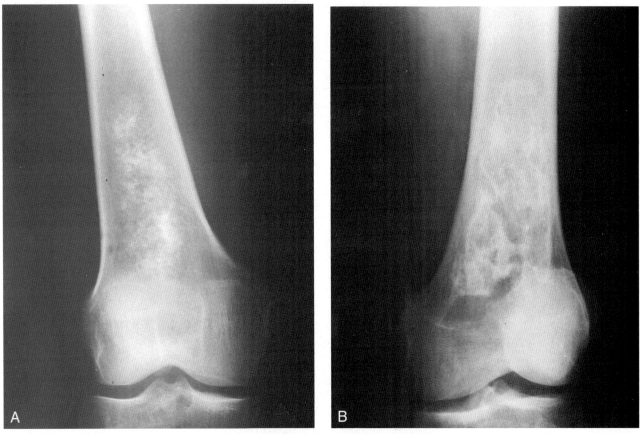

Figure 11.66. Difference between matrix and heterotopic calcification. A. Enchondroma of the distal femur demonstrates flocculent matrix resembling rings, or *C*s and *O*s. It is concentrated in the *center* of the lesion. **B.** Heterotopic calcification in a bone infarct. The calcification is mainly in the *periphery* of the lesion and has a wavy or serpentine appearance.

Figure 11.67. Lipoma of the antecubital fossa (*arrows*). The lucency within this large mass indicates that a major component is fat.

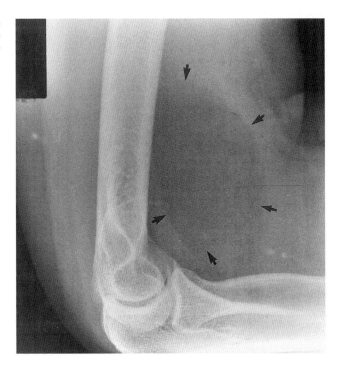

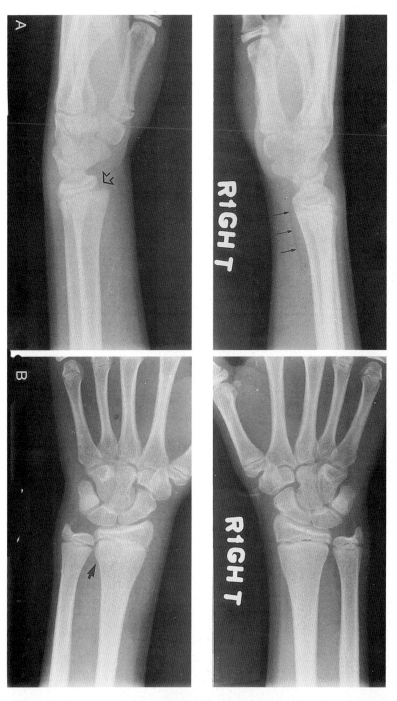

Figure 11.68. Soft tissue changes in a patient with a Salter-Harris-Ogden type 2 fracture of the distal radius. A. Lateral views show the normal pronator quadratus fat stripe (*small arrows*) on the right. Notice the obliteration of this line and overall soft tissue swelling on the left. There is widening of the physis on the left (*open arrow*). **B.** Frontal views show buckling of the ulnar cortex of the distal radius on the left (*arrow*). Notice the differences in soft tissue compared with the right. The changes on the frontal views are even more subtle than those on the lateral views.

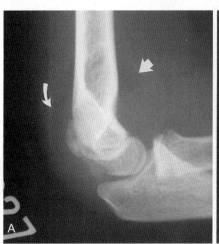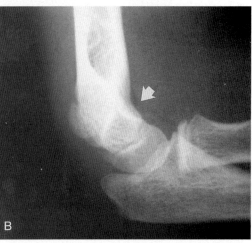

Figure 11.69. Elbow fat pad. A. Lateral radiograph shows elevation of the anterior (*large arrow*) and posterior (*curved arrow*) in a patient with a subtle fracture of the distal humerus. **B.** Lateral radiograph of the opposite side shows the normal position and appearance of the anterior fat pad (*arrow*). The posterior fat pad is never visible under normal circumstances.

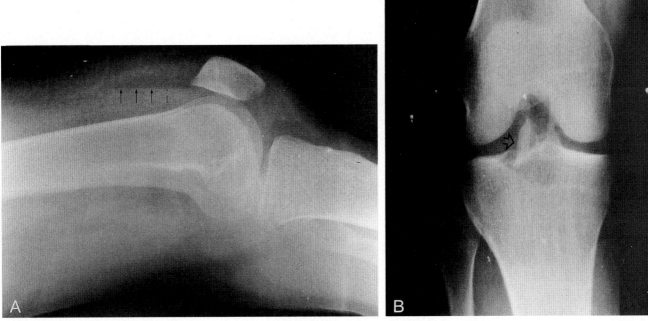

Figure 11.70. Tibial plateau fracture. A. Horizontal beam lateral film shows a fat-fluid level (lipohe-marthrosis, *arrows*) in the suprapatellar space. **B.** Frontal view shows avulsion of the tibial intercondylar spines (*arrow*).

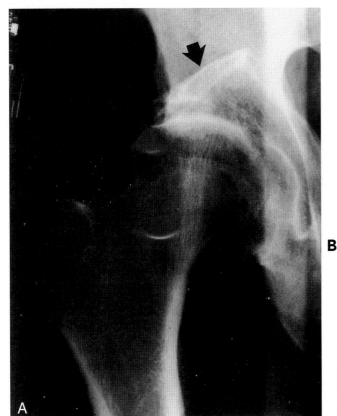

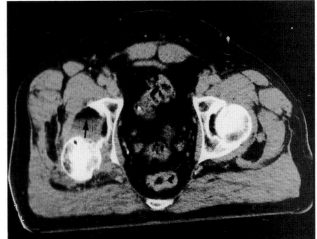

Figure 11.71. Femoral head dislocation and acetabular fracture. A. Detail frontal view shows superior migration of the femoral head in association with a fracture of the acetabulum (*arrow*). **B.** CT image using soft tissue windowing shows the right femoral head to be displaced posteriorly. There is a lipohemarthrosis within the hip joint capsule (*arrow*).

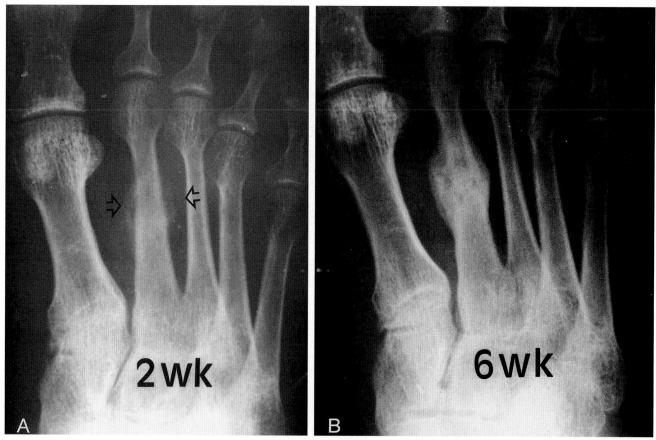

Figure 11.72.   Stress fracture of the second metatarsal. A. Frontal radiographs made 2 weeks after onset of symptoms shows irregular periosteal reaction along the midshaft of the second metatarsal (*arrows*). The underlying bone appears moth eaten. **B.** Six weeks after onset of symptoms, healing has occurred. Notice the solid periosteal reaction across the fracture site. There has been some bony resorption of the fracture margins with the healing and remodeling process.

Gas in the tissues indicates trauma, recent surgery, infection, or gas gangrene. Other soft tissue findings include the presence of foreign bodies, abdominal aortic aneurysm, or renal calculi in patients being evaluated for back pain.

History of Trauma or Surgery

Because trauma constitutes the most common bone "disease" you will encounter, it is very important to elicit a history of trauma whenever possible. A stress fracture (Fig. 11.72) may be misdiagnosed as a malignant bone tumor unless a specific history of trauma (pain with an unusual activity, condition worsening with that activity, and relief achieved by rest) is obtained. Occasionally, however, a history of trauma will be deliberately withheld, as in the case of child abuse or of a child or adult who, prior to injury, was doing something prohibited or illegal.

Similarly, it is important to know whether the patient has had surgery on a particular bone or joint. Healing surgical sites, particularly those used for bone graft donation (Fig. 11.73), may have ominous radiographic appearances. It is therefore imperative to know about any previous operations.

It is also important to know whether a patient has undergone radiation therapy to an area of bony abnormality. Radiation may produce bizarre findings of mixed lucency and bony sclerosis (Fig. 11.74). Some bone sarcomas are the result of previous radiation (Fig. 11.75). In addition, radiation of bones makes them more susceptible to the insufficiency type of stress fracture, particularly in the pelvis and sacrum (Fig. 11.76).

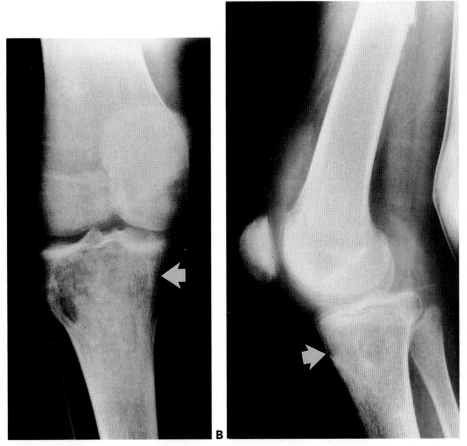

Figure 11.73. Bone graft donor site. Frontal **(A)** and lateral **(B)** radiographs show a large, lucent lesion in the proximal tibia (*arrows*). Giant cell tumor or chondrosarcoma might be suspected unless given the history that 3 months before, the patient underwent surgical plating and bone grafting for multiple long bone fractures. The proximal tibia was the site for the donor bone. Radiographs of this area were normal at that time.

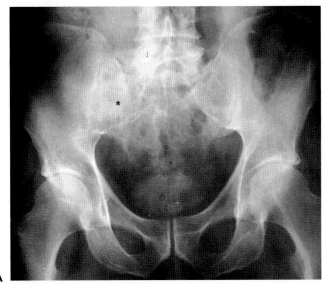
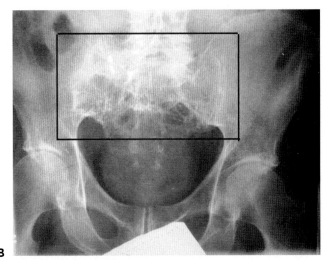

Figure 11.74. Radiation changes in the pelvis in a patient who was treated for multiple myeloma. A. Pelvic radiograph shows a bubbly destructive lesion in the right side of the sacrum (*). Compare with the left. **B.** Pelvic radiograph 1 year later shows sclerosis in the sacrum. Notice that the abnormal bone is confined to the area subtended by the radiation portal (*rectangle*).

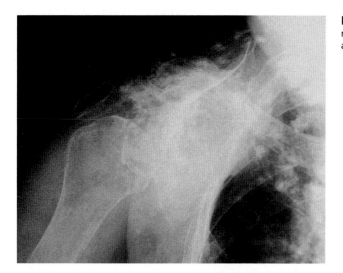

Figure 11.75.   Radiation-induced chondrosarcoma. Shoulder radiograph shows flocculent tumor matrix. The patient had been irradiated for breast carcinoma.

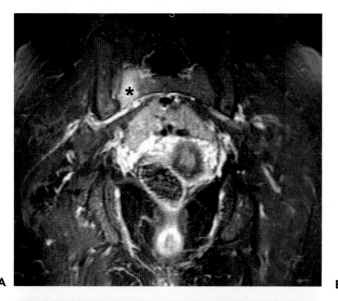

A

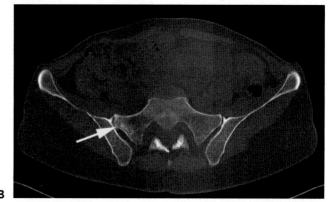

B

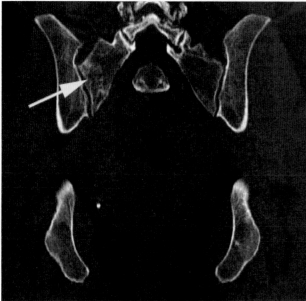

C

Figure 11.76.   Insufficiency stress fracture of the sacrum.
A. Coronal short T1 inversion recovery MR image shows a linear area of increased signal in the body of the sacrum on the right (*). A radionuclide bone scan (not shown) had increased tracer activity in this area. **B.** Axial CT image shows a linear area of sclerosis in the same area of the sacrum (*arrow*). **C.** Coronal reconstructed CT image shows the same finding (*arrow*). Radiographs (not shown) were normal.

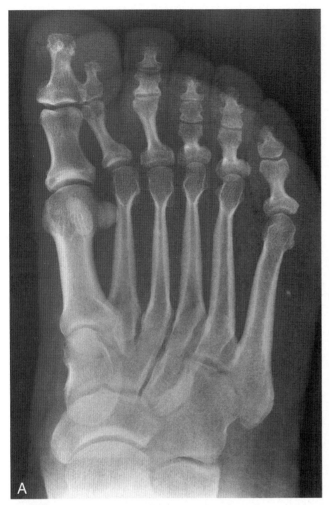
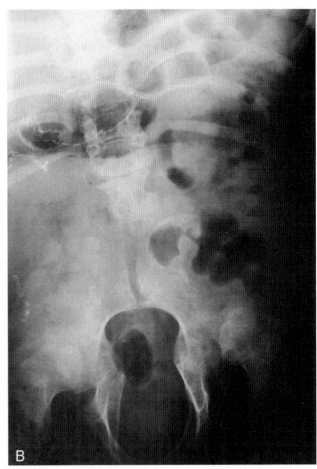

Figure 11.77. Congenital deformities. A. Polydactyly in a patient with six toes. **B.** Sacral agenesis in a patient with caudal regression syndrome.

Additional Observations

Abnormalities of Bony Anatomy and Alignment

Deformities in bone generally indicate a congenital abnormality (Fig. 11.77). However, they may also occur as a result of poorly treated trauma (Fig. 11.78). Two types of malalignment may occur in joints: subluxations and dislocations. *Subluxation* is a partial loss of continuity between articulating surfaces; *dislocation* is the complete loss of continuity at that joint space. These are illustrated in Figure 11.79. Shoulder, hip, and finger dislocations are the most commonly encountered. Artificial joints occasionally dislocate (Fig. 11.80).

Abnormalities of Bony Mineralization and Texture

The degree of mineralization of a bone is directly related to the patient's age, the physiologic state, and the amount of activity or stress being placed on that bone. Furthermore, the texture of the trabeculae (thin, delicate, coarsened, smudged) may tell you something about the patient's metabolic state. It is important to differentiate the terms osteopenia and osteoporosis. *Osteopenia* is a term used to define a decrease in mineralization of bones as demonstrated on radiographs. *Osteoporosis* is a term that defines a specific pathologic state in which there is diminution of bone substance. It may be determined by either bone densitometry or by biopsy and mineral analysis.

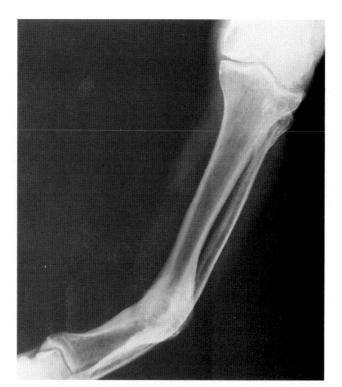

Figure 11.78. Deformity of the distal tibia and fibula secondary to poorly managed fractures.

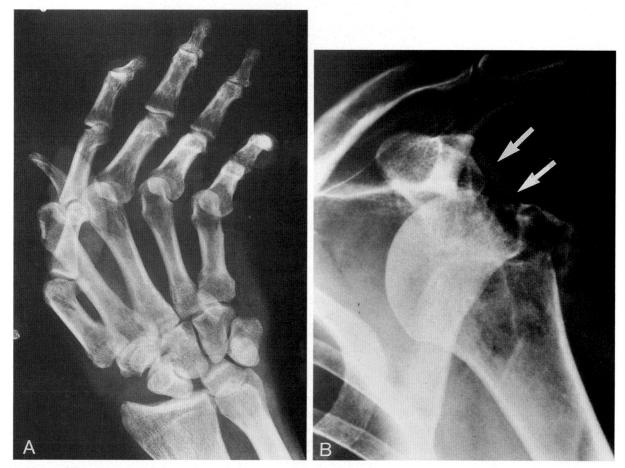

Figure 11.79. Subluxation and dislocation. A. Ulnar subluxation of the carpus and metacarpophalangeal joint subluxations in a patient with systemic lupus erythematosus. **B.** Anterior inferior humeral dislocation. There is complete loss of continuity between the joint surfaces. Also evident are a naked glenoid (*arrows*) and a fracture of the humeral head (Hill-Sachs deformity). *(continued on page 423)*

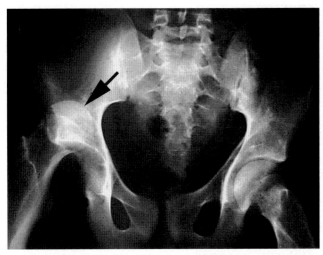

C

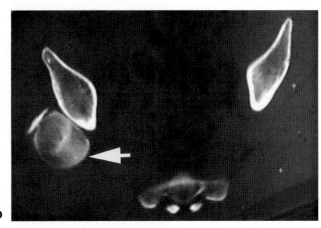

D

Figure 11.79. *(continued)*   **C.** Hip dislocation. Pelvic radiograph shows superior displacement of the femoral head (*arrow*). **D.** CT image shows the dislocated femoral head to be posterior as well as superior (*arrow*). A small sliver of bone from the acetabulum sits just lateral to the femoral head.

Figure 11.80. Dislocated total hip implant. The femoral component is dislocated superiorly and posteriorly.

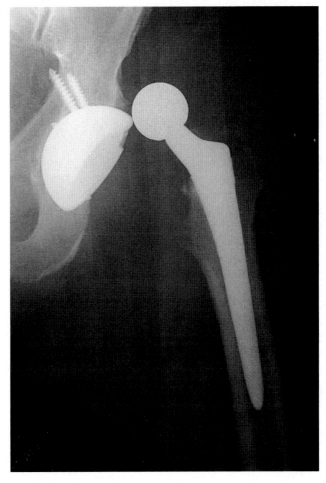

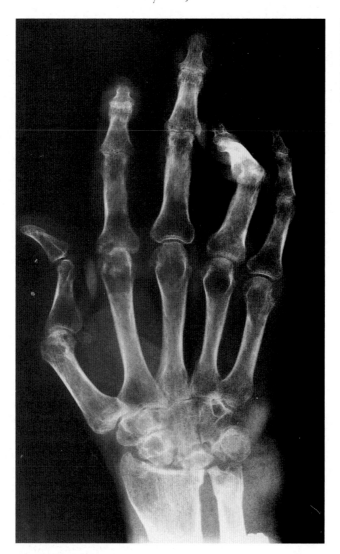

Figure 11.81. Advanced rheumatoid arthritis. This disease primarily involves the wrist joint, the metacarpophalangeal joints, and the proximal interphalangeal joints. Notice the erosive changes in these locations.

Osteoporosis commonly occurs in elderly patients and in postmenopausal women. However, an acute form of osteoporosis may occur after a limb is immobilized. Diminished mineralization is also a common manifestation of inactivity as well as of certain diseases such as renal osteodystrophy, rheumatoid arthritis (Fig. 11.81), and scurvy. *Renal osteodystrophy* is a complex of several metabolic conditions with four prominent radiographic manifestations: osteoporosis, coarsening of bony trabeculae, osteomalacia, and hyperparathyroidism. It is most often encountered in patients with chronic renal failure. The radiographic picture may feature one of the components more prominently than others or simply be a combination of all four. Features of osteomalacia include osteoporosis, *smudged and indistinct trabeculae*, resorption about the physes in the skeletally immature (Fig. 11.82), and a curious appearance in the vertebral column of alternating horizontal bands of osteoporosis centrally with osteosclerosis along the vertebral end plate termed *"rugger jersey spine"* (Fig. 11.83) because it resembles the horizontal stripes on a rugby jersey. Hyperparathyroidism, on the other hand, produces osteoporosis, resorption of the tufts of the distal phalanges, subperiosteal resorption along the radial borders of phalanges, resorption about the distal clavicles (see Fig. 11.41B) and other symphyseal joints, as well as along *entheses* (tendinous insertion points), and a curious mixed pattern of osteopenia and fluffy sclerosis in the skull called *salt and pepper skull* (see Fig. 11.41C).

It is sometimes difficult to differentiate osteoporosis from permeative bone destruction on either radiographs or CT. In these situations, MR imaging can help make the differentiation. Osteoporosis produces a scan that shows fatty replacement of marrow that is high on T1-weighted images. Infiltrative disorders generally produce low signal in the marrow spaces on T1-weighted studies (Fig. 11.84). Furthermore, osteoporotic vertebral fractures, if recent, usually

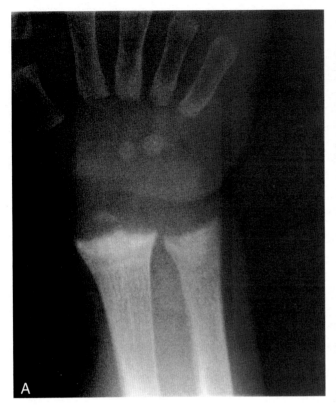

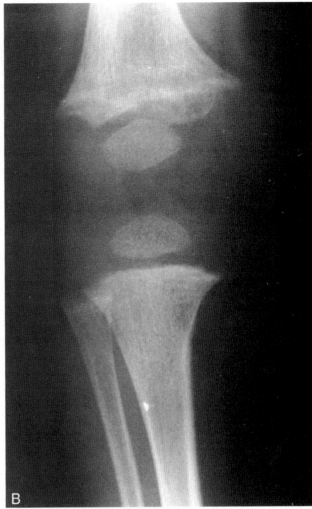

Figure 11.82. Rickets in a child. A. Wrist radiograph shows irregular frayed metaphyses and coarsened trabeculae. **B.** Knee radiograph shows similar findings.

Figure 11.83. "Rugger jersey spine" in a patient with chronic renal failure and osteomalacia. Notice the striped appearance from the alternating areas of osteosclerosis along the disc plates with central osteoporosis. The relatively lucent disc spaces also contribute to the striped appearance.

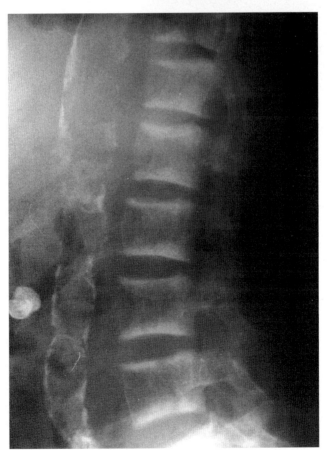

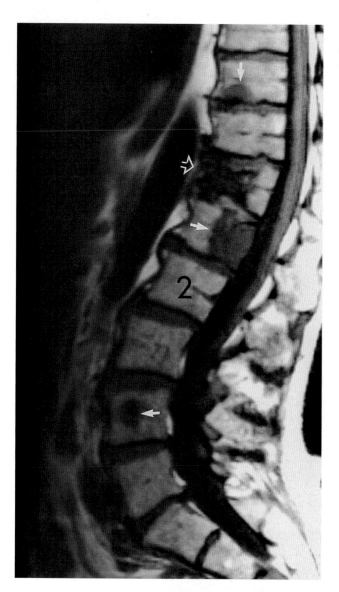

Figure 11.84.   Metastases (*solid arrows*) and pathologic collapse (*open arrow*) of T12 as demonstrated on a T1-weighted MR image. The abnormal signal in the collapsed vertebra extends throughout the vertebra, typical of metastases. Compare with Figure 11.85.

have more of a linear distribution of abnormal signal than does that associated with infiltration (Fig. 11.85). In some instances, biopsy may be necessary to establish the proper diagnosis.

Patients with osteoporosis (of any origin) are subject to *insufficiency* stress fractures. These fractures result from the effect of normal muscle activity on bone that is deficient in mineral. In contradistinction, *fatigue* stress fractures result from excessive muscular activity on bones of normal mineralization. The typical patient with an insufficiency stress fracture is an elderly woman who has engaged in some low-impact activity, such as walking through a mall, with sudden onset of sacral, groin, or lower limb pain (see Fig. 11.76). Typically, the pain is worse with activity and is relieved by rest. In many instances, the patient's clinical picture may be clouded by a history of previous malignancy and radiation therapy.

For an excellent in-depth discussion of bone mineral physiology and pathology, consult Resnick's *Diagnosis of Bone and Joint Disorders.*

Joint Space Abnormalities

The width of the joint space and the appearance of the distal ends of articulating bones are important in the diagnosis of arthritis. The distribution, location, and erosive patterns produced by the various arthritides allow considerable accuracy in radiologic diagnosis, particularly when correlated with clinical and laboratory findings. You should familiarize yourself with the changes in the three most common types of arthritis you will encounter: rheumatoid, degenerative, and gouty. The salient features of these diseases are summarized here.

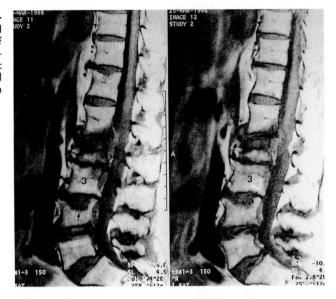

Figure 11.85. Osteopenic collapse of L2. Two T1-weighted images show collapse of the body of L2. There is low signal in a *linear* distribution, typical of nonpathologic collapse. Notice the central Schmorl node of L4 (*arrow*). Compare with Figure 11.84.

Rheumatoid arthritis. The radiographic findings of rheumatoid arthritis depend on the stage of the disease. Early findings include fusiform pericapsular swelling, joint effusion, and subtle demineralization of the subarticular bone. As the disease progresses, marginal erosions occur, usually associated with narrowing of the joint space (Fig. 11.86). The degree of osteopenia has also progressed. In the late form of the disease, considerable destruction has taken place about the joints, and subluxations occur. In the end stage, ankylosis occurs (Fig. 11.87). Ankylosis is the common end point of all severe joint disorders, regardless of the cause. Rheumatoid arthritis affects the cervical vertebral column in at least 50% of patients with the disease; most of these patients have no cervical symptoms. This is an important fact to know because the most serious complication of cervical rheumatoid arthritis is atlantoaxial subluxation (Fig. 11.88). In the large joints, such as the hips and knees, joint space loss is severe but without the extensive proliferative changes that occur with osteoarthritis.

Juvenile rheumatoid arthritis (JRA). This disease is one of the chronic polyarthritides of childhood that is similar in pathology to its adult counterpart. However, the involvement of growing bones produces clinical and radiologic features that are uniquely different. Unlike the adult form of the disease, which primarily affects the smaller joints, the clinical and radiologic manifestations of JRA are found early on in larger joints (knee, ankle, shoulder) as well as in the smaller joints of the hands, wrists, and cervical vertebral column. Typical radiologic changes include soft tissue swelling, overgrowth and squaring of the epiphyses because of hyperemia, and early ankylosis. Erosive changes that are the hallmark of the adult disease are seldom found in JRA. Figure 11.89 shows typical features of JRA.

Degenerative arthritis (osteoarthritis). Osteoarthritis may be primary or secondary. The primary form results from the aging process and the "wear and tear" that process inflicts on joints. The secondary form is the result of any injury or disease that disrupts articular cartilage or interferes with the normal motion of the affected joint(s). There are three salient features of degenerative arthritis: narrowed joint spaces, subarticular reactive sclerosis, and spur formation (Fig. 11.90). Mineralization generally remains normal. In severe forms, subarticular cysts or *geodes* occur. There may also be chondrocalcinosis, particularly in the knees. A particularly aggressive form of this disease that affects middle-aged and elderly women is known as *erosive osteoarthritis*. It primarily affects the distal interphalangeal joints of the hands (see Fig. 11.46).

Gout. This disorder arises from abnormal urate metabolism. In the early stages of this disease, soft tissue swelling is the only radiographic finding. Indeed, the disease must be present for 5

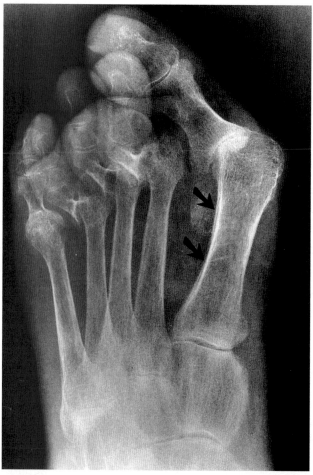

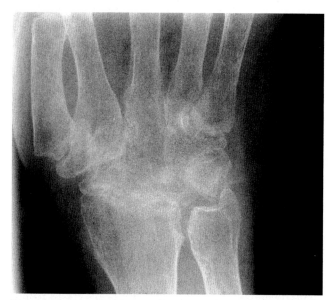

Figure 11.86. Rheumatoid arthritis of the foot with lateral subluxations of the metatarsophalangeal joints. There are erosive changes in the second through fifth metatarsophalangeal joints. There is periosteal reaction (*arrows*) along the shaft of the first metacarpal.

Figure 11.87. End stage rheumatoid arthritis with bony ankylosis in the wrist. Normal anatomic margins of the carpal bones cannot be identified. Notice the severe osteopenia.

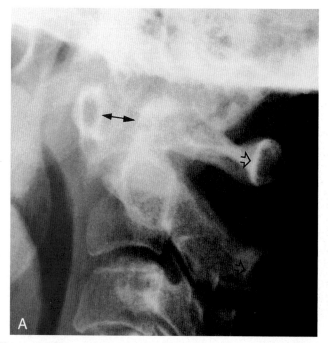

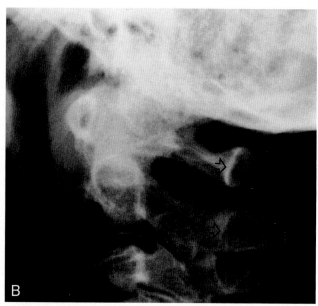

Figure 11.88. Atlantoaxial subluxation in a patient with rheumatoid arthritis. A. Lateral radiograph in flexion shows anterior subluxation of C1 on C2. Notice the widening of the predental space (*double arrow*) and malalignment of the spinolaminar lines of C1 and C2 (*open arrows*). **B.** Lateral radiograph in extension shows the subluxation to have reduced nearly completely. The spinolaminar line (*open arrows*) is still not anatomically aligned.

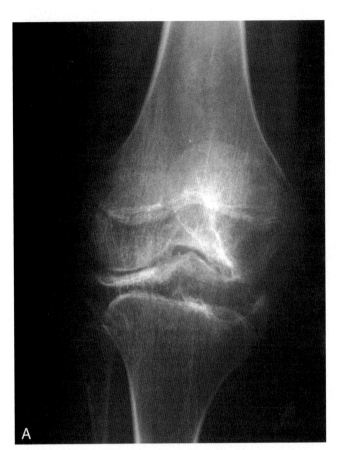 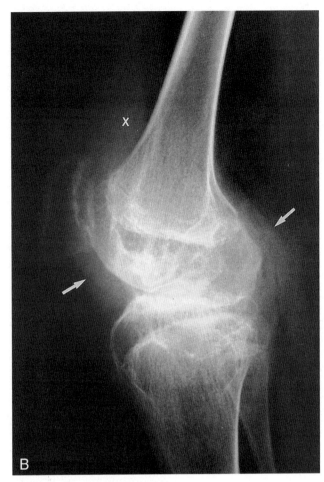

Figure 11.89.   Juvenile rheumatoid arthritis of the knee. A. Frontal view shows hypertrophy of the epiphyses and joint space narrowing. **B.** Lateral view shows epiphyseal hypertrophy with erosions along the joint surface. There is a suprapatellar effusion (*X*) and evidence of synovial hypertrophy anteriorly and posteriorly (*arrows*).

Figure 11.90.   Osteoarthritis of the knee. There is subchondral sclerosis (*straight arrows*) and a large marginal osteophyte (*curved arrow*) laterally.

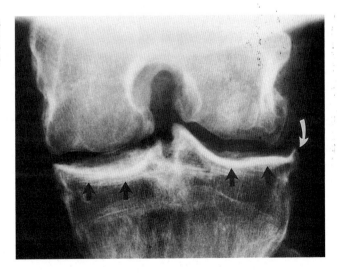

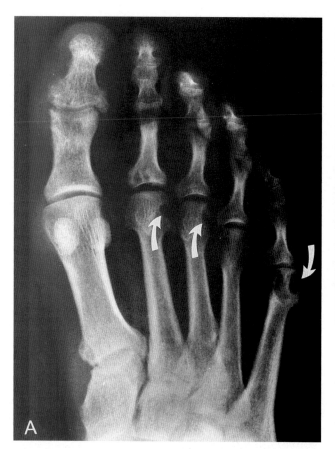

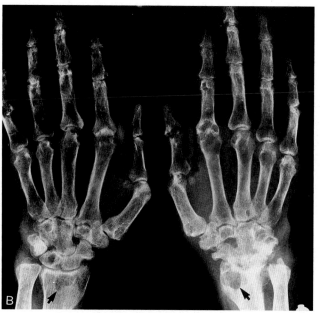

Figure 11.91.   Gout. A. Detail view of a foot shows para-articular punched-out lesions in the distal metatarsals (*arrows*). Other joints are involved as well. **B.** Involvement of the hands and wrists in the same patient shows multiple lesions. Notice the asymmetry, predominantly para-articular involvement and overall preservation of mineralization around the joints. There are intraosseous tophi in the distal radii (*arrows*). Compare the findings here with Figure 11.81, rheumatoid arthritis.

to 7 years before erosive changes and large punched-out lesions are seen. These erosions may be articular or para-articular (more common) and result from *tophus* formation; often they have overhanging edges (Fig. 11.91) and have the appearance of a rat bite. The erosions are more common in the "bare" (para-articular) areas. The degree of mineralization is usually normal except in an acute attack.

Calcium pyrophosphate deposition disease (CPPD). This common disorder, often termed *pseudogout,* is another of the crystalline arthropathies. The clinical picture of this disease is identical to that of an acute gouty attack. However, aspiration of the affected joint(s) reveals pyrophosphate crystals instead of urate crystals. CPPD, unlike gout, responds to treatment with nonsteroidal anti-inflammatory drugs. Radiographically, the hallmark of CPPD is chondrocalcinosis of both hyaline and fibrocartilage and the paucity of large osteophytes. The knee and the wrist are the two joints most commonly involved (Fig. 11.92).

Neuropathic osteoarthropathy (Charcot joint). This disorder is the result of denervation of joints caused by pre-existing diseases such as diabetes mellitus, syringomyelia, or neurosyphilis (tabes dorsalis). In the United States, diabetes is the most common etiology. Denervation of the joints allows the microfractures that occur in everyone as the result of daily "wear and tear" on the bones to go undetected by the patient. Continued activity on those compromised bones and joints results in propagation of the fractures. Ultimately, the affected part disintegrates into a "bag of bones." The main radiographic features of neuropathic disease are severe fragmentation, dislocation, and reactive changes (Fig. 11.93). The appearance has been described by skeletal radiologist Frieda Feldman as "osteoarthritis with a vengeance." Often there will be the appearance of previous surgical resection with straight margins (Fig. 11.94). The foot is the most common location in diabetics; the shoulder, in patients with syringomyelia. Vertebral neuropathic joints are not uncommon. Charcot joints from neurosyphilis are a medical curiosity today and radiographs of them are found only in teaching files.

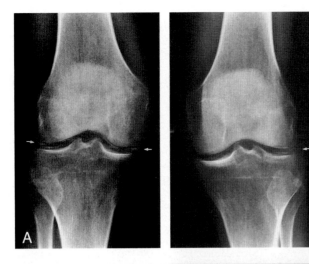

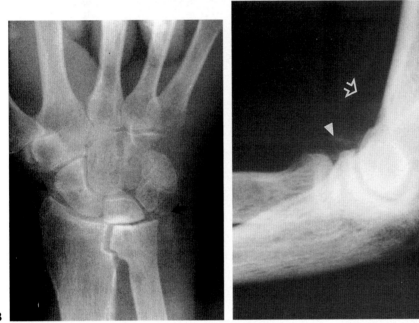

Figure 11.92. Calcium pyrophosphate deposition disease (CPPD, pseudogout). A. Frontal radiographs of the knees show bilateral chondrocalcinosis of the menisci (*arrows*). **B.** Frontal radiograph of a wrist shows chondrocalcinosis (*arrows*) as well as narrowing of the radiocarpal joint. The squaring of the distal radiocarpal joint is also typical for this disorder. **C.** Lateral radiograph of the elbow in the same patient shows chondrocalcinosis (*arrowhead*) and elevation of the anterior fat pad (*arrow*) indicating a joint effusion.

Trauma

As previously mentioned, skeletal trauma is the most common bone disorder. *A fracture is really a soft tissue injury in which a bone is broken.* In most instances, the bone, if left by itself, will heal. However, in dealing with fractures, you must be concerned with associated soft tissue injuries. For example, a fracture of the skull itself may be trivial. However, if there is damage to the underlying meningeal vessels or brain, the injury is significant. Similarly, vertebral fractures are often associated with neurologic deficit from damage to the spinal cord. Therefore, in evaluating a patient who has sustained skeletal trauma, it is important to also assess the status of the adjacent soft tissue structures. In patients who have suffered severe multisystem trauma, the goal of imaging should be to diagnose those abnormalities that are most likely to be life threatening, such as cranial, thoracic, visceral, or vascular injuries. Often radiographic assessment of the skeleton will have a lower priority.

In trauma patients, views other than those considered routine may be necessary to demonstrate suspected fractures. Furthermore, *comparison views* with the opposite, uninjured limb may be necessary, particularly in evaluating possible epiphyseal injuries in children (Fig. 11.95). I recommend selective use of comparison views—that is, only in special circumstances and never routinely (with the exception of the pediatric elbow, where there are six growth

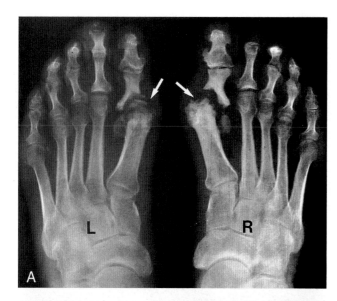

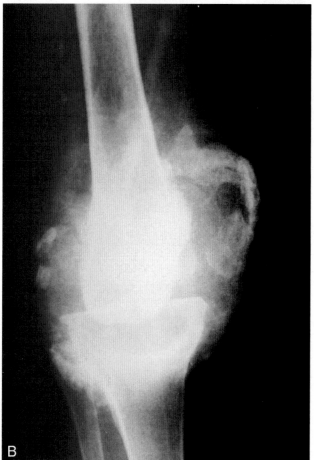

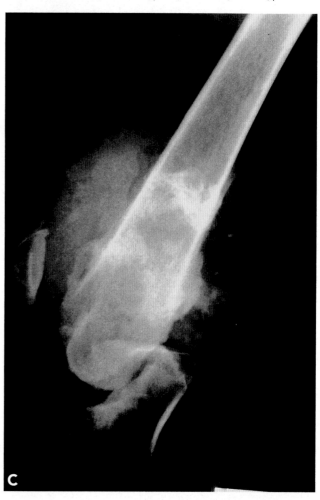

Figure 11.93. Neuropathic (Charcot) joints in two diabetic patients. A. Radiographs of both feet show bilateral neuropathic joints at the first metatarsophalangeal joints (*arrows*). On the left there is periarticular osteopenia, indicating superimposed infection. Frontal **(B)** and lateral **(C)** knee radiographs of another patient show disintegration of the knee joint with considerable bony debris ("bag of bones") and a large joint effusion. In the past, involvement of this joint was typically caused by neurosyphilis.

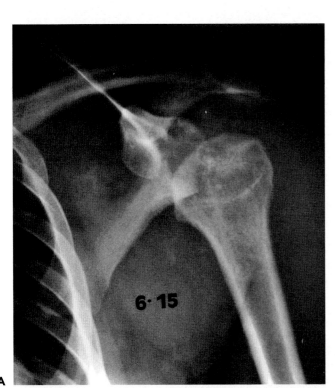
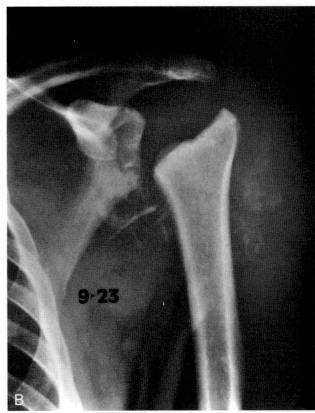

Figure 11.94.   Neuropathic (Charcot) joint disease of the shoulder in a patient with syringomyelia. A. Frontal radiograph shows irregularity of the joint surfaces and bony debris within the joint capsule. **B.** Three months later, the joint shows signs of further destruction. The humeral head appears to be amputated. The amount of periarticular debris has increased.

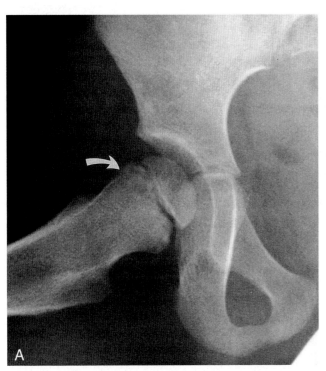
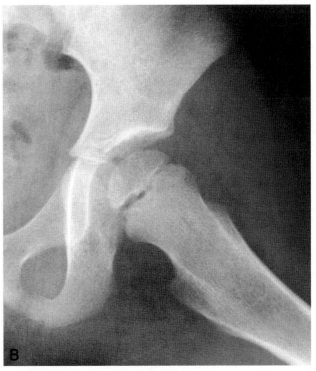

Figure 11.95.   Use of comparison views in trauma. A. Frog-leg lateral view of the right hip in a child demonstrates buckling of the metaphyseal cortex (*arrow*). **B.** Comparison view of the left side is normal.   *(continued on page 434)*

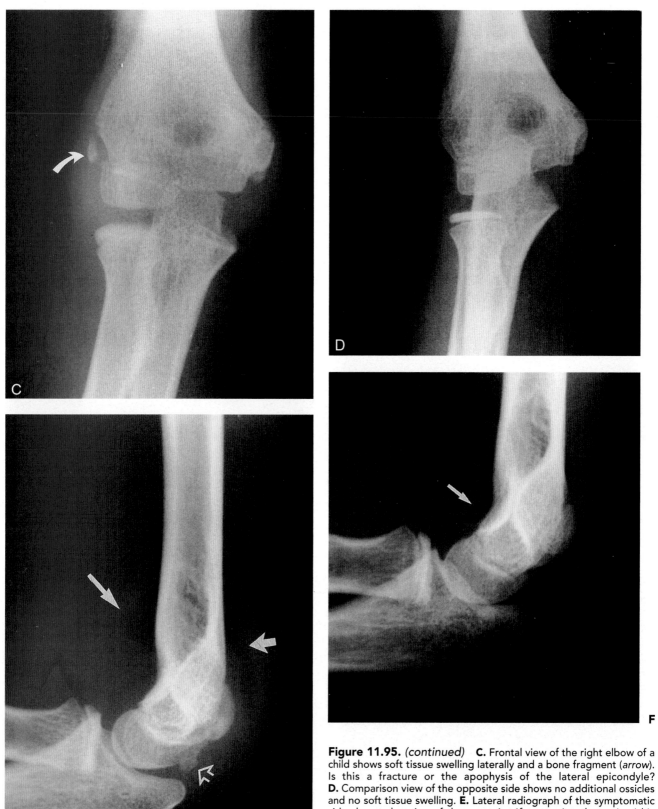

Figure 11.95. *(continued)* **C.** Frontal view of the right elbow of a child shows soft tissue swelling laterally and a bone fragment (*arrow*). Is this a fracture or the apophysis of the lateral epicondyle? **D.** Comparison view of the opposite side shows no additional ossicles and no soft tissue swelling. **E.** Lateral radiograph of the symptomatic side shows elevation of the posterior (*fat arrow*) and anterior (*thin arrow*) fat pads in addition to the avulsed bone fragment (*open arrow*). **F.** Comparison view of the opposite side shows a normal anterior fat pad (*arrow*) and no avulsed bone fragment. The lateral epicondylar apophysis usually ossifies around age 12; this patient is considerably younger.

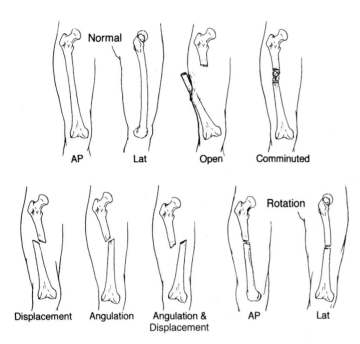

centers). Occasionally, stress views to test ligamentous stability and arteriography to investigate the possibility of vascular injury may be necessary.

The *descriptive terminology* of fractures is important; the referring clinician, orthopaedic surgeon, and radiologist must all speak the same language. Fractures are described by location within the bone (head, neck, shaft, etc.); type (spiral, comminuted, oblique, green-stick); and position of the fragments (degrees of angulation, displacement, overriding, distraction; Fig. 11.96). Figure 11.97 shows several common types of fractures and their descriptive terminology. For a further discussion of terminology, refer to *The Handbook of Fractures*, by Koval and Zuckerman.

Fractures in children occur in two distinct patterns, depending on whether the injury is near the physis or the shaft. Injuries about the physis are classified according to the *Salter-Harris-Ogden (S-H-O)* classification, which is based on the degree of involvement of the epiphysis, physis, or metaphysis. The type 1 injury is a pure epiphysiolysis. Type 2, the most common, involves the epiphysis and a small metaphyseal fragment. The type 3 injury is a vertical fracture of the epiphysis with epiphysiolysis of the fracture fragment. Type 4 is a vertical epiphyseal fracture with metaphyseal involvement. Type 5, the rarest, is uniform compression of the physeal plate. Type 6 is a compression of part of the physeal plate with lysis of the other part. Type 7 is an osteochondral fracture of the epiphysis. Type 8 injuries affect the metaphyseal growth and remodeling areas. Type 9 injuries are those of periosteal portions of the diaphysis. Figure 11.98 illustrates the S-H-O classification. Types 1 and 2 are said to produce little or no growth disturbance; types 3 through 6 have a higher potential for growth disturbance, and type 7 has no potential for disturbance but can produce joint problems from the intra-articular loose fragments. Type 8 injuries may result in epiphysiolysis caused by ischemia from disruption of the blood supply in the metaphysis. Type 9 injuries may result in failure of remodeling because of the periosteal injury. Colloquially, these injuries are usually called Salter-type fractures.

Slipped capital femoral epiphysis (SCFE) is a S-H-O type 1 injury that occurs most frequently in boys in their early teens. In many instances, the child is overweight. At least half of the patients report some history of trauma. Hip pain and limp are the most common presenting symptoms; however, up to one-fourth of patients may present with knee pain. In some instances the slip may be bilateral. The radiographic manifestations are often subtle on an anterior-posterior projection. A line drawn along the lateral border of the femoral neck should normally intersect the femoral capital epiphysis with approximately 20% of the diameter of the head lying lateral to this line. With SCFE, too much or too little of the femoral head will lie lateral to this line (Fig. 11.99). Frog-leg lateral views often show the slippage better than the

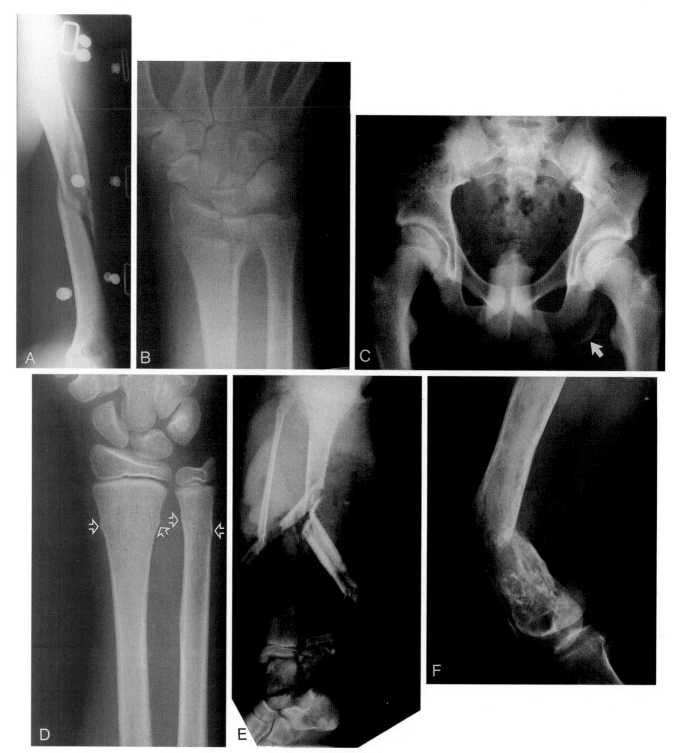

Figure 11.97.   Fractures and their descriptive terminology. A. Spiral comminuted fracture of the midshaft of the humerus. **B.** Comminuted, intra-articular compression fracture of the distal radius. There is also a fracture of the ulnar styloid. **C.** Avulsion fracture (*arrow*) of the ischial apophysis. **D.** Green-stick (torus) fractures of the distal radius and ulna (*arrows*). The torus fracture presents as a bulge along the surface of the otherwise smooth bone. **E.** Comminuted open fractures of the distal tibia and fibula. **F.** Pathologic fracture of the distal femur in a patient with a malignant bone tumor. Notice the bone destruction around the fracture.   (continued on page 437)

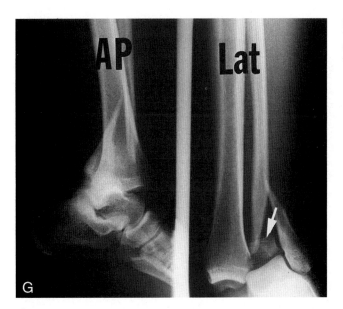

Figure 11.97. *(continued)* **G.** Fracture-dislocation of the ankle. There are fractures of the distal fibula and posterior lip of the tibia *(arrow)*. The foot is dislocated *and* rotated laterally. Notice the orientation markers on the radiographs. AP, anterior-posterior; Lat, lateral.

frontal views (see Fig. 11.99B). Complications of this injury include avascular necrosis and chondrolysis. The former condition may result from damage to the blood supply to the femoral head at the time of injury or as a result of surgical pinning to treat the disorder.

Fractures of the shafts of bones may be either complete or of the green-stick variety. Three types of green-stick fractures are recognized: *classic green-stick* (fracture on one side of the bone, bent on the other); *torus,* resembling the base of a Greek column (buckling of cortex on both sides of the bone); and *"lead pipe"* (one side buckled, one side cracked). Of these, the torus variety (see Fig. 11.97D) is the most common.

Stress fractures are the result of increased muscle activity on normal bone (*fatigue fracture*) or of normal muscle activity on bone with compromised mineral content (*insufficiency fracture*). In the typical fatigue fracture, the activity is new or in excess of the structural tolerance of the patient's bone(s). The activity is usually vigorous and repetitive. The typical history in a patient with a stress fracture (any type) is of pain with activity that is relieved by rest and made worse by resuming the activity. Tumors and infections typically produce pain at rest as well as with activity. *Stress fractures are common injuries that occur at predictable sites with specific activities.* For example, running typically produces fractures of the proximal posterior medial tibia (Fig. 11.100) or of the distal fibula (Fig. 11.101). Other common sites include the metatarsal shafts in military recruits ("march fractures"), calcaneus in people engaged in jumping activities, and pars interarticularis of the lumbar vertebrae in gymnasts.

Figure 11.98. Salter-Harris-Ogden classification of growth region injuries. See text for description.

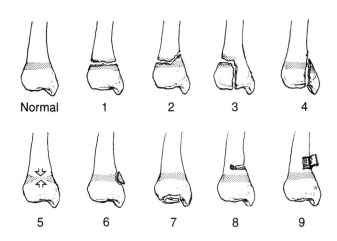

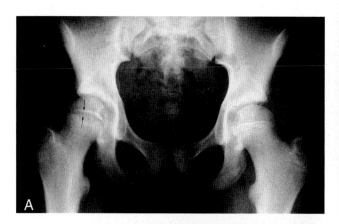

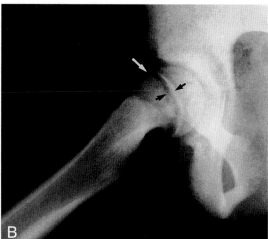

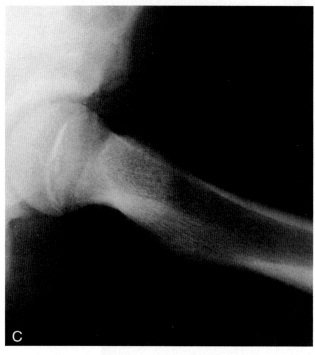

Figure 11.99.   Slipped femoral capital epiphysis (SCFE). A. Pelvic radiograph shows asymmetry of the physes with widening on the right (*arrows*). **B.** Frog-leg lateral view of the right hip shows widening of the physis (*short arrows*) and malalignment of the epiphysis with the metaphysis laterally (*long arrow*). **C.** Frog-leg view of the left is normal.

Insufficiency fractures were discussed under abnormalities of bone mineralization. Common locations for this type of stress fracture are the sacrum, pubic arches, and femoral necks. The initial radiographs of a patient with a stress fracture may be normal; the patient should be treated symptomatically and return for a repeat radiographic examination in 7 to 10 days. For elderly patients in whom a diagnosis needs to be made immediately, as well as in elite athletes or persons in whom rest will interfere with their jobs, MR imaging may be performed because it will show the abnormalities before the radiographs (Fig. 11.102). If time is not of the essence in making such a diagnosis, a radionuclide scan may be performed instead.

Although an in-depth description of fractures is beyond the scope of this book, you should follow some of the principles listed here when evaluating patients with skeletal trauma:

■ *Assume a fracture is present if there is pain, swelling, and discoloration over a bony surface in a child.* It is best to treat patients for fractures and bring them back in 7 to 10 days for follow-up radiographs rather than let them leave the emergency department with untreated fractures.

■ Comparison views should be made only when you and your radiologist are uncertain about the presence or absence of a fracture (particularly in small children whose physeal lines could be confused for a fracture).

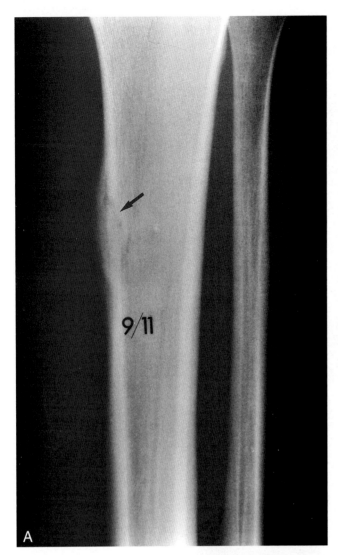

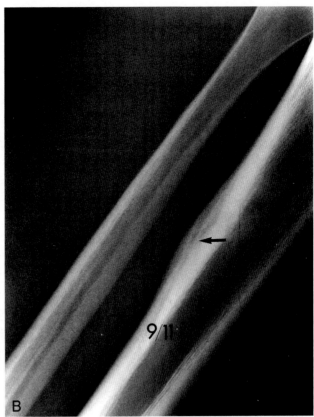

Figure 11.100. Tibial stress fracture in a runner. A. Detail view of a frontal radiograph of the tibia shows the fracture along the medial cortex (*arrow*). Laminated periosteal reaction indicates the patient continued to run despite the pain. **B.** Lateral view shows the fracture involves the posterior cortex (*arrow*). This is the typical site for a stress fracture caused by running.

Figure 11.101. Stress fracture (*arrow*) of the distal fibula in runner.

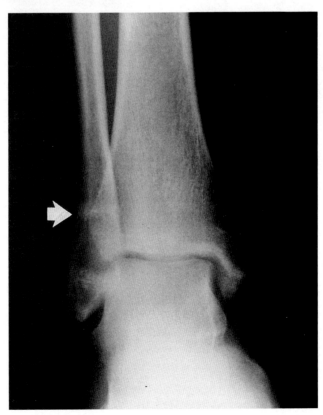

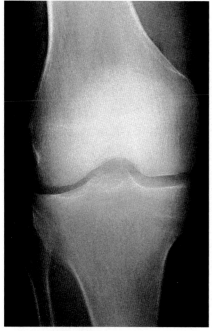

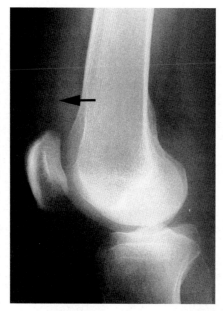

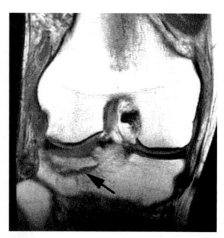

A,B

C

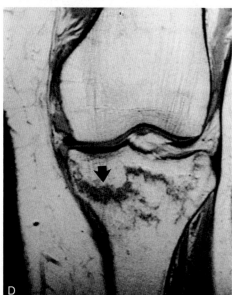

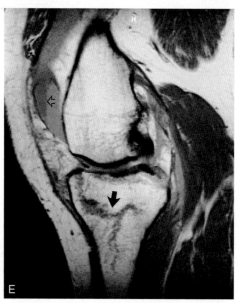

D

E

Figure 11.102. MR imaging for diagnosing occult fractures. A. Frontal radiograph of the knee is normal. **B.** Lateral radiograph is normal except for a lipohemarthrosis in the suprapatellar bursa (*arrow*). **C.** Coronal T1-weighted MR image shows a depressed fracture of the lateral tibial plateau (*arrow*). Coronal (**D**) and lateral (**E**) T1-weighted images of the knee in another patient show serpentine linear areas of low signal representing an occult fracture (*solid arrows*). There is a lipohemarthrosis (*open arrow*) in E. The radiograph (not shown) was normal.

- Acute fractures typically have irregular margins that resemble the pieces of a jigsaw puzzle. You can mentally put the pieces together even if they are displaced (Fig. 11.103). Old, ununited fractures or accessory ossicles have smooth, rounded margins and do not have the "jigsaw puzzle effect."
- A CT scan is useful for evaluating fractures of certain joints such as the shoulder, knee (Fig. 11.104), and ankle. It is also the best method of assessing pelvic fractures (Fig. 11.105) and in establishing the extent of vertebral fractures.
- MR is useful in assessing the extent of spinal cord compression in vertebral fractures (Fig. 11.106). It is also helpful in determining whether or not an occult fracture is present, particularly in the elderly (see Fig. 11.102 D, E). In these instances, we perform a limited examination consisting of T1-weighted images in two planes only.

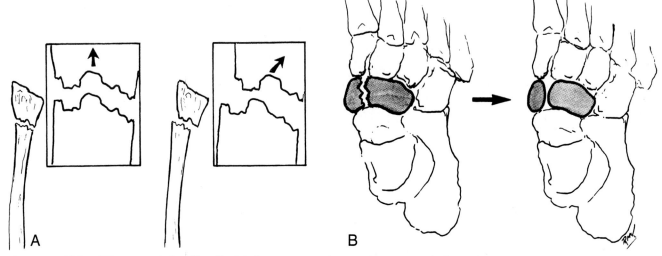

Figure 11.103. "Jigsaw puzzle effect" with fractures. A. The irregular margins of a fracture may be matched perfectly, like the pieces of a jigsaw puzzle, even if there is displacement (indicated by arrows). Accessory ossicles or old ununited fractures do not match perfectly. **B.** Drawing showing a fracture of the tarsal navicular bone on the left that went to nonunion. Notice the change in configuration of the margins of the ossicles.

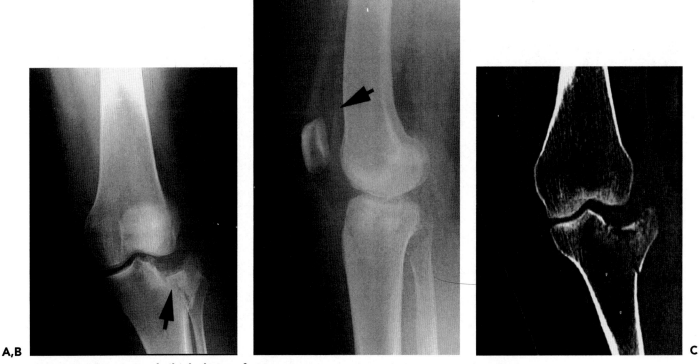

A,B   **C**

Figure 11.104. Lateral tibial plateau fracture. A. Frontal radiograph shows a severely comminuted depressed fracture of the lateral tibial plateau (*arrow*). **B.** Lateral radiograph (made with a horizontal beam) shows a lipohemarthrosis in the suprapatellar space (*arrow*). **C.** Coronal reconstructed CT image shows the fracture in detail.   (continued on page 442)

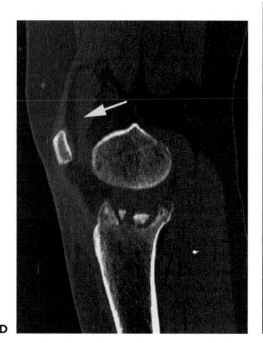

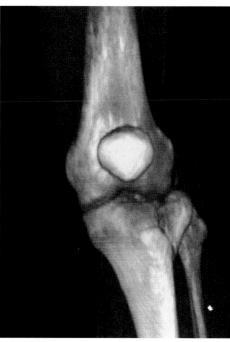

Figure 11.104. *(continued)*
D. Sagittal reconstructed CT image shows the lipohemarthrosis *(arrow)*. **E.** Three-dimensional volumetric reconstructed image shows the fracture from the vantage point that the orthopaedist would see at the time of surgery.

D

E

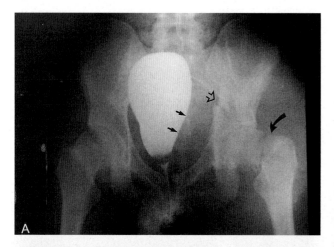

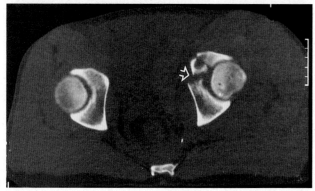

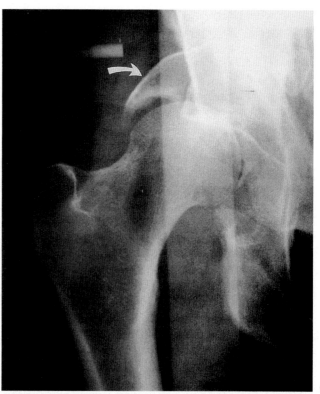

A

B

C

Figure 11.105.   Pelvic fractures. A. Frontal radiograph shows fractures involving the left acetabulum *(open arrow)* and left femoral neck *(curved arrow)*. A large pelvic hematoma compresses and displaces the contrast-filled bladder to the right *(small arrows)*. There is extravasated contrast just below the pubic symphysis as a result of a urethral injury. The floor of the bladder is elevated as another manifestation of this injury. **B.** CT image through the hips shows the severely comminuted acetabular fracture on the left *(arrow)*. **C.** Acetabular fracture of the right hip *(arrow)* in another patient with posterior and superior dislocation of the femoral head.   *(continued on page 443)*

Figure 11.105. *(continued)* **D.** CT image shows the posterior dislocation of the femoral head. There is an intra-articular bone fragment (*arrow*).

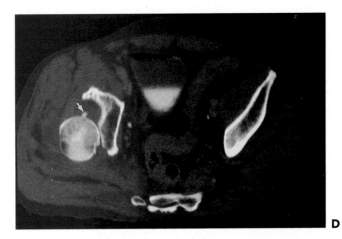

D

Postoperative Changes

A large number of joint implants and appliances are used in orthopaedics today. You should familiarize yourself with the more common of these and their appearance in bone (see Fig. 11.107). Furthermore, the sites of previous screw holes, osteotomies, or implants may present a variety of bony defects that are easily recognizable if you are familiar with the types of procedures used in orthopaedic surgery (Fig. 11.108). Remember, straight lines and rectangular margins are human made (Fig. 11.109); nature prefers curves and circles.

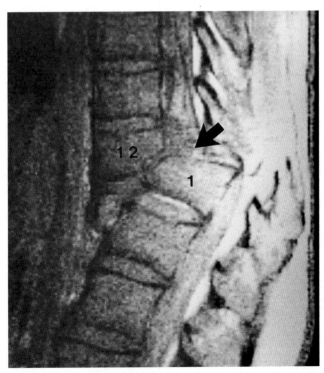

Figure 11.106. **Fracture dislocation of T12 on L1.** An MR image shows the dislocation. Notice the cord transection (*arrow*).

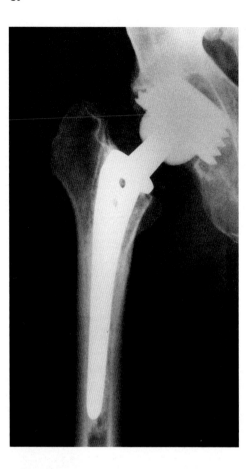

Figure 11.107. Normal postoperative appearance of a total hip implant.

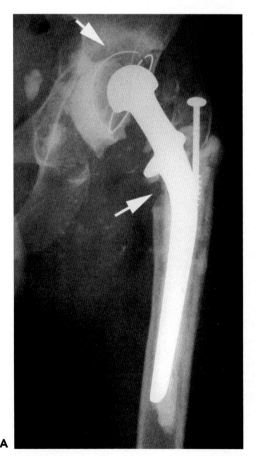

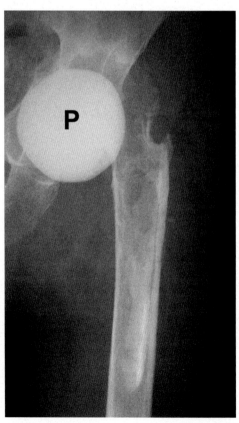

Figure 11.108. Antibiotic cement in place after removal of joint implants. A. Radiograph shows loosening of a total hip implant. Notice the spaces between the acetabular component and the femoral component and their respective bones (*arrows*). **B.** After removal of the device, a large puck (*P*) of antibiotic methyl methacrylate cement has been inserted as a spacer until a new device is implanted. *(continued on page 445)*

A

B

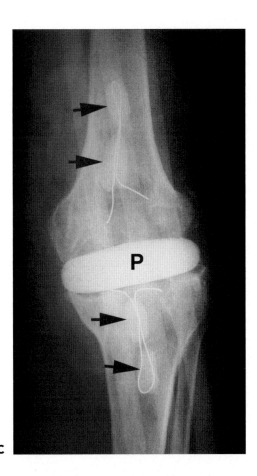

C

Figure 11.108. *(continued)* **C.** Knee radiograph following removal of a total joint implant in insertion of a puck (*P*) and intramedullary beads (*arrows*) of cement. The beads are connected by wire to make removal easier.

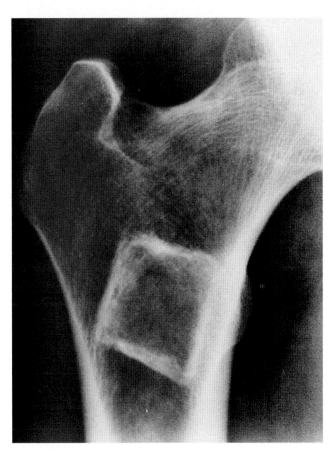

Figure 11.109. Residuum of an excisional bone biopsy. The square margins of this sclerotic lesion are the clue to the iatrogenic nature of the lesion.

SUMMARY AND KEY POINTS

- Bone abnormalities are among the most common you will encounter. Of these, fractures and arthritic conditions occur most frequently.
- Most bone lesions fall into one of six basic pathologic categories: congenital, inflammatory, metabolic, neoplastic, traumatic, and vascular.
- By recognizing patterns of destruction and the use of a series of predictor variables, it is possible to reduce the complexities of skeletal radiology to a workable format.
- The application of the mnemonic **ABCS** was introduced to describe the analysis of bone and joint lesions: **A**natomy and alignment abnormalities, **B**ony mineralization and texture abnormalities, **C**artilage (joint space) abnormalities, and **S**oft tissue abnormalities.
- A number of common entities were discussed, as were the principles of fracture diagnosis.

SUGGESTED ADDITIONAL READING

Brower AC, Flemming DJ. Arthritis in Black and White. 2nd Ed. Philadelphia: WB Saunders, 1997.

Chew FS. Bui-Mansfield LT, Kline MJ. The Core Curriculum: Musculoskeletal Imaging. Philadelphia: Lippincott Williams & Wilkins, 2003.

Helms CA. Fundamentals of Skeletal Radiology. 3rd Ed. Philadelphia: WB Saunders, 2005.

Kang HS, Ahn JM, Resnick DL. Internal Derangements of Joints: Emphasis on MR Imaging. 2nd Ed. Philadelphia: WB Saunders, 2002.

Kleinman PK. Diagnostic Imaging of Child Abuse. 2nd Ed. St. Louis: Mosby, 1998.

Koval KJ, Zuckerman JD. Handbook of Fractures. 2nd Ed. Philadelphia: Lippincott Williams & Wilkins, 2001.

Laor T, Jaramillo D, Oestreich AE. Musculoskeletal system. In: Kirks DR, Griscom NT, eds. Practical Pediatric Imaging: Diagnostic Radiology of Infants and Children. 3rd Ed. Philadelphia: Lippincott-Raven, 1998:327–510.

Manaster BJ, Disler DG, May DA. Musculoskeletal Imaging: The Requisites. 2nd Ed. St. Louis: Mosby, 2002.

Ogden JA. Skeletal Injury in the Child. 2nd Ed. Philadelphia: WB Saunders, 1990.

Ozonoff MB. Pediatric Orthopedic Radiology. 2nd Ed. Philadelphia: WB Saunders, 1992.

Resnick DL. Diagnosis of Bone and Joint Disorders. 4th Ed. Philadelphia: WB Saunders, 2002.

Resnick DL, Kransdorf MJ. Bone and Joint Imaging. 3rd Ed. Philadelphia: WB Saunders, 2005.

Rogers, LF. Radiology of Skeletal Trauma. 3rd Ed. New York: Churchill Livingstone, 2002.

Stoller DW, Tirman P, Bredella MA. Diagnostic Imaging: Orthopaedics. Philadelphia: WB Saunders, 2004.

Swischuk LE. Imaging of the Newborn, Infant, and Young Child. 5th Ed. Philadelphia: Lippincott Williams & Wilkins, 2004: 747–755.

Van Holsbeeck MT, Introcaso JT. Musculoskeletal Ultrasound. 2nd Ed. St. Louis: Mosby, 2001.

Weissman BNW, Sledge CB. Orthopedic Radiology. 2nd Ed. Philadelphia: WB Saunders, 1999.

Cranial Imaging

12

Neuroradiology is the subspecialty concerned with radiologic investigation and intervention of the brain and spinal cord. It is this area that has been most dramatically changed by the technical developments in imaging of the past 30 years. Computed tomography (CT), magnetic resonance (MR) imaging, digital subtraction angiography (DSA), and positron emission tomography (PET) scanning have been major breakthroughs in the imaging of the brain and spinal cord. Although abnormalities in other areas of the body may be grossly evident, the changes present on studies of the central nervous system are often subtle. The student or house officer who is confronted with a neuroradiologic study is often frustrated and feels insecure. Remember, however, that neuroradiology is founded on the same principles of anatomy, physiology, and pathology as any other diagnostic area. This chapter begins the discussion of neuroradiology by focusing on cranial imaging; Chapter 13 continues the discussion with its focus on vertebral and spinal cord imaging. Because of the complexity of neuroradiologic examinations, detailed descriptions of the various entities are beyond the scope of this book. However, the pertinent aspects of each type of study, their indications, and a basic discussion of the main pathologic entities is included to provide you with the foundation you need to select the appropriate studies for your patients.

TECHNICAL CONSIDERATIONS

The cranial contents are studied by CT, MR, angiography, and nuclear imaging. Prior to the development of cross-sectional imaging, cranial evaluations were performed to display the effects of certain intracranial abnormalities on structures that could be opacified. Hence, the main purpose of skull radiographs was to detect enlargement of the sella turcica, intracranial calcifications, and shifts in the calcified pineal. Cerebral angiography was a primary tool to detect *neovascularity* (new tumor vessels) and to show displacement and encasement of vessels by intracranial masses. It was also used to show brain compression from extracerebral masses such as subdural and epidural hematomas. *Pneumoencephalography* was performed to outline the cerebral ventricular system and to show the effects of neoplasms and other lesions on those structures. Of these modalities, only angiography has as important a role today, as discussed later in the chapter.

Although CT and MR are the prime investigative tools for cranial imaging, there is still a limited role for skull radiography: penetrating injury, destructive lesions, metabolic bone disease, congenital anomalies, and postoperative changes. In addition, facial radiographs are still effective for screening for suspected facial fractures. In penetrating injuries, such as a gunshot wound (GSW), the skull radiograph is cost-effective. It is a well-known fact that any GSW that crosses the midline of the cranium is fatal. In our practice, we routinely obtain an anterior-posterior (AP) skull radiograph on all cranial GSW patients to determine whether the bullet has traversed the midline. If this is the case, no additional studies are performed; if not, we proceed with cranial CT.

Except as already noted, a *CT examination* of the brain and surrounding tissue is usually performed as the initial study for evaluation of patients with suspected intracranial abnormalities. This study is generally done first without and then with intravenous contrast enhancement to demonstrate vascular structures or abnormalities, extra-axial hematomas, or enhancement of lesions. CT of the face and sinuses is also performed to evaluate patients with suspected trauma or infection, respectively. Although radiographs of those areas are valuable, CT provides more information, particularly about displacement of bone fragments in trauma and about possible bone destruction in sinusitis.

Cranial MR imaging is one of the greatest technological improvements for evaluating suspected intracranial lesions. It is the primary investigative tool for suspected intracranial abnormalities, such as tumors and multiple sclerosis, because it can display the brain in exquisite detail in axial, coronal, and sagittal planes. Cranial MR is performed using T1- and T2-weighted spin echo sequences as well as various gradient echo, and inversion recovery (STIR and FLAIR) sequences. The scanning parameters of these studies are adjusted to optimize the characteristics of certain intracranial lesions. In addition, MR angiography is now commonly performed either alone, or after intravenous contrast enhancement, as a relatively noninvasive procedure for evaluating the carotid, vertebral, and cerebral arteries.

Cerebral angiography is used to evaluate vascular lesions such as atherosclerotic occlusive disease, aneurysms, and arteriovenous malformations. It is also used to supplement CT and MR imaging in patients with tumors to aid the surgeon in their removal and to identify the major vessels feeding brain tumors. Interventional vascular procedures (see Chapter 3) are now commonly performed to occlude those abnormalities (see Fig. 3.13). DSA allows the neuroradiologist to perform the studies using minimal amounts of contrast media.

Nuclear imaging of the brain was the only noninvasive cranial procedure before the development of CT and MR imaging. The current role of brain scintigraphy is one of defining brain function and blood flow. Four types of nuclear studies are performed: conventional scintigraphy with blood-barrier agents, cerebral perfusion, cisternography, and PET scanning.

Conventional scintigraphy was used in situations where the brain CT was negative or equivocal, such as suspected subacute or chronic subdural hematomas, encephalitis, or suspicion of lymphoma versus toxoplasmosis in immunodeficient patients. Nuclear imaging was more sensitive than CT for these applications. However, with the advent of MR imaging, most of these diagnoses are now better addressed with MR imaging.

Cerebral perfusion imaging with single photon computer emission tomography (SPECT) technology is still used for patients who are being considered for carotid endarterectomies or intracranial vascular aneurysm occlusion. By placing an intraluminal balloon in the diseased carotid artery, subsequent radioisotope injection can provide information about cerebral cortex perfusion on the ipsilateral side. This allows the physician to determine whether sacrificing a carotid artery will compromise cortical perfusion and function.

Indium-111 radionuclide cisternography is used to identify sites of cerebrospinal fluid leakage, evaluate shunt patency, and diagnose normal pressure hydrocephalus. Studies for cerebrospinal fluid leakage are usually performed in collaboration with neurosurgeons. Using indium-111–labeled radiotracers, imaging is possible up to 3 days after the initial time of administration, allowing imaging at multiple time points.

PET scanning is used primarily for brain perfusion and metabolism evaluation. The conventional isotope is F-18 fluoro-2-deoxyglucose (F-18 FDG), which is produced by cyclotron. By injecting F-18 FDG and performing multiplanar imaging, information regarding gray and white matter perfusion can be obtained. Clinical applications include differentiating radiation necrosis from residual tumor, localizing seizure foci for planning of surgery, and diagnosing Alzheimer disease. Currently, radioisotopes that will specifically target dopaminergic systems are in development that may help diagnose Parkinson disease.

Finally, radionuclide imaging is also used in providing visual corroboration of a clinical diagnosis of brain death. By injecting technetium-99m–tagged diethylenetriamine pentaacetic acid (DTPA) and performing immediate flow images in the region of the head and neck, intracranial perfusion is assessed. Absence of arterial flow on early images as well as lack of pooling in the venous system on subsequent "blood pool" images is consistent with brain death.

ANATOMIC CONSIDERATIONS

Skull radiographs, as previously mentioned, are used whenever there is a history of penetrating trauma, facial fracture, sinus disease, destructive lesion, or metabolic problem. Most commonly, skull films are obtained as part of a metastatic or metabolic bone survey. Their analysis should be conducted in a logical, orderly fashion using the *ABCS* method described in Chapter 11; however, for skull radiographs, the *C* stands for calcifications. The order of examination, therefore, should be bony vault, sella turcica, facial bones, basal foramina, sinuses, calcifications, and soft tissues.

Skull anatomy is complex. However, the symmetry of the skull provides, in most instances, a ready "comparison view" of the unaffected side. For this reason, it is necessary to review the more common radiographic views used and their pertinent anatomy. The standard radiographic views of the skull are the posterior-anterior (PA), lateral, AP half-axial (Towne), and base. Each view is designed to demonstrate particular areas of the skull. The *PA view* shows the frontal bones, frontal and ethmoid sinuses, nasal cavity, superior orbital rims, and mandible (Fig. 12.1). The *lateral view* demonstrates the frontal, parietal, temporal, and occipital bones, the mastoid region, the sella turcica, the roofs of the orbits, and the lateral aspects of the facial bones (Fig. 12.2). The *modified half-axial projection* (Towne, occipital view; Fig. 12.3) shows the occipital bone, the mandibular condyles and temporomandibular (TM) joints, the mastoid and middle ear regions, the foramen magnum, and the zygomatic arches. The *base view*

Figure 12.1. PA skull radiograph. The following structures are visible: falx cerebri (F_x), frontal sinus (F_s), internal auditory canal (I_A), sphenoid sinus (S_s), and maxillary sinus (M_s).

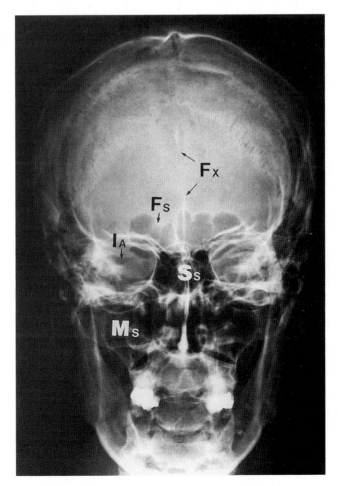

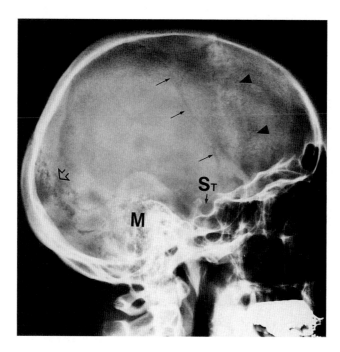

Figure 12.2. Lateral radiograph of the skull. The following structures are visible: coronal suture (*arrowheads*), occipital suture (*open arrow*), middle meningeal vascular grooves (*straight arrows*), sella turcica (S_T), and mastoid air cells (*M*).

(Fig. 12.4) shows the major basal foramina and the zygomatic arches. This view is not as useful as thin CT sections through the skull base, because the latter examination portrays the anatomy in greater detail (Fig. 12.5). The occipitomental (*Waters*) projection (Fig. 12.6) is used primarily to study the facial bones and sinuses. Dentists and oral surgeons also use a *panoramic* type of tomogram to study the mandible and facial bones (Fig. 12.7). The TM joints are best studied by CT and MR imaging.

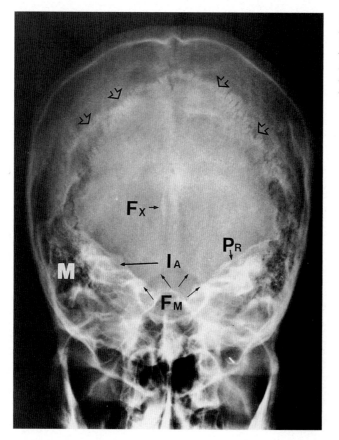

Figure 12.3. Modified half-axial projection (Towne). The following structures are visible: occipital sutures (*open arrows*), mastoid air cells (*M*), falx cerebri (F_X), internal auditory canal (I_A), petrous ridge (P_R), and foramen magnum (F_M).

Figure 12.4.   Base view. The following structures are visible: mastoid air cells (*M*), mandible (*M$_N$*), maxillary sinus (*M$_s$*), sphenoid sinus (*S$_s$*), foramen magnum (*F$_M$*), and temporomandibular joint (*T$_M$*).

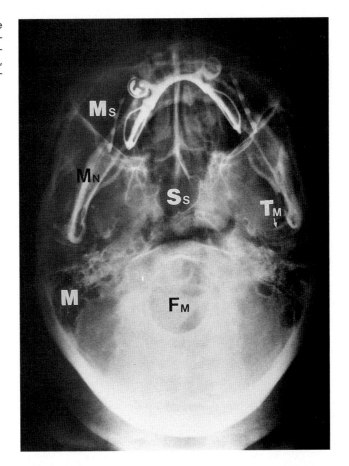

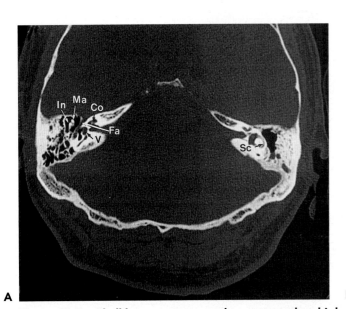

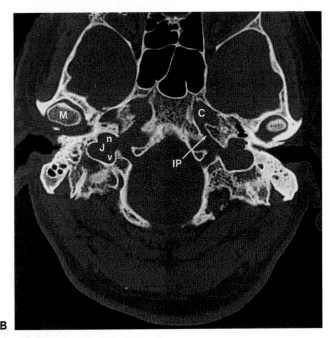

Figure 12.5.   Skull base anatomy as demonstrated on high-detail CT. A. Level of the mastoids.
B. Level of the mandibular condyles.   *(continued on page 452)*

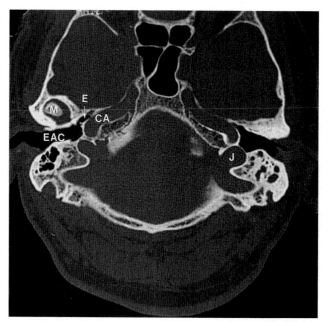

Figure 12.5. *(continued)* **C.** Level of the external auditory canals. The following structures are visible: incus (*In*); malleus (*Ma*); cochlea (*Co*); facial nerve canal (*Fa*); vestibule (*V*); semicircular canal (*Sc*); mandibular condyle (*M*); jugular foramen (*J*) with its anterior pars nervosa (*n*, containing cranial nerve IX) and pars vascularis (*v*, containing cranial nerves X and XI); inferior petrosal sinus (*IP*); carotid-cavernous sinus (*C*); carotid artery (*CA*); opening of the eustachian tube (*E*); and external auditory canal (*EAC*).

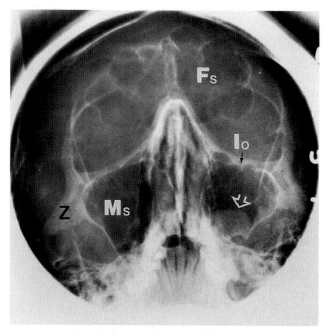

Figure 12.6. Occipitomental (Waters) projection. The following structures are visible: zygomatic arch (*Z*), maxillary sinus (*M*$_s$), frontal sinus (*F*$_s$), and inferior orbital rim (*I*$_o$ and *small arrow*). A mucous retention cyst (*open arrow*) is in the left maxillary sinus.

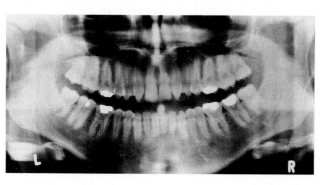

Figure 12.7. Panoramic tomogram of the mandible.

Figure 12.8. Prominent vascular groove (*curved arrow*) that ends in a venous lake (*large black arrow*). Notice the branch (*open arrow*).

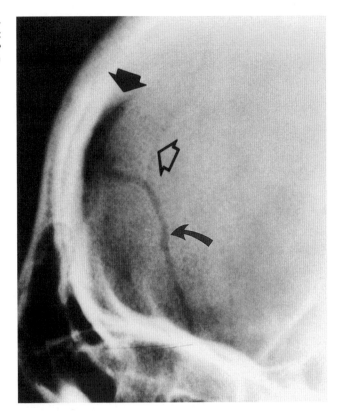

A large variety of normal structures and conditions may cause diagnostic concern. These include prominent vascular grooves (Fig. 12.8), hyperostosis frontalis interna (Fig. 12.9), calcified falx cerebri (Fig. 12.10), and persistent anomalous sutures (Fig. 12.11). When in doubt, review the films with a radiologist.

Evaluation of the brain with CT and MR produces transverse images that are remarkable in their similarity. MR has the advantage of producing images that clearly distinguish gray from

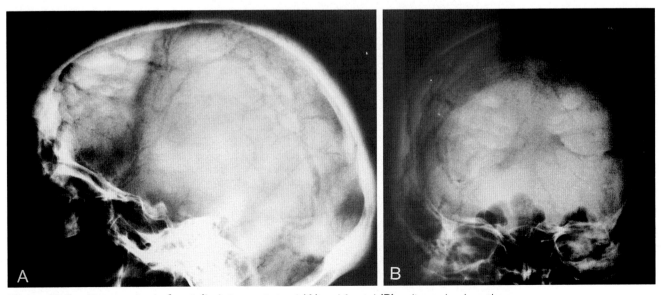

Figure 12.9.   Hyperostosis frontalis interna. Lateral **(A)** and frontal **(B)** radiographs show the thickened internal table of the skull. This is a normal variant.

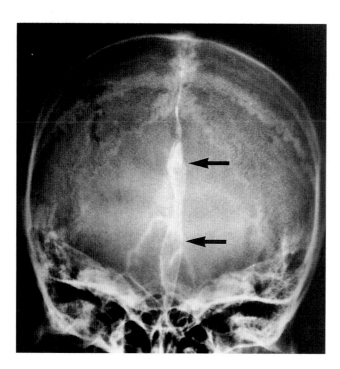

Figure 12.10.   Calcified falx cerebri (*arrows*).

white matter, and it has the additional advantage of being able to portray the brain in sagittal and coronal as well as in axial planes. Enhancement of vascular structures may be accomplished by using intravenous gadolinium DTPA. CT images are filmed at both brain (soft tissue) and bone windows.

Figures 12.12 through 12.15 show representative CT images and their MR counterparts of the various normal intracranial structures.

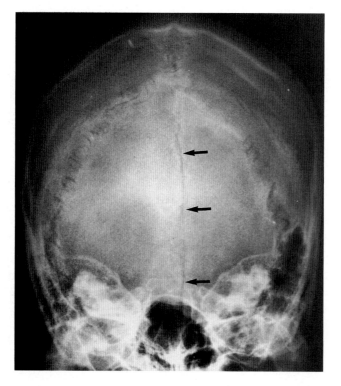

Figure 12.11.   Persistent metopic suture (*arrows*). This could be mistaken for a fracture.

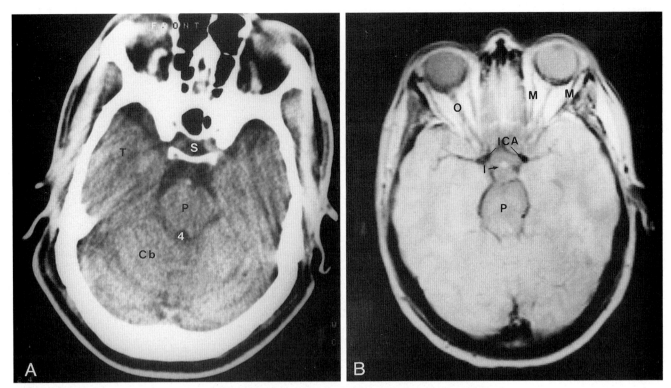

Figure 12.12.   Normal structures of the brain near the skull base. A. CT scan. **B.** Comparable MR image. Notice the greater detail compared with the CT. The following landmarks are visible: cerebellum (*Cb*), fourth ventricle (*4*), pons (*P*), temporal lobe (*T*), sella turcica (*S*), infundibulum of the pituitary (*I*), internal carotid arteries (*ICA*), optic nerve (*O*), and ocular muscles (*M*).

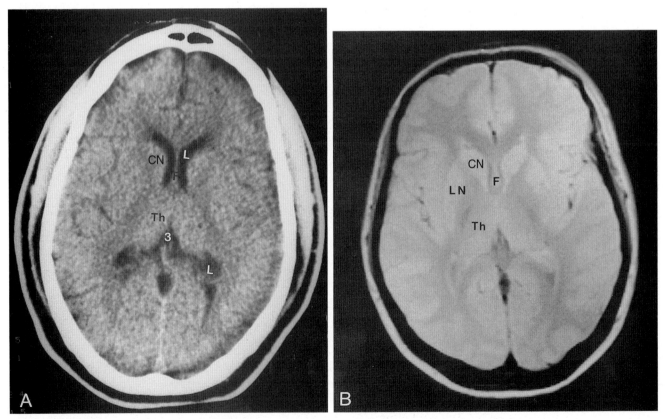

Figure 12.13.   Normal midbrain structures. A. CT scan. **B.** Comparable MR image. The following structures are visible: caudate nucleus (*CN*), lateral ventricle (*L*), fornix (*F*), thalamus (*Th*), third ventricle (*3*), and lentiform nucleus (*LN*).

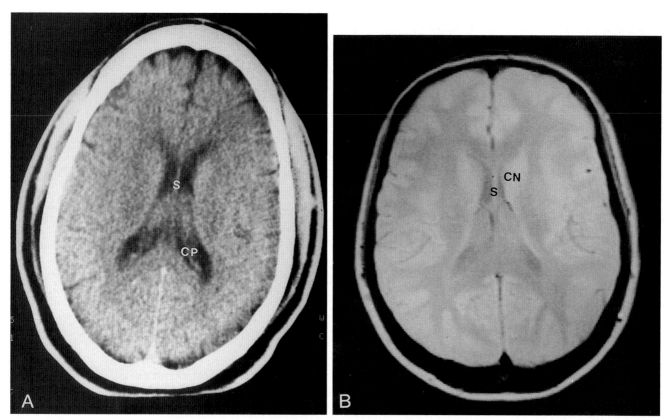

Figure 12.14. **Normal cerebral anatomy.** These views are slightly higher than those in Figure 12.13. **A.** CT scan. **B.** Comparable MR image. The following structures are visible: interventricular septum (*S*), choroid plexus (*CP*), and caudate nucleus (*CN*).

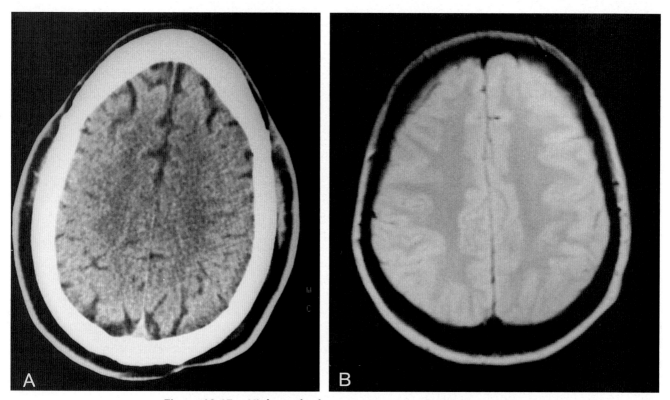

Figure 12.15. **High cerebral cortex. A.** CT scan. **B.** MR image. Notice the improved differentiation between gray matter and white matter by MR.

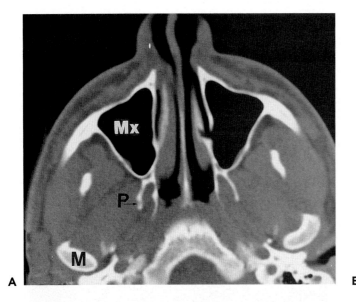

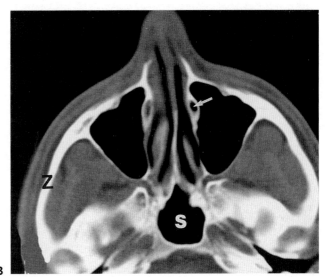

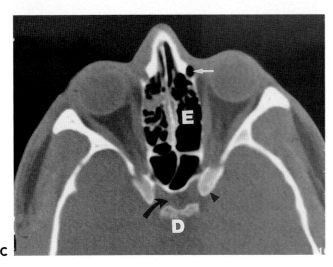

Figure 12.16.   Normal facial anatomy as demonstrated by axial CT imaging. A. Image through the lower maxilla shows the following structures: maxillary sinus (*Mx*), pterygoid plates (*P*), and mandibular condyle (*M*). **B.** Image through mid-maxilla shows the following structures: zygomatic arch (*Z*), sphenoid sinus (*S*), and nasolacrimal duct (*arrow*). **C.** Image through mid-orbits shows the following structures: nasolacrimal duct (*straight arrow*), ethmoid sinus (*E*), sella turcica (*curved arrow*); dorsum sellae (*D*); anterior clinoid process (*arrowhead*). In addition, notice the intraocular muscles in each eye.

Facial CT is now the primary investigative tool for evaluating facial fractures as well as sinus disease. Thin section (2-mm) axial and direct coronal images are routinely obtained. If direct coronal images are precluded by the patient's condition, coronal reconstruction is used instead. Figures 12.16 and 12.17 show normal facial anatomy in axial and coronal planes, respectively. Oral, maxillofacial, and plastic surgeons have found three-dimensional reconstruction of facial images to be extremely useful (Fig. 12.18). Interestingly, radiographs of the face (Waters and lateral views) are still very accurate in identifying fractures.

PATHOLOGIC CONSIDERATIONS

The most common pathologic states you will encounter radiologically in the nervous system are trauma, neoplasms, vascular disease, multiple sclerosis, infections, and cerebral atrophy and hydrocephalus.

Trauma

As previously mentioned, fractures of the skull and their sequelae are the best examples of the statement, "A fracture is a soft tissue injury in which a bone is broken." Indications for CT

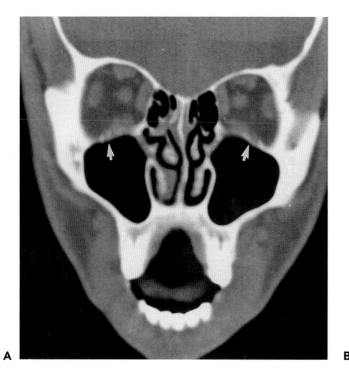

A

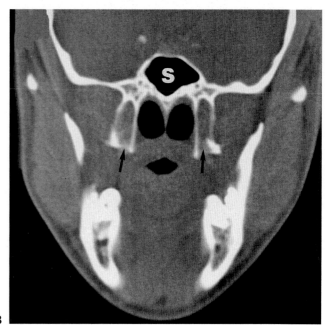

B

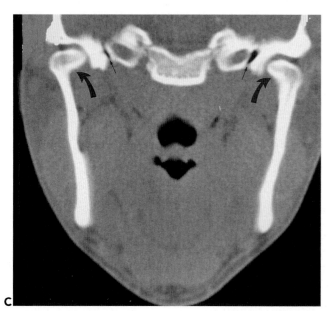

C

Figure 12.17.   Normal facial anatomy as demonstrated by direct coronal CT imaging. A. Image through the posterior orbits shows the orbital floors (*arrows*). Notice the intraocular muscles and the optic nerves within the orbits. **B.** Image through the back of the maxilla shows the pterygoid plates (*arrows*) and the sphenoid sinus (*S*). **C.** Image through the skull base shows the mandibular condyles (*curved arrows*) and eustachian tubes (*small straight arrows*).

examination after trauma include signs and symptoms of neurologic abnormality: loss of consciousness and abnormal neurologic findings on examination. Because the treatment of skull fractures, with two notable exceptions, is directed toward treating the neurologic abnormality, the presence or absence of a fracture itself makes little difference in the management of the patient. You will encounter many patients in whom a skull fracture is present without neurologic findings or sequelae, as well as patients with head injury without fracture where significant neurologic damage has occurred.

Two situations in which the *skull fracture* itself is significant are the depressed fracture and the fracture associated with penetration of a bullet or other foreign object. However, in both

Figure 12.18. Value of three-dimensional CT in a patient with bilateral mandibular fractures (*arrows*). This is the view that the surgeon would see at the time of surgery.

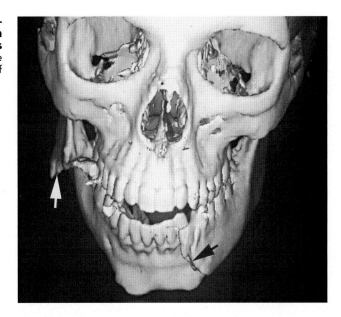

these instances, associated neurologic abnormalities are usually present and will dictate CT examination before corrective therapy. Brain injury is indicated by brain edema or hemorrhage. On CT, brain edema is manifest as an area of low density; acute hemorrhage as an area of high density. Figures 12.19 to 12.22 illustrate skull fractures and their associated findings. MR portrays brain edema as areas of low signal intensity on T1-weighted images and increased signal intensity on T2-weighted and short T1 inversion recovery (STIR) images.

There are three types of posttraumatic intracranial bleeding: intracerebral hemorrhage and epidural and subdural hematomas. Intracerebral hemorrhage presents on CT as areas of increased density in the acute stage. Frequently, intracerebral hemorrhages are associated with

Figure 12.19. Depressed skull fracture in the right frontal region (*arrows*).

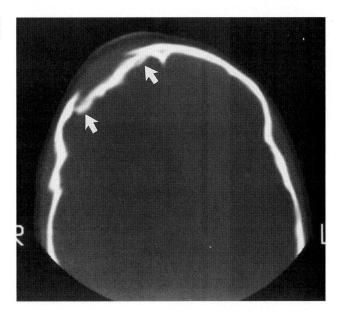

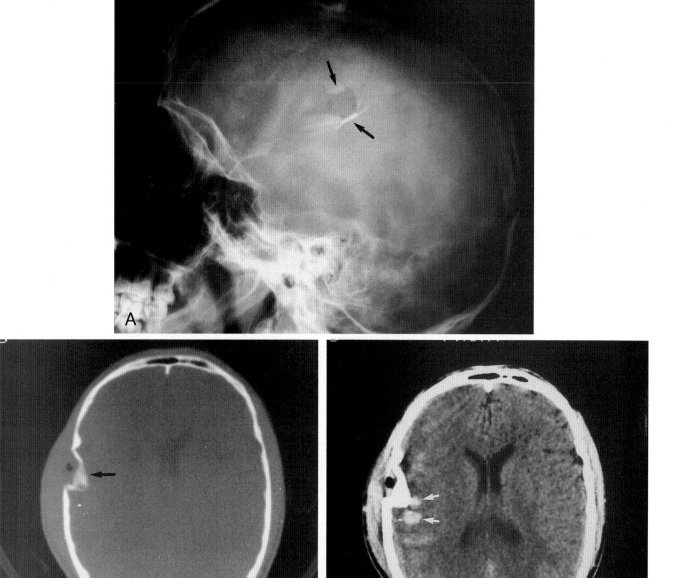

Figure 12.20.   Depressed skull fracture with intracerebral hemorrhage. A. Lateral radiograph
shows a comminuted depressed fracture in the parietal region (*arrows*). **B.** CT image at bone window
shows the depressed fragment (*arrow*). **C.** Same image using brain windows shows multiple areas of
intracranial hemorrhage (*arrows*) adjacent to the fracture.

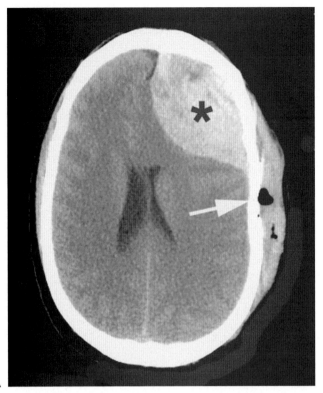
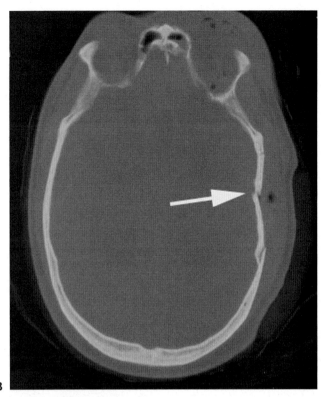

Figure 12.21.   Skull fracture in the left temporal region with epidural hematoma. A. CT image at brain window shows the lentiform epidural hematoma (*) in the left frontal region. Notice the superficial hematoma and gas in the left temporal region (arrow). **B.** CT image slightly lower at bone window shows the depressed fracture (arrow). Epidural hematomas are not always over fractures.

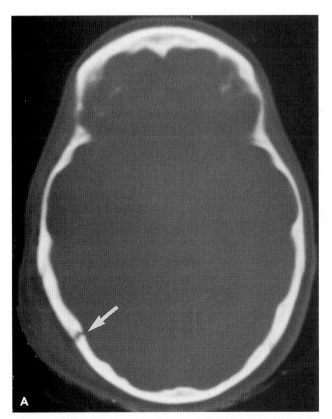
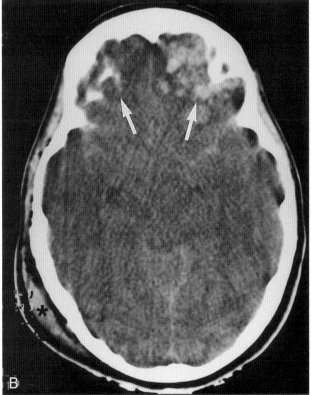

Figure 12.22.   Contrecoup brain injury. A. CT image at bone window shows a fracture in the right posterior parietal bone (arrow). **B.** Same image at brain window shows areas of intracerebral hemorrhage in the frontal lobes (arrows). Notice the scalp hematoma (*) in the right occipital area.

bleeding into the ventricles (Fig. 12.23A, B). On MR imaging, the signal of the hemorrhage depends on its age and may range from low to high intensity (see Fig. 12.23C). Epidural and subdural *hematomas* may result from cranial trauma. *Epidural hematomas* are usually the result of fractures that involve one of the meningeal arteries. These hematomas characteristically have a *lentiform* shape (Fig. 12.24 and 12.25; see Fig. 12.21). *Subdural hematomas* result from injury, often trivial, to the meningeal veins. They are especially common in elderly patients

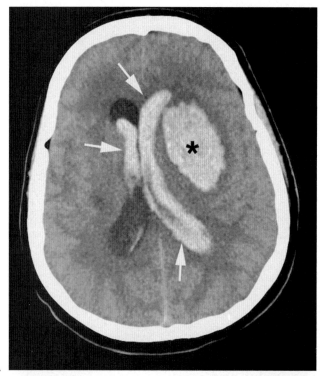

A

Figure 12.23.   MR image of intracranial hemorrhage. A and B. CT images show a large parietal lobe hemorrhage (*). Notice the intraventricular blood (*arrows*). **C.** Coronal T1-weighted MR image shows a hematoma in the right parietal lobe (*) in another patient. (MR image courtesy of James M. Provenzale, MD, Department of Diagnostic Radiology, Duke University Medical Center.)

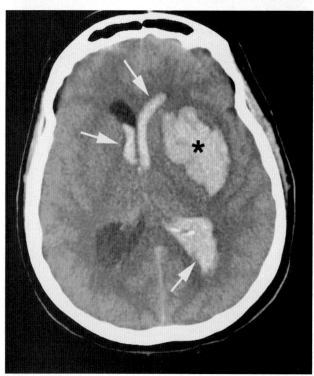

B

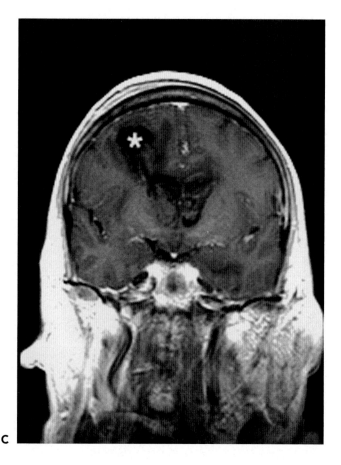

C

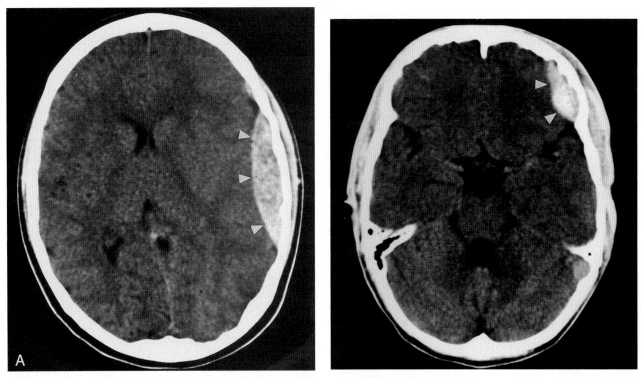

Figure 12.24. Acute epidural hematomas in two patients. Notice the typical lentiform shape to the hematomas (*arrowheads*).

Figure 12.25. MR image of epidural hematoma. An intracerebral hemorrhage (*arrowheads*) and an occipital epidural hematoma (*arrow*) are evident. Notice the lentiform shape to the epidural.

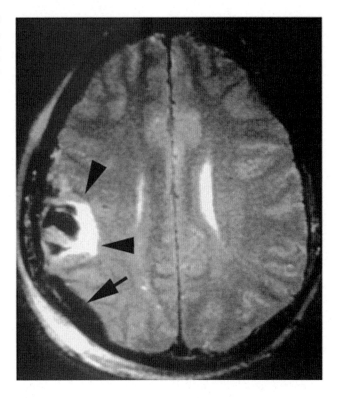

and may cause dementia. In the acute stage, they conform to the contour of the brain and have a *crescentic* shape (Figs. 12.26 and 12.27). When they become chronic, they assume a lentiform shape (Fig. 12.28).

Facial fractures are common injuries. At our level I trauma center, facial fractures occurred in approximately 15% of the 25,000 trauma patients seen over the past decade. Facial fractures occur in various patterns that produce characteristic radiographic and CT abnormalities reflecting the distinctive type of injury. For example, a direct blow to the eye (usually from a fist) is likely to result in an *orbital blowout fracture* (Fig. 12.29) of either the floor or medial wall. Similarly, a blow to the malar region (from a fist) is most likely to produce a *zygomaticomaxillary complex* fracture, characterized by fractures of the zygomatic arch, the frontozygomatic suture, the anterior inferior orbital rim, and the anterior maxillary wall (Fig. 12.30). This fracture is sometimes erroneously called a *tripod fracture* because it produces a triangular bone fragment. Other more severe forms of facial trauma include various

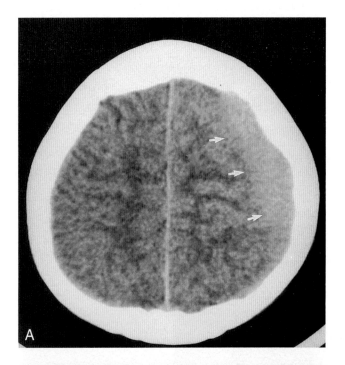

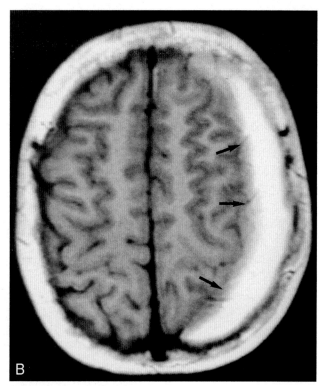

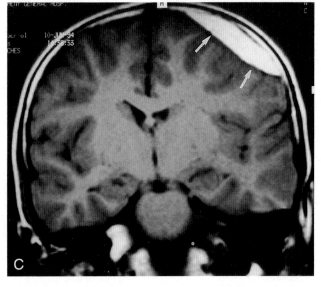

Figure 12.26. Acute subdural hematoma. A. CT image shows a faint area of increased density on the left (*arrow*). Axial **(B)** and coronal **(C)** T1-weighted MR images show the lentiform hematoma (*arrows*) to greater advantage than does the CT image. Notice the compression of the brain and distortion of the left lateral ventricle in C.

Figure 12.27. MR image of subdural hematoma. T2-weighted MR image shows a frontal subdural hematoma (*arrows*) that has separated into cellular and serum components. (Courtesy James M. Provenzale, MD, Department of Diagnostic Radiology, Duke University Medical Center.)

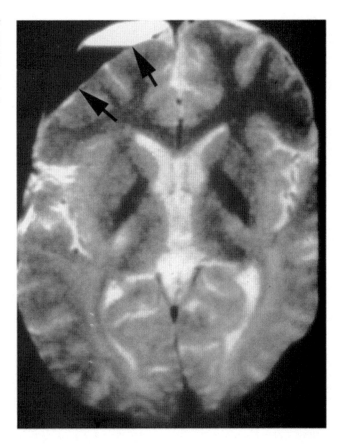

Figure 12.28. Chronic subdural hematoma. CT image shows compression of the left side of the brain by a large extracerebral hematoma (*open arrows*). The blood products have separated, and a fluid level is visible (*solid arrows*).

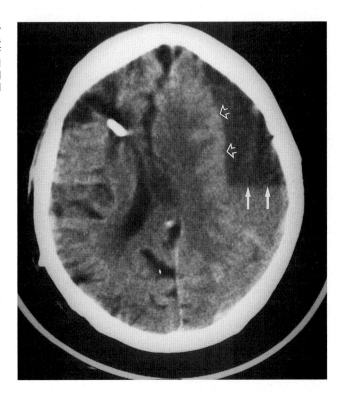

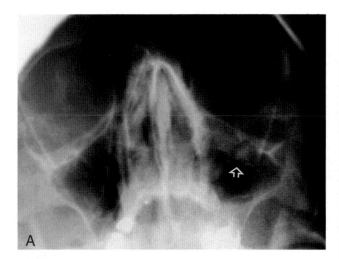

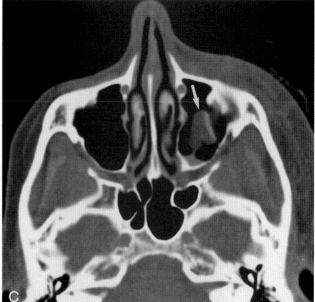

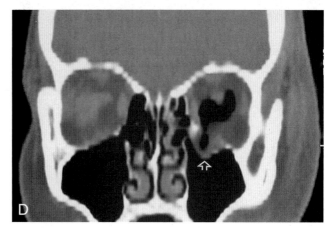

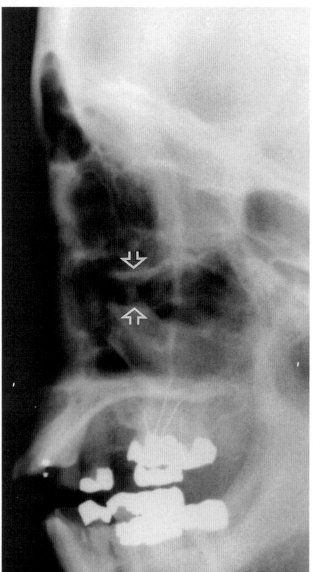

Figure 12.29.   Blowout fracture of the left orbital floor.
A. Waters view shows a double density at the roof of the left maxillary sinus (*arrow*) as well as an air-fluid level. **B.** Lateral facial radiograph shows a "double floor sign" (*arrows*). The lower arrow points to the depressed floor of the left orbit. **C.** Axial CT image shows a soft tissue density (*arrow*) projecting into the maxillary sinus on the left. This represents the orbital content herniated through the fracture. **D.** Coronal tomographic reconstruction shows the fractured orbital floor and the downward herniation of orbital content (*arrow*).

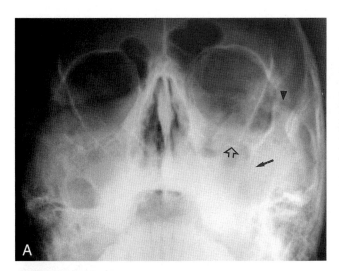

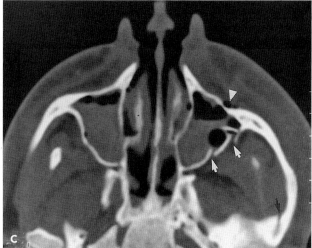

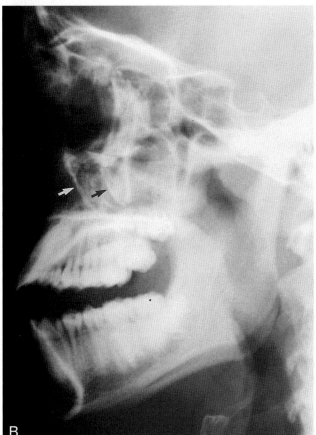

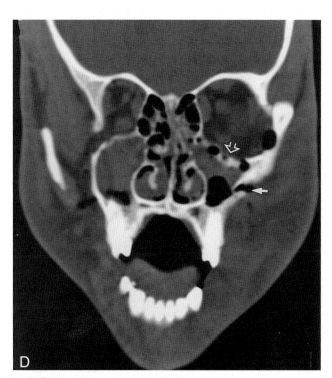

Figure 12.30.   Zygomaticomaxillary complex fracture on the left. A. Waters view shows soft tissue swelling over the entire face. However, there is asymmetry between the bony structures. Notice the fractures of the floor of the orbit (*open arrow*), lateral maxillary wall (*long arrow*), and lateral wall of the orbit (*arrowhead*) on the left. **B.** Lateral radiograph shows a "double strut sign" (*arrows*). The posterior arrow points to the malar strut on the left that has been displaced posteriorly as a result of the fracture. **C.** Axial CT image demonstrates fractures of the posterior wall of the maxillary sinus (*white arrows*), fracture of the zygomatic arch (*black arrow*), and gas in the malar soft tissues on the left (*arrowhead*). Notice the asymmetry between the zygomatic bones. **D.** Direct coronal CT image demonstrates fractures through the floor of the orbit (*open arrow*) and lateral wall of the maxilla on the left (*solid arrow*).

degrees of maxillofacial separation (the *LeFort fractures*; Fig. 12.31). CT imaging, which often is three-dimensional, is required for complete evaluation of these patients (Fig. 12.32). CT is also extremely useful for postoperative evaluation of patients with facial fractures.

An associated abnormality that often occurs in patients with skull or facial trauma is *cervical vertebral trauma*. A direct blow to the skull or face is usually of sufficient force to produce enough stress on the cervical vertebrae in flexion, extension, or lateral flexion to cause a fracture or ligamentous disruption. At our medical center, every patient evaluated for skull or facial trauma is considered "at high risk" for vertebral injury (see Chapter 13) and, therefore, undergoes cervical CT examination at the same time the cranial examination is obtained.

Neoplasms

The diagnosis of primary or metastatic brain tumors has been greatly aided by CT and MR imaging. Although some of your patients will have these lesions, the actual interpretation of their imaging studies will be performed by neuroradiologists, neurologists, and neurosurgeons.

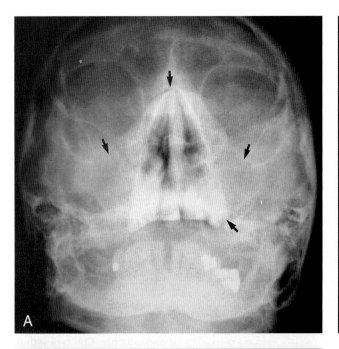

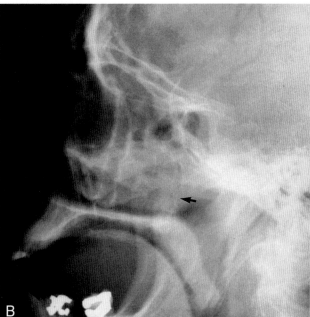

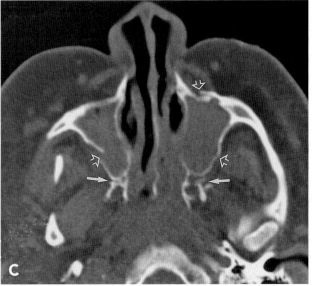

Figure 12.31.   LeFort II fracture. A. Waters view demonstrates extensive soft tissue swelling and distortion of the facial anatomy. Fractures are visible through the floors of both orbits, bridge of the nose, and lateral maxillary wall on the left (*arrows*). In addition, note the malocclusion between the maxilla and the mandible. **B.** Lateral radiograph shows fractures through the pterygoid plates (*arrow*). **C.** Axial CT image shows bilateral maxillary fractures (*open arrows*) as well as fractures through the pterygoid plates (*solid arrows*). Notice the opacification of the maxillary sinuses.

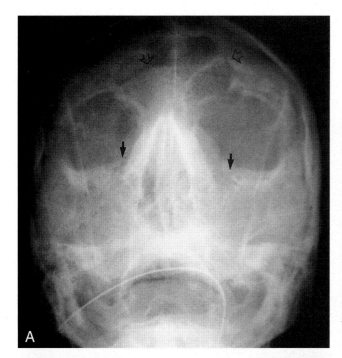

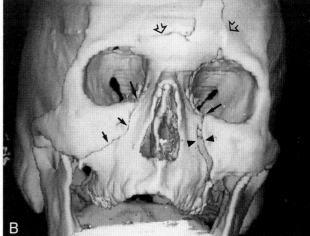

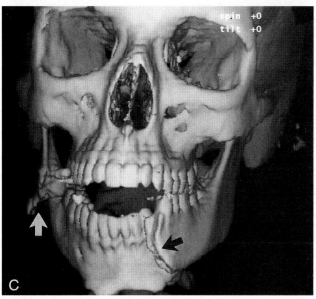

Figure 12.32.   Value of three-dimensional CT for facial fractures. A. Waters view of a patient with a LeFort II fracture. Notice the fracture lines through the medial inferior walls of both orbits (*solid arrows*) and across the frontal bone (*open arrows*). In addition, massive soft tissue swelling is evident. **B.** Three-dimensional CT reconstruction shows the fractures of the orbits (*long arrows*) and frontal bone (*open arrows*), as well as fractures of the anterior wall of the maxilla. The right-sided maxillary fracture (*short arrows*) has not separated as the fracture on the left (*arrowheads*) has. Compare with A. **C.** Three-dimensional CT reconstruction in another patient with bilateral mandibular fractures (*arrows*). Notice the malocclusion as well as the displacement of the fracture fragments.

For this reason, the discussion of neoplasms here is brief, concentrating on the CT and MR appearance.

Intracranial tumors may be axial: in brain substance, such as gliomas; extra-axial, such as meningiomas; or rarely, a bone tumor. Imaging findings include delineation of the tumor mass on CT (Fig. 12.33) or MR (Fig. 12.34). In addition, edema is produced by intracerebral tumors in various degrees. On MR studies, edema is manifest as low signal intensity on T1-weighted images and high signal intensity on T2-weighted images. The mass itself or the edema may result in displacement of the ventricles as well as compression of adjacent normal brain tissues (Fig. 12.35). Multiple masses suggest metastases as the etiology. Similarly, metastasis is suggested if a large amount of edema is surrounding the tumor (Fig. 12.36).

Vascular changes of tumors include displacement of vessels (Fig. 12.37) and the presence of *neovascularity* (tumor vessels). One of the features of many brain tumors, because of their vascularity, is that they often enhance on CT or MR imaging when the patient has had an intravenous injection of contrast material (Fig. 12.38).

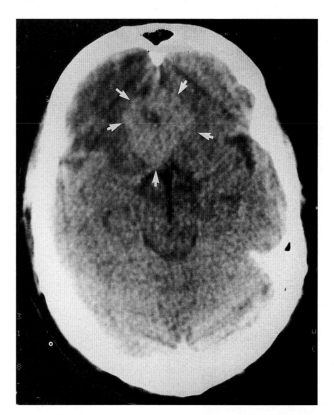

Figure 12.33. **Frontal meningioma.** CT image shows a mass in the frontal region (*arrows*).

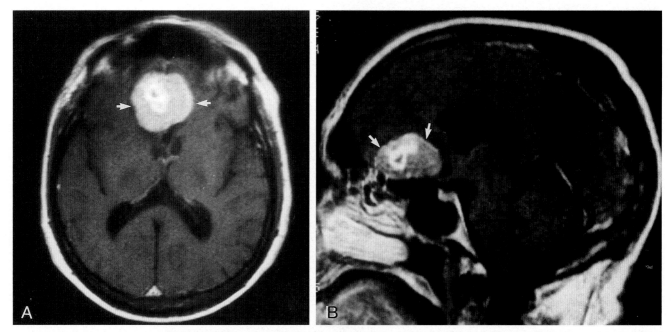

Figure 12.34. **Frontal meningioma.** (This is the same patient as in Fig. 12.33.) **A.** Axial T1-weighted MR image shows the mass to better advantage (*arrows*) than does the CT. Notice the extremely high signal in the center of the mass. **B.** Direct sagittal T1-weighted MR image shows similar findings (*arrows*).

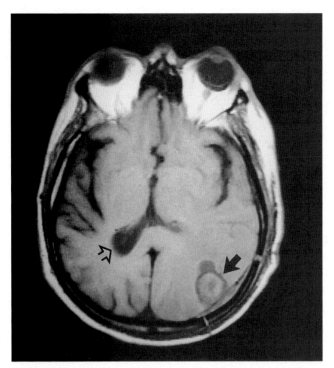

Figure 12.35.   Metastatic lesion showing ventricular compression. T1-weighted MR image shows that the metastatic lesion (*solid arrow*) in the left occipital lobe has compressed the posterior horn of the left lateral ventricle. Compare with the normal right ventricle (*open arrow*).

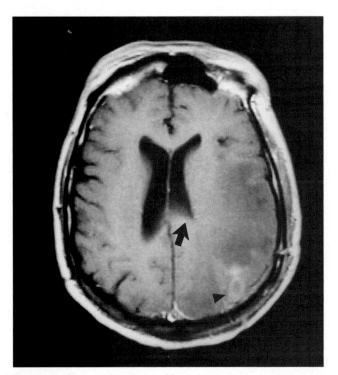

Figure 12.36.   Metastatic lesion showing edema. (This is the same patient as in Figs. 12.35 and 12.38.) T1-weighted MR image shows the edema as an area of lower signal than a normal brain. Notice the loss of convolutional markings on the left, ventricular compression (*arrow*), and the tumor itself (*arrowhead*).

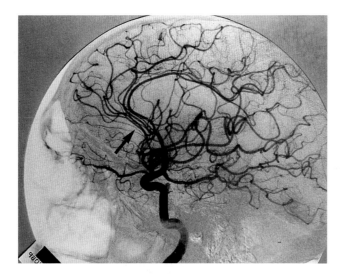

Figure 12.37. Cerebral arteriogram in a patient with frontal meningioma. (This is the same patient as in Figs. 12.33 and 12.34.) The tumor elevates both anterior cerebral arteries (*arrow*).

One of the newer developments in neurosurgery makes use of stereotactic biopsy of brain tumors using CT guidance to identify the exact location for the neurosurgeon. To perform this type of examination, a stereotactic template is clamped to the patient's skull before CT examination. Location coordinates of the lesion are obtained through measurements from the relationships of the tumor to the template. This has resulted in more accurate localization of tumors with subsequent loss of less normal brain tissue during the surgical procedure.

Intraoperative ultrasound is also used to locate brain lesions for the neurosurgeon. The ultrasound probe is placed directly on the dura or brain surface after surgical exposure. As with stereotactic guidance, the ultrasonic examination provides both location and depth information to the surgeon.

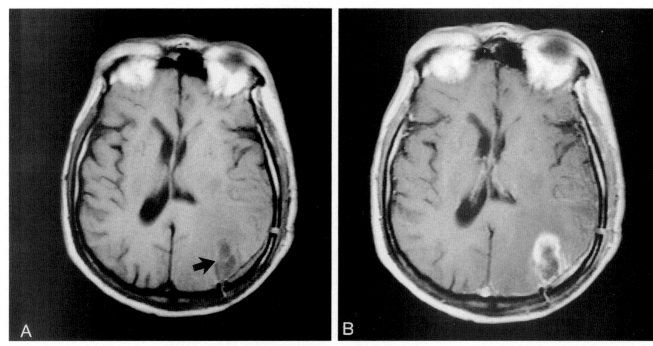

Figure 12.38. Metastatic brain tumor showing contrast enhancement. (This is the same patient as in Figs. 12.35 and 12.36.) **A.** T1-weighted MR image without contrast shows the tumor as a multilobular area of low signal (*arrow*). **B.** After intravenous contrast enhancement with gadolinium, the tumor is much more prominent. The unenhanced portion of the tumor represents necrosis. *(continued on page 473)*

Figure 12.38. *(continued)* **C.** Coronal T1-weighted image after intravenous contrast enhancement in another patient shows multiple metastatic nodules that are hypervascular. Notice the edema surrounding many of them.

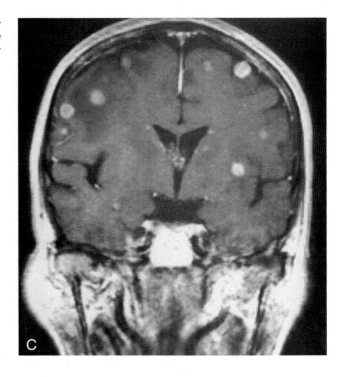

Vascular Disease

Vascular-related abnormalities are common in the head and neck. This group of disorders includes infarction secondary to atherosclerotic or embolic occlusion (Fig. 12.39), intracerebral hemorrhage (Fig. 12.40), arteriovenous malformations (AVMs), aneurysms (Figs. 12.41 and 12.42), and extracerebral hemorrhages (Fig. 12.43). All these may be readily diagnosed by CT and/or MR examinations. Furthermore, examination of the carotid arteries in the neck by Doppler ultrasound (Fig. 12.44) is used to evaluate patients with suspected ischemic cerebral problems. Positive studies are followed up with arteriography if carotid angioplasty is contemplated.

Figure 12.39. Brain infarcts. A. T2-weighted MR image shows bilateral areas of high signal (*arrows*). Notice the ventricular dilation in this elderly patient. *(continued on page 474)*

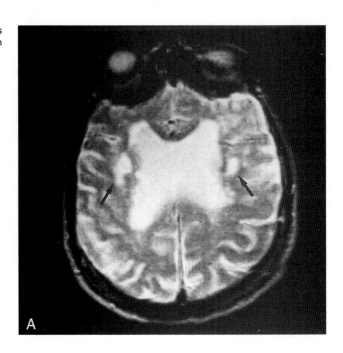

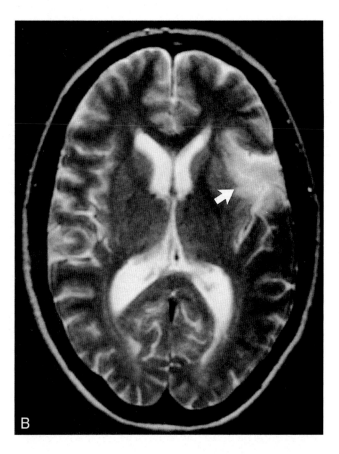

Figure 12.39. *(continued)* **B.** T2-weighted image in another patient shows a large area of high signal in the left parietal region (*arrow*).

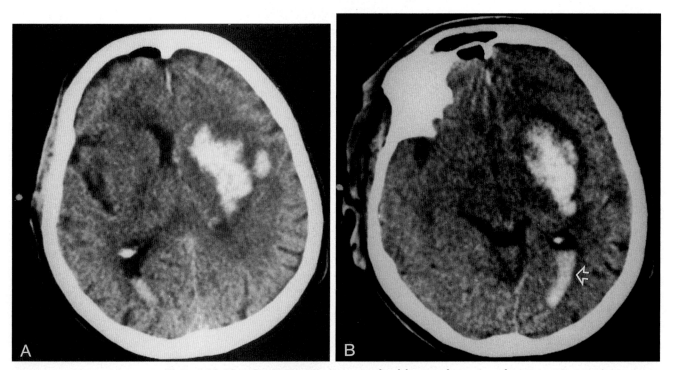

Figure 12.40. Spontaneous intracerebral hemorrhage in a hypertensive patient. A. CT image shows increased density of the hemorrhage in the left periventricular region. **B.** At a slightly lower level, blood layers out in the posterior horn of the lateral ventricle (*arrow*).

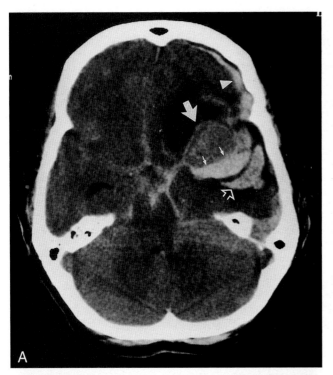

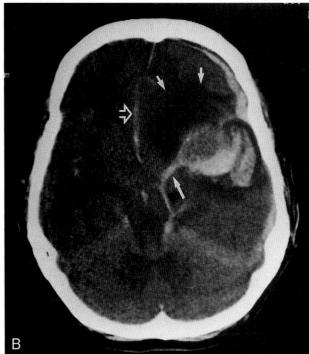

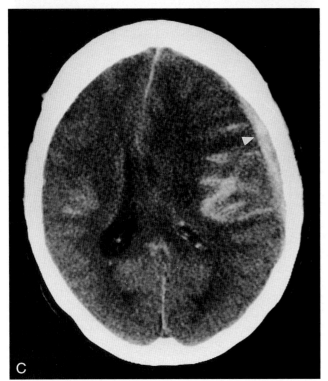

Figure 12.41. Bleeding intracerebral aneurysm. A. CT image near the circle of Willis demonstrates a large left-sided aneurysm (*large arrow*). The lower portion of the aneurysm is filled with fresh blood (*small arrows*), the upper with clot. A subarachnoid hemorrhage (*open arrow*) and a subdural hematoma (*arrowhead*) are evident. **B.** CT image slightly higher shows a large area of edema anterior to the aneurysm (*small solid arrows*). There is bowing of the falx to the left (*open arrow*). The origin of the aneurysm from the internal middle cerebral artery (*long solid arrow*) is visible. **C.** CT image slightly higher demonstrates intracerebral hemorrhage as well as the subdural hematoma (*arrowhead*).

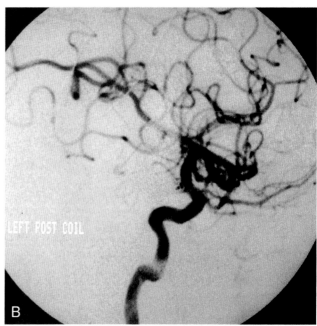

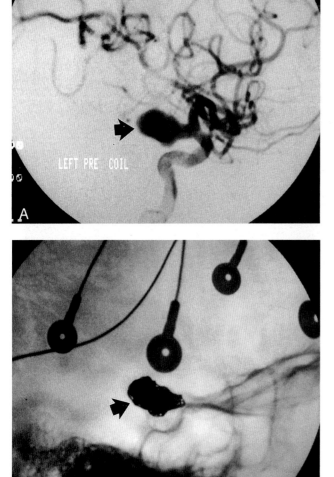

Figure 12.42.   Aneurysm of the intracranial portion of the internal carotid artery. A. Digital subtraction angiogram shows a large saccular aneurysm (*arrow*). **B.** Angiogram after successful occlusion of the aneurysm by a coil. The subtraction technique obscures the coil. **C.** Digital image shows the coil (*arrow*) just above the sella turcica. Notice the similarity in shape between the coil and the aneurysm, as demonstrated in A.

Premature infants are prone to intracerebral hemorrhages. Transcranial ultrasound of the newborn skull can detect these hemorrhages and identify ventricular changes that indicate developing hydrocephalus (Fig. 12.45).

AVMs and aneurysms are another cause of intracerebral and subarachnoid hemorrhages. These lesions have imaging characteristics identical to their counterparts found in other parts of the body. Furthermore, these lesions often present with subarachnoid hemorrhage, which on CT and MR imaging shows blood collections in the subarachnoid space, basal cisterns, and ventricles (Figs. 12.46 and 12.47). Many of these lesions can be treated using the interventional techniques described in Chapter 3.

Although nuclear imaging historically had a role in evaluating patients with suspected cerebrovascular problems, with the advent of CT angiography and MR imaging, use of

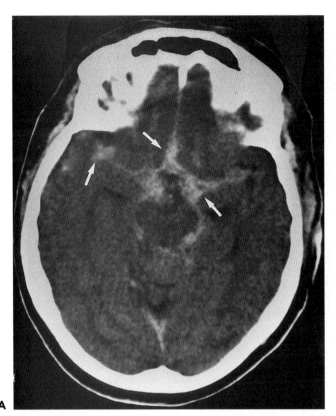

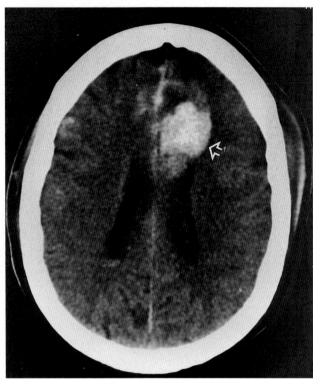

A   B

Figure 12.43.   Subarachnoid hemorrhage. A. CT image without intravenous contrast enhancement shows blood outlining the stellate basal cisterns (*arrows*). **B.** CT image higher shows intracerebral hemorrhage as well (*arrow*).

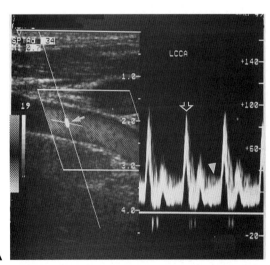

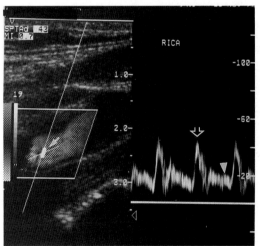

A   B

Figure 12.44.   Carotid Doppler ultrasound examination. A. Normal left common carotid artery (LCCA). The gray-scale image of a portion of the LCCA shows the vessel to be widely patent. The vessel walls are smooth, without visible atheromatous plaques. The rectangle within the vessel lumen (*small arrow*) is the Doppler sample site from which the flow characteristics and velocities generate the Doppler waveform tracing shown to the right of the gray-scale image. There is a normal peak systolic flow velocity of approximately 90 cm/sec (*open arrow*; normal <125 cm/sec) as well as antegrade blood flow velocity of 40 cm/sec at the end of diastole (*arrowhead*). **B.** Significant stenosis in the right internal carotid artery (RICA). The gray-scale image of a portion of a RICA shows gross vessel wall irregularity with significant stenosis near the Doppler sample site (*small arrow*). The peak systolic flow velocity is only 45 cm/sec (*open arrow*). The antegrade blood flow velocity at the end of diastole is 20 cm/sec (*arrowhead*). Compare with the flow velocities in A.

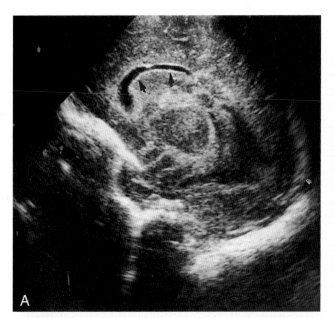

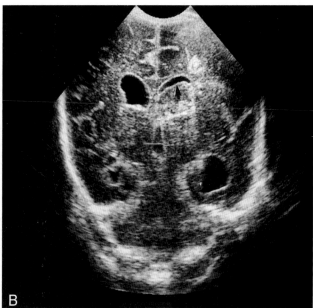

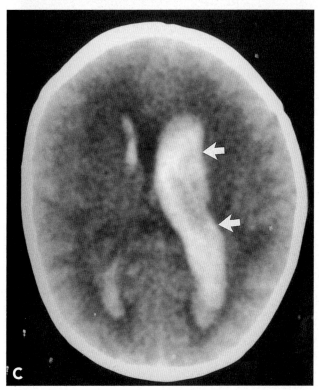

Figure 12.45.   Intracranial hemorrhage in a premature newborn. A. Sagittal transcranial ultrasound image demonstrates a mass within the lateral ventricle (*arrows*). **B.** Coronal image shows the clot within the left lateral ventricle (*arrow*). Compare with the opposite side. **C.** CT image shows blood in both lateral ventricles. On the left, it has formed a ventricular cast (*arrows*).

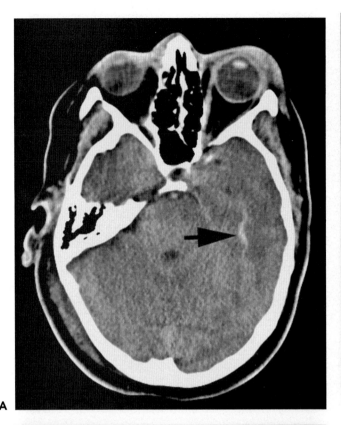

A

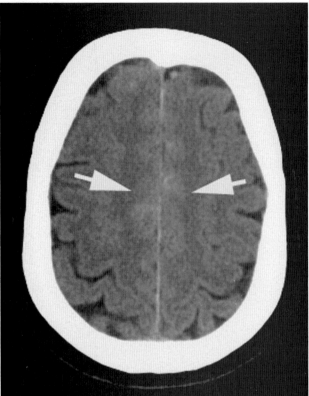

B

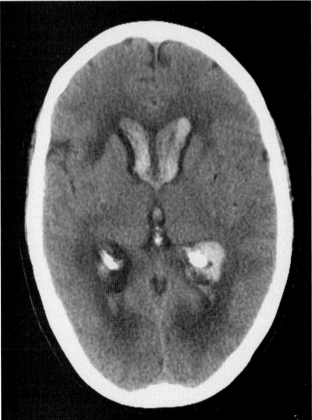

C

Figure 12.46.   CT of subarachnoid hemorrhage. A. CT image shows a high-density streak (*arrow*) representing blood in the Sylvian fissure. **B.** CT image in another patient shows blood in the sulci along the central fissure (*arrows*). **C.** CT image in another patient showing intraventricular hemorrhage, which appears as white areas in the ventricles. (Courtesy of James M. Provenzale, MD, Department of Diagnostic Radiology, Duke University Medical Center.)

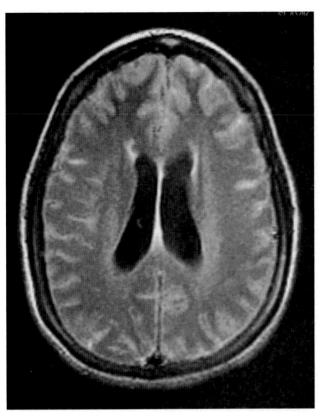
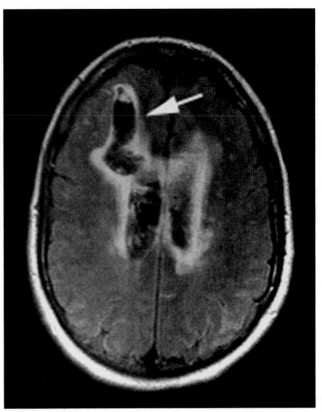

A   B

Figure 12.47.   MR of subarachnoid hemorrhage. (This is the same patient as in Fig. 12.46.C.) **A.** Fluid-attenuated inversion recovery (FLAIR) MR image shows high-signal material in the cerebral sulci, representing fresh blood. **B.** FLAIR image shows blood in the ventricle as increased signal due to the state of oxyhemoglobin. A secondary area of hemorrhage in the right frontal lobe (*arrow*) was iatrogenic, resulting from placement of a ventriculostomy. (Courtesy of James M. Provenzale, MD, Department of Diagnostic Radiology, Duke University Medical Center.)

radionuclide studies to assess entities such as AVMs or aneurysms has declined. Radionuclide flow studies are most likely to be used today to confirm brain death (Fig. 12.48).

Multiple Sclerosis

The development of MR imaging has provided a new method of evaluating patients with suspected multiple sclerosis. This insidious and severely debilitating disease that affects primarily young adults previously defied all imaging methods to establish a correct diagnosis. MR imaging clearly demonstrates the plaques that form within the white matter of the brain (Fig. 12.49).

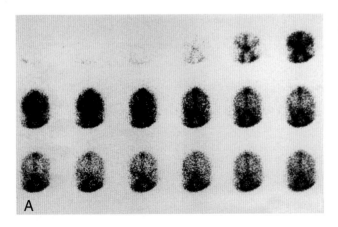

A

Figure 12.48.   Brain death. A. Normal radionuclide isotope flow study shows normal flow to the brain.   *(continued on page 481)*

Figure 12.48. *(continued)* **B.** In brain death, there is no circulation to the brain. Isotope is seen in the carotid vessels and the face. Compare with A. **C.** Delayed image shows no intracerebral isotope and concentration of isotope in the nasal cavity ("hot nose sign"). This pattern is considered pathognomonic for brain death.

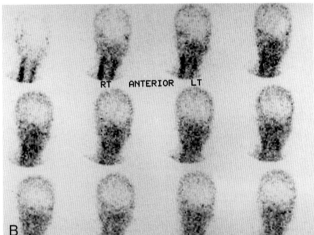

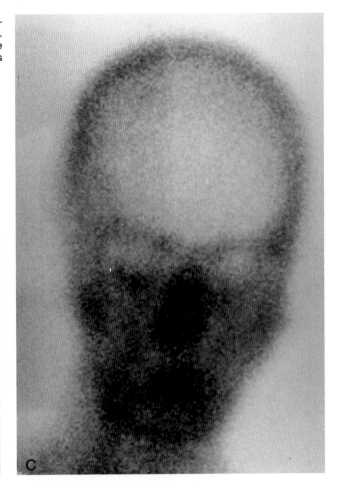

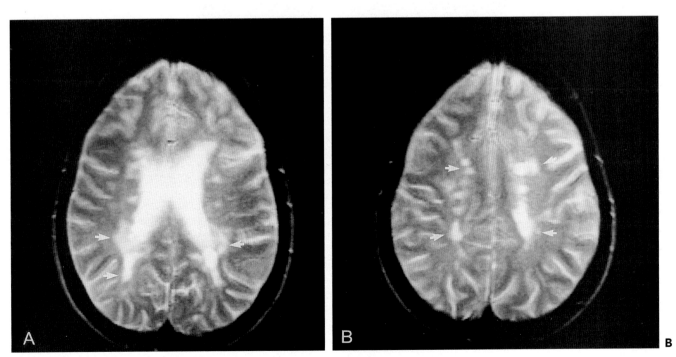

Figure 12.49.   Multiple sclerosis. A and B. Contiguous T2-weighted MR images show areas of ventricular plaques of high signal (*arrows*).   *(continued on page 482)*

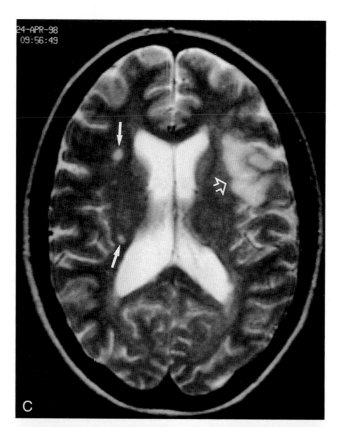

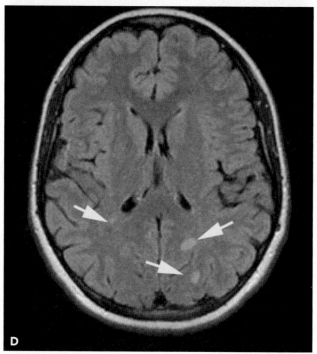

Figure 12.49. *(continued)* **C.** (This is the same patient as in Fig. 12.39B.) T2-weighted image in another patient shows small periventricular plaques *(solid arrows)* as well as an area of left parietal infarction *(open arrow).* **D.** T1-weighted image in another patient shows plaques in the white matter *(arrows).*

Although the disease remains incurable, an earlier accurate diagnosis is essential first to rule out other significant diseases and second to begin therapy. Furthermore, once the diagnosis is established, MR imaging may be used to follow the progress of the disease.

Brain Abscesses and Encephalitis

A brain abscess often presents as a mass. The clinical history is not always one of acute onset of neurologic symptoms. Nearly every patient has an established focus of infection elsewhere in the body. The finding on CT and MR is a mass, usually with an enhancing rim representing the capsule around it (Figs. 12.50 and 12.51). The mass may be difficult to differentiate from a necrotic tumor.

Encephalitis caused by the type 1 herpes simplex virus affects the inferior frontal lobes as well as the temporal lobes. Early diagnosis is important because of the availability of antiviral therapy with acyclovir, which must be administered within the first few days of the illness. The typical features include increased signal intensity on T2-weighted images in the affected gyri (Fig. 12.52). Gyral enhancement with gadolinium compounds is also characteristic.

As many as two-thirds of patients with HIV infection commonly develop neurologic symptoms. In most instances these symptoms are from vascular insults, direct HIV neurotoxicity, or opportunistic infections. Toxoplasmosis is the most common opportunistic organism to involve HIV patients. The typical toxoplasma lesion is that of one or more enhancing masses throughout the brain (Fig. 12.53). The diagnosis is confirmed by biopsy of the lesion. The lesions are almost identical, from an imaging standpoint, with lymphoma, a tumor that commonly affects the same group of patients.

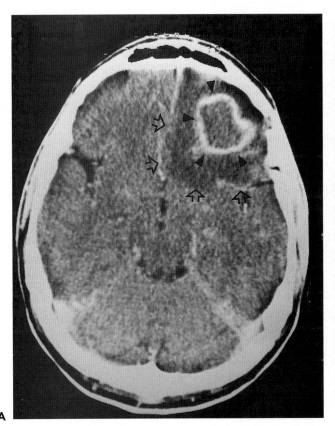
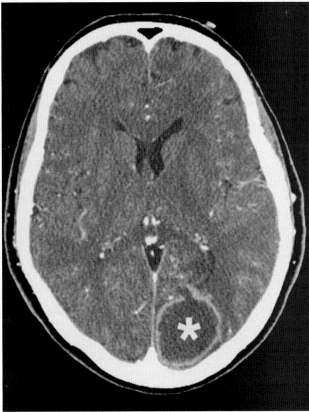

A

B

Figure 12.50.   Brain abscesses. A. Left frontal brain abscess. CT image after intravenous contrast enhancement shows the rim of the abscess to enhance (*arrowheads*). Notice the surrounding edema (*open arrows*). **B.** Left occipital lobe abscess (*) following contrast enhancement.

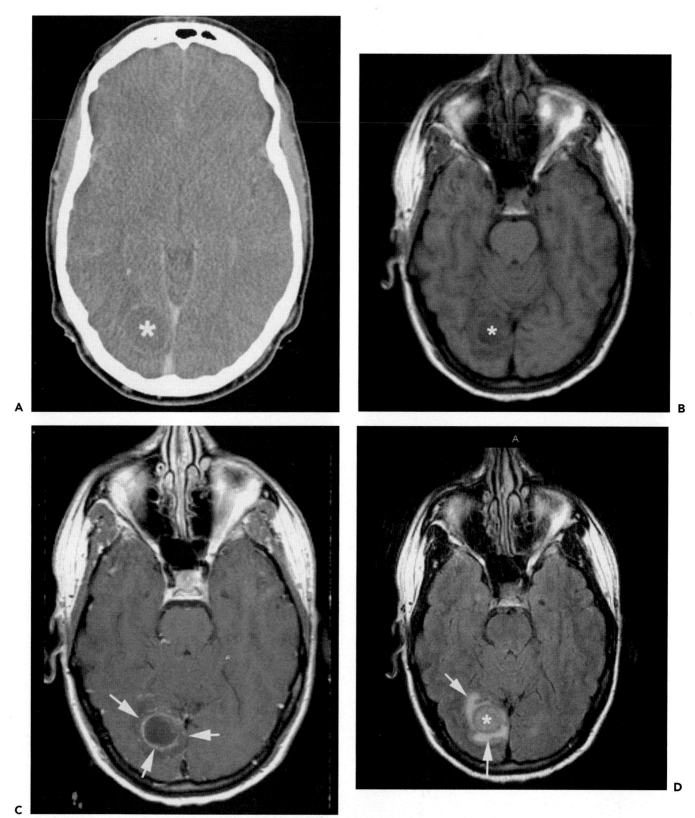

Figure 12.51.   MR of brain abscess. A. CT image shows an area of low density surrounded by a dense ring in the right occipital lobe (*). **B.** T1-weighted MR image shows similar findings (*). **C.** T1-weighted MR image following contrast shows enhancement of the wall of the abscess (*arrows*). **D.** T2-weighted MR image before contrast shows the ring of edema (*arrows*) surrounding the abscess (*).

Figure 12.52. Herpes encephalitis. T2-weighted MR image shows the entire left temporal lobe to be swollen and to show abnormal hyperintensity of cortex and white matter from edema (*open arrow*). In addition, notice similar but less extensive changes on the right (*small arrow*).

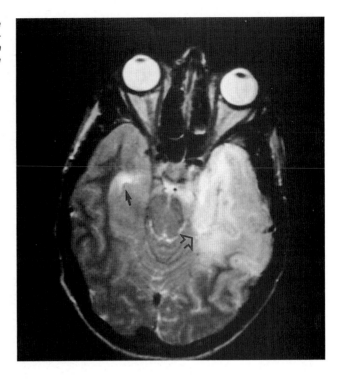

Cerebral Atrophy and Hydrocephalus

Cerebral atrophy occurs as a result of many causes, including infarction, previous trauma, and aging. The typical CT and MR appearance of this disorder is deepening of the sulci and widening of the ventricles (Fig. 12.54). A certain amount of cerebral atrophy is part of the normal aging process. Patients with Alzheimer disease also demonstrate these findings. PET scanning is particularly helpful in confirming the diagnosis (Fig. 12.55).

Figure 12.53. Toxoplasmosis in a patient with HIV infection. CT image shows a ringlike abscess (*arrows*) surrounded by edema.

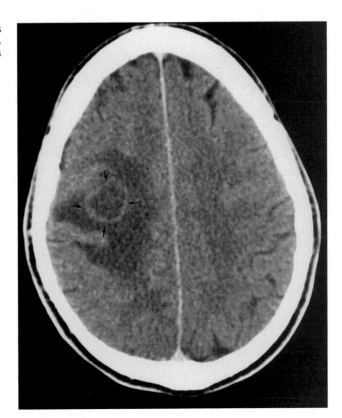

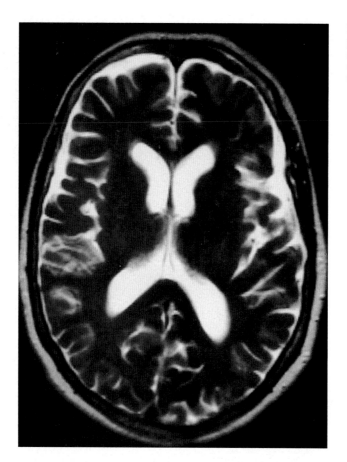

Figure 12.54. Cerebral atrophy. Inversion recovery MR image shows enlargement of the ventricles and deepening of the intracerebral sulci.

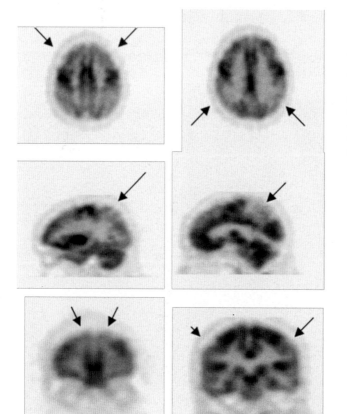

A

Figure 12.55. PET scan of patient with Alzheimer disease compared with normal. A. Focal decrease in perfusion with F-18 FDG of parieto-temporal as well as frontal and posterior cingulate cortex (arrows), with preservation of cortical perfusion in motor cortex and temporal lobes, is characteristic for the diagnosis of Alzheimer disease. (continued on page 487)

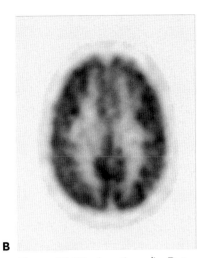
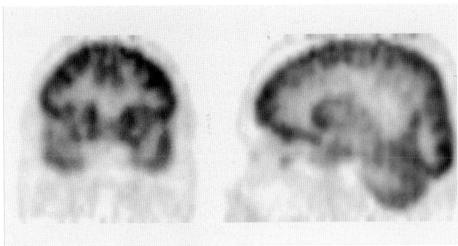

B

Figure 12.55. *(continued)*   **B.** Symmetric cortical perfusion in a normal patient.

Massive dilation of the ventricular system produces *hydrocephalus*. This dilation compresses other brain structures and impairs function. Hence, the necessity for early diagnosis and shunting. Hydrocephalus may be congenital or acquired. Congenital hydrocephalus is usually the result of a syndrome that includes brain abnormalities such as the Arnold-Chiari malformation of the hindbrain and spina bifida. These conditions may be identified in the prenatal period through obstetric ultrasound (see Fig. 10.10A). On CT or MR imaging, hydrocephalus appears as massive dilation of the ventricular system (Fig. 12.56).

Figure 12.56. Hydrocephalus. T1-weighted MR image shows massive dilation of the lateral ventricles with blunting of their apices. The cortex is shallow and the sulci are effaced.

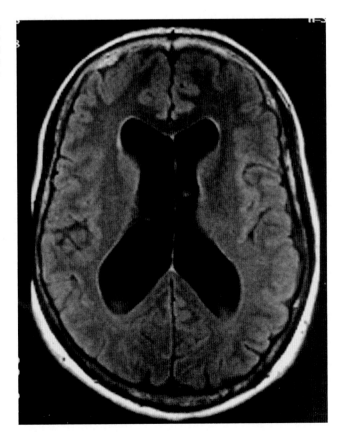

SUMMARY AND KEY POINTS

- This chapter emphasizes the impact that cranial CT, MR, and PET scanning has had on neuroradiology.
- Six pathologic entities—trauma, tumor, vascular disease, multiple sclerosis, infections, and cerebral atrophy and hydrocephalus—were discussed briefly.
- Most of these studies will be interpreted by a neuroradiologist, neurologist, or neurosurgeon.

SUGGESTED ADDITIONAL READING

Daffner RH. Imaging of facial trauma. Curr Prob Diag Radiol 1997;26:159–184.

Gaensler EHL. Head and neck imaging. In: Brant WE, Helms CA, eds. Fundamentals of Diagnostic Radiology. 2nd Ed. Philadelphia: Lippincott Williams & Wilkins, 1999:25–231.

Grossman RI, Yousem DM. Neuroradiology: The Requisites. 2nd Ed. St. Louis: Mosby, 2003.

Harnsberger HR, Hudgins PA, Wiggins RH, et al. Diagnostic Imaging: Head and Neck. Philadelphia: WB Saunders, 2005.

Latschaw RE, Kucharczyk J, Moseley M. Imaging of the Nervous System. Diagnostic and Therapeutic Applications. St. Louis: Mosby, 2005.

Osborne AG, Blaser SI, Salzman KL. Diagnostic Imaging: Brain. Philadelphia: WB Saunders, 2004.

Robertson RL, Ball WS Jr, Barnes PD. Skull and brain. In: Kirks DR, Griscom NT, eds. Practical Pediatric Imaging. Diagnostic Radiology of Infants and Children. 3rd Ed. Philadelphia: Lippincott-Raven, 1998:65–200.

Som PM, Curtin HD, eds. Head and Neck Imaging. 4th Ed. St. Louis: Mosby-Year Book, 2003.

Timmins JH. Central nervous system scintigraphy. In: Brant WE, Helms CA, eds. Fundamentals of Diagnostic Radiology. 2nd Ed. Philadelphia: Lippincott Williams & Wilkins, 1999:1333–1343.

Vertebral Imaging

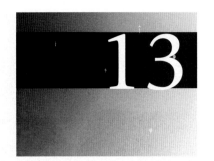

The vertebral column is an integral part of two anatomic systems. The vertebrae themselves are an important skeletal link between the cranium, upper limbs, and lower limbs. The spinal cord, including its meninges, vascular supply, and peripheral nerves, is part of the nervous system. Disease or injury to one part of this complex often affects both components. This chapter discusses using various imaging techniques to evaluate the vertebral column and its contents.

TECHNICAL CONSIDERATIONS

Four types of imaging examinations are used to evaluate the vertebral column and its contents: radiography, computed tomography (CT), magnetic resonance (MR) imaging, and myelography. Image-guided interventional procedures performed on the spine include biopsy and aspiration, discography, nerve block, and vertebroplasty.

Radiography is still the mainstay for the diagnosis of diseases affecting the vertebral column. Radiographs should be obtained before any special examination because often abnormalities not only will be apparent on a plain film but also may have findings characteristic enough to allow for diagnoses. Furthermore, the radiograph serves as a road map to aid in interpreting a CT or MR study. The standard examination of the cervical vertebral column consists of lateral, frontal (anterior-posterior [AP]) views of the lower column and occipitoatlantoaxial region ("open mouth"), and oblique views. Flexion and extension views may be obtained if necessary. For suspected trauma in our hospital, we use only a single lateral cervical radiograph to demonstrate C2. The definitive evaluation of the cervical spine is with CT (as discussed later in this section). In the thoracic and lumbar regions, standard frontal and lateral radiographs are obtained. We also obtain a "swimmer view" of the cervicothoracic junction.

A review of the normal radiographic anatomy of the cervical region shows similarities that may be applied throughout the vertebral column (Fig. 13.1). On the lateral view, the anterior and posterior aspects of the vertebral bodies are aligned. The *spinolaminar line,* a dense white line that represents the junction of the laminae to form the spinous process, also is normally aligned. The facet or *apophyseal* joints overlap in an orderly fashion (*imbrication*). The distances between spinous processes and between the laminae are uniform and should not vary by more than 2 mm. The disc and joint spaces are also uniform. The prevertebral soft tissues are normal. A ringlike density over the central portion of the body of C2 is an important radiologic landmark. This so-called Harris ring is actually a confluence of radiographic shadows from the superior articular facet of C2 superiorly, the posterior vertebral body line posteriorly, the transverse foramen inferiorly, and the anterior vertebral body anteriorly. This ring is often disrupted in fractures through the body of C2.

The frontal view shows normal alignment of the lateral margins of the vertebrae. The pedicles are normally aligned, and the distance between them does not vary more than 2 mm from

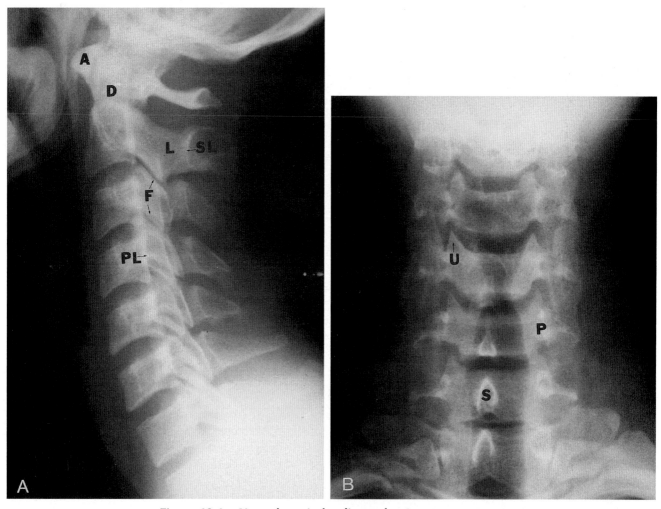

Figure 13.1. Normal cervical radiographs. A. Lateral view. Notice the normal alignment of the anterior and posterior portions of the vertebral bodies. The posterior vertebral body line (*PL*) is solid. The spinolaminar line (*SL*) is also aligned. The facet joints (*F*) are uniform and symmetric. The spaces between the laminae (*L*) are uniform with the exception of C2–C3, a normal variant. Notice the position of the dens (*D*) and its relation to the anterior arch of the atlas (*A*). The width of the body of C2 does not exceed that of C3. Notice the ring-like structure immediately below the dens. This structure is actually a composite of normal images. Disruption of this "ring" is an important finding in trauma. **B.** Frontal view. Notice the alignment of the spinous processes (*S*), the pedicles (*P*), and the uncinate processes (*U*).

level to level. The interspinous (interlaminar) spaces are uniform, and the distance between them should also not vary by more than 2 mm from level to level. The uncinate processes are small, pointed projections along the posterolateral margins of the cervical vertebrae only.

CT is one of the most frequently used examinations for evaluating the vertebral column and its contents. CT scans are more sensitive for finding cervical fractures than are radiographs and do so with considerable time savings. CT is particularly advantageous for areas that do not lend themselves well to diagnosis, such as the articular pillars, the cervicothoracic junction, and the upper thoracic column. In addition to providing transverse images of the vertebrae and showing the surrounding soft tissues, a CT scan provides a further dimension to evaluation of vertebral disease and injury (Fig. 13.2). Sagittal, coronal, and three-dimensional reconstructions may be obtained as well as the axial images (Fig. 13.3). CT is also used to evaluate herniated intervertebral discs (Fig. 13.4). In this regard, it may be combined with myelography to enhance a diagnosis. CT is also used in various infectious and neoplastic disorders to show not only the extent of destruction but also the spread of the lesion into the soft tissues (Fig. 13.5).

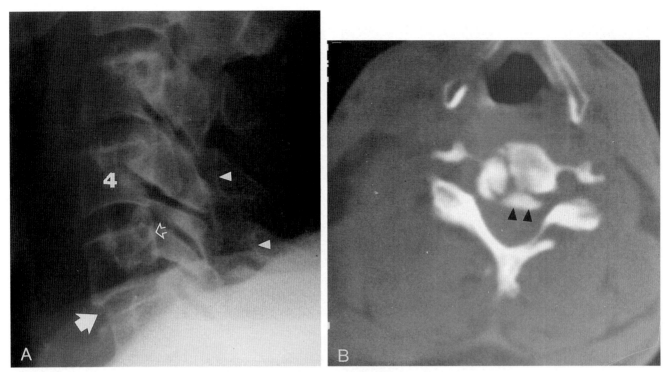

Figure 13.2.   C5 burst fracture. A. Lateral radiograph shows anterolisthesis of C5 on C6 (*large arrow*). There is bowing of the posterior vertebral body line (*open arrow*) and disruption of the spino-laminar line (*arrowheads*). The fact that the spinolaminar line of C5 is not forward indicates that there are bilateral laminar fractures at that level. **B.** CT image shows fractures of the body of C5 with retropulsion of a bone fragment into the vertebral canal (*arrowheads*).

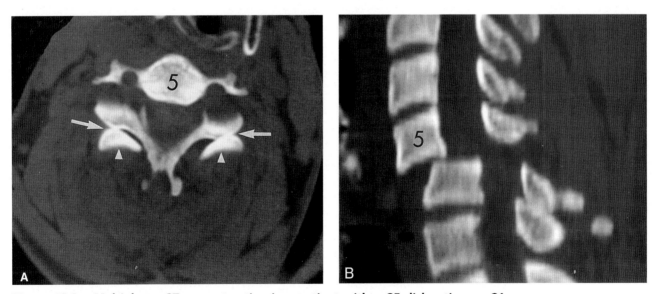

Figure 13.3.   Multiplanar CT reconstruction in a patient with a C5 dislocation on C6.
A. Axial CT image shows bilateral jumped and locked facets at C5–C6 (*arrows*). Notice the "naked" facets of C6 (*arrowheads*). **B.** Midline sagittal tomographic reconstruction shows the degree of dislocation. Left
(continued on page 492)

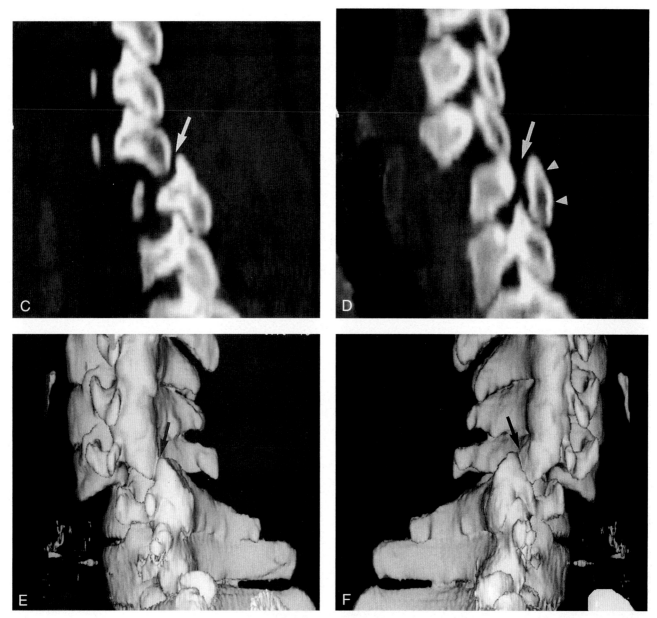

Figure 13.3. *(continued)* **(C)** and right **(D)** parasagittal reconstructions of the facets show the locked facets (*arrows*). In D, a fracture of the articular pillar has resulted in a separate fragment (*arrowheads*). Left **(E)** and right **(F)** three-dimensional reconstruction images show the locked facets (*arrows*) and provide another dimension of the injury for the surgeon.

MR imaging is used for vertebral abnormalities almost as much as for cranial abnormalities. The advantage of MR over CT and radiographs is that it demonstrates the spinal cord in addition to portraying the data in axial, sagittal, and coronal planes. Thus, it is useful for demonstrating herniated intervertebral discs (Fig. 13.6), infections (Fig. 13.7), and tumors (Fig. 13.8), as well as trauma (Fig. 13.9).

Myelography was used more extensively before the development of MR for evaluating compressive lesions involving the spinal cord. It is used now when there is a contraindication to MR, such as the presence of a cardiac pacemaker. Myelography is performed by introducing water-soluble, low-osmolar contrast media into the subarachnoid space. Radiographs are then made after the patient is placed in the appropriate position to allow the contrast to fill the area of interest. Following the radiographic portion of the exam, the patient is typically sent for a

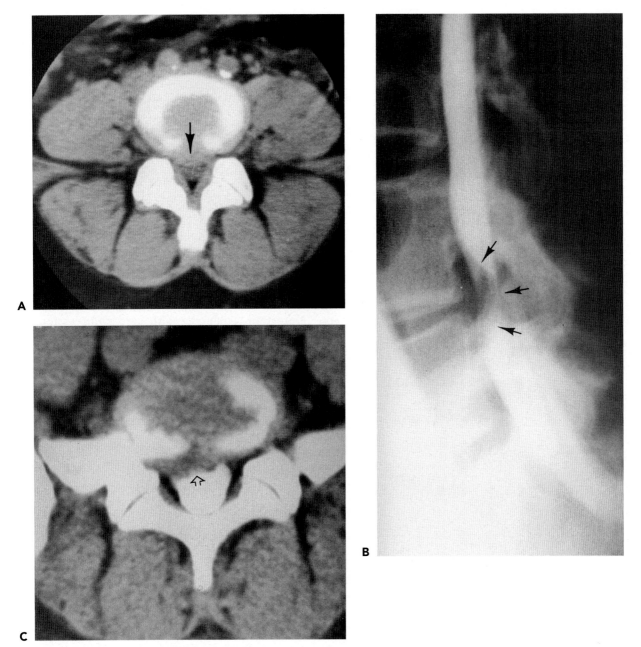

Figure 13.4.   Herniated nucleus pulposus. A. CT image shows a soft tissue density (*arrow*) encroaching the thecal sac. **B.** Myelogram shows extradural compression of the contrast-filled thecal sac (*arrows*) in the same patient. **C.** CT myelogram in a different patient shows herniated disc material compressing the contrast-filled thecal sac (*arrow*).

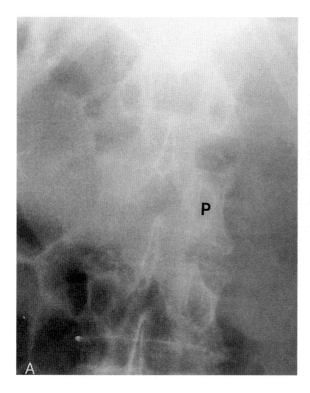

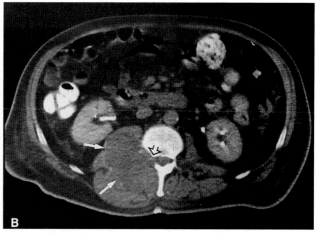

Figure 13.5.   Metastatic carcinoma with cord compression.
A. Frontal radiograph shows destruction of the pedicle and body of L2 on the right. Notice the normal pedicle (*P*) on the left. **B.** CT image through the same area shows a large paraspinal mass (*solid arrows*). Notice the destroyed pedicle on the right (*open arrow*).

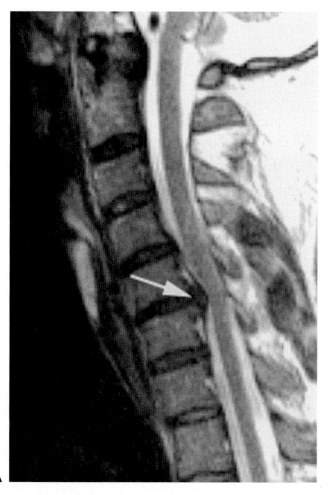

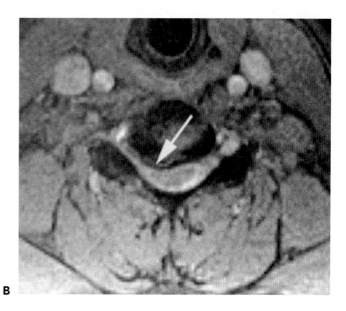

Figure 13.6.   Herniated nucleus pulposus. Sagittal (**A**) and axial (**B**) T2-weighted images show a herniated cervical disc (*arrows*). (continued on page 495)

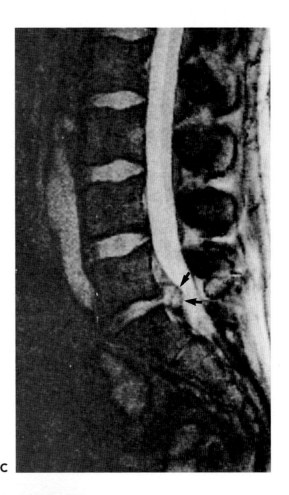

Figure 13.6. *(continued)* **C.** Herniated lumbar disc in another patient. Sagittal gradient echo MR image shows the herniated nuclear material (*arrows*) impinging the thecal sac.

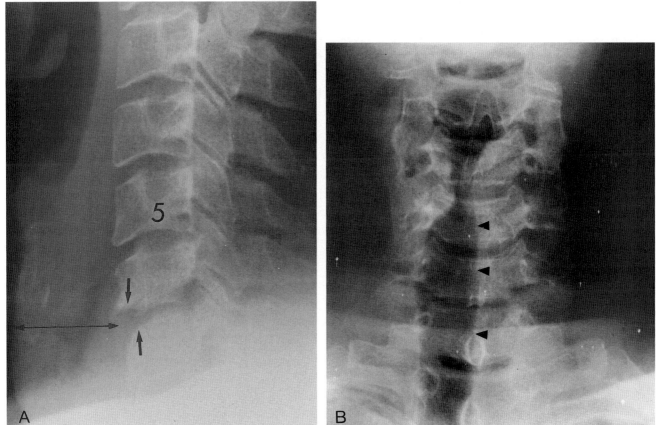

Figure 13.7.   Disc space infection. A. Lateral radiograph shows erosions along the C6 disc space (*single arrows*). Notice the increased width of the prevertebral soft tissues (*double arrow*). **B.** Frontal radiograph shows displacement of the trachea (*arrowheads*) to the right of the large prevertebral soft tissue mass. (continued on page 496)

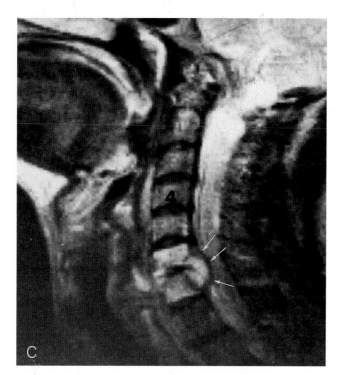

Figure 13.7. *(continued)* **C.** Gradient echo MR image shows an epidural abscess *(arrows)* compressing the thecal sac at C6 and C7.

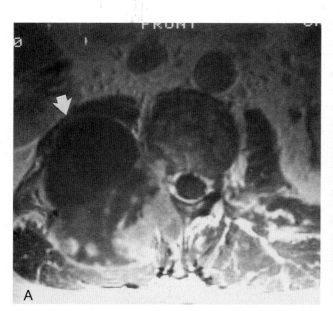

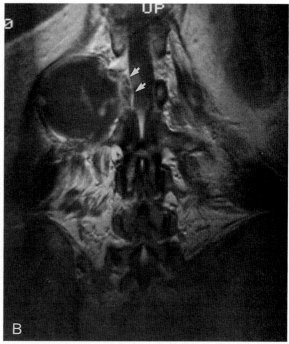

Figure 13.8.   Metastatic tumor invading vertebral canal. (A and B are same patient as in Fig. 13.5.) **A.** Axial gradient echo MR image shows a large paraspinal mass *(arrow)*. **B.** Direct coronal image shows compression of the epidural space *(arrows)* by the large mass. *(continued on page 497)*

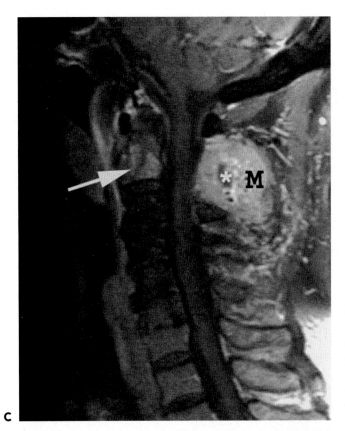

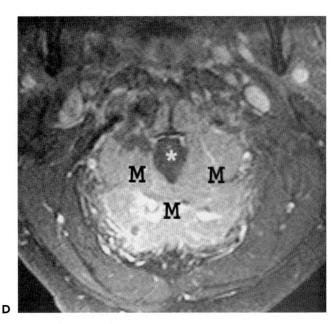

D

C

Figure 13.8. *(continued)* **C.** Contrast-enhanced T1-weighted sagittal image in another patient with metastatic renal carcinoma. Notice the involvement of the body of C2 by tumor *(arrow)* as well as replacement of the C2 posterior elements by a tumor mass *(M)*. There is a central zone of necrosis (*) in this mass. **D.** Axial image of same patient as in C shows the spinal cord (*) compressed by the surrounding mass *(M)*, which has virtually replaced C2.

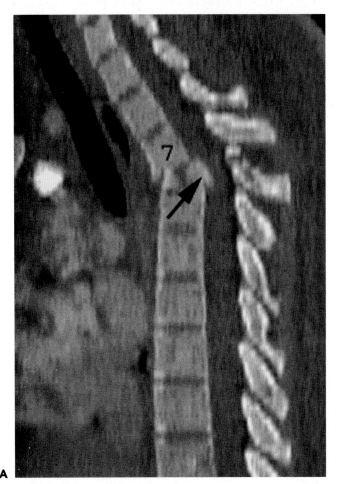

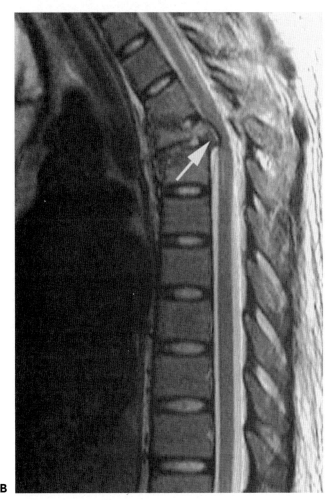

A

B

Figure 13.9.   Utility of MR imaging in vertebral trauma. A. Sagittal reconstructed CT image shows a burst fracture of T1 with retropulsion of a bone fragment into the vertebral canal (arrow). **B.** T2-weighted sagittal MR image shows the cord compression (arrow). *(continued on page 498)*

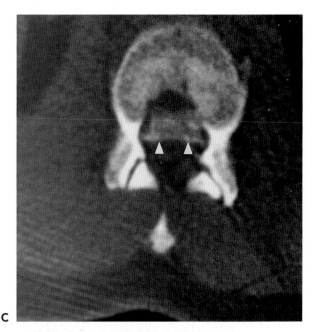

C

Figure 13.9. *(continued)* **C.** CT image in another patient with a burst fracture of L2 shows a large bone fragment in the vertebral canal (*arrowheads*). **D.** T1-weighted MR image shows the fragment (*arrow*) compressing the thecal sac. **E.** Sagittal proton density image of the patient shown in Figure 13.3 demonstrates dislocation of C5 on C6, rupture of the posterior longitudinal ligament (*long arrow*), and stripping of the anterior longitudinal ligament (*short arrows*) from C6. In addition, notice the signal change in the swollen spinal cord at the injury site.

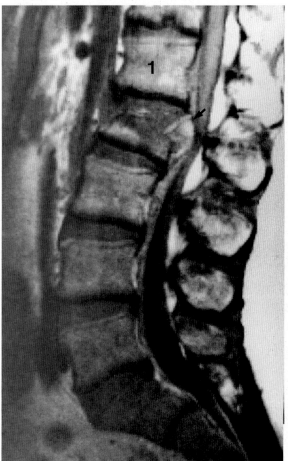

D

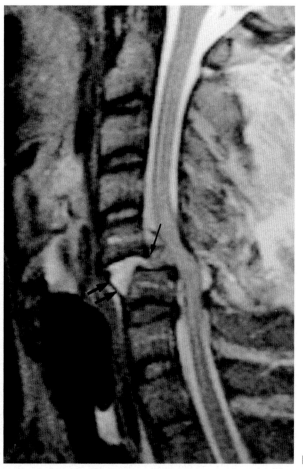

E

CT examination (Fig. 13.10; see Fig. 13.4C). It is used most often to evaluate herniated nucleus pulposus (see Fig. 13.4B) Myelography is also used in trauma patients to evaluate for suspected nerve root avulsions (Fig. 13.11).

Diagnostic ultrasound is used intraoperatively to evaluate spinal cord lesions. This technique allows a special ultrasound transducer to be placed directly on the dura to determine the exact location of a spinal cord tumor.

Among the *interventional procedures* performed on the spine are biopsy and aspiration, discography, nerve blocks, and vertebroplasty. A *biopsy and aspiration* of a suspected area of infection is performed under CT guidance. It is, in all respects, identical to a biopsy and aspiration performed anywhere else on the skeleton. The only caveat is that there must be a safe path for the needle to traverse.

Discography is occasionally used for symptomatic patients who have several levels of disc abnormality on MR studies. Asymptomatic disc herniations are common in patients over age 40 years. Discography is used to determine which abnormal disc is causing the patient's symptoms. Under fluoroscopic or CT guidance, a needle is placed into the nucleus pulposus, and contrast is injected not only to outline the margins of the nucleus and show herniation but also to reproduce the patient's symptoms.

Nerve blocks are performed under fluoroscopic or CT guidance to relieve pain from impingements of osteophytes or disc herniations (Fig. 13.12). The injections are a mixture of a long-acting local anesthetic (mepivacaine) and prednisone. Similarly, epidural blocks can also be performed.

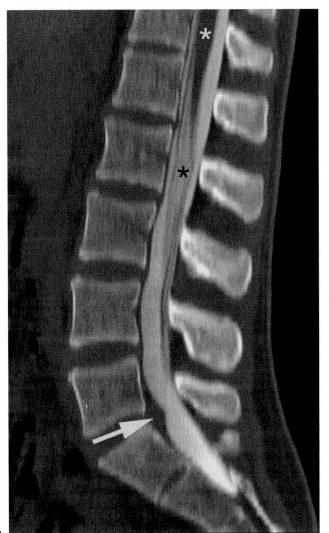

A

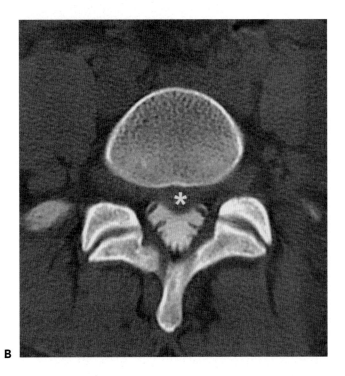

B

Figure 13.10. Herniated intervertebral disc. A. Sagittal reconstructed view of a CT myelogram shows a herniated disc compressing the contrast-filled thecal sac (*arrow*). Notice the spinal cord (*white* *) ending at the filum terminale (*black* *). **B.** Axial CT image shows the central herniated disc (*) compressing the thecal sac. The filling defects in the periphery represent branches of the filum terminale.

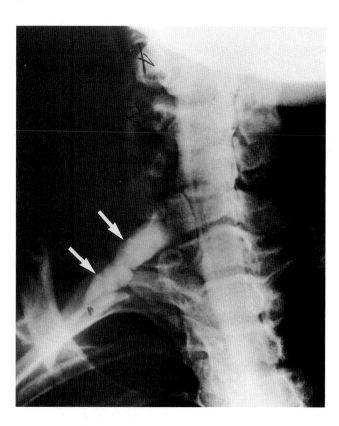

Figure 13.11. Nerve root avulsion after trauma. Myelogram shows extravasation of contrast along the root sheath (*arrows*).

Vertebroplasty and *kyphoplasty* are interventional procedures in which methylmethacrylate is injected into vertebral bodies to relieve pain, reestablish the anatomic height of vertebrae, or treat bone destruction caused by a tumor. These procedures are performed primarily by neurosurgeons and orthopaedic spine surgeons as well as by interventional neuroradiologists.

ANATOMIC CONSIDERATIONS

The vertebral column is a collection of 33 irregular bones extending from the base of the skull through the entire length of the neck and trunk. Because of the attached muscles, ligaments, and intervertebral discs, the vertebral column is a strong flexible support for the body that also protects the spinal cord. The upper 24 presacral vertebrae remain separate throughout life. The remaining five sacral and four coccygeal segments are fused and thus called the fixed vertebrae.

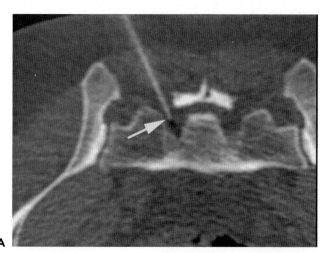
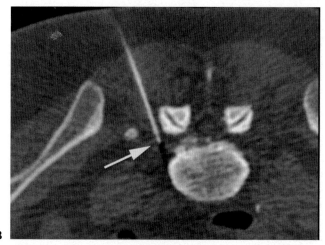

A   **B**

Figure 13.12. CT-guided nerve blocks. A. S1 root. **B.** L5 root. Arrows show the needle placements adjacent to the neural foramina.

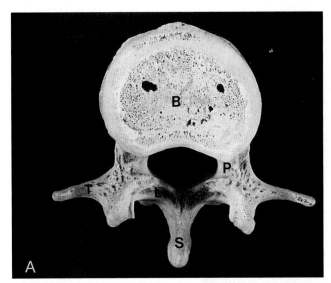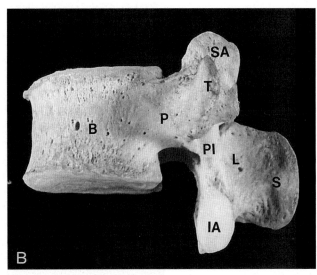

Figure 13.13. "Typical" vertebra (L2). A. Top view. The following structures are visible: *B,* vertebral body; *P,* pedicle; *S,* spinous process; *L,* lamina; *T,* transverse process. **B.** Side view. The following additional structures are visible: *SA,* superior articular facet; *IA,* inferior articular facet; *PI,* pars interarticularis. All vertebrae, with the exception of C1, have these structures.

There are certain common characteristics of all the moveable presacral vertebrae. With the exception of the atlas (C1) and the axis (C2), all these "typical" vertebrae include an anterior *body* that serves a weight-bearing function and a *vertebral arch* located posterior to the body that acts as a protective shell for the spinal cord, meninges, peripheral nerves, and blood vessels (Fig. 13.13). The vertebral arch comprises two *pedicles* and two *laminae.* The pedicles join the arch to the vertebral body; the laminae join the pedicles to form the posterior wall of the vertebral foramen, which encloses the spinal cord. Seven projections or processes are attached to the vertebral arch: two *transverse processes,* one *spinous process,* and four *articular processes.* The transverse processes and spinous process serve as the attachment points for muscles. In the cervical region, the transverse processes point downward; in the thoracic, they point upward. This difference allows for accurate distinctions between the cervical and thoracic vertebrae on a frontal radiograph. The articular processes determine the direction and degree of motion permitted by the particular segment of the vertebral column. The cervical articular processes are called *articular pillars.*

The posterior vertebral body line is an important radiographic structure to recognize on all lateral radiographs. In the cervical and upper thoracic regions, it is a single, uninterrupted vertical line along the posterior margin of the vertebral body (see Fig. 13.1). In the lower thoracic and lumbar regions, this line is interrupted centrally by the nutrient vessels (Fig.13.14). At C2, the posterior vertebral body line continues with the dens. *Any displacement, rotation, angulation, bowing, or absence of this line is abnormal* (Fig. 13.15).

Differences in the structure of the vertebrae occur at each level. All *cervical vertebrae* have, as distinguishing features, transverse foramina in each transverse process. The atlas, C1, has no body. The axis, on the other hand, has a toothlike projection from the upper portion of its body—the dens or odontoid process. C3 through C7 also have uncinate processes along the posterolateral margin of the upper surface of the vertebral body that develop during adolescence and provide additional stabilization. Degenerative changes along the articulations (*Luschka joints*) that these uncinate processes form with the vertebrae above are a common cause of neck pain in older individuals.

The *thoracic vertebrae* all have one or more paired facets to accept the ribs. The upper thoracic vertebrae more closely resemble cervical vertebrae, and the lower thoracic vertebrae more closely resemble lumbar vertebrae. The spinous processes of the thoracic vertebrae point downward.

Lumbar vertebrae lack both the transverse foramina and costal facets. Their spinous processes are large and rectangular. Their main function is support. The area between the facets is called the *pars interarticularis,* or simply the *pars.* This area is composed of bone that is thinner than the remainder of the vertebra and is subject to shearing and torsional stresses. For this reason, fractures called pars interarticularis defects (or *spondylolyses*) are not uncommon (Fig. 13.16).

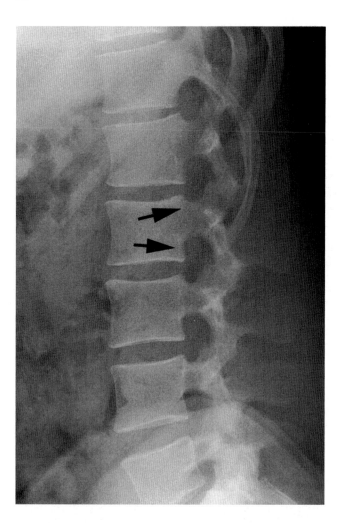

Figure 13.14. Normal lateral view of lumbar vertebra. The posterior vertebral body line (*arrows*) is interrupted centrally by a nutrient vessel.

The vertebrae are separated and articulated by a series of joints and supporting ligaments. There are basically two types of joints: slightly movable *symphyseal* joints (the intervertebral discs), and freely movable *synovial* (facet or apophyseal) joints. Motion in these joints is of a gliding nature. The intervertebral disc comprises a laminated outer portion called the *annulus fibrosis* and an inner portion called the *nucleus pulposus.* The nucleus pulposus is eccentrically located with the shorter distance toward the vertebral canal. Therefore, herniation of this material into the vertebral canal is more common than herniation anteriorly. The supporting ligaments (Fig. 13.17) serve to stabilize the vertebral column and restrict motion.

Motion permitted in the cervical region is flexion, extension, and rotation. Most rotation occurs with lateral flexion. At C1 and C2, the maximum allowable range in flexion and extension is 20° and 40° of rotation, respectively. The remainder of the cervical column has a maximum allowable range of flexion and extension of up to 20°. The thoracic region is relatively restricted by the attached ribs. A minimal amount (at 5°) of flexion occurs in the upper thoracic vertebrae. However, at the thoracolumbar junction (T11–L2), a greater degree of flexion and minimal extension is allowed (12°). In the lumbar region, flexion and extension, to a lesser degree than that in the cervical region, are also allowed. A minor degree of rotation is also permitted predominantly at the thoracolumbar junction. The reason for the allowable motion relates to the orientation of the facet joints at each level. In the cervical region, the joints are oriented at 45°; in the thoracic, at 60°. However, at the thoracolumbar junction, the facets are oriented at 90° to each other. This arrangement greatly restricts motion and accounts for the high incidence of injuries to these levels. The greater degree of allowable motion in the cervical region accounts for the incidence of injuries in that region. As one ages, the craniovertebral junction becomes the most mobile segment, accounting for the higher incidence of injuries to this region in the elderly.

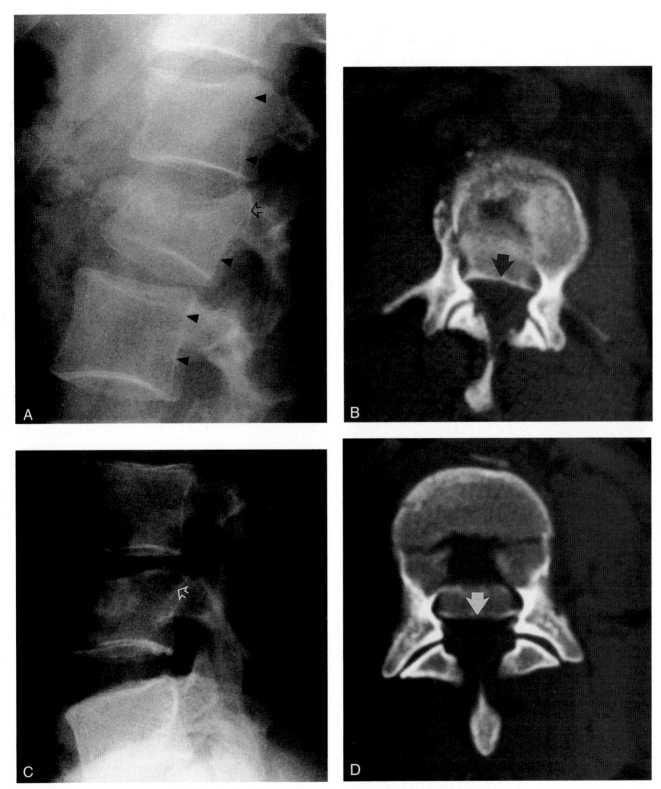

Figure 13.15. Posterior vertebral body line (PVL) disruption in two patients with burst fractures. A. Lateral radiograph shows posterior bowing of the upper PVL at L2 (*open arrow*). The normal PVL of the neighboring vertebrae are straight (*arrowheads*). **B.** CT image shows a large fragment of the PVL displaced posteriorly into the vertebral canal (*arrow*). **C.** Lateral radiograph in another patient shows posterior angulation of the upper portion of the PVL of L4 (*arrow*). Compare with the neighboring vertebrae. **D.** CT image shows a large fragment of the PVL displaced posteriorly into the vertebral canal (*arrow*). Any displacement, rotation, angulation, bowing, or absence of a portion of or all of the PVL is abnormal.

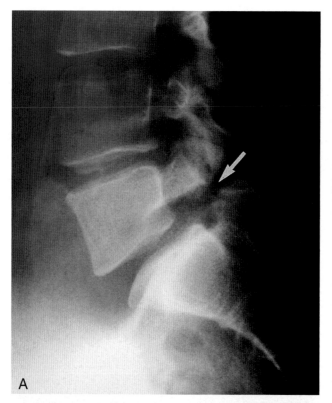

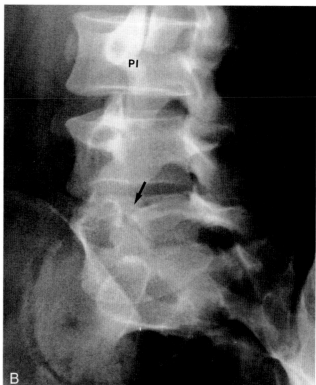

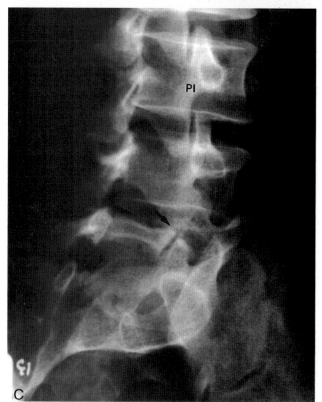

Figure 13.16. Bilateral pars interarticularis defects. A. Lateral radiograph shows complete interruption of the pars at L5 (*arrow*). Compare with L4 and Fig. 13.13B. Right **(B)** and left **(C)** oblique radiographs show absence of the pars at L5 (*arrows*). Notice the normal appearance of the pars (*PI*) above.

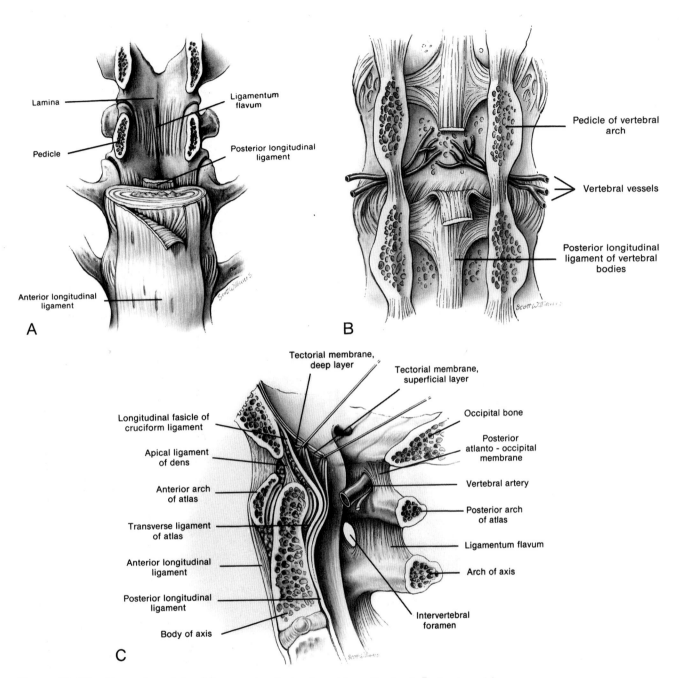

Figure 13.17.   Normal vertebral ligaments. A. As viewed from the front. **B.** As viewed from behind. **C.** Sagittal view of the craniovertebral junction. (Reproduced with permission from Daffner RH. Imaging of Vertebral Trauma. 2nd Ed. Philadelphia: Lippincott-Raven, 1996.)

PATHOLOGIC CONSIDERATIONS

In your practice, you will encounter six categories of abnormalities involving the vertebral column:

1. Developmental
2. Degenerative and arthritic
3. Traumatic
4. Neoplastic
5. Infectious
6. Postoperative

Developmental Abnormalities

Developmental abnormalities occur primarily within the vertebral column. It is estimated that 1 in 1,000 live births results in a significant developmental abnormality of the vertebral column. These may range from nothing more serious than an unfused spinous process (*spina bifida occulta;* Fig. 13.18A) to a severe form of spinal dysraphism, usually with multiple associated abnormalities (see Fig. 13.18B). Often these anomalies produce scoliosis. Other anomalies include hemivertebrae, congenital fusions, and cervical ribs. Among the plethora of associated findings are neurologic abnormalities such as hydrocephalus and urinary tract problems. Because of advancements in medical, surgical, and rehabilitation therapy, patients with severe spinal abnormalities can survive into adulthood and lead productive lives.

More common are segmentation anomalies occurring in the lumbar region and producing either *lumbarization* of S1 or *sacralization* of L5 (Fig.13.19). If surgery is to be performed, it is important for the correct level to be identified. Therefore, it is imperative that radiographs be obtained to accompany all vertebral CT and MR studies.

Degenerative and Arthritic Abnormalities

Degenerative disease (*spondylosis*) of the vertebral column is one of the most common entities that you will encounter. The extent of degenerative disease may range from mild disc space narrowing and spur formation (Fig. 13.20) to severe *spondylosis deformans*, in which there is disc space narrowing, facet joint narrowing, and spur formation (Fig. 13.21). These spurs may encroach on either the intervertebral foramina or the vertebral canal to produce stenosis of those structures. Impingement on the spinal cord or peripheral nerves is best evaluated by CT,

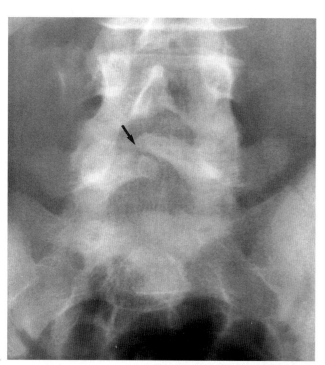

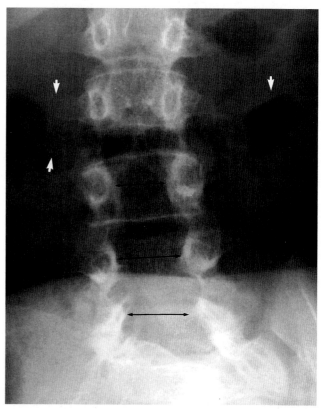

A   B

Figure 13.18.   Vertebral dysraphism. A. Spina bifida occulta. There is failure of fusion of the laminae of L5, producing a cleft (*arrow*). This is a normal variant with no associated neurologic or clinical findings. **B.** Severe spina bifida. There is wide dysraphism with congenital absence of the laminae of L3, L4, and L5 (*double arrows*). This anomaly is usually associated with a myriad of neurologic abnormalities including hydrocephalus. Notice the ventriculoperitoneal shunt catheter (*small arrows*).

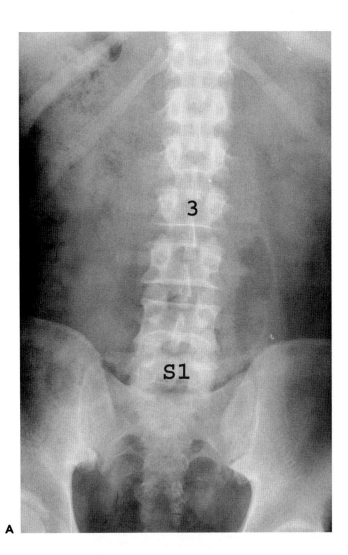

A

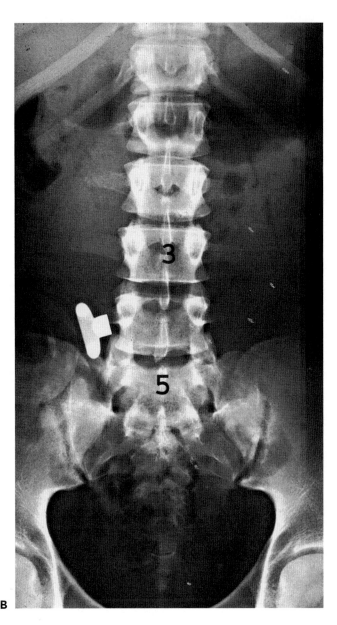

B

Figure 13.19. Segmentation anomalies of the lumbar spine. A. Lumbarization of S1. **B.** Sacralization of L5. The transverse processes of L3 are usually the longest. Furthermore, a line drawn horizontally across the iliac crests should pass through or very close to the L4 disc space.

MR, or myelography (Fig. 13.22). Degeneration of the intervertebral disc frequently results in herniation of the semisolid nucleus pulposus into the vertebral canal. In addition, minor degrees of anterolisthesis or retrolisthesis may occur.

Herniated intervertebral discs in the lumbar region are found very commonly as incidental findings in asymptomatic patients. However, once a patient becomes symptomatic, evaluation with CT, MR, and/or myelography is indicated. These examinations are extremely accurate in locating the extent of the herniated nuclear material (Fig. 13.23) as well as determining whether free disc fragments are within the vertebral canal. The noninvasive features of CT and MR make them particularly appealing as the first form of imaging to be performed in these patients.

A common variation of disc herniation is the *Schmorl node*. This condition results from herniation of disc material into the vertebral body, producing a "die punch" deformity (Fig.13.24). Anterior herniations may produce a corner fracture of the vertebral body—the so-called *limbus deformity* (Fig. 13.25). Both of these lesions are associated with narrowing of the affected disc space.

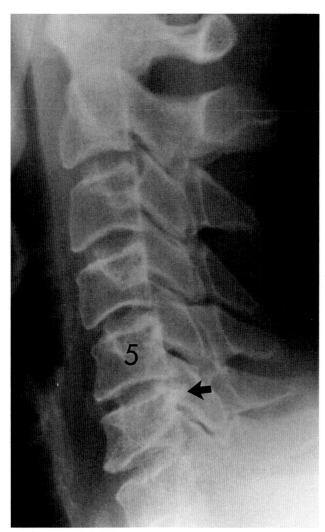

Figure 13.20. Mild cervical spondylosis. Lateral radiograph shows narrowing of the C5 disc space. Posterior spurs (*arrow*) impinge on the vertebral canal.

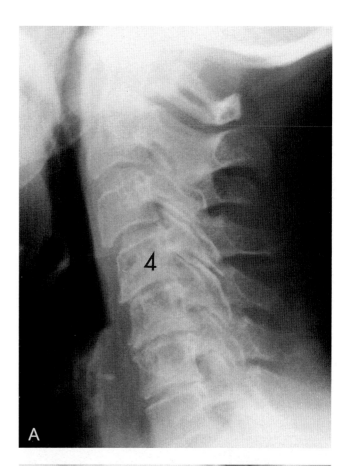

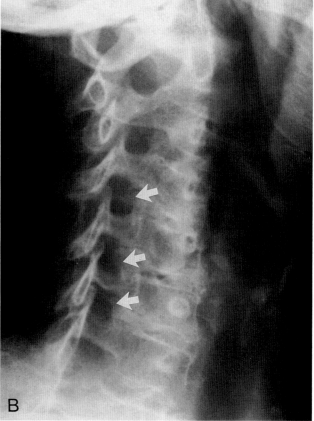

Figure 13.21. Severe cervical spondylosis. A. Lateral radiograph shows narrowing of all the disc spaces below C4. Spurs encroach the vertebral canal at the disc level. Notice the sclerosis of the facet joints. **B.** Oblique view shows spurs encroaching the intervertebral foramina at multiple levels (*arrows*).

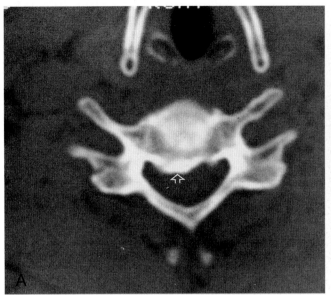

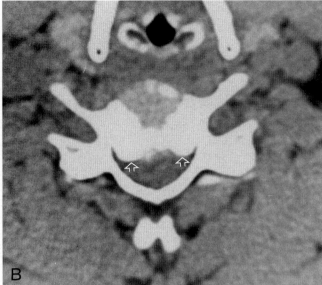

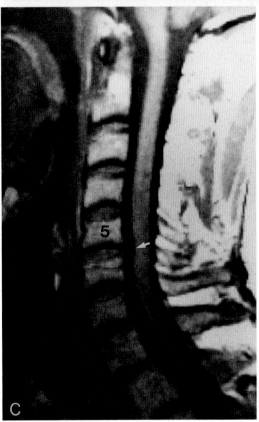

Figure 13.22.   Cervical spondylosis. (This is the same patient as in Fig. 13.20.) **A.** CT image at bone window shows a large osteophyte narrowing the vertebral canal (*arrow*). **B.** CT image at soft tissue windows at a level slightly lower than A shows bilateral narrowing (*arrows*). **C.** Sagittal T1-weighted MR image shows encroachment of the vertebral canal by a herniated disc and spurs at C5 (*arrow*). The cord is not compressed in this view.

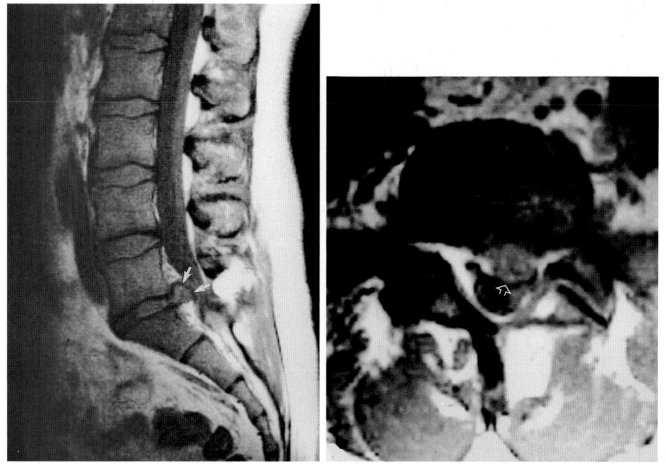

A

B

Figure 13.23. Herniated nucleus pulposus. A. T1-weighted sagittal MR image shows impingement of the thecal sac by the herniated nuclear material (*arrows*). **B.** Axial sagittal gradient echo MR image shows the herniation (*arrow*) is more to the left.

Arthritis commonly involves the vertebral column. It is estimated that as many as 50% of patients with rheumatoid arthritis have cervical involvement. The diseases known as the *seronegative spondyloarthropathies* test negative for the HLA B-27 antigen and cause peripheral and vertebral arthritic changes. These disorders include ankylosing spondylitis (Fig. 13.26), psoriatic arthropathy, reactive arthritis, and the arthropathy of inflammatory bowel disease. These conditions are characterized by involvement of the sacroiliac joints and the formation of syndesmophytes rather than osteophytes (see Fig. 13.27). Syndesmophytes represent ossification of the anulus fibrosis and are oriented vertically; osteophytes represent ossification of Sharpey fibers at the margin of the disc and are oriented horizontally at their points of origin (Fig. 13.27).

Trauma

Trauma to the vertebral column, unfortunately, occurs frequently. Motor vehicle accidents account for most vertebral injuries. Falls from a height of 10 feet or more are the second most common source. Usually, vertebral injuries could have been prevented by the proper use of seat belts or other restraining devices in motor vehicles. A patient with injuries resulting from one of the following categories should be considered as having a cervical vertebral injury until proven otherwise: high-velocity motor vehicle accident; motorcycle accident; significant head or facial injury; fall from 10 feet or greater; drowning; electrocution; altered mental status (alcohol, drugs, or loss of consciousness); evidence of direct cervical injury (cervical pain, spasm, or obvious deformity); evidence of rigid vertebral disease (ankylosing spondylitis or

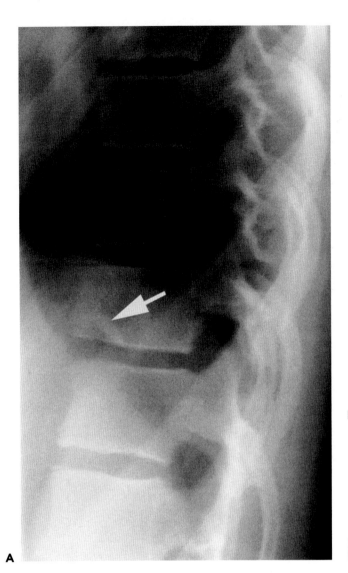

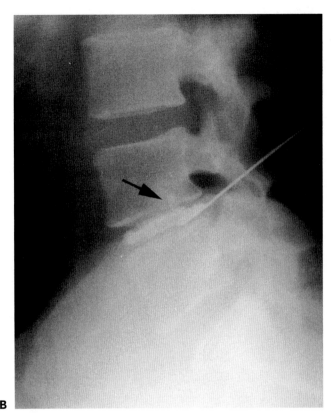

Figure 13.24. Schmorl nodes. A. Anterior node (*arrow*). **B.** Discogram showing extravasation into a Schmorl node (*arrow*).

A

diffuse idiopathic skeletal hyperostosis); age greater than 65 years; or thoracic or lumbar fractures. In my experience and that of other investigators, the incidence of multilevel noncontiguous vertebral fractures is 25%.

Throughout history, no injury has produced greater anxiety in health care workers than vertebral fractures and dislocations. The physician who must deal with a spine-injured patient often feels incapable of interpreting radiographic studies that can show the full extent of injury. Following some basic principles of interpretation, however, can allow you to determine whether a significant abnormality is present and if additional special imaging studies are necessary. Radiography was the mainstay of the evaluation of any patient with suspected vertebral trauma. However, radiographic studies are time consuming. In a study I conducted, the average time for a six-view cervical radiographic study was 22 minutes. In addition, in 70% of patients, at least one film was inadequate and had to be repeated. In the United States, radiography has largely been supplanted by CT. Multidetector CT scanners allow rapid data acquisition. In our level 1 trauma center, the cervical CT scan is obtained immediately following the cranial scan. Thoracic and lumbar images are obtained from data gathered by the thoracic, abdominal, and pelvic scan. All studies undergo multiplanar reconstruction (MPR) to produce sagittal and coronal images. In addition, the workstations in our picture archiving and communications system allow additional MPR if necessary. We still obtain a single lateral cervical radiograph to see C2, because we have found that horizontal fractures of the dens may not

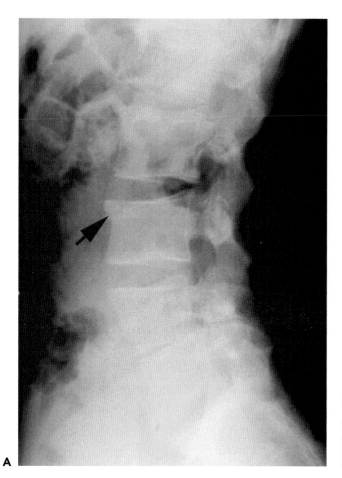

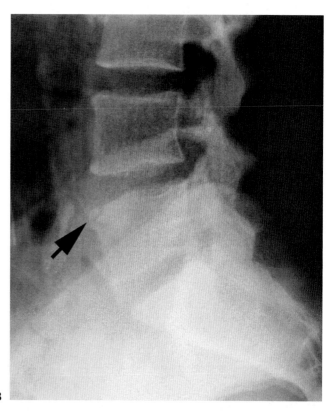

Figure 13.25.   Limbus deformities (*arrows*) from anterior disc herniations. Notice the narrow disc space at the affected level in B. These may be distinguished from fractures by virtue of their sclerotic margins.

A

always be demonstrated by CT. Furthermore, we have found that artifacts caused by dental fillings may obscure dens fractures. Rather than taking thoracic or lumbar radiographs, we use CT.

The interpretation of those studies demands that a logical system be followed in their interpretation. I prefer the ABCS system, introduced in Chapter 11:

Alignment abnormalities
Bony integrity abnormalities
Cartilage (joint space) abnormalities
Soft tissue abnormalities

The normal anatomic relations were listed in the previous section. The principles discussed here apply to CT studies as well as to radiographs. *Abnormalities of alignment* that may indicate fracture are disruption of the anterior or posterior vertebral body lines (Fig. 13.28), disruption of the spinolaminar line, jumped and locked facets and rotation of spinous processes (Fig. 13.29), widening of the interpedicular distance, widening of the predental space, and kyphotic angulation.

Numerous minor variations and discrepancies of alignment measurements occur between various vertebral structures. As a rule, 2 mm is the normal upper limits of difference for the following measurements: interspinous or interlaminar space, interpedicle distance (transverse or vertical), unilateral or bilateral atlantoaxial offset, anterolisthesis or retrolisthesis with flexion or extension, facet joint width, and the difference in the height of the anterior and posterior thoracic and lumbar vertebral bodies. This important *rule of 2s* will hold you in good stead in most instances.

Abnormalities of bony integrity include any obvious fracture (Fig. 13.30), disruption of the "ring" of C2, widening of C2 (the so-called fat C2 sign; Fig. 13.31), widening of the interpedicle distance, and disruption of the posterior vertebral body line.

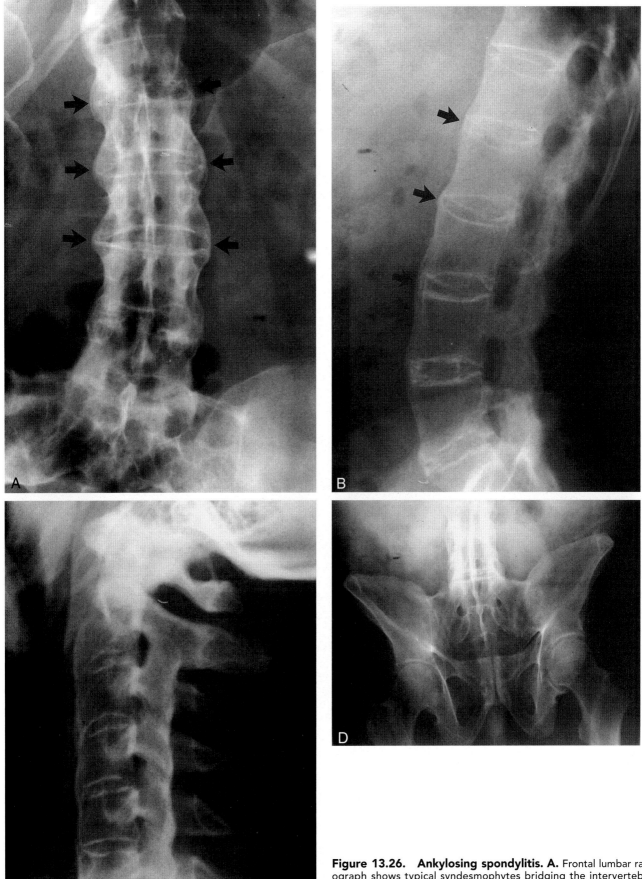

Figure 13.26. Ankylosing spondylitis. A. Frontal lumbar radiograph shows typical syndesmophytes bridging the intervertebral disc spaces (*arrows*). This gives the vertebral column a distinct "bamboo" appearance. **B.** Lateral lumbar radiograph shows the delicate anterior syndesmophytes (*arrows*). Notice the squaring of the disc margins of the vertebral bodies. **C.** Lateral cervical radiograph shows complete ankylosis anteriorly as well as of the facet joints posteriorly. **D.** Pelvic radiograph shows ankylosis of the sacroiliac joints in a symmetric manner, typical of this disease.

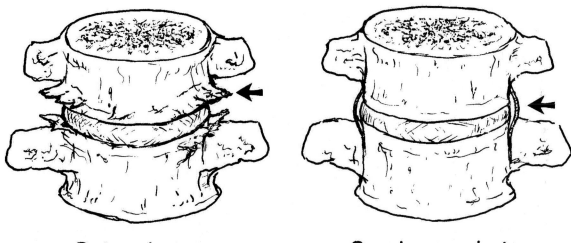

Osteophytes   Syndesmophytes

Figure 13.27. Syndesmophytes vs. osteophytes. The syndesmophyte extends vertically across the disc space (*arrow*). Osteophytes initially extend horizontally from the affected disc (*arrow*). Later, vertical bridging occurs.

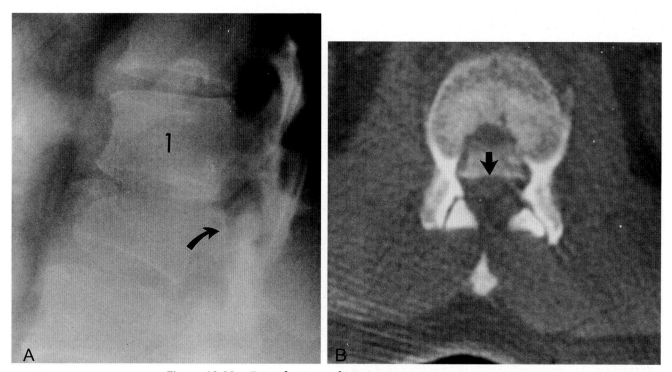

Figure 13.28. Burst fracture of L2. A. Lateral radiograph shows burst fracture of L2 with retropulsion of a bone fragment (*arrow*) from the posterior vertebral body line. **B.** CT image shows the fragment (*arrow*) narrowing the vertebral canal.

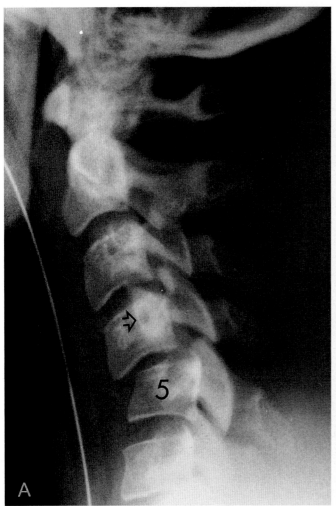

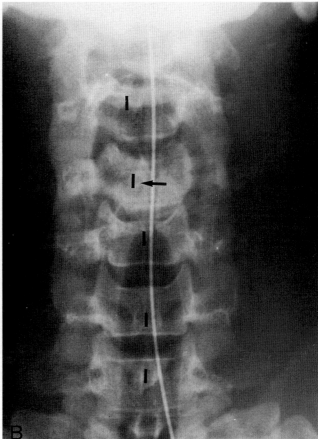

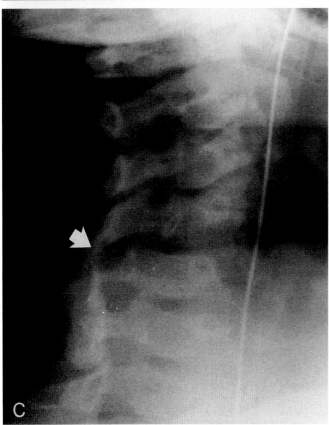

Figure 13.29. Unilateral facet lock. A. Lateral radiograph shows anterolisthesis of C4 on C5. Notice the widening of one facet joint (*solid arrow*). The rotated pillar of C4 (*open arrow*) may be seen through the body of C4 as part of a "bow tie." **B.** Frontal radiograph shows malalignment of the spinous processes (*solid vertical lines*). The spinous processes of C3 and C4 are displaced to the right (*arrow*), indicating that it is the right facet that is locked. **C.** Supine oblique view shows the locked facet (*arrow*).

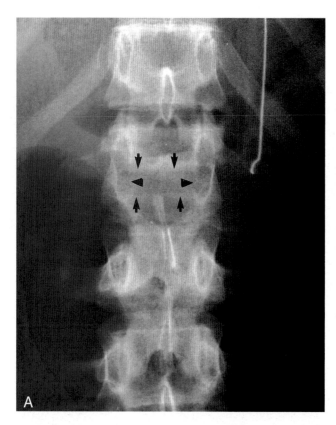

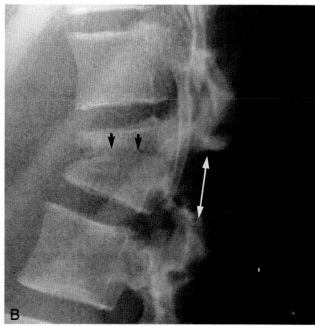

Figure 13.30. Chance fracture of L1. A. Frontal radiograph demonstrates a horizontal fracture that involves the lamina (*arrows*) as well as the pedicles (*arrowheads*) of L1. **B.** Lateral radiograph demonstrates the horizontal fracture line (*short arrows*) as well as the posterior distraction (*double arrow*) that occurs with this injury.

Cartilage or joint space abnormalities include widening of the predental space (more than 3 mm in an adult and 5 mm in a child), abnormally wide intervertebral disc space (Fig. 13.32), widening of the facet joints (or "naked" facets; Fig. 13.33), and widening of the interspinous or interlaminar distance.

Soft tissue abnormalities are encountered primarily with cervical injuries. These include widening of the prevertebral soft tissues in the cervical region (Fig. 13.34), the loss of the psoas stripe, and paraspinal soft tissue masses (Fig. 13.35). The finding of any or all of the previously mentioned signs on radiographs should be sufficient reason to perform CT and/or MR exami-

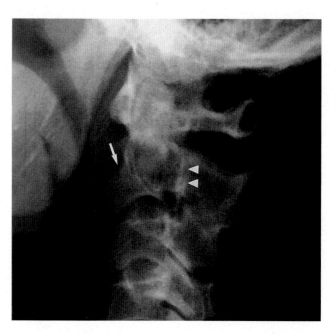

Figure 13.31. Subtle C2 fracture. Widening of the body of C2 in relation to C3 is apparent. Notice the fracture along the anterior margin (*arrow*). The posterior vertebral body line is displaced posteriorly (*arrowheads*). Notice the disruption of the spinolaminar line.

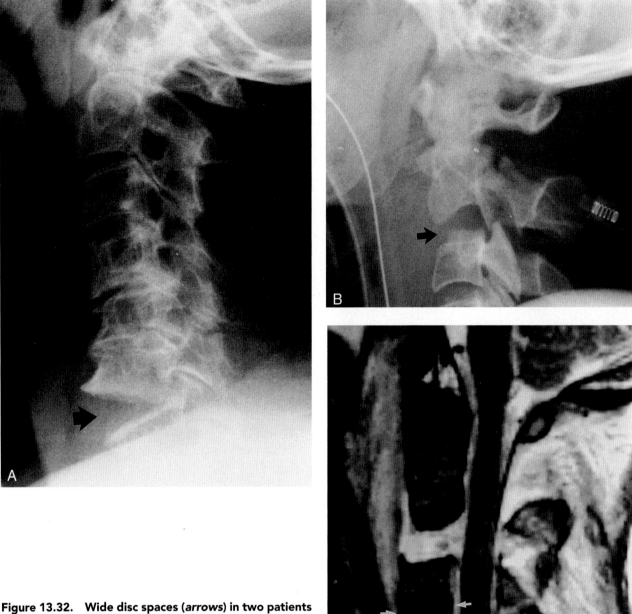

Figure 13.32.   Wide disc spaces (*arrows*) in two patients with extension injuries. A. Elderly patient with an extension sprain. The C6 disc space is much wider than its mates. **B and C.** Patient with a "hanged man" fracture of C2. In B, notice the wide disc space compared with that at C3. T2-weighted MR image in C shows the anterior and posterior longitudinal ligaments torn at the C2 disc level. Compare with the normal ligaments at C3 (*arrows*). Notice the high signal from edema and hemorrhage at the damaged C2 disc.

nations on a patient with suspected vertebral injuries. It should go without saying, however, that a patient with known neurologic deficit should undergo MR examination as soon as possible to determine the full extent of injury (Fig. 13.36).

How reliable are these radiologic signs? Based on my experience over a 15-year period at a level 1 major trauma center, the most reliable signs of underlying (cervical) vertebral injury are widening of the interspinous space, widening of the facet joints, widening of the retropharyngeal space (more than 7 mm in adults and children), and loss of the prevertebral fat stripe. These findings *never* occurred normally or as the *sole* manifestation of injury in my experience. Loss of lordosis, kyphotic angulation, and tracheal deviation also occurred in high incidence but were always associated with one or more of the signs in the first group.

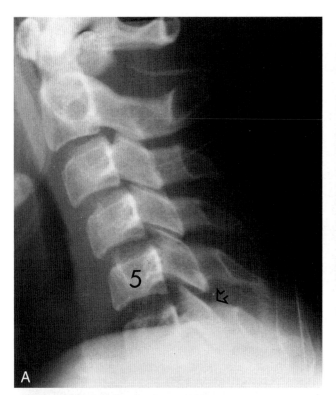

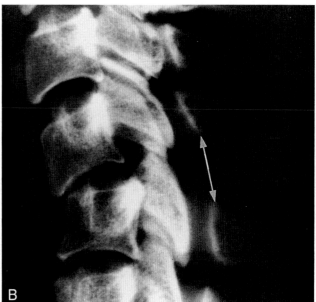

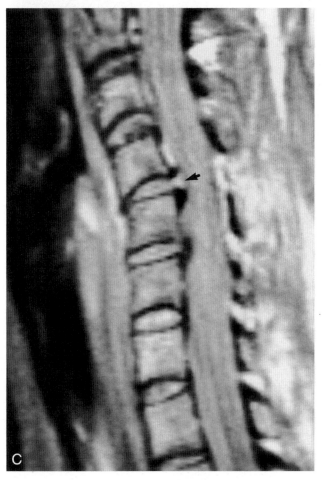

Figure 13.33. Widened facet joints in two patients with flexion sprains. A. Lateral radiograph in a patient with a mild flexion sprain shows the wide facet joint at C5 (*arrow*). **B and C.** Patient with a severe flexion sprain. Lateral radiograph in B shows, in addition to the wide facet joint at C4, widening of the interspinous space (*double arrow*). Sagittal MR image in C demonstrates rupture of the posterior longitudinal ligament (*arrow*).

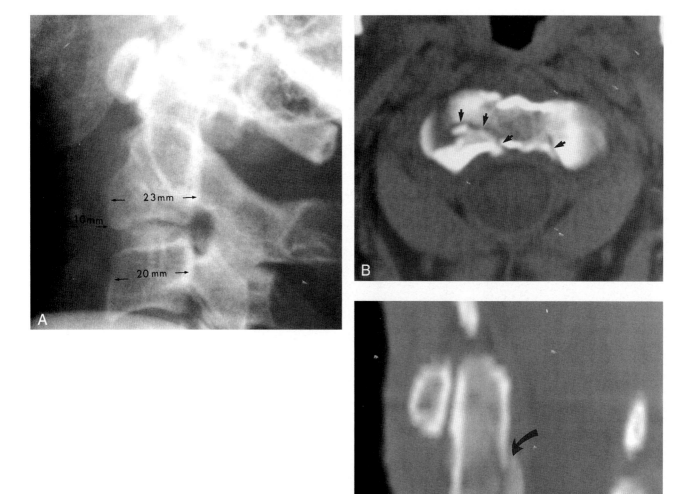

Figure 13.34. Wide retropharyngeal space and "fat C2" sign in a patient with a subtle fracture. A. Lateral radiograph demonstrates an increase in the retropharyngeal soft tissues to 10 mm (<7 mm is normal). The body of C2 measures 23 mm compared with 20 mm at C3. **B.** CT image through C2 shows multiple fractures (*arrows*). **C.** Sagittal CT reconstruction demonstrates the fracture of C2 (*arrow*).

Why is it still necessary to obtain radiographs if CT is both easier to obtain and more sensitive in identifying fractures? There are three reasons. First, as previously discussed, limited radiography is still needed to find some fractures, particularly at C2. Second, partial-volume averaging, a physical phenomenon in CT scanning, produces images with data from two levels. The junction point may appear lucent and be misdiagnosed as a fracture. Radiographs will clarify the problem. Finally, a motion artifact may produce a bizarre reconstructed image that has the appearance of a fracture (Fig. 13.37). In this situation, radiographs will also clarify the problem. Remember that for all cases, your consulting radiologist will be in the best position to answer questions about real or suspected abnormalities on plain films.

Neoplasms

The vertebral column has a rich vascular supply. In addition, it is also rich in red marrow. As such, it is one of the most frequent sites for metastases to occur. The evaluation of patients for suspected metastases of the vertebral column usually includes radiographs, radionuclide bone

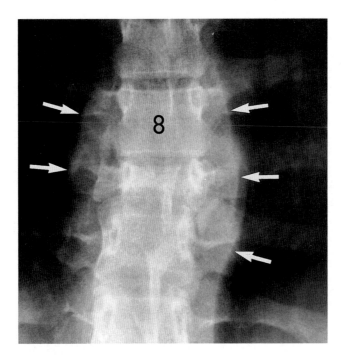

Figure 13.35. Wide paraspinal line. Frontal radiograph shows widening of the paraspinal lines (*arrows*) bilaterally in this patient with a T9 fracture-dislocation.

scanning, MR, and CT. MR is most sensitive because it shows changes in the water content of the marrow that occur as the result of metastases (Fig. 13.38). Often these abnormalities will be detected on MR imaging and not by radionuclide bone scan, particularly in patients with myeloma. In addition, MR has the distinct advantage of delineating areas of spinal cord compression. Radiographs are not as sensitive as MR or radionuclide bone scanning. It has been

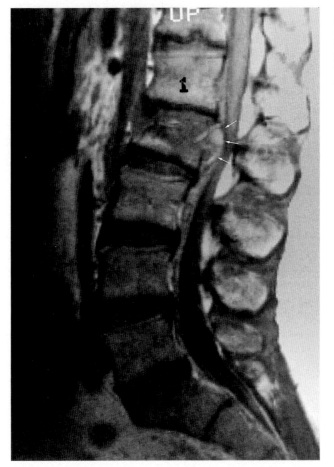

Figure 13.36. Burst fracture of L2. (This is the same patient as in Fig. 13.28.) Sagittal T1-weighted image shows the burst fracture of L2 with retropulsion of a bone fragment encroaching the thecal sac (*arrows*).

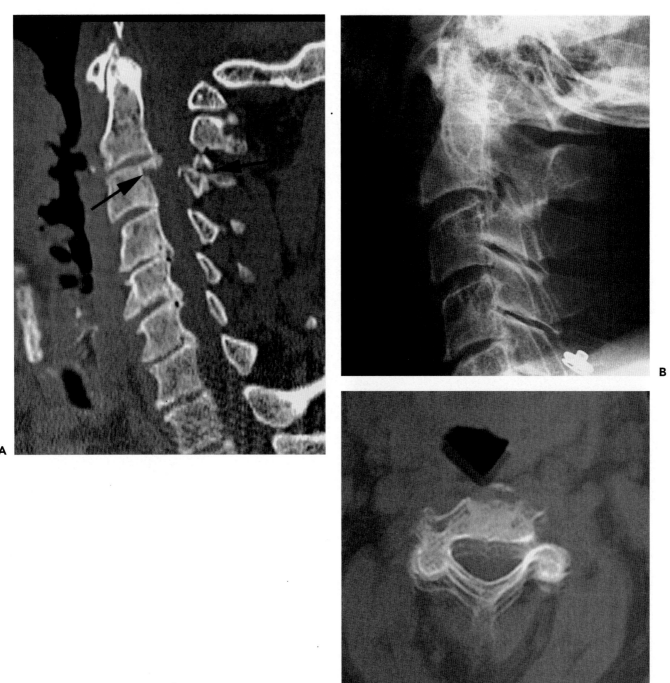

Figure 13.37.   Motion artifact. A. Sagittal reconstructed image shows an apparent fracture through C3 (*arrows*). **B.** Lateral radiograph shows no fracture. **C.** CT image shows the motion causing the artifact.

estimated that up to 50% of cancellous bone must be destroyed before the lesion is visible on plain films. In this regard, CT has some advantages.

Infections

Infections often affect the vertebral column either as a direct consequence of surgery or from hematogenous seeding. The region adjacent to the intervertebral discs are most commonly involved. For most infections, radiographs will reveal bony destruction along both sides of bony margins of disc space. A CT scan will show the lytic areas to better advantage and may delineate an associated soft tissue mass. MR imaging shows the inflammatory mass as well as any involvement of the vertebral canal with epidural abscess. Figure 13.39 shows a typical disc space infection.

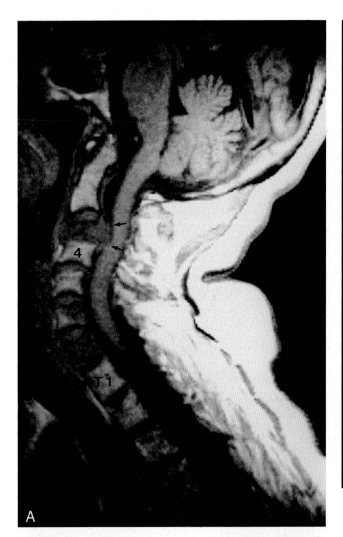

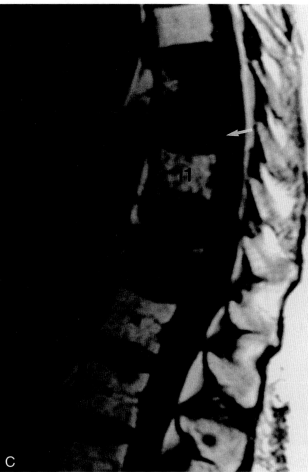

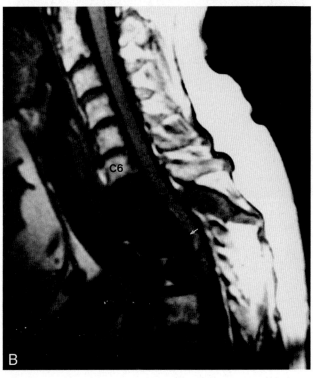

Figure 13.38.   Metastases invading the vertebral canal.
A. Sagittal T1-weighted MR image shows a destructive process involving C3. There is extradural compression of the spinal cord (*arrows*). Additional metastatic lesions are present at C6 and C7, as evidenced by the low signal (*darkness*) in those vertebrae. **B.** Sagittal T1-weighted MR image in another patient shows extensive involvement of C7 through T3. Notice the canal involvement at T2 (*arrow*) and the spinous process involvement at T1. **C.** Thoracolumbar metastases in another patient. T1-weighted sagittal MR image shows pathologic collapse at T12 and L1. There is posterior breakthrough of tumor at T10 (*arrow*).

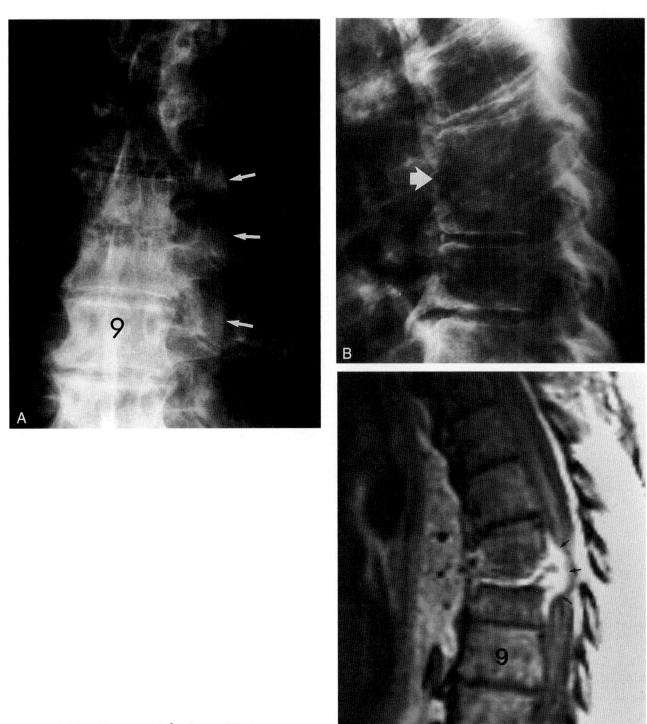

Figure 13.39. Disc space infection at T7. A. Frontal radiograph shows loss of the disc margin along the T7 disc space. Compare with the levels above and below. In addition, a paraspinal mass is evident on the left (*arrows*). **B.** Lateral radiograph shows loss of the disc margins at the T7 disc level (*arrow*). Again, compare with the levels above and below. **C.** Sagittal gradient echo MR image shows a high-signal epidural abscess compressing the spinal cord at the T7 disc level (*arrows*).

Postoperative Changes

The most common postoperative change you will encounter is in the patient who has undergone a *laminectomy*. In these patients, segments of lamina of various sizes will be missing at the involved level(s) (Fig. 13.40). Other postoperative changes will include the presence of various types of *stabilizing devices* used to correct abnormalities as the result of trauma (Fig. 13.41) or scoliosis. When reviewing films that have surgical hardware, it is important to compare them with the previous studies to determine whether loosening or fracture of the components has occurred (Fig. 13.42).

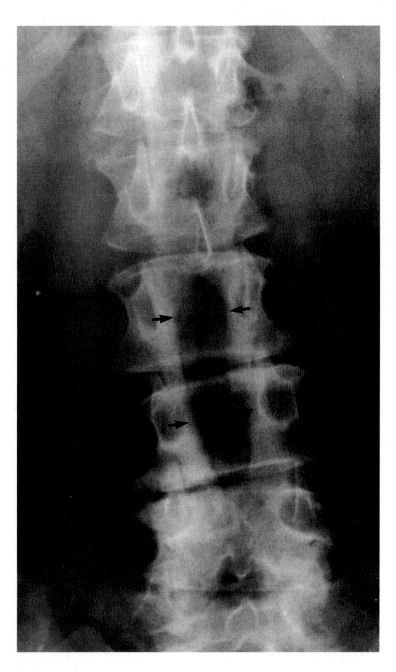

Figure 13.40. Appearance after laminectomy. Notice the absence of the laminae and spinous processes of L3 and L4. The lucency represents the surgical margins (*arrows*).

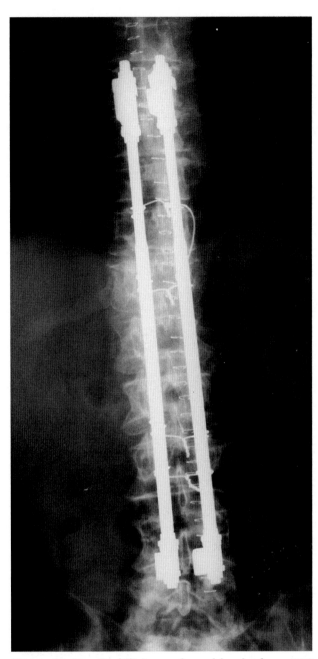

Figure 13.41.   Stabilizing rods and hooks for a T12 fracture. The rods extend from T8 to L4.

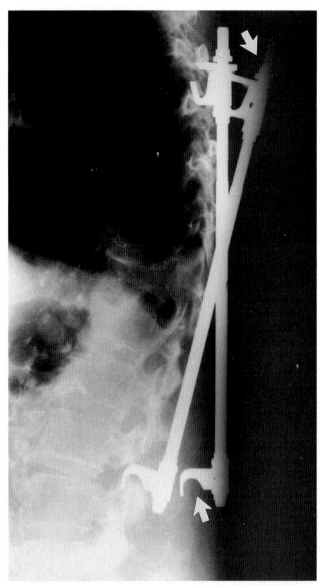

Figure 13.42.   Unhooking of stabilizing rods. (This is the same patient as in Fig. 13.41.) One rod has unhooked on top; one on the bottom (*arrows*).

SUMMARY AND KEY POINTS

■ This chapter reviewed vertebral anatomy and the various techniques for evaluating the vertebral column.

■ CT has become the prime screening method for patients with suspected vertebral trauma.

■ MR imaging provides the clinician with a direct view of the spinal cord.

■ Despite the advantages of CT and MR imaging of the spine, radiography is still necessary.

■ The assessment of developmental, degenerative and arthritic, traumatic, neoplastic, infectious, and postoperative abnormalities was discussed.

SUGGESTED ADDITIONAL READING

Daffner RH. Cervical radiography for trauma patients: a time-effective technique? AJR 2000;175:1309–1311.

Daffner RH. Helical CT of the cervical spine for trauma patients: a time study. AJR 2001;177:677–679.

Daffner RH. Imaging of Vertebral Trauma. 2nd Ed. Philadelphia: Lippincott-Raven, 1996.

Fenton DS, Czervionke LF. Image-Guided Spine Intervention. Philadelphia: WB Saunders, 2003.

Latschaw RE, Kucharczyk J, Moseley M. Imaging of the Nervous System: Diagnostic and Therapeutic Applications. St. Louis: Mosby, 2005.

Poussaint TY, Barnes PD, Ball WS Jr. Spine and spinal cord. In: Kirks DR, Griscom NT, eds. Practical Pediatric Imaging. Diagnostic Radiology of Infants and Children. 3rd Ed. Philadelphia: Lippincott-Raven, 1998:259–325.

Renfrew DL. Atlas of Spine Injection. Philadelphia: WB Saunders, 2004.

Ross JS, Brant-Zawadzki MN, Chen MZ, et al. Diagnostic Imaging: Spine. Philadelphia: WB Saunders, 2005.

Appendix

In my many years in diagnostic radiology, I have had the good fortune of observing many interesting and helpful signs. Some are based on common sense, some on radiologic lore, and all on fact. Here are 37 of my favorites, in no particular order. Note that many of these signs relate to the musculoskeletal system, one of my favorite areas of diagnostic radiology. I invite readers to send me their own pearls for possible inclusion in a future edition of this work.

Daffner's Diagnostic Pearls

1. Common things occur more commonly, even in unusual locations.
2. A common thing in an unusual location still looks like the original entity.
3. Ninety-nine percent of lytic bone lesions in patients over age 50 are metastases.
4. If a bone lesion looks like nothing you have ever seen before, think of fibrous dysplasia.
5. Infection can look like virtually anything.
6. Tuberculosis is, unfortunately, not rare.
7. Tuberculosis and eosinophilic granuloma are great imitators.
8. With odd-looking lytic bone lesions in a child, think of eosinophilic granuloma.
9. In common type 1 lateral compression pelvic fractures, severe blood loss will be from the liver or spleen, not the pelvis.
10. Be careful of injured hips in elderly patients—femoral neck fractures can be invisible initially, and lawyers love them.
11. Femoral shaft fractures may be associated with occult hip fractures.
12. In expanded lytic bone lesions in older patients, do not forget brown tumors.
13. For any patient with trauma to the knees, look carefully at the lateral view for an effusion. No effusion virtually guarantees no significant injury.
14. Never, ever, forget the edges or corners of the image.
15. Think stress (toddler) fracture of the tibia in any toddler who refuses to bear weight on a limb.
16. Anything with straight lines is human made. Nature prefers curves.
17. Any trauma cervical spine that "looks funny" or just doesn't look right isn't. Look for the signs of unilateral jumped and locked facets.
18. If you perform enough studies, you will eventually find something you cannot explain.
19. If you perform enough studies, you will eventually find something you will wish you had not.
20. With a "common" bone lesion in an unusual location, mentally transfer that lesion to the knee. The diagnosis should be more apparent.
21. Contrary to how we are taught, patients are entitled to and often have more than one disease.
22. A fracture is a soft tissue injury in which a bone is broken.
23. A positive bone scan in a patient with known malignancy does not always mean metastases. Frequently, there will be multiple etiologies to account for the abnormalities—and none may be due to metastases!
24. Never forget to look at the teeth—you may be surprised at what you find.
25. Absence of evidence of a disease is not evidence of absence of that disease.
26. The distribution of surgical clips should be noted. A realignment indicates a growing mass or abscess.
27. Opaque foreign bodies that change position are sitting in fluid.
28. Never forget the "blood" behind the "silver." Every imaging study represents a person who has feelings just as you do.
29. Old films are your best friends. Never forget to call on them.
30. Cut a corner today, pay for it tomorrow.
31. Imaging is no substitute for a careful history and physical examination.
32. Ninety percent of trauma victims are committing an illegal act, are high on alcohol and/or drugs, or are guilty of extreme stupidity. The other 10% are victims of the first group.
33. Anything blue on an hematoxylin and eosin stained pathology slide is bad.
34. Sinusitis is a clinical diagnosis. Sinus images frequently bear no relationship to the patient's symptoms.
35. Never allow a diagnostic study to replace your brain in dealing with a patient.
36. While you can't kill a "gomer" or an old farmer, remember that "crocks" die, too.
37. Although radiology may seem complicated, it is not rocket science.

Index

Page numbers in *italics* denote figures; those followed by t denote tables.